P9-CKV-247

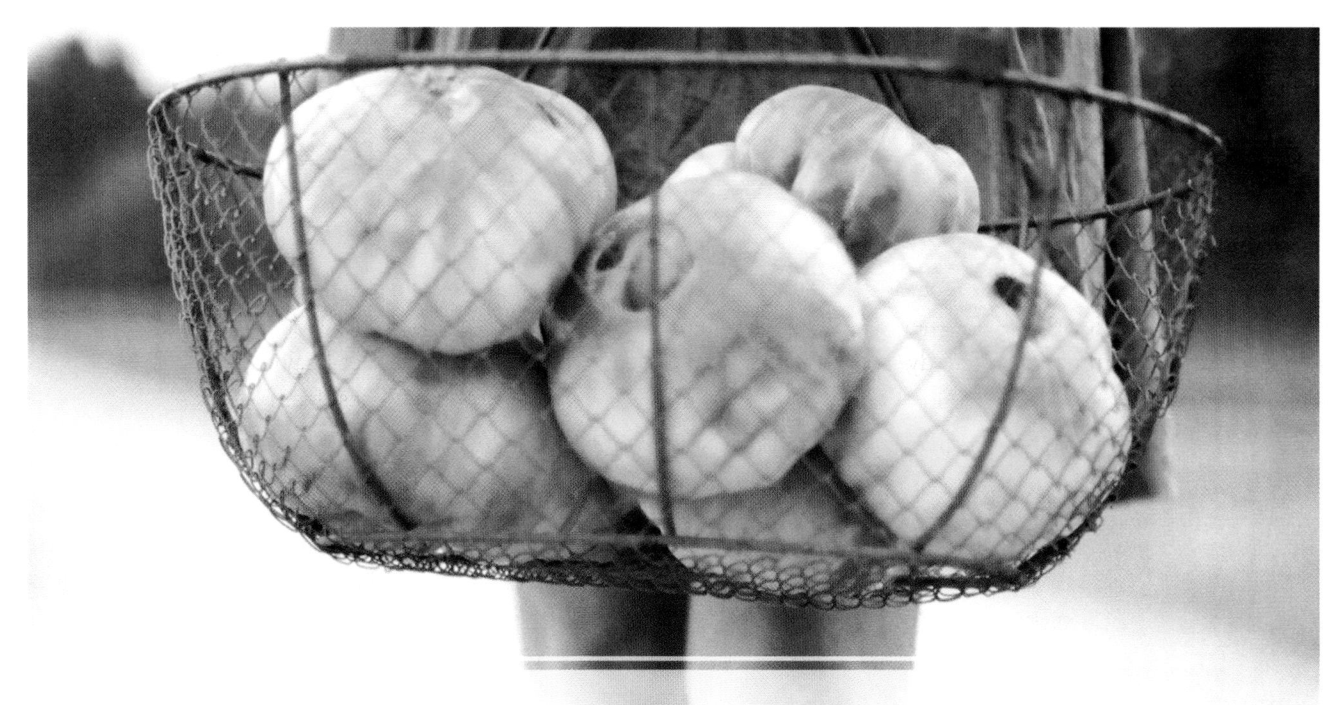

The Homegrown Paleo Cookbook

Over 100 Delicious,
Gluten-Free, Farm-to-Table Recipes, and
A Complete Guide to Growing Your Own Healthy Food

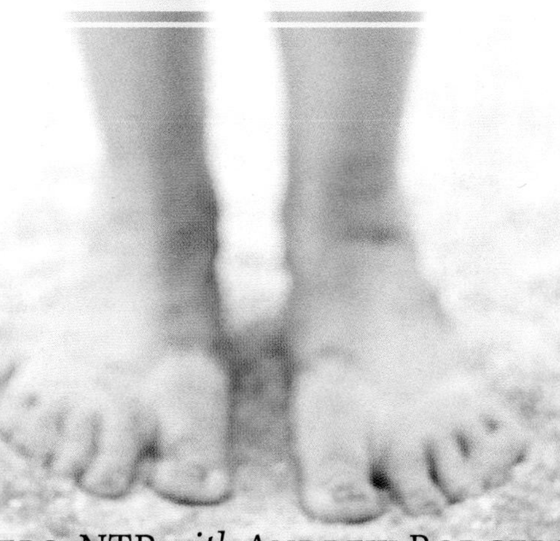

Diana Rodgers, NTP *with* Andrew Rodgers

Victory Belt Publishing, Inc.
Las Vegas

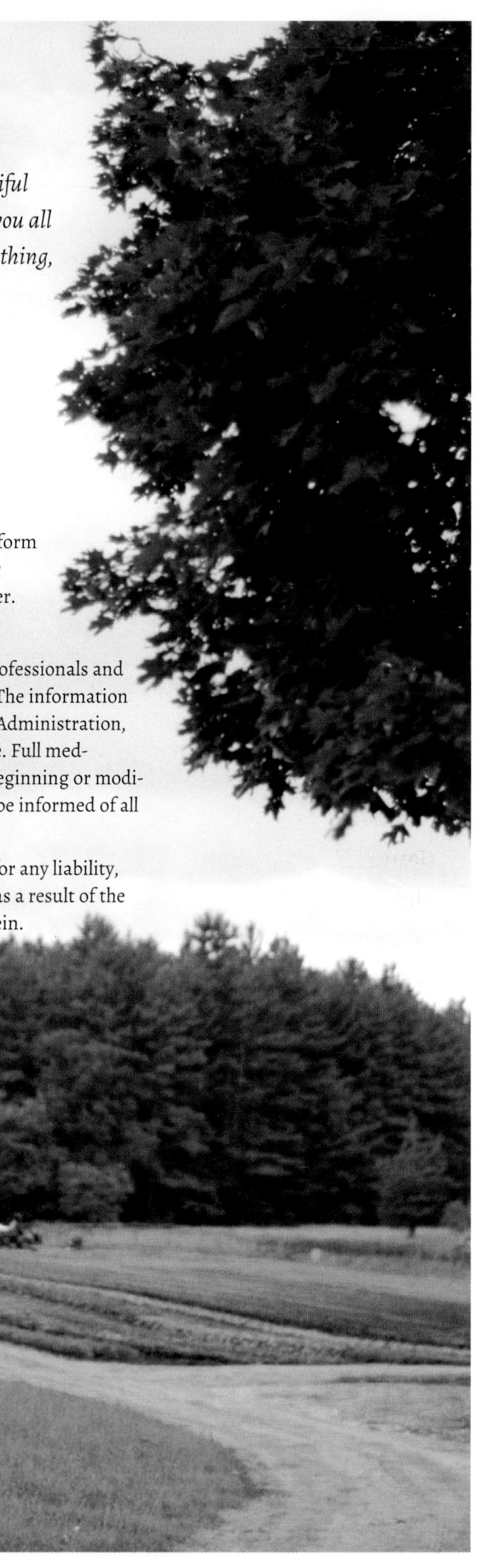

Dedication

My love goes out to our future generation and to my beautiful and intensely inquisitive children, Anson and Phoebe. May you all grow up to be passionate and open-minded, to question everything, and to make the world a better place.

First Published in 2015 by Victory Belt Publishing Inc.

ISBN 13: 978-1-628600-62-9

Printed in the U.S.A.

RRD 0115

Book design by: Yordan Terziev and Boryana Yordanova

Cover design by: Melissa Schwab

Photography by: Heidi Murphy

Contents

More Praise for *The Homegrown Paleo Cookbook*

A beautiful book that unites the Paleo diet with the sustainable homefront. Don't read this book to change your diet. Read it to change your life.

—Shannon Hayes, author of *Radical Homemakers*

Diana makes wholesome, fresh food both accessible and a lot of fun. She shows how to integrate sustainable eating into the life of a busy family. A perfect resource for a working mom like me.

—Emily Deans, MD, Clinical Instructor, Harvard Medical School

The way we farm animals, the impact of farming systems on the environment, and the nutritional quality of the meat, milk, and eggs they produce are all intrinsically linked. If we manage animals according to their needs, we know they produce better-tasting, healthier meat, milk, and eggs, and we don't have to rely on things like routine antibiotics and other chemical inputs. And we know that managing animals on pasture—rather than in confinement—can actually have a positive impact on the environment and could help to mitigate climate change.

In *The Homegrown Paleo Cookbook*, Diana Rodgers not only articulates the reasons we urgently need to change the way we farm and feed ourselves in a clear, candid, and accessible way, but she empowers the reader, offering uncomplicated guidance and support so we can all achieve a truly sustainable, healthful, and rewarding diet—one meal at a time.

—Andrew Gunther, Program Director, Animal Welfare Approved

The shift in agriculture, from one based on biology to one based on chemistry, and the resulting shift in consumption from whole foods to highly processed foods have resulted in nutrition-related disease, obesity, and environmental destruction. We can change this frightening and unnecessary situation. And we can start by changing what our own families eat. Diana provides an excellent, easy-to-follow road map for changing our diets and regenerating the health of our families, the environment, and the planet.

—Allan Savory, founder of the Savory Institute and author of *The Grazing Revolution: A Radical Plan to Save the Earth*

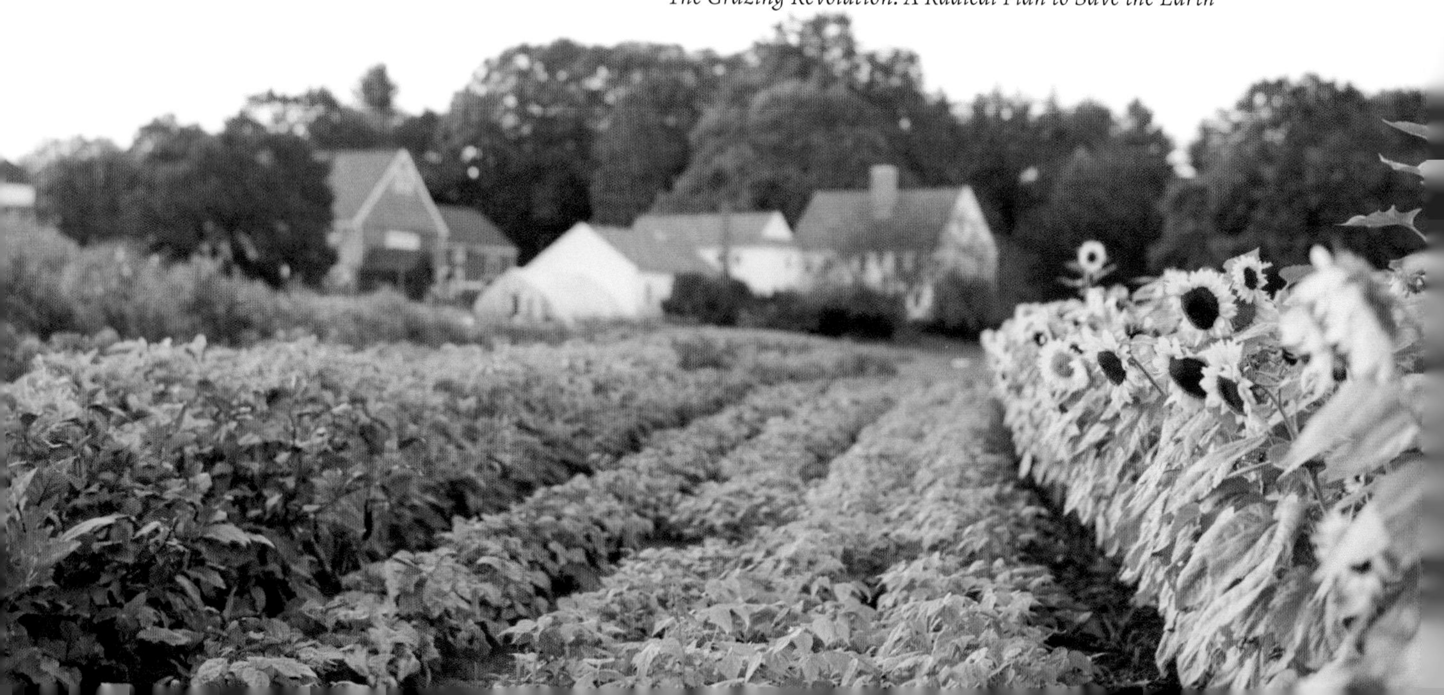

Preface
by Joel Salatin

Before supermarkets, cattle feedlots, chicken factories, takeout, and the moldboard plow, people acquired most of their diet proximate to where they lived. They hunted, fished, and tended food plots right outside their door—or tent or yurt or hut. While often they suffered from infectious diseases due to unhygienic or smoky living conditions, they otherwise enjoyed excellent health, and many lived to ripe old age.

In this readable and practical book, Diana Rodgers shows us how to re-create the healthful living and nutritious food of our ancestors, without re-creating their living conditions. Using our techno-glitzy culinary gizmos with ancient food stocks, we can certainly live in the best of times. Highly developed civilizations need not succumb to a new generation of non infectious ailments like type II diabetes and cancer.

We can enjoy unprecedented health, but only if we participate. We cannot build a healthy future on potato chips, fast food, and convenience.

When people ask me, "What can I do to join the integrity food movement?" I respond with three action steps. First, get in your kitchen to prepare, process, package, and preserve whole foods acquired directly from producers or from your own personal production. Second, take all your recreational and entertainment budget for one year and spend that time and money info-taining yourself into the food treasures in your area. Join the tribe that gets it. Third, do something yourself, whether keeping a beehive on the roof, a container garden on the patio, or two chickens in the space formerly occupied by the boa constrictor, gerbil, dog, or cat. Every single person can actively join a visceral relationship with their body's fuel.

Overcoming our societal ignorance requires guidebooks, hand-holding, and cheerleaders. Diana is a cheerleader for a healthy future; a future with ecological, economic, and emotional integrity. If you find yourself yearning for an abundant future, a healthy future, a vibrant relationship with your ecological umbilical, this handbook will lead you to that place. Thank you, Diana, for adding your experience and wisdom to integrity living. I hope this inspires many people to come down out of the stands and begin playing the most exciting game—life.

Foreword
by Robb Wolf

I was first introduced to Diana several years ago by a mutual acquaintance, Mat Lalonde. Diana and I have since become great friends, copresenting at a number of conferences, and we have really bonded on the sustainability story she develops so well in this book.

To give you an idea of the importance of sustainability, let me relate a conversation I had with Mat on the topic. First, you have to understand that Mat is usually the smartest person in the room—he has a PhD from Harvard in one of the most prestigious organic chemistry labs in the world—and even though he is a dear friend, if I put forward something he regards as lame, he will give me a verbal pummeling only slightly less uncomfortable than being submerged in concentrated sulfuric acid. His nickname is "the Kraken," because when the Kraken is released, cities, towns, and poorly conceived thoughts are summarily destroyed. So broaching the topic of the Paleo diet and sustainability with Mat was . . . stressful. I tried to butter him up by first talking about some training ideas and then his favorite Ramones song, and then I blurted out something like this: "So, I've been thinking about all this Paleo stuff in the context of sustainability. When you think about stable, dynamic ecologies, don't we see an interaction of plant and animal consumers? Is Planet of the Vegans really sustainable? How do we build a long-term sustainable food system on government subsidies and ever more expensive oil?"

At this point I braced for my acid bath. Much to my surprise, however, Mat responded with something like this: "Yeah, the current system is totally unsustainable, and the vegan model is perhaps even worse than what we have now. Five hundred years from now food production will look like a hybrid of what Allan Savory and Joel Salatin have developed."

Not only did I survive my encounter with the Kraken, he actually agreed with me! Now, I can be an idiot on a variety of topics, but if Mat actually saw things as I did, I had to think I was on to something. It was at that point that I started to talk more openly about sustainability.

I'll be honest, for most folks who follow my work on diet and nutrition, this was a tough pill to swallow. All kinds of emotionally loaded things are dragged to the surface when we talk about sustainability, including politics and values. I built my following as a strength coach and nutrition geek—why on earth would I get into the quagmire of food politics? Well, because it's really important, and in my opinion, if we don't explore these ideas, our society (and perhaps the world) could face some very difficult times in the future.

Diana and I both arrived separately at the same idea: that we need to get more people producing food in a decentralized, sustainable fashion. Easy(ish) to say; quite another thing to actually get folks doing this. We've talked about ways to train farmers, land trusts, political action groups, and the need for a basic manual to help people like me who have a strong interest in all this to actually start putting ideas into action. *The Homegrown Paleo Cookbook* is that manual.

The Homegrown Paleo Cookbook is your field guide to changing the world. That may sound like a lofty goal for a book, but think about it this way: Some of you reading this will maintain a modest garden at home, supplementing your family's food with fresh, nutritious produce, and possibly even raise a few chickens, goats, and other critters. For some of you, however, this book will be your gateway drug to changing what you are doing with your life and opting to become part of the sustainable food system.

Almost fifteen years ago, I came to believe that the Paleo diet would transform medicine. By all accounts, that process is well underway, and we are all the better for it. I am similarly convinced that a decentralized, sustainable food system will largely supplant the current factory farm–based model. It will take time and there will be significant pushback, but like the Paleo diet, it makes sense. The Paleo diet works so well because it takes its cue from nature and human genetics and focuses on the foods we were designed to eat. Similarly, biodynamic, sustainable food production emulates how ecology has functioned since the beginning of time.

I am incredibly excited for this book because it not only offers an important perspective on the Paleo diet, it also is an introduction to how to integrate the healthiest food we can eat with the healthiest and most sustainable practices of production.

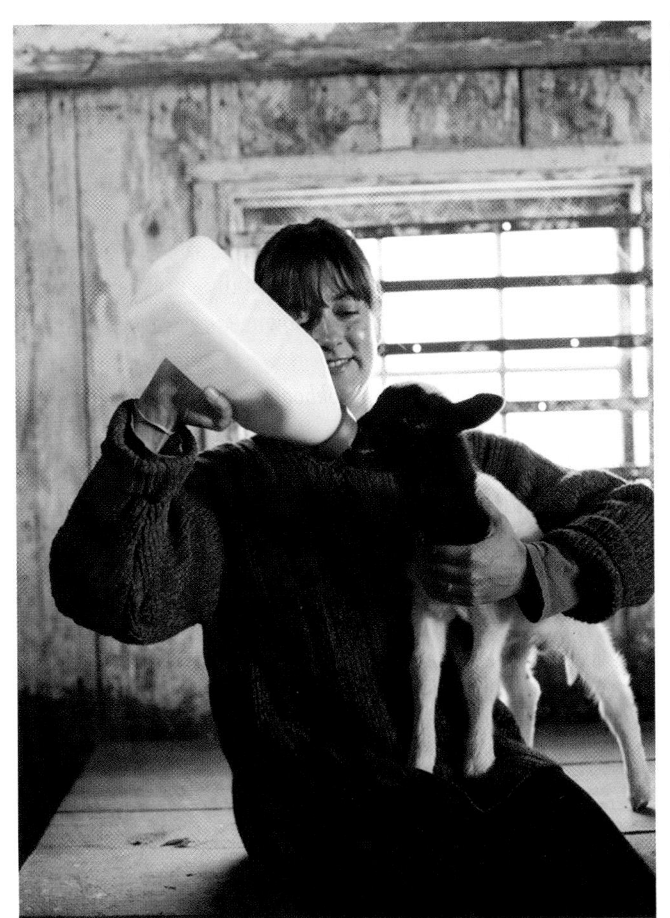

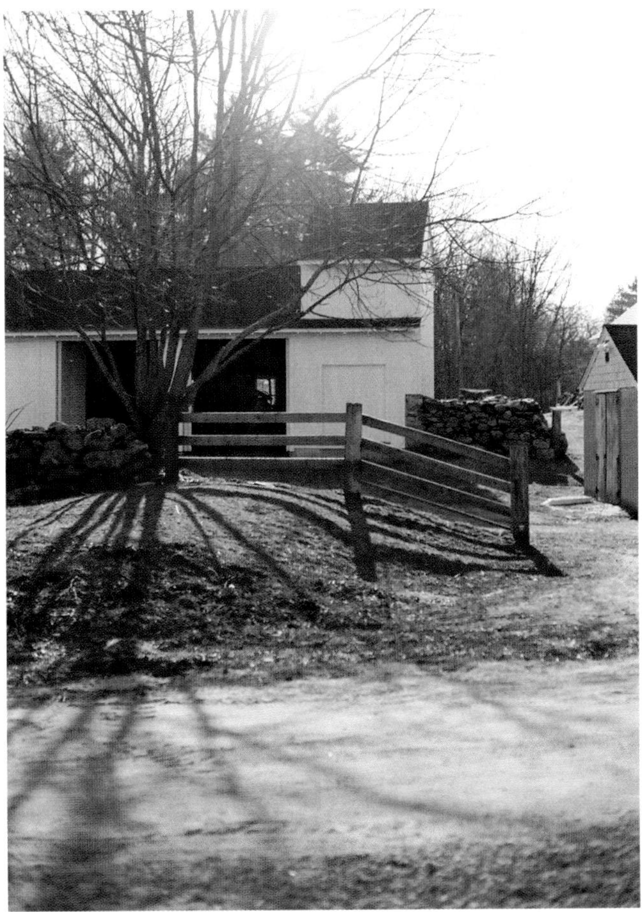

Introduction

As a culture, we have become so detached from real food—food that doesn't come prepackaged or wrapped in plastic, with bright labels advertising how good it is.

We're so busy. Convenience has overtaken the value of homegrown and homemade, nutrient-dense food. We rely on marketing messages from a handful of powerful industry giants to tell us what's good for us, instead of choosing the types of food that we were designed to thrive on. Our modern lives may be vastly different from those of our Paleolithic ancestors, but I believe that through modern research, technology, and old-fashioned common sense, we can develop a better connection with how we were meant to eat and live.

With this book, my goal is to help you understand how the food you consume is produced and give you the tools to make more sustainable choices. Even if you're not in a position right now to have a vegetable patch or raise chickens, this book will make you a much more informed consumer. You'll know why it's so important to seek out fresh, local food from farmers markets, Community-Supported Agriculture (CSA) programs, and local farms, and you'll know what to look for at each of these places and what questions to ask.

It's my hope to see lawns turned into grazing pasture or vegetable gardens, fruit trees replacing decorative shrubs, more people spending time outdoors, and folks cooking homemade, seasonal, and healthy meals with locally produced ingredients. This book is about explaining why that's so important, and how to make it happen.

My Story

Throughout my childhood, I was plagued with digestive distress, low muscle tone, and chronic nosebleeds. I was hospitalized numerous times for dehydration, and the only answer my doctor gave my parents was to give me soy milk instead of cow's milk. Despite all that, my mother thought she was doing everything right. Marketing messages had convinced her generation that anything made by science was far superior to what nature could grow. Breastfeeding was only for people who couldn't afford formula. Making home-cooked meals was a thing of the past. We had packaged cereal for breakfast, bought school lunches, and enjoyed frozen dinners in front of the television.

During high school and college summers, I worked on an organic farm. I loved being outdoors, with the sun on my skin and my hands in the soil. I met my husband, Andrew, when I was nineteen. At the time, he had just returned from a fall semester camping expedition in the Rocky Mountains with the National Outdoor Leadership School. (He survived with no tents—pretty hard-core. I was in love!) He was an English major with a strong interest in the environment, and I loved getting my degree in art education, but we both felt lost when it came to answering the perennial question, "What do you want to be when you grow up?" While we were students, we started a small business called The Indentured Students, which let people hire college kids for odd jobs like landscaping, walking dogs, and moving furniture. It was a great experience in entrepreneurship, and we got the bug for running our own business.

When it came time to decide whether to expand the business or try something new, we opted for something new: we moved to the West Coast and got "real jobs." Andrew was quickly hired by a major market research company to conduct focus groups for high-tech companies. I took a job at an advertising agency, also focusing in high tech. While it was nice to be able to pay the bills, we both knew there was more to life. On the weekends, we often took small road trips to get into the country. We especially loved spending time on Sauvie Island, an island in the Columbia River about half an hour from Portland. It's mostly farmland, and the time we spent there hooked Andrew on the idea of becoming a professional farmer. Not only would he not have to wear a tie and work in a gray cubicle, but he'd also be doing something that could save land from being developed.

We moved back to Massachusetts and got married. Andrew entered a graduate program in soil science and began working on a farm to learn the hands-on skills he'd need as a farmer. He soon became the manager of Green Meadows Farm in Hamilton, Massachusetts. I kept my job in marketing for a while, but after a few years I joined him to help run the farm.

Meanwhile, in a quest for better health, I decided to adopt a low-fat, mostly vegetarian diet full of fried tofu and lots of whole grains. My health went downhill fast. When I was twenty-six, I was diagnosed with celiac disease, an autoimmune condition in which gluten provokes an immune response that damages the lining of the small intestine. I had to go on a gluten-free diet, which at the time felt like the most restrictive, evil diet ever created. However, after just two weeks gluten-free, my GI symptoms had mostly disappeared.

Rather than really changing how I ate, though, I was just buying gluten-free versions of the foods I was already eating on my low-fat, nutrient-poor, high-carbohydrate diet. For many years following my diagnosis, this was my routine: gluten-free toast with a banana and a glass of orange juice for breakfast; a sandwich made with gluten-free bread, diet soda, and chips for lunch; and gluten-free pasta for dinner, with a gluten-free cookie for dessert and maybe a gluten-free beer. I was on a blood sugar roller coaster. I got tunnel vision and the shakes if I went for more than two hours without eating, so I started carrying a bag full of gluten-free granola bars in my purse. But I didn't really understand what was going on or why my diet was causing me so much trouble.

When I left my marketing job to manage the farm store at Green Meadows Farm, I learned more about the Weston A. Price Foundation, an organization that works to educate the public about nutrition and the benefits of whole food, which really changed my thinking about fats and traditional foods. We hosted a raw milk co-op through the farm, and I brought in nutrient-dense foods like coconut oil and started to render the fat from our pasture-raised pork. But I was struggling to come up with intelligent answers to visitors' questions about nutrition, such as "Why exactly is coconut oil good for you?" So I decided to enroll in the Nutritional Therapy Association's program to learn more about why the Standard American Diet was failing so many people. It was an eye-opening experience. Towards the end of the program, I decided to try the thirty-day Paleo challenge described in Robb Wolf's *The Paleo Solution*. It completely changed my life. No longer did I need to eat every two hours. My blood sugar spikes were under control, and my blood work showed the ideal markers for a completely healthy person. I also joined a CrossFit gym and found a very smart trainer who understood what kind of workouts my body needs, and I became much stronger than I had ever been in my life.

I was so excited about the changes I saw in myself, thanks to my new lifestyle, that I decided to dedicate my life to helping others make similar changes. I opened my nutrition practice and continued to investigate which foods are optimal not only for human health but also for the environment.

After nearly a decade at Green Meadows Farm, we decided to move to Clark Farm in Carlisle, Massachusetts, in 2012. A dairy farm for many years, it had recently been sold to Marjie Findlay and Geoff Freeman, who wanted to revive it as a family-run farm. Andrew and I were delighted to move our family to the farm and take over its day-to-day management. Today, we operate a vegetable CSA; raise pigs, sheep, goats, and chickens; and run educational programs for local schoolchildren.

I also run my nutrition practice out of our farmhouse and write about sustainable food options for health and the environment on my blog, Sustainable Dish, and I cohost a podcast called *Modern Farm Girls* with fellow dirt lover and nutritionist Liz Wolfe. Additionally, I have started a video series featuring different aspects of farm life that is posted on my YouTube channel, Sustainable Dish, and on my blog. As I write this, I'm nearing the completion of my program to become a registered dietitian (RD), so that I can work more closely with the medical community and help people regain their health through dietary changes. I haven't lost my love of art, though, and I'm thrilled to have creative outlets in developing recipes using stunning food from our farm and, of course, in creating this beautiful book.

I'm on a mission. I sincerely hope to inspire others to choose sustainably grown, nutrient-dense foods, and to slow down from the hectic pace of our technology-driven, overly scheduled lives and get back to a more sustainable existence. Whether you choose to buy from a local farmer, grow containers of herbs on your porch, start homesteading on your land, or perhaps become a farmer yourself, this book will help you launch a more grounded, healthier lifestyle.

Diana Rodgers

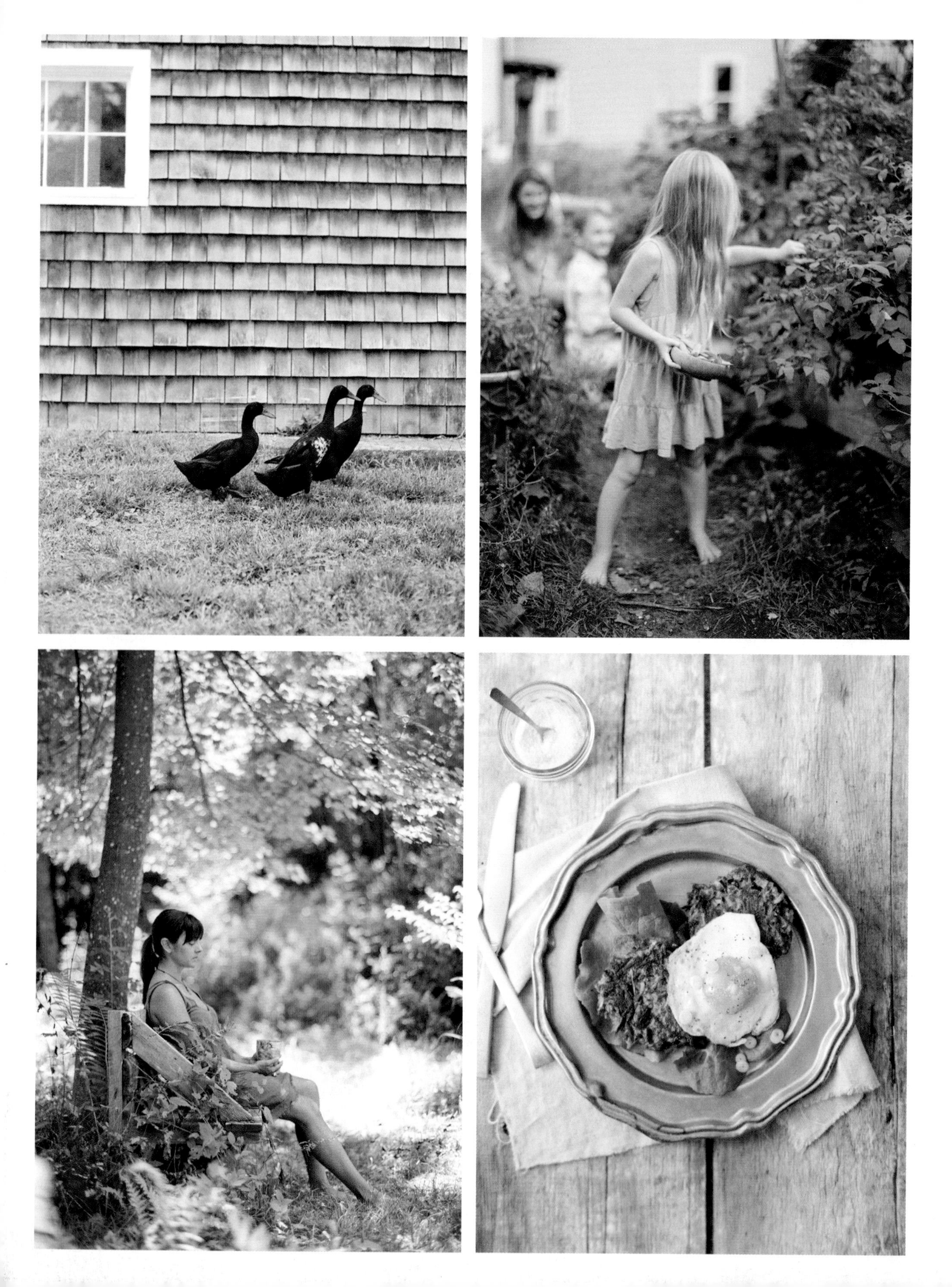

The Case for Sustainable Paleo Living

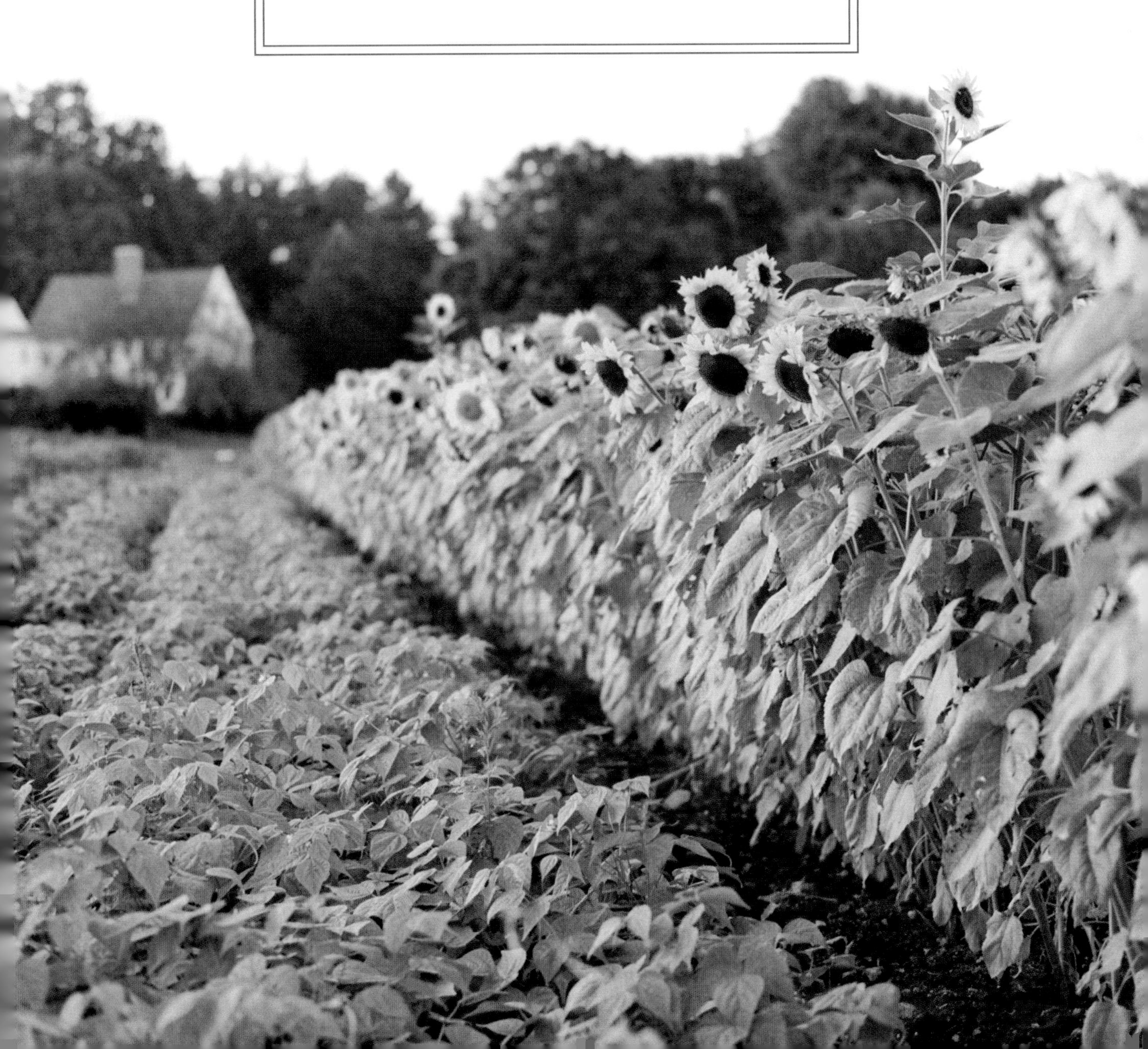

"To be interested in food but not in food production is clearly absurd."

– Wendell Berry

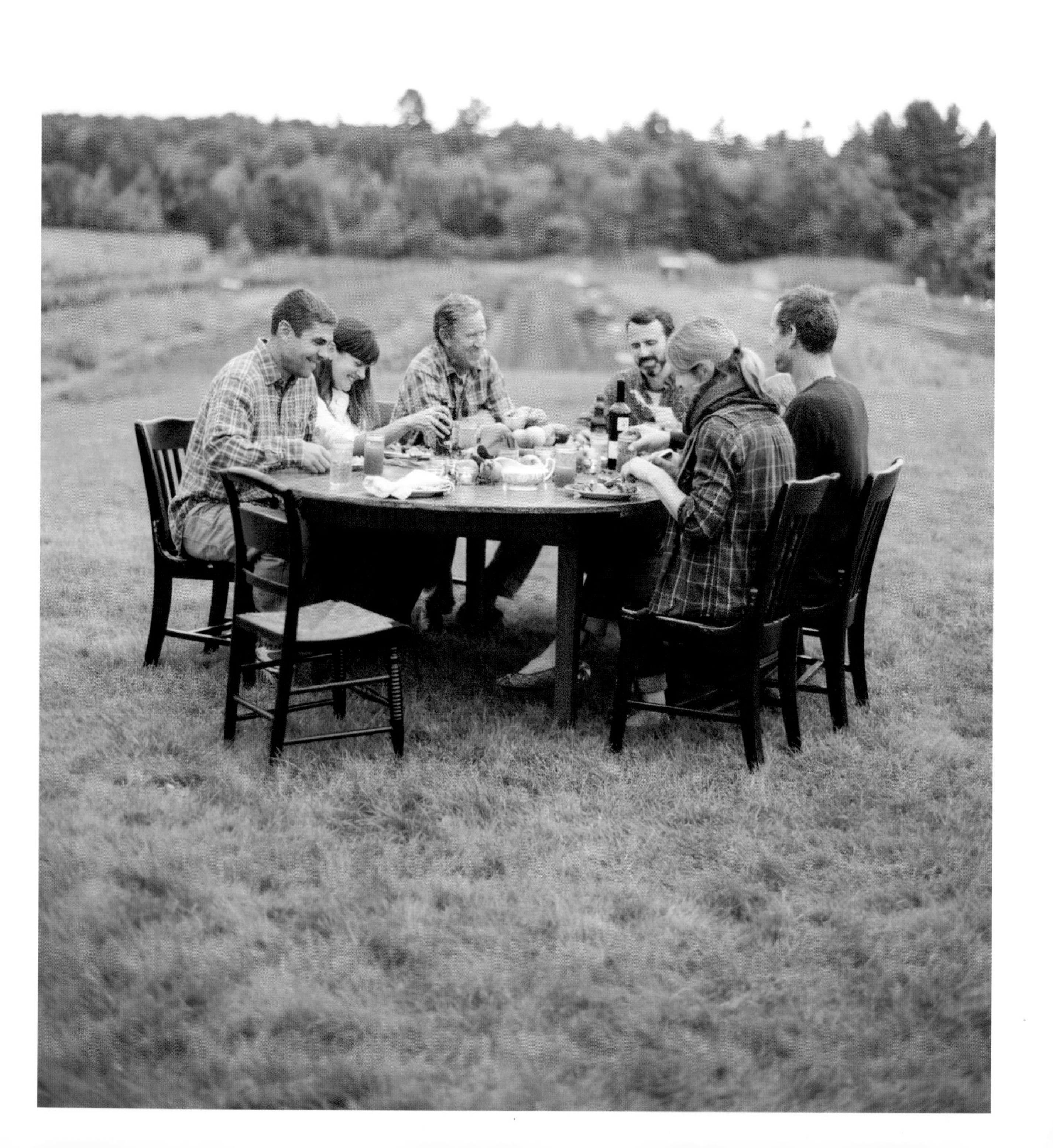

The Problems with Modern Eating

Despite all of our technology, social conventions, art, cities, and all the other trappings of civilization, at our core, humans are animals. And just like other animals, we have a species-specific diet and environment in which we thrive. Veer too far from our natural setting and nutritional needs, and you'll start to see some major problems. In fact, right now we're seeing some really major problems because we've strayed from the foods and lifestyle our bodies need. Our physical and mental health is suffering because of our modern lifestyle.

We live in a world that is far removed from the one our hunter-gatherer ancestors knew. Some people liken our modern environment to an unnatural, zoo-like setting. We work long hours, mostly sitting down under florescent lights, and commute long distances in gas-guzzling cars to come home to our toxic dwellings, which are wrapped in plastic siding, to watch a box of flickering images that tells us why we want the next cool gadget and how brand X packaged food will save us so much time in the kitchen and has "a taste kids love." We exercise indoors on a hamster wheel–like contraption while watching more flickering images of how our bodies should look. The toxic pollution we breathe in; the chemicals that surround us in our homes, offices, and lawns; pharmaceutical and recreational drugs; and alcohol are all foreign stressors to our bodies. We aren't sleeping enough and are addicted to caffeine to keep us going. We're in over our heads financially with mortgages, car loans, and student loans, yet we've never before had such a high standard of "living."

The food we eat is as far from nature as our lifestyle. We consume animals that were raised in factories and vegetables that were sprayed with chemicals and harvested by people who can't afford to eat what they pick. Many people are grossed out by the sight of a bone in their meat. We want our meat nicely wrapped, with a clean label telling us how much protein and how little fat it has. Our cattle are mostly raised in Concentrated Animal Feeding Operations (CAFOs), and when I drive through very urban settings and watch peoples shuffling to work with stressed, unsmiling faces, I wonder if we, too, are living in CAFOs.

"I am losing precious days. I am degenerating into a machine for making money. I am learning nothing in this trivial world of men. I must break away and get out into the mountains to learn the news."

– John Muir

The home is a pit stop where we plunk our stuff. Homemakers are largely a thing of the past, reserved for the rich and those stuck in the past. Households are forced to have two incomes to keep up with our ever-growing economic strains. Because of this, we've lost our skills as home economists and have created a culture of nine-to-five (and then some) office work. Inexpensive, industrially produced convenience food, loaded with chemicals and health claims, has moved in to relieve us of the burden of cooking.

BREAKDOWN OF MONEY SPENT ON GROCERIES

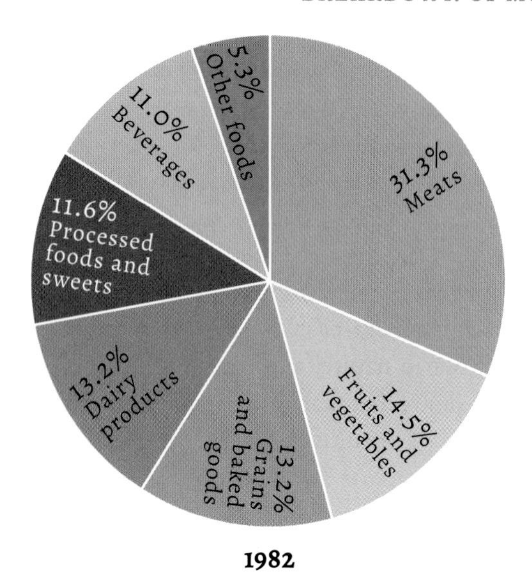

1982

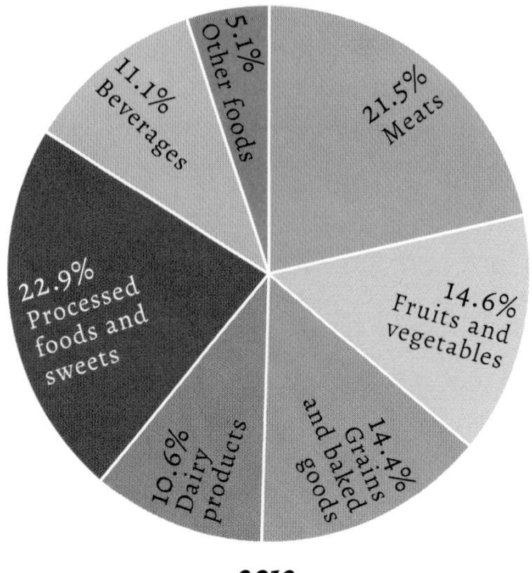

2012

Source: Bureau of Labor Statistics

Take a look at how much the Bureau of Labor Statistics says we spend today on processed foods and sweets plus beverages. That 34 percent is terrifying.

Our children are being shaped by an unnatural diet, lack of sleep, and too much screen time. Seventeen percent of American children ages two to nineteen are obese. And healthy, active, and naturally curious children are being overmedicated to become complacent, obedient, lethargic drones. According to the CDC, the percentage of children ages four to seventeen who were on medication for attention-deficit/hyperactivity disorder increased from 4.8 percent in 2007 to 6.1 percent in 2011. (Interestingly, some studies on dietary treatments for ADHD have had promising results.) Of course, some kids do benefit from medication for ADHD, but all kids benefit from plenty of healthy activity and a diet of real, whole foods.

Adults are faring even worse. In spite of all of our modern medical care, our state of health is deplorable. Here are some of the latest data from the CDC and American Cancer Society:

- 35.7 percent of Americans over the age of twenty are obese, and an additional 33.1 percent are overweight.
- 25.8 million people in the U.S.have diabetes. 90 to 95 percent of diabetes in adults is type II diabetes.
- 86 million American adults ages twenty or older have prediabetes.
- Between the costs of medical care, loss of work, and early death, diabetes cost Americans $245 billion in 2012.
- In high-income countries like the U.S., 25 to 33 percent of cancers are related to lifestyle factors such as poor nutrition, physical inactivity, and excess weight.
- Each year, over 200,000 deaths from heart and lung diseases, cancer, and stroke could be prevented with lifestyle and environmental changes.

Not only are we sick, we're also sad. According to the American Academy of Child and Adolescent Psychiatry, in the U.S., about 9 percent of adults and 5 percent of children and adolescents suffer from depression. It's easy to assume that this has nothing to do with food, but a study published in *Psychosomatic Medicine* found "lower rates of depression, anxiety, and bipolar disorder among those who consumed a traditional diet of meat and vegetables than people who followed a modern Western diet heavy with processed fast foods or even a health-food diet of tofu and salads."

We're dying of preventable, diet- and lifestyle-related diseases that were largely nonexistent during the Paleolithic times, such as type II diabetes.

"IN THE UNITED STATES AND MOST WESTERN COUNTRIES, DIET-RELATED CHRONIC DISEASES REPRESENT THE SINGLE LARGEST CAUSE OF MORBIDITY AND MORTALITY. THESE DISEASES ARE EPIDEMIC IN CONTEMPORARY WESTERNIZED POPULATIONS AND TYPICALLY AFFLICT 50–65% OF THE ADULT POPULATION, YET THEY ARE RARE OR NONEXISTENT IN HUNTER-GATHERERS AND OTHER LESS WESTERNIZED PEOPLE . . . AND CAN LARGELY BE BLAMED ON EXCESSIVE CONSUMPTION OF MODERN FOODS (CEREALS, REFINED SUGARS, PROCESSED VEGETABLE OILS, INDUSTRIALLY RAISED MEATS)."

—From a study titled "Origins and Evolution of the Western Diet: Health Implications for the 21st Century" in the *American Journal of Clinical Nutrition*

We're inflamed, swollen ticks, and we keep looking for the next pill that will save us when the answer is actually simple: we need to look back at how humans lived for thousands of years, eating nonindustrialized foods and moving much more than we do now. This is the essence of the Paleo lifestyle.

Many wrongly assume that our hunter-gatherer ancestors lived shorter lives, and they jump to the conclusion that it's dangerous to eat like them. But our ancestors weren't dying of chronic, inflammatory diseases like obesity, diabetes, heart disease, and autoimmune disease. Their lifespans were shortened by lack of emergency medical care and modern sanitation, a higher infant mortality rate, and tribal warfare. When these factors are taken into account, their lifespans were roughly equivalent to our own.

Modern life isn't without its joys. I love my hot showers, my refrigerator, and, of course, my smartphone. I'm not saying we all need to go back to caveman life, but we do need to strive to find a balance between what modern life has to offer and what we can learn from our past. We need to move more often, get out in nature, and consume foods that are nutrient-dense and that benefit, not harm, the body. Foods that were cultivated after the Paleolithic era can still be good for you. Broccoli, for example, was not around during the Paleolithic era (it was bred later from wild cabbage), but it's a nutrient-dense food, and when it's sustainably grown—by which I mean that it does not come from a large-scale, industrial farm that uses pesticides and chemical fertilizers, trucks the produce across the country or overseas, and treats its workers badly—it's healthy for the environment, too.

Cows did not exist during the Paleolithic era, either (they evolved from wild oxen over 10,000 years ago). But humans have hunted large ruminant animals for hundreds of thousands of years, and beef is a nutrient-dense food. Today, though, something has gone terribly wrong. Movies like *Food, Inc.* have done a great job of highlighting the tragedy of industrially produced meat, and the moral and ethical outrage over CAFOs has prompted many people to turn to veganism and vegetarianism. So how can those of us who believe that meat is an essential part of the human diet answer those concerns? Is there a moral, sustainable way to eat meat?

The Modern Debate on Eating Meat

I really do understand where vegetarians and vegans are coming from when they make the moral argument that no animals should have to die to feed us. It's a compelling point, for sure. However, what they often don't realize is that many animals are still dying to feed them.

In 2003, Steven L. Davis of Oregon State University published an article in the *Journal of Agricultural and Environmental Ethics* whose thesis was stated in its title: "The Least Harm Principle May Require that Humans Consume a Diet Containing Large Herbivores, Not a Vegan Diet." In it, Davis explains that many insects, field mice, birds, and frogs are killed by intensive crop production. If all of the 120 million hectares (about 300 million acres) of cropland harvested in the U.S. each year were used to grow foods suitable for a vegan diet, Davis estimates, 1.8 billion animals would be killed annually to support a plant-based diet. The exact figure may be debatable because there's little data on exactly how many mice, birds, frogs, and other field animals are in each hectare, but the point remains: the vegan diet is not a bloodless one.

It's fair to ask if there's a difference between killing field animals like bunnies, field mice, gophers, raccoons in order to consume a vegan diet, and killing farm animals like chickens, pigs, sheep, and cows to consume an omnivore diet. But if our goal is simply to minimize the number of animal deaths, then the more moral choice is to consume larger herbivores, like cows, that have been raised on pasture instead of grains, so that fewer fields need to be cultivated and fewer field animals are killed.

The animal's quality of life is also important to consider. Was that pig raised in confinement on a cement floor, or was it allowed to "express its pigness," as Joel Salatin would say, and given space to roam, romp, and play? Was it treated well and respected when it died? Did it suffer, or was its slaughter humane? If we want to make a moral choice about eating meat, we need to think about these questions and seek out humanely raised meat. Labels like "Animal Welfare Approved" and other independent certifications for humanely raised meat are starting to make that a bit easier.

In addition to the moral question, we need to consider whether eating meat is sustainable. It requires a lot more resources to produce a diet heavy in grain than a diet whose protein comes from pasture-based livestock. In a healthy, sustainable system, livestock—unlike grains—require very little from us in the form of heavy machinery, irrigation, chemical fertilizers, herbicides, and pesticides. Grains also need heavy processing, unsustainable packaging, and transport. Finally, don't forget "enrichment"—all the vitamins and minerals that have been stripped out during processing need to be added back in when grains are transformed into white bread, pasta, flour, cookies, cakes, and more.

There's another environmental benefit to consuming pastured-raised animals: they do not need to compete with humans for cropland. Goats, pigs, chickens, cows, and many other animals can thrive on marginal land that is unsuitable for vegetable or grain production.

Finally, it's simply not possible to have a healthy vegetable farm without any animal inputs. We need decomposing animal products for healthy soil. We need animals' poop, urine, blood, and bones for vital bacteria, calcium, nitrogen, iron, and other elements required for life. Grazing animals provide all of this.

Healthy, sustainable land isn't the same as untouched land. I live in a town where a huge percentage of land is in conservation. Although the fallow fields and vast forests, which are purely for hiking and preserving songbirds, are beautiful to look at, it's important to realize that in order to stay healthy, those pastures need herbivores to break down the grasses and fertilize the soil. Land needs to be used, not locked up. We can't simply fence off pastoral views and expect them to stay healthy when there are no grazing animals to complete the nutrient cycle.

The diet that's best for both us and the environment is one that's mainly focused on nonindustrialized food: the sustainable Paleo diet.

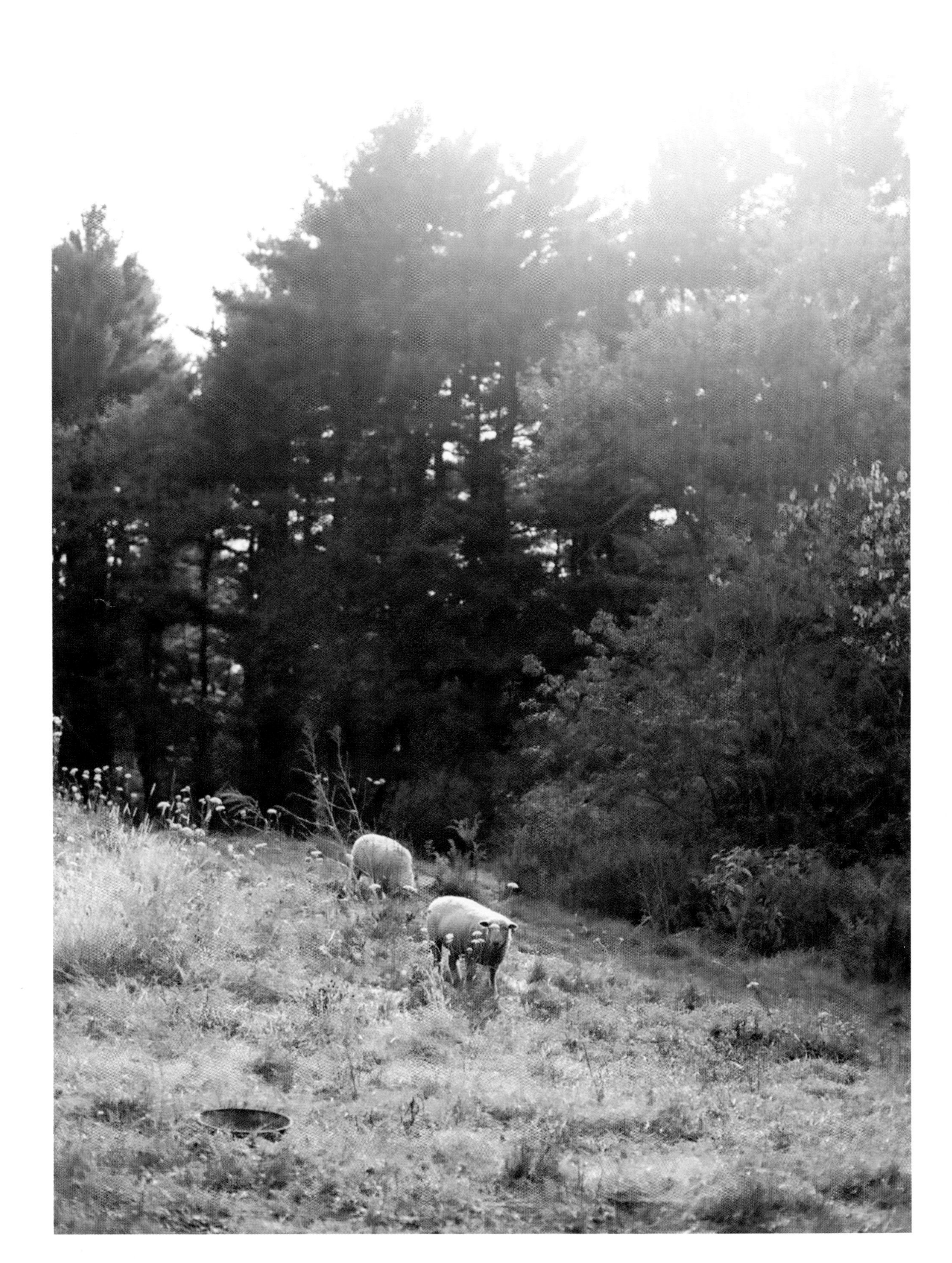

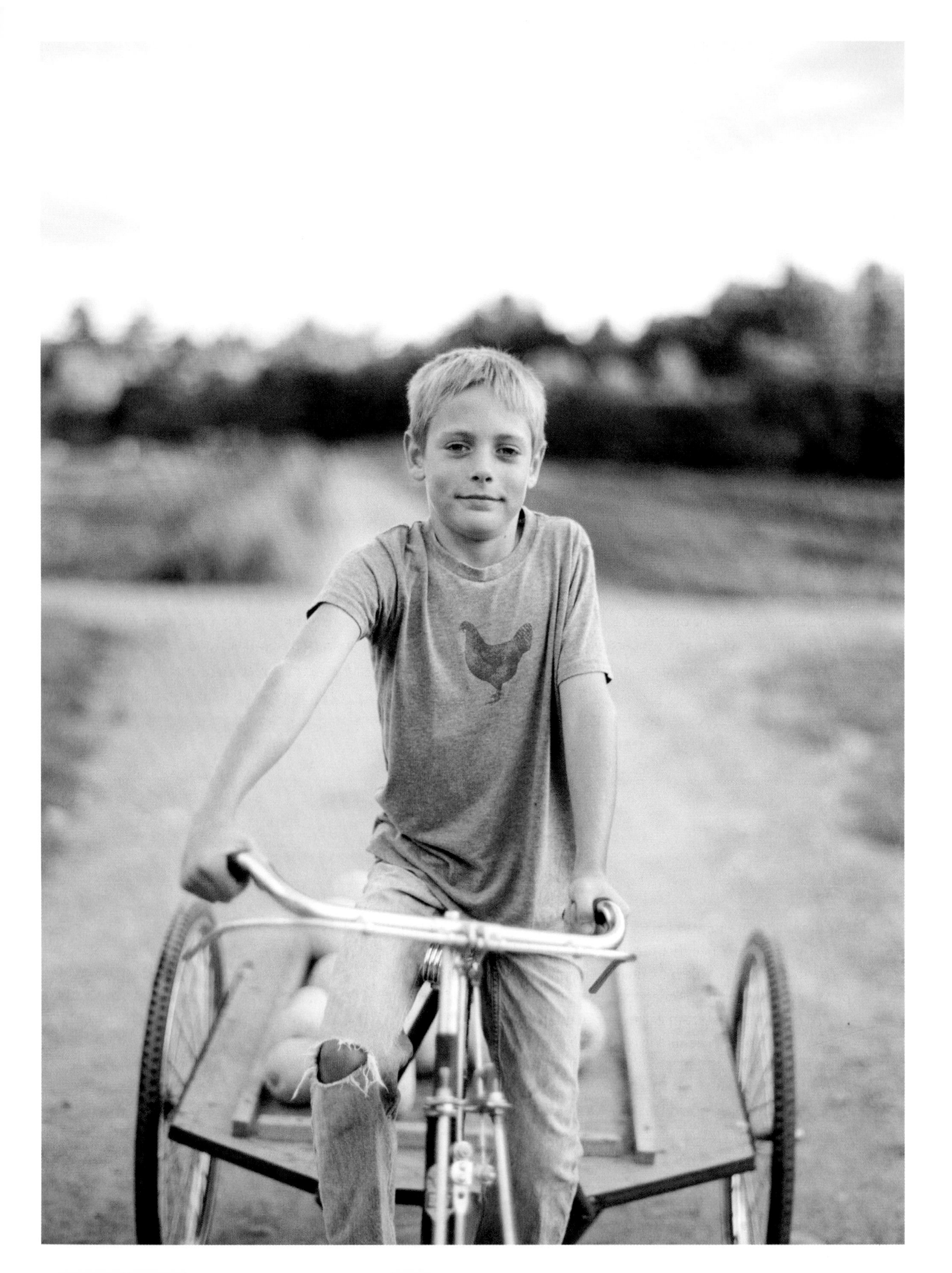

The Sustainable Paleo Diet

The Paleo diet is simple at its core: It's a way of eating that focuses on the foods the human body was designed to thrive on, primarily meats, vegetables, and fruit. It eliminates all refined sugars, grains, legumes, and most dairy products.

Most folks turn to the Paleo diet to improve their health or athletic performance, or for weight loss. As a nutritional therapist, I've seen firsthand how Paleo can help with all of these issues. It's not even necessary to be strict about it to get the benefits—like many people, I follow what's known as the 80/20 rule, where 80 percent of the foods are Paleo and 20 percent are healthy but not, strictly speaking, Paleo—dairy and certain starches, for example. (There's more on dairy and its place in a Paleo diet on page 18.) The main goal is always to focus on nutrient-dense foods for optimal health.

Unfortunately, what isn't always taken into consideration is how our food is grown and raised. Is a meal healthy if it is composed of CAFO chicken breast with a side of conventionally grown, pesticide-laden asparagus from Mexico and conventionally grown sweet potatoes harvested by underpaid and exploited workers? This is where the idea of sustainable Paleo comes into play. The quality of our food is very important, but so is its source. I believe that in order to be truly Paleo, the majority of our food needs to be sustainably produced. Food that truly nourishes is food that is grown in a manner that can be sustainable for the environment, for the farm workers, the consumers, and their communities.

The 80/20 rule is also a good guideline when considering the source of your food: aim for more organic and sustainably raised food. Maybe 80 percent sustainable seems overwhelming at first, but by making small changes, you'll be surprised at how easy it can be to get there.

Transitioning to Paleo

For those who are new to Paleo, I recommend following a strict Paleo diet for thirty days and then following the 80/20 rule: 80 percent Paleo foods, 20 percent healthy but non-Paleo foods.

This can be a *big* shift in eating for many people. If a strict Paleo diet seems too overwhelming, consider trying what I call the "baby step protocol": eliminate all gluten and refined sugar from your diet for thirty days. Just taking this step can result in amazing health benefits.

After thirty days, transition your breakfast to Paleo for the next two weeks. Then, for the next two weeks, make both your breakfast and lunch Paleo. Finally, start the thirty-day challenge of squeaky-clean Paleo—no grains, legumes, dairy, or sweeteners.

Decide what makes the most sense for you, whether diving right into the full Paleo challenge or transitioning more gradually, and then make it happen!

real food challenge
Farmers Ranchers Fisherfolk
family, immigrant & minority farmers, farmers abroad
Climate
alternative energy, emissions, climate change
Animals
fisheries, animal welfare, habitat loss
Natural Resources
soil, water, seeds, biodiversity
Access
affordability, hunger relief
Health
safety, nutrition
Celebration
taste, awareness, connection to food
Economics
urban & rural economies, fair trade, food policy
Control
self-sufficiency, food sovereignty & security, food justice
Education
youth development, leadership
Culture
traditions, relationships, public space, spirituality
Farmworkers
wages, health, living & working conditions
Food Chain Workers
processing plant, distribution, food service workers
Producers . Earth . Consumers . Communities

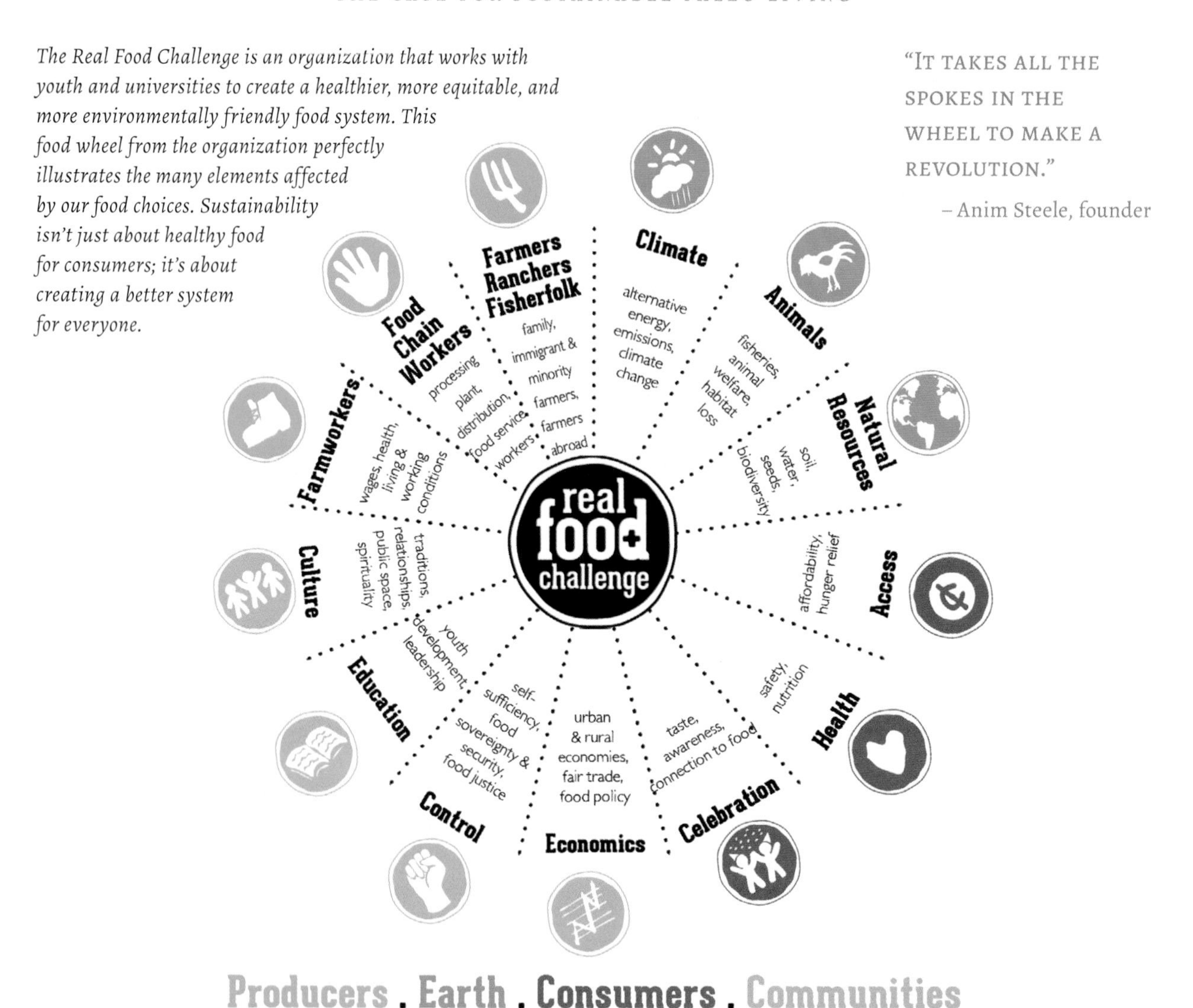

The Real Food Challenge is an organization that works with youth and universities to create a healthier, more equitable, and more environmentally friendly food system. This food wheel from the organization perfectly illustrates the many elements affected by our food choices. Sustainability isn't just about healthy food for consumers; it's about creating a better system for everyone.

"IT TAKES ALL THE SPOKES IN THE WHEEL TO MAKE A REVOLUTION."

– Anim Steele, founder

Paleo Foods and Sustainable Sources

Fat

Olive oil, which is full of healthy monounsaturated fats, is great for salads and low-heat cooking, but saturated fat—found in butter, ghee, and tallow from grass-fed cows, and bacon fat and lard from pastured pork—is ideal for high-heat cooking. (For more on butter and other dairy products, see page 18.) Coconut oil is another fantastic saturated fat that's a favorite among Paleo chefs, but for most of us it's not a locally produced item, so I limit my use of coconut oil. Foods that are good sources of fat include avocados, egg yolks from pastured chickens, and fatty cuts of meat from pastured animals.

Protein

Pasture-raised meat is always best. Compared to grain-fed meat, it has more vitamins and minerals and a much higher ratio of omega-3 to omega-6 fatty acids, which is associated with lower rates of heart disease, cancer, and autoimmune diseases. Grass-fed, locally produced beef, lamb, goat, and pork are fantastic, and if you live near the coast, seek out sustainable, local seafood. Chicken and other poultry are generally harder to source sustainably than larger herbivores and most wild fish, but eggs from pastured chickens are great sources of protein. Game meats, like venison and elk, are also excellent. Organ meats, such as liver, are very rich sources of vitamins and are a great addition to your weekly diet. Sausage and bacon are great, but pay attention to what's in the sausage—sometimes breadcrumbs are added to Irish sausages, and if you see "hydrolyzed vegetable protein" on the label, it really means gluten. I prefer to make my own sausages (such as my Cinnamon-Basil Breakfast Sausages, page 204) so I know exactly what goes into them.

Vegetables

Nonstarchy vegetables are great at making you feel full without consuming a lot of calories, which is useful if you're looking to lose weight, but their real benefit is in their vitamin and antioxidant content. Some vegetables, like lettuce and other easily digestible greens, can be eaten raw, but cruciferous vegetables like kale, collards, cabbage, bok choy, and broccoli should usually be cooked in order to lower their goitrogens, which can affect the thyroid. If weight loss is your goal, consume starchy root vegetables and squashes in moderation. CSAs and farmers markets are your best bets for purchasing vegetables if you're not growing them yourself.

ON WHITE POTATOES

I know many advocates of the Paleo diet were originally against eating white potatoes, but happily, most leaders in the community have now embraced them. White potatoes are an excellent source of starch for replenishing glycogen stores after exercise, and they're rich in many vitamins and minerals. White potatoes are higher in calories than sweet potatoes and winter squash, but most people without an active autoimmune disease can tolerate peeled white potatoes very well. But if you prefer to avoid them, feel free to substitute sweet potatoes for the white potatoes in my recipes.

EGGS: KNOW YOUR TERMS

There are lots of different ways to raise chickens, and when it comes to labeling eggs, some of the terms can be confusing. They're important, though. If you don't see a label that says otherwise, that carton of eggs probably comes from chickens that were given antibiotics and raised in cramped cages where the air is thick with dust and ammonia.

Pasture-raised
Eggs from chickens that are raised in pasture, where they're free to graze and peck for insects and get lots of sunshine. These are a significantly better source of long-chain omega-3 fatty acids—which are anti-inflammatory and have a ton of health benefits—than eggs from grain-fed chickens.

Organic
Eggs from chickens that have been fed organic grain. This doesn't necessarily mean that they've eaten their natural diet of grass and bugs, which is what pastured chickens consume.

Cage-free
Eggs from chickens that were not kept in small cages. However, these chickens are usually still raised indoors in crowded conditions, and there's no guarantee that they weren't given antibiotics or fed anything other than GMO grain.

Fed vegetarian feed/All-natural
These labels just mean the chickens were fed grains and possibly other vegetable matter, but they did not have access to the outside (where they would have consumed bugs and even mice, which is what chickens love to eat). In fact, these words mean nothing in terms of the welfare of the chickens.

Omega-3
Eggs with an "omega-3" label might have more omega-3s because the chickens got additional flax seeds in their grain mix, but that doesn't mean that the birds ever saw the light of the outdoors.

THERE'S SUCH A THING AS TOO LOW-CARB

Many people avoid roots and tubers on a Paleo diet because they are trying to reduce their carbohydrate intake. Carbohydrates do have benefits: they lower cortisol, fuel intense workouts (like CrossFit), and act as a prebiotic in your intestines by feeding your good bacteria. And if you restrict carbs too much—usually under 50 grams per day—you may experience sleeplessness, anxiety, depression, low energy, dry eyes, gastrointestinal distress, and weight gain. (Yes, you can actually gain weight from being too low-carb!) If you're experiencing any of these symptoms and have been limiting your intake of roots and tubers, please consider adding them back to your diet.

Fruit

Local, in-season fruits and berries are an ideal choice for treats—they're both nutritious and sustainable. However, if you're trying to lose weight, it's a good idea to moderate your fruit intake because it is high in sugar. Look for local berries and tree fruit at your local markets during the summer months.

Salt

Of all the different varieties of salt, natural sea salt has the best profile of minerals and trace elements, including magnesium, phosphorus, bromine, boron, zinc, iron, manganese, and copper. Surprisingly, though, it has very little iodine. Eating seaweed once a week or so is a great way to replace the iodine in your diet. I buy sheets of nori to use as wrappers for "sandwiches" and dulse or kelp flakes (we have local Atlantic sources!) to sprinkle in my soups and stews.

Nuts and Seeds

Although nuts and seeds are great sources of nutrients, they are very calorically dense and easy to eat in excess, especially when they're salted. Also, nuts contain large amounts of phytic acid, which interferes with the enzymes that break down our food. Soaking and then dehydrating them reduces their phytic acid. (For soaking instructions, see page 211.)

Sweeteners

Try to avoid sweeteners. They're strictly off-limits if you're on a thirty-day Paleo challenge, but even after, use only natural sweeteners, such as honey or maple syrup, and use those only sparingly. Artificial sweeteners can actually alter gut microbes, leading to metabolic issues.

In general, be careful of overconsuming sweetened foods, even when they are marketed as "Paleo." Paleo cookies, muffins, and cakes are still cookies, muffins, and cakes, and they don't have a place in your daily meals. Please consider them occasional treats. In my nutrition practice, I've found that clients who consistently eat sweets crave them more, and my feeling is that the easiest way to combat your sweet tooth is simply to avoid eating sweets.

Condiments, Herbs, and Spices

This is definitely an area where I include some non-local items in my diet. It is possible to cut out all spices—which are rarely from local sources here in the U.S.—and focus on seasonal herbs, but spices and condiments greatly enhance the flavor of my meals, so I'm willing to be a little flexible here. If you're trying to cut out sugar, it can be especially helpful to use spices that have sweet flavors, such as allspice, anise, cinnamon, cloves, ginger, and nutmeg. I also frequently use cumin, coriander, cardamom, thyme, fresh ginger, basil, and paprika, as well as Paleo-friendly condiments like Thai red curry paste, Dijon mustard, and coconut aminos, which are a great substitute for soy sauce. I also love garden-fresh herbs like basil, cilantro, and fresh tarragon. Avoid spice blends that have added sugars or chemical additives, and if you're purchasing non-local spices, seek out organically grown, fair trade–certified brands.

Grains

Grains are not part of the Paleo diet. They contain antinutrients, which can block the absorption of vitamins and minerals, and they're nutrient-poor, especially compared to organically grown roots and tubers, another source of carbohydrates. If you compare the nutrients in one cup of cooked whole wheat cereal to those in one cup of a baked sweet potato,

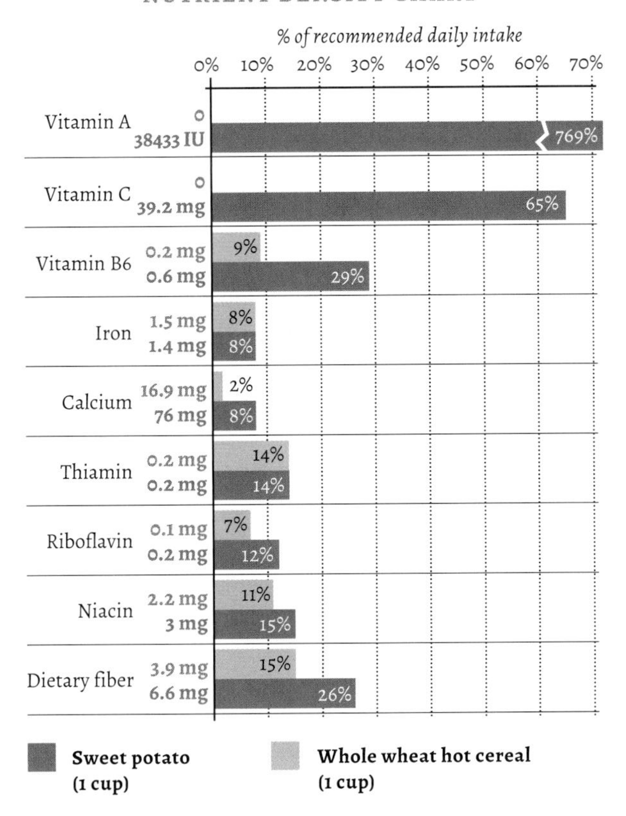

the sweet potato wins the nutrient density contest by a long shot, with 769% of the recommended daily intake of vitamin A and 65% of the recommended daily intake of vitamin C. In comparison, one cup of cooked, whole wheat cereal has no vitamin A or C, and very little of other nutrients.

Sweet potatoes, and vegetables in general, are also a fantastic source of fiber, so you don't need to worry that eliminating grains will reduce your fiber intake. In fact, as you can see in the chart, sweet potatoes have nearly twice as much dietary fiber as whole wheat hot cereal.

There are other problems with grains, too. They have a very high ratio of omega-6 to omega-3, which, along with other components in grains, can cause inflammation and is associated with a ton of illnesses, including heart disease, cancer, diabetes, and more. Many people also find that if they try grains again after cutting them out of their diet, they have a clear, immediate reaction to them, with symptoms that range from gastrointestinal distress to rashes, headaches, and "brain fog." Gluten, a protein found in wheat, rye, and barley, is particularly problematic for many people and can cause a host of difficulties, including celiac disease, in which gluten triggers the immune system to attack the small intestine. Traditional testing for celiac disease only screens for certain antibodies, and some people who have tested negative nevertheless feel better when they are gluten-free. In fact, non-celiac gluten sensitivity is gaining more attention in the medical community. What's more, even if you don't experience symptoms after ingesting gluten, it could still be causing inflammation in your system and decreasing the absorption of nutrients. In general, I've found that most folks feel much better when they eliminate gluten from their diet.

All that said, I do think that the occasional consumption of gluten-free grains may work for some folks. While grains are completely off-limits on a thirty-day Paleo challenge, after that, you can try reintroducing them to your diet if you wish, taking note of how your body responds when you eat them. But keep in mind that if you're following the 80/20 rule, they're part of the 20 and need to be consumed in moderation.

Environmentally speaking, however, grains are not an ideal crop. They are generally grown in a large-scale, monocrop method (more on the problems with that on page 23). When you combine the sustainability and nutrition concerns, it just doesn't make sense for humans to be eating a grain-heavy diet.

Legumes

Like grains, legumes contain antinutrients, and they aren't very nutrient-dense to begin with. However, soaking and cooking legumes can help inactivate their antinutrients, and if you tolerate them well, it's fine to eat the occasional bowl of split pea soup or add garbanzo beans to your salad.

Legumes have an important environmental advantage over grains, however: they fix nitrogen and improve soil quality. On our farm, we plant them as a cover crop when a field is fallow to reduce soil erosion and increase soil nitrogen.

Flours

Since grains are generally off-limits on a Paleo diet, many people turn to Paleo-friendly flours such as blanched almond flour, coconut flour, tapioca starch, potato starch, and arrowroot flour. I have to admit that I rarely use these flours. When I do, I avoid nut flours, which are highly caloric and contain delicate polyunsaturated fats, which can be damaged in the high heat of an oven. Instead, I stick to coconut flour, tapioca starch, and potato starch.

But more importantly, my caution about sweeteners applies to flours, too, since both are mostly used in baked goods. It can be really hard to resist that plate of cookies sitting on the kitchen counter, but they're just not good for you (even if they are "Paleo" cookies). Especially if you're trying to lose weight, please consider striking baked goods from your diet.

Dairy

When it comes to consuming dairy on a Paleo diet, there's a lot of disagreement. It wasn't consumed during the Paleolithic era, but there's much to be said for it nutritionally. Plain whole-milk yogurts, crème fraîche, and raw-milk cheeses from grass-fed cows are great sources of fat-soluble vitamins and conjugated linoleic acid (CLA), which can help regulate glucose levels. Dairy is also a good source of protein. (However, low-fat, ultra-pasteurized milk; American cheese; and low-fat, fruit-flavored yogurts are processed foods with poor nutrient density and should be avoided.)

In some people, though, dairy can cause weight gain, acne, congestion, or digestive issues. Try eliminating all dairy during your thirty-day Paleo challenge. If you would like to reintroduce it after that period, add it back to your diet slowly and take note of how your body responds.

Sustainability is a particular concern with the dairy industry. Routine antibiotics, conventional grain feeding, and manure lagoons are commonplace on big dairy farms, which, unsurprisingly, are not the happiest places for the cows, nor the healthiest systems for the animals or the environment. Small-scale, pasture-based dairies are a much better option for the cows, for the environment, and for a more nutritious product.

A PALEO CHEAT SHEET

It can be difficult to remember exactly which foods are Paleo and which aren't. In his "The Paleolithic Solution" seminar, Robb Wolf showed a chart similar to the one below, which I found very helpful. When you mix and match all of these options, you end up with over 45,000 possible combinations. That means you don't have to repeat the same dinner for 127 years!

PROTEIN	NONSTARCHY VEG	STARCHY VEG*	FAT/OIL	SPICE	HERB
Lamb chops	Kale	Sweet potatoes	Ghee	Ginger	Basil
Wild salmon	Broccoli	White potatoes	Coconut oil	Paprika	Thyme
Ground beef	Bok choy	Carrots	Lard	Cinnamon	Chives
Venison	Spinach	Beets	Tallow	Black pepper	Parsley
Chicken	Cabbage	Parsnips	Olive oil	Mustard	Rosemary
Scallops	Bell peppers	Winter squash	Duck fat	Curry	Cilantro

**Starchy vegetables should be consumed in moderation. Aim for about 50 to 125 grams per day, depending on your activity level.*

How Much Should You Eat?

After I talk with my nutrition clients about the kinds of foods they should be eating, their next question is always "How much should I eat?" I suggest eating three meals a day, and for each meal, here are some great starting points:

- **Protein:** About 4 to 8 ounces (about the size of your palm or a little larger), depending on your size and needs
- **Nonstarchy vegetables:** Piled high on your plate
- **Starchy vegetables:** About 4 ounces (the equivalent of one small sweet potato), or 8 ounces for athletes
- **Healthy fat:** About 1 tablespoon

If you get hungry between meals, try snacking on a handful of nuts (just a handful!) and a piece of fruit.

Remember, just because a food is allowed on the Paleo diet doesn't mean that portion size doesn't matter. Bacon is great, but not ten pounds of it in one sitting. Although you should eat enough that you don't feel hungry, you don't want to eat to overcapacity, either.

And keep in mind that everyone is different. The macronutrient combination and calorie load that works for a twenty-five-year-old athlete may not work for a fifty-year-old who's recovering from hip surgery. It's best to consider your weight loss goals, stress level, and activity level. For weight loss, consider consuming the bulk of your daily starch intake in a post-workout meal. Also, since eating a nutrient-dense diet can sometimes mean consuming more calories than you need, tracking your total calories can be very helpful. Those who are highly stressed or have certain health issues, such as thyroid disease, may not do well on a very low carbohydrate diet. Athletes, who need more energy, should consume more starchy vegetables, such as carrots, parsnips, and sweet potatoes. Everyone is unique, so please tinker with your own diet until you find what works for you.

When Paleo Just Isn't Enough

What if you've been following the Paleo diet and are still not feeling great? The culprit could be an unhealthy lifestyle (overtraining, poor sleep, stress), other food intolerances, poor digestion, parasites, or even just an unhealthy microbiome in your gut. It's worth it to take a good look at all of these components. If you have an autoimmune disease, the autoimmune protocol, which eliminates foods like eggs, nuts, and nightshades, maybe helpful. Foods containing large amounts of FODMAPs (fermentable oligo-di-monosaccharides and polyols) can also cause digestive distress in some people. I recommend seeking out a health-care practitioner to run a stool test, which can identify any overgrowth of pathogenic bacteria or parasites. Also, the resources section at the end of this book includes some great books and blogs that can help you investigate the autoimmune protocol and low FODMAPs diet.

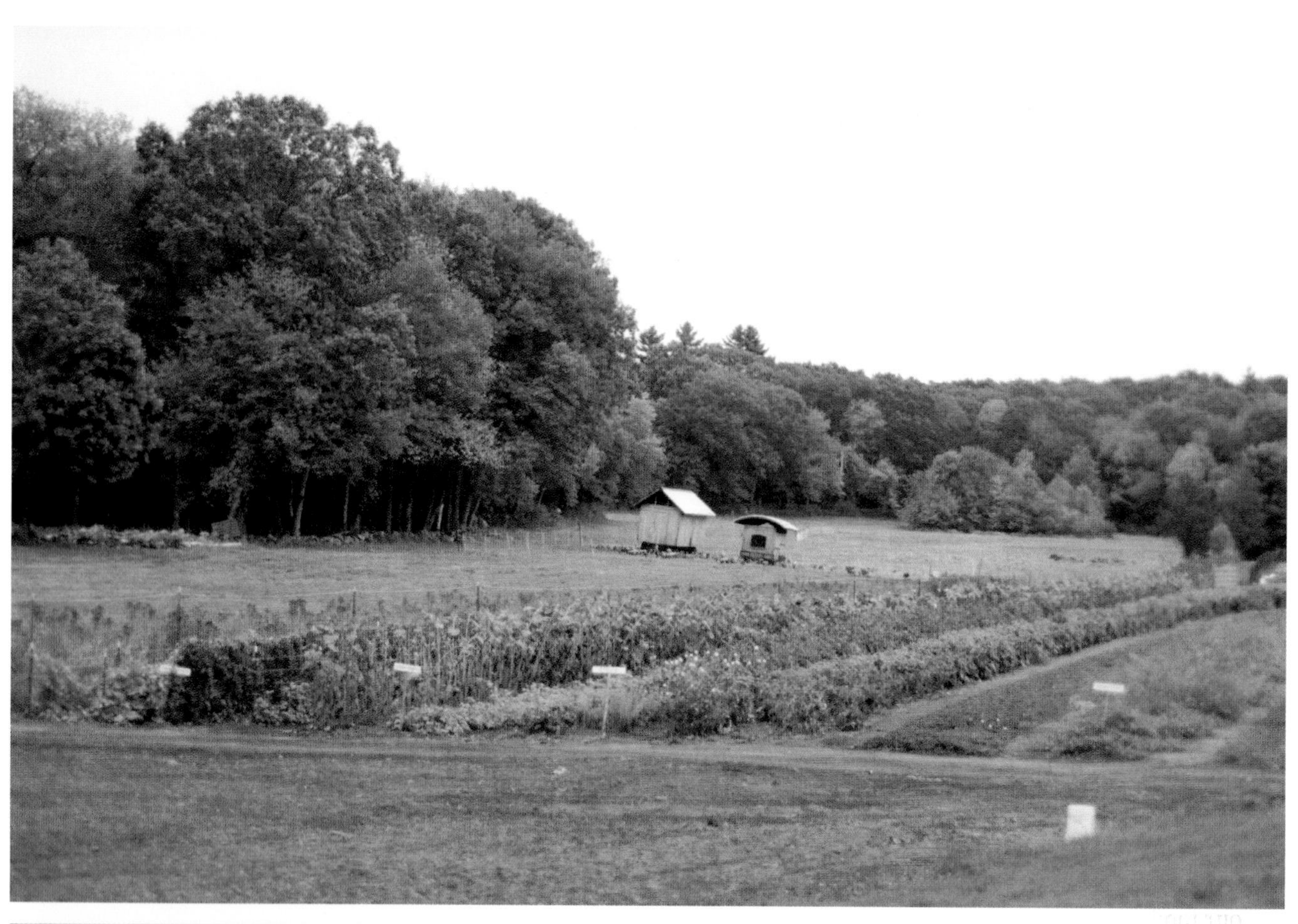

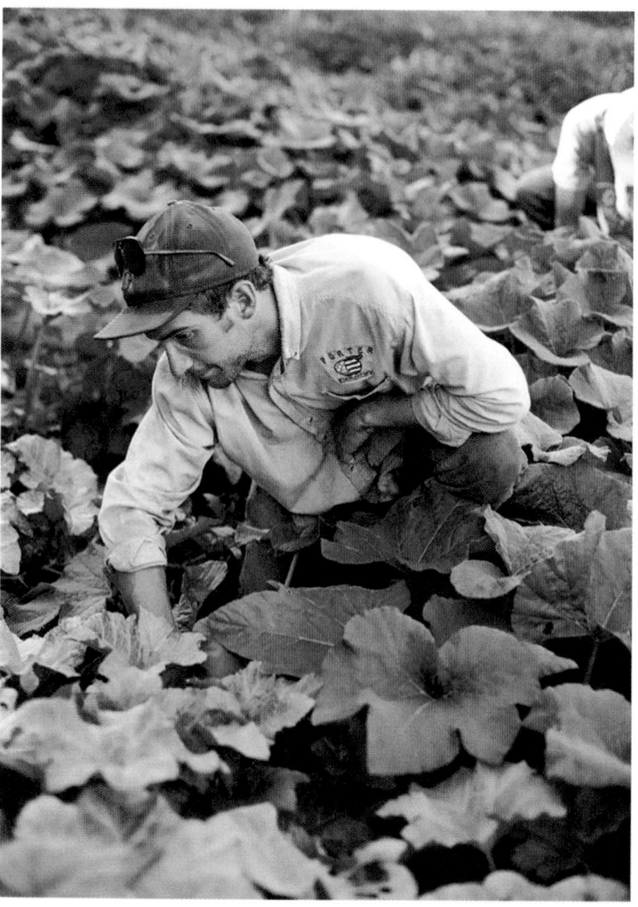

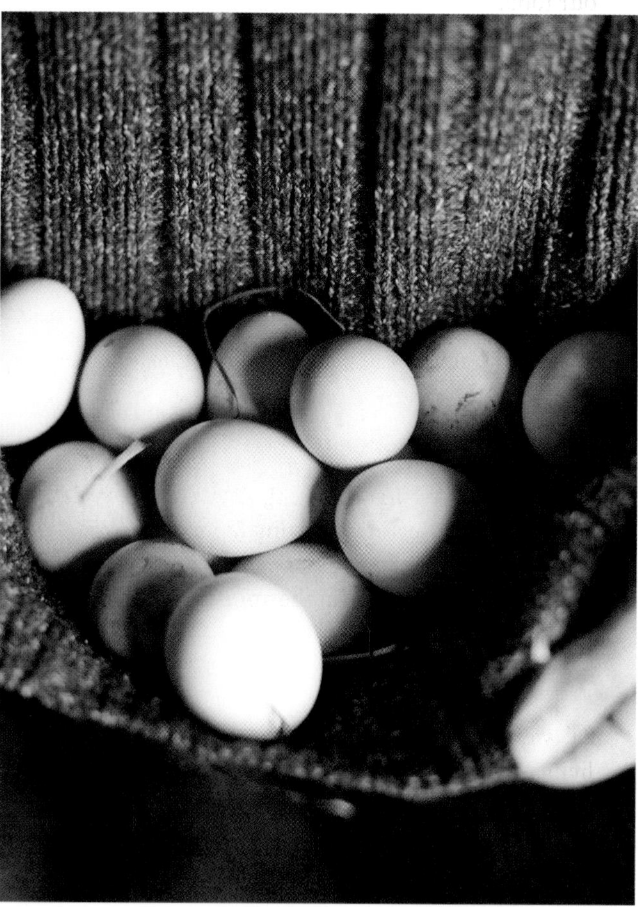

UNDERSTANDING FOOD PRODUCTION AND SUSTAINABILITY

GROWING FOOD AND RAISING ANIMALS OURSELVES IS, I THINK, THE BEST OPTION FOR TRULY UNDERSTANDING WHERE OUR FOOD COMES FROM. BUT THAT'S NOT POSSIBLE FOR EVERYONE, AND EVEN IF YOU CAN'T RAISE YOUR OWN CHICKENS AND HAVE A VEGETABLE GARDEN, UNDERSTANDING FOOD PRODUCTION IS ESSENTIAL FOR ONE SIMPLE REASON: BUYING FOOD IS A POLITICAL ACT.

Every time you purchase food, you are casting your vote for the future of farming. You can choose to encourage industrial food institutions, or you can buy food that supports small-scale, sustainable farming. Either way, to be an informed consumer, it's important to understand how the food you eat is produced.

Of course, I strongly recommend seeking out small-scale, sustainable farms (I'll explain why in a moment), and understanding sustainability is vital when it comes to making the best food choices for yourself, the environment, and the people who grow our food.

Sustainable agriculture is about growing produce and raising farm animals in a way that maintains the health and viability of the land and its resources, reuses and recycles material in order to make the most efficient use of it, treats animals humanely, pays workers a living wage, supports local communities, and keeps the farm economically self-sustaining.

Ultimately, all that leads to a decentralized food system, in which consumers buy directly from local farmers.

THE HALLMARKS OF SUSTAINABILITY

Pastured animals
Keeping animals on pasture, where they can graze freely and get plenty of sunshine and exercise, is best for the animals. It also makes their meat more nutritious for us.

Rotational grazing
Pasture does best when grazing animals are moved from section to section, allowing the manure to fertilize the soil and the grass to recover. It also helps reduce the parasite load in the animals. (See more on page 61.)

Happy farm workers
All workers should be treated with respect and paid a living wage.

Composting
An essential part of organic gardening, composting is the best way to make the most of all the scraps and waste that are inevitable on any farm (or in any household, for that matter).

Organic growing practices
Avoiding chemical fertilizers and toxic pesticides is crucial for healthy produce, and a healthy environment.

Humane slaughter
Caring for animals includes making sure their slaughter is as quick and pain-free as possible, and it shouldn't frighten the animals unnecessarily.

Small Is Beautiful: The Benefits of a Decentralized Food System

It's probably no surprise that fresh, local produce is more nutrient-dense than produce that was harvested a week ago, sat on a truck for days, and then waited in a supermarket bin before you brought it home. But the reasons to buy from small-scale, local farmers who use sustainable practices go far beyond nutrition.

It supports local communities

When you spend your money at a small local farm, more of your dollars stay in the community, since small-scale farmers generally purchase their supplies (seeds, machinery, tools, and so on) from local businesses. That helps to generate local jobs and stimulates the economy right in your community.

It's better for the farm workers

According to the National Farm Worker Ministry, the average income of a crop worker is between $10,000 and $12,499 a year. To give you some perspective, the 2014 federal poverty line was $11,670 for an individual and $23,850 for a family of four. Cropworkers are often paid "piece rate" wages, which are based on how much they pick, instead of an hourly wage. The piece rate for oranges in Florida, for instance, is $0.85 per 90-pound box of oranges. The average productivity for a worker is eight boxes per hour. This means that during an eight-hour workday, a worker picks about sixty-four boxes of oranges, 5,760 pounds. For that day, the worker receives $54.40— $6.80 per hour, which is less than the minimum wage. Paying workers this way also creates an incentive for them to take fewer much-needed water breaks, and on large farms, rent for housing for farm workers (which often means overcrowded trailers) is automatically deducted from their paychecks.

Children are particularly vulnerable when it comes to farm work. There are an estimated 500,000 farm workers under the age of eighteen in the U.S. Farms are exempt from many labor laws, and these children suffer extreme working conditions: infrequent water and food breaks, high temperatures, pesticide exposure, and dangerous machinery (70 percent of all tractor injuries involve children). The kids are also often subjected to intense emotional strain due to unstable home lives, as families follow the harvest and pull kids from school. Young girls are especially in danger of sexual abuse from their bosses in the fields. And all that's just in the U.S.—working conditions in other countries can be far worse.

Small-scale farms are much more likely to offer fair wages, paid time off, and opportunities for advancement. In addition, they often train future farmers through apprenticeships and internships. This is critical for the future of farming. On our farm, for instance, we employ a mix of local teens, young adults who want to get into farming, and adults who volunteer their labor in exchange for food. We pay fair (not piece rate) wages, and take the time to ensure proper training and safety precautions are being met.

It's better for the animals

Livestock raised on small farms are generally subjected to less-stressful living conditions, fewer antibiotics, and more peaceful slaughter than those raised on Concentrated Animal Feeding Operations (CAFOs). Instead of spending their whole lives in cramped spaces under fluorescent lights, eating a strictly grain-based diet, cattle on small, sustainable farms spend their lives on pasture, with sunshine, green grass, and the freedom move comfortably.

But just because a farm is small doesn't necessarily mean the animals are grass fed or treated well. I highly encourage you to do your homework and visit the farm you purchase your meat from. Do the animals look happy? Do they seem healthy and have enough space? Are there signs of vermin or disease? Ask where they are slaughtered and see if any complaints have been filed against the slaughterhouse. When we start considering the treatment of animals, we're in a much better position to buy humanely raised meat, which is healthier for us, too.

For their products to be labeled "Certified Organic" or "Animal Welfare Approved," farms and slaughterhouses must meet strict guidelines for the care and end-of-life process for farm animals. Not all farms that treat animals humanely have these certifications, but if you aren't able to visit a farm firsthand, these labels are a good way to make sure you're supporting a humane, sustainable operation. (For more on slaughterhouses, see page 75.)

It encourages biodiversity

When you join a CSA or shop at a farmers market, you'll see all kinds of produce and meat from heritage animal breeds and heirloom produce varieties. These older breeds and varieties are dying out as a few commercial ones dominate agribusiness, and as they go extinct, their genetic lines—and valuable traits that let them thrive in different habitats—are lost forever. It's critical that we support biodiversity when it comes to our food consumption to keep these breeds and varieties thriving year after year, and small-scale farms offer the best way to do that.

Large, industrial-scale agricultural operations tend to use monocropping, in which a single crop is grown on the same piece of land year after year. Monocropping reduces biodiversity and damages the soil. Small-scale farms, on the other hand, tend to diversify and rotate their crops, and to allow parts of the land to remain fallow and rest between seasons. It keeps native and heirloom varieties alive and improves the health of the soil.

Large industrial farms also destroy the many native species of plants and animals that once thrived on their land. Seek out farms that encourage small ecosystems like wetlands, ponds, woodland, and fallow fields, so that the whole farm is a living system, not only a place to plant seeds.

Preserving heritage breeds of animals, and crossing them for hybrid vigor, is also important. Factory farming has led a handful of breeds of pigs, cows, and chickens to dominate our food system. Those breeds, which do well in indoor conditions and put on weight quickly but aren't adapted for life outside factory farms, have supplanted heritage breeds, and as these go extinct, their adaptations for different environments are lost. The best way to ensure that heritage breeds survive is to create a demand for them by eating them.

It's environmentally responsible

When we purchase inexpensive, conventionally grown bananas from the grocery store, we don't see their real cost. We don't see the devastating effects of toxic pesticides that are sprayed over the monocrop plantations and land on neighboring schools, making the children sick, or the environmental effects of shipping bananas around the world.

THE NEXT BIG THING: REGIONAL AGGREGATION

More and more sustainable farmers are joining together in co-ops to offer consumers a wider variety of sustainable food. Our farm partners with others that are great at growing certain crops, like squash, or that offer food, like goat cheese, that we don't have the time or capacity for. Our customers love the extra variety, and it means more sales for us and the other producers.

Similarly, companies across the country have begun sourcing produce, meats, and other local foods from responsible growers and compiling them on one website—sort of like a virtual farmers market. You can go to the website, click on the item to find out more about the farm it came from, and make your purchases. The food is delivered to a drop-off point in your area, or even right to your house. In some cases, not all of the products are from small farms or are sourced locally (some sites carry items like bananas and grain-fed beef), but it's certainly a step in the right direction. Two great examples are Relay Foods in the Washington, DC/Charlottesville, North Carolina, area, and Polyface Yum, a division of Joel Salatin's Polyface Farms that serves Virginia, Maryland, and the District of Columbia. It's convenient for consumers, and since the farmers don't have to leave their farms to sell their products or worry about marketing, they can focus on growing.

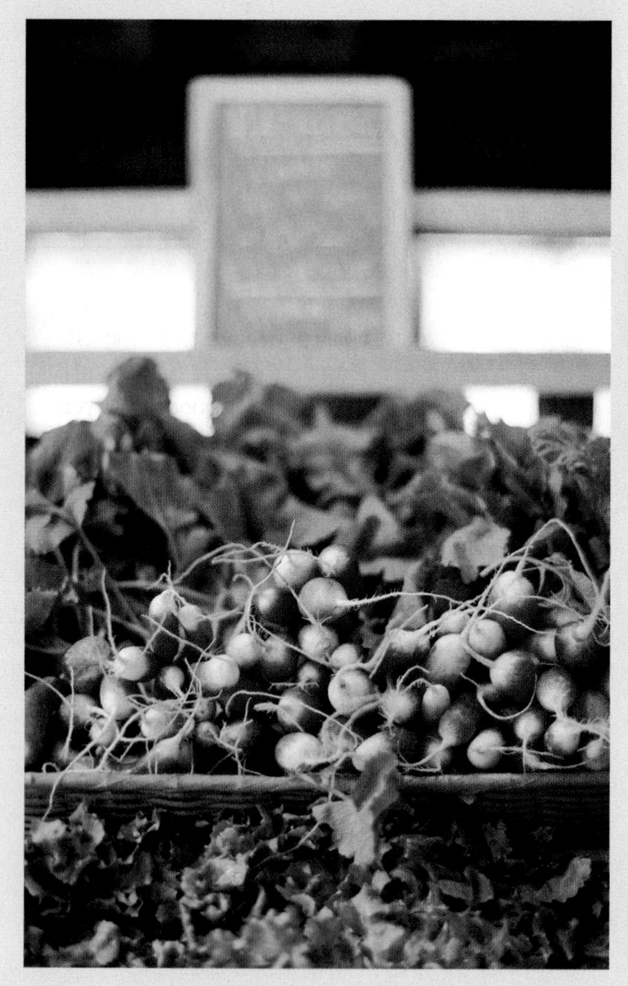

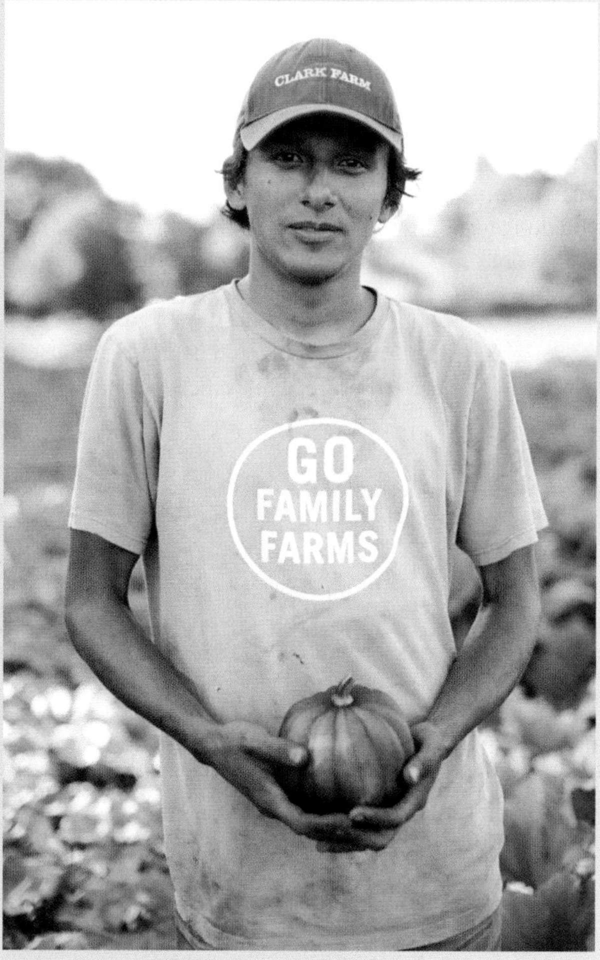

10 QUESTIONS TO ASK A FARMER

BEFORE YOU BUY DIRECTLY FROM A LOCAL FARMER, IT'S ALWAYS A GOOD IDEA TO INTERVIEW THEM. I CAN TELL YOU FIRSTHAND, AS SOMEONE WHO SPENT YEARS ATTENDING FARMERS MARKETS, THAT SOME FARMERS ARE MUCH MORE RESPONSIBLE AND ETHICAL ABOUT THEIR GROWING PRACTICES THAN OTHERS. HERE ARE SOME GOOD STARTER QUESTIONS TO HELP YOU IDENTIFY A RESPONSIBLE GROWER.

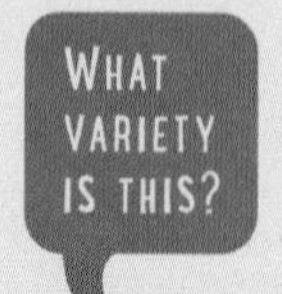

It's ideal to buy directly from the farmer who grew the crop, but sometimes it's hard to tell if the person you're taking to at a farmers market actually grew the crop or if they bought it from another farm to sell. If they did grow the crop, they'll probably know the variety of every seed they grew. Another good question to ask is, "When was this picked?"

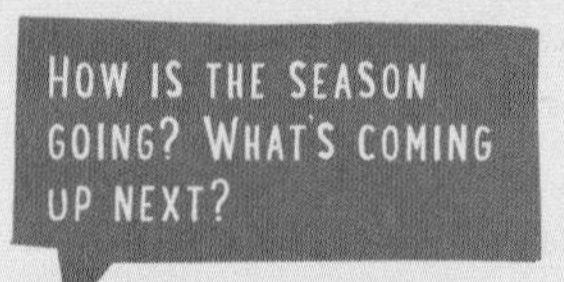

These are fantastic questions to engage a farmer in conversation. Those who are growing their own produce will probably have a lot to say about weather conditions and will know what crops will be at the market next week.

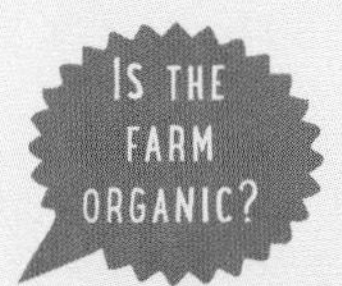

Getting certified as an organic farm can be a headache of paperwork and costly for small producers. But even if a farm isn't advertising as organic, it could be using sustainable growing practices. If they answer "no," ask how they handle pests and disease—you don't want anything grown with pesticides.

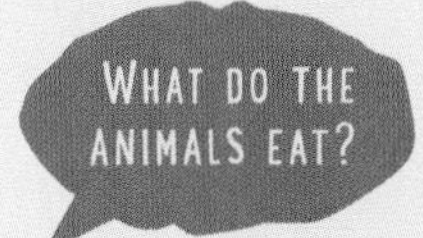

Herbivores like sheep, goats, and cows should be mostly on pasture, while chickens and pigs are okay with some supplemental grain. If you're talking to a beef farmer, ask how the cows are "finished." Many grass-fed beef farms finish their cows on corn, which is hard for the cows to digest. If some of the animals are fed grain, is it organic and soy-free? If not, why not? It can be really hard for farmers to get their hands on bulk organic, soy-free grain, but the more questions they get from customers, the more likely they will be to seek it out.

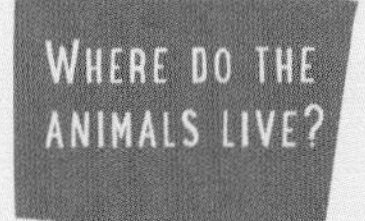

The answer should be that they live outside and are rotationally grazed. Follow up with "How often are they rotated?" Herbivores and chickens that are pastured on the same patch of grass each day are not as healthy as those who are moved often.

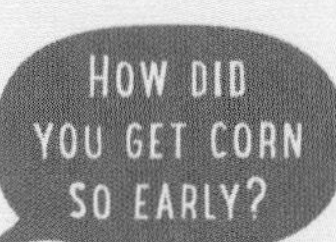

Be aware of what's in season in your area and ask about anything that seems out of place. If you see a farmer selling corn or tomatoes in June in Maine, something's not right. Although some growers may start their plants in a greenhouse, usually those who have a certain crop very early actually purchased it from out of state. Look behind the farm's table for produce boxes with labels identifying other states—if you're at a market in Michigan, you don't want to see a box of blueberries with a New Jersey label. Keep in mind, too, that most farmers in a region will generally have the same items at the same time, so anything out of the ordinary is worth a second glance.

How many different types of produce do you grow?

The variety of a farm's produce is usually a good indicator of whether the farm is truly sustainable. A farm that grows only a handful of crops is less likely to rotate crops and allow fields to lay fallow so the soil can recover.

Can I visit the farm?

No matter how many questions you ask a farmer, seeing the farm firsthand is really the best way to tell if it's good fit for you. From the minute you step out of your car, you'll be able to tell how well the farm is run. Are the fields full of weeds? Do the animals look healthy? Do they have enough room? Are the tools put away and the machines in good repair? Do the workers seem happy? Don't be surprised if the farm has specific visiting hours or only a couple of open houses a year. Some farms are more visitor-friendly than others.

Can I volunteer?

Some farmers are open to bartering for services in exchange for produce. Plus, volunteering at a farm is fun, a great workout, an opportunity to meet people, and a way to connect with how your food is grown.

Maybe the farmer you're talking to has a big sweet potato harvest coming up and could use your help. Are you a great cook? Maybe you could prepare lunch for the farm crew one day. Are you great with computers? Maybe the farmer could use a hand with their website. But be aware that not all farms accept volunteers—there can be liability issues, and they may not have the time or staff needed to train volunteers.

Do you have more of that delicious (fill in the blank)?

Let the farmer know how much you loved the zucchini from last week, or how the lettuce made the most delicious salad you've ever had. Farming pays little and is really hard work, and manning a table at a farmers market can be exhausting. Make someone's day by showing how much you appreciate them.

We also don't see the real cost of conventional meat, dairy, and egg products at the supermarket. The negative consequences of CAFOs—which affect all of us, whether we choose to buy the products or not—are known in economics as "externalities," and they include massive waste, from toxic sludge to poisonous chemicals, that have the potential to heat up the atmosphere, poison fisheries, pollute drinking water, contaminate the soil, and damage recreational areas. Ultimately we taxpayers foot the bill for CAFOs with hundreds of billions of dollars in subsidies, medical expenses, insurance premiums, declining property values, and cleanup costs.

Even organic growing practices aren't really enough, although they're important—they eliminate the toxic effects of synthetic pesticides and fertilizers, but that's only one piece of the puzzle. An organic Cavendish banana is still grown in a monocrop environment and shipped to the U.S. from far away. We need to seek out more varieties of bananas, so that it's impossible for one disease to wipe out the entire supply. An even better choice would be to seek out locally grown fruit instead—apples in Washington and New York, for instance, oranges in Florida, or pawpaws in Ohio. Many of the problems of large industrial farms exist at large-scale organic farms that produce bagged spinach, broccoli, and peppers: they're still growing monocrops and using fossil fuels to package and ship them all over the country, creating pollution.

Small-scale sustainable farms that use organic growing techniques are better for the planet. They improve the soil through crop rotation and rotational grazing. They avoid petrochemical fertilizers and pesticides and instead use products like fish emulsion, a fertilizer made from seafood industry by-products that adds nutrients to the soil. And because they're mostly selling to local residents, less fossil fuel is needed to package and transport food.

SUSTAINABILITY COULD SAVE THE WORLD

When you consider that the majority of the world's landmass is so dry and arid that it is unsuitable for growing crops, the idea that we should try to feed everyone with grain, or grain-fed animals, seems terribly flawed—especially since unsustainable farming practices are a major cause of desertification. The Savory Institute, a nonprofit organization founded by Allan Savory, has proposed a system of strategic, intensive rotational grazing that could allow marginal land to support herd animals.

"It helps to think of soil as a living organism covered with skin like a human. We can live with a certain percentage of our skin damaged, but if too high a percentage is damaged, we die. So, too, does soil and thus most life."

– Allan Savory

Marginal areas can be brought back to life with herds of wild or domestic herbivores, like cattle, sheep, goats, horses, and camels, that mimic the herds of wild grazing animals that used to roam the land. When they eat grasses, herbivores trim down the plants to stimulate healthy growth, and their feces is a rich fertilizer for the soil that also helps improve its water-holding capacity. The key is balance: the herds need to be the right size, and they need to spend the right amount of time on a patch of land so that they neither overgraze nor undergraze the plants.

With more water and more organic matter from feces in the soil, the land is better suited for growing crops—and providing economic stability for those who depend on it. And the meat of grazing herbivores provides highly bioavailable protein and other nutrients for humans. It's a win-win.

This idea fits beautifully with the nutritional philosophy of Paleo. Restoring grazing animals to their natural, wild ways, roaming and grazing on grassland, actually heals the land.

A NOTE ON FAIR TRADE

You've probably seen the "fair trade" label applied to coffee and chocolate found in higher-end markets. It can also be applied to other products, including tea, bananas, sugar, honey, rice, flowers, and cotton.

The original intent of the label was to support sustainability among small-scale producers in developing countries. Chocolate, in particular, has been associated with problems that the fair-trade label was intended to address. Many African cacao farmers use child labor to harvest their crops. Most of the children cannot speak the local language, are fed a terrible diet of only corn paste and bananas, have no access to medical care, and breathe in harsh chemical pesticides. A 2011 Tulane University study found that a "projected total of 819,921 children in Côte d'Ivoire and 997,357 children in Ghana worked on cocoa-related activities" in 2007 and 2008.

The fair-trade label has indeed helped curb these problems. According to an analysis by the International Institute for Sustainable Development, coffee farms whose products are fair trade–certified appear to perform distinctly better in occupational health and safety, employee relations, and labor rights than their noncertified counterparts.

However, as an article in *Stanford Social Innovation Review* put it, "Fair Trade coffee has evolved from an economic and social justice movement to largely a marketing model for ethical consumerism." Some fair trade organizations have been criticized for creating uneven economic advantages for coffee growers. A new movement called "Authentic Fair Trade" or even "Direct Trade" appear to be addressing some of the flaws within the original fair trade movement.

All in all, although fair-trade labels have done a lot to bring awareness of sustainability issues to the food industry, the system is not without its flaws.

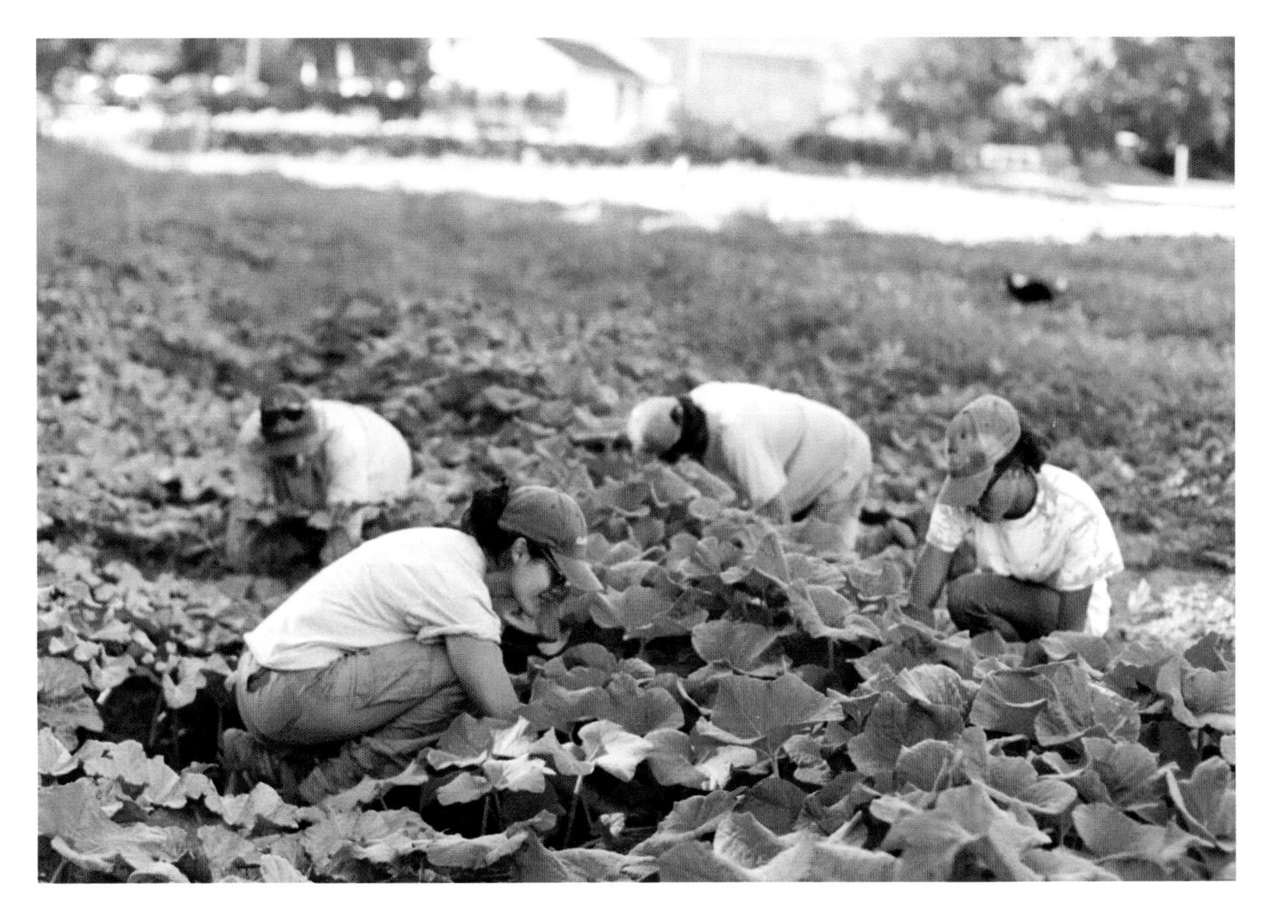

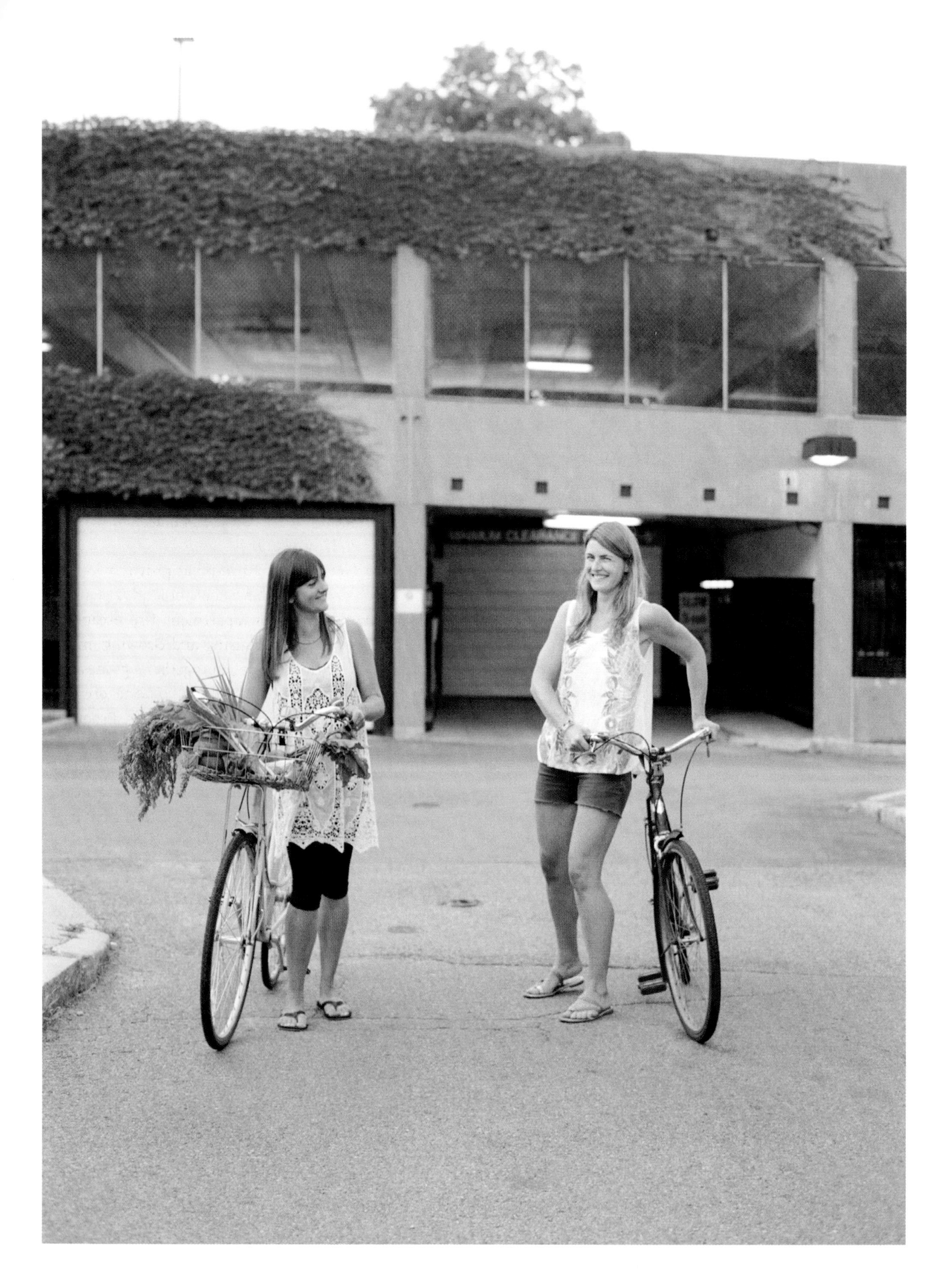

What You Can Do

The rewards of homesteading go even beyond the benefits for the animals and the environment. Growing your own food is liberating, and a great way to teach your children where food comes from and the value of hard work. It's also the best way to understand our connection to the land and other animals, and it deepens that connection at the same time. Plus, food you've grown yourself tastes better than anything you can buy.

During World War I and World War II, the U.S. and U.K. governments encouraged citizens to grow "victory gardens" to help reduce food shortages. Ordinary citizens rallied to grow their own food, turning sports fields into pasture for sheep and creating vegetable gardens in vacant lots and on apartment rooftops. The victory gardens advertising campaigns were very successful and made a big difference in the production of food during both wars.

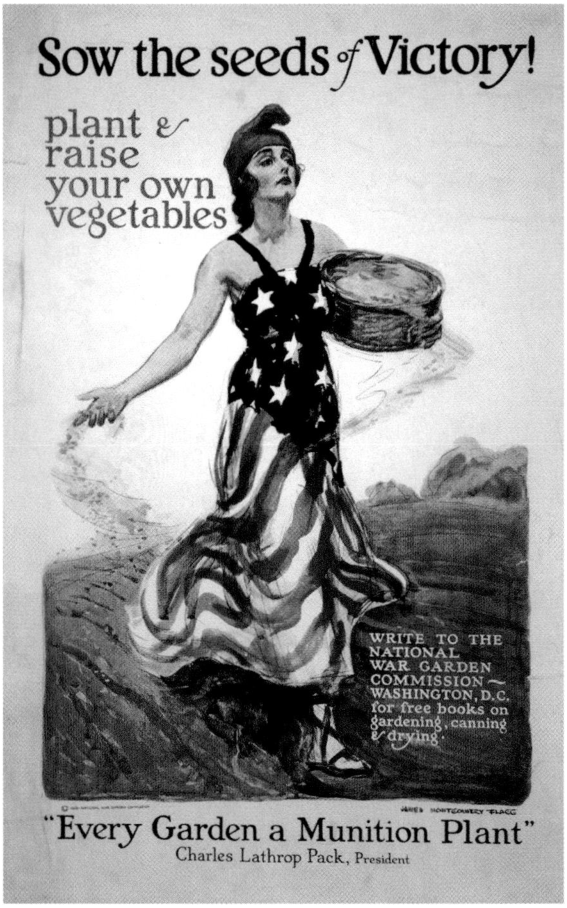

Victory gardens had a specific wartime purpose in preventing food shortages, but the campaigns' slogans and energy could just as easily apply to growing your own food today—and they proved that it really is possible for ordinary people to grow their own food, even in cities. In fact, the victory gardens campaign inspired Paleo guru Robb Wolf to create a "liberty gardens" campaign, a program that I now help oversee. The goal is to encourage people to change the existing food system in the U.S. by growing their own food and being more eco-conscious about their food purchases in general. I'd love to see advertisements for liberty gardens in magazines and billboards across the country!

I hope that you'll try your hand at growing your own food—whether you have acres of land, a small backyard, or even just an apartment fire escape. In the next two sections, Raising and Growing, my husband, Andrew, and I have put together a guide to help you get started with any level of homesteading, from container gardening on your patio in Brooklyn to keeping chickens and a few beehives in your backyard to creating a full, small-scale farm with animals as well as crops. Andrew has brought farms back from the financial brink, and he knows what it takes to have a thriving and sustainable farming operation, or just a healthy backyard garden. Try it for yourself, and you'll understand why nothing tastes better than fresh eggs from your own chickens and tomatoes just off the vine.

Frances Roberts / Alamy

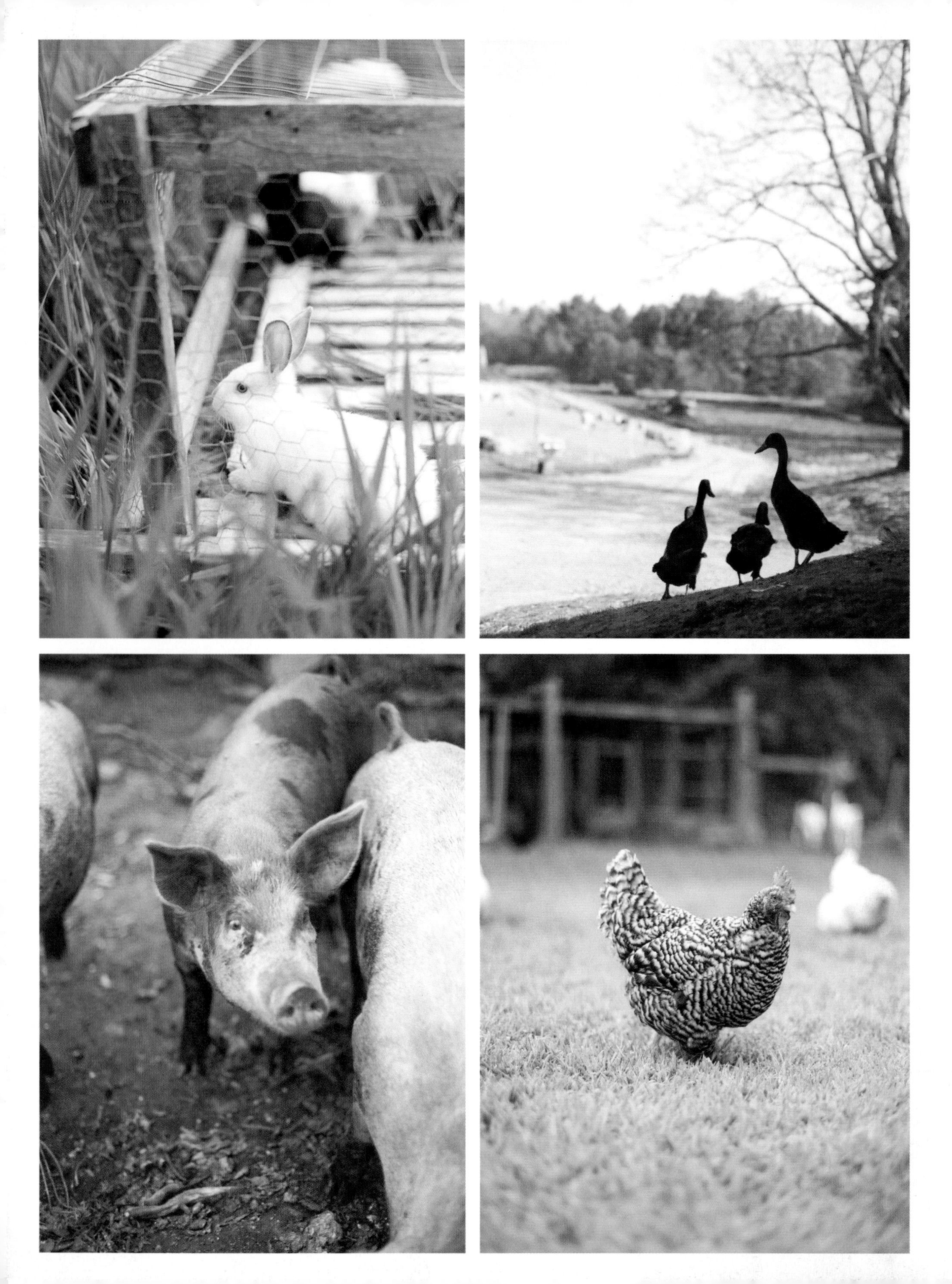

Raising

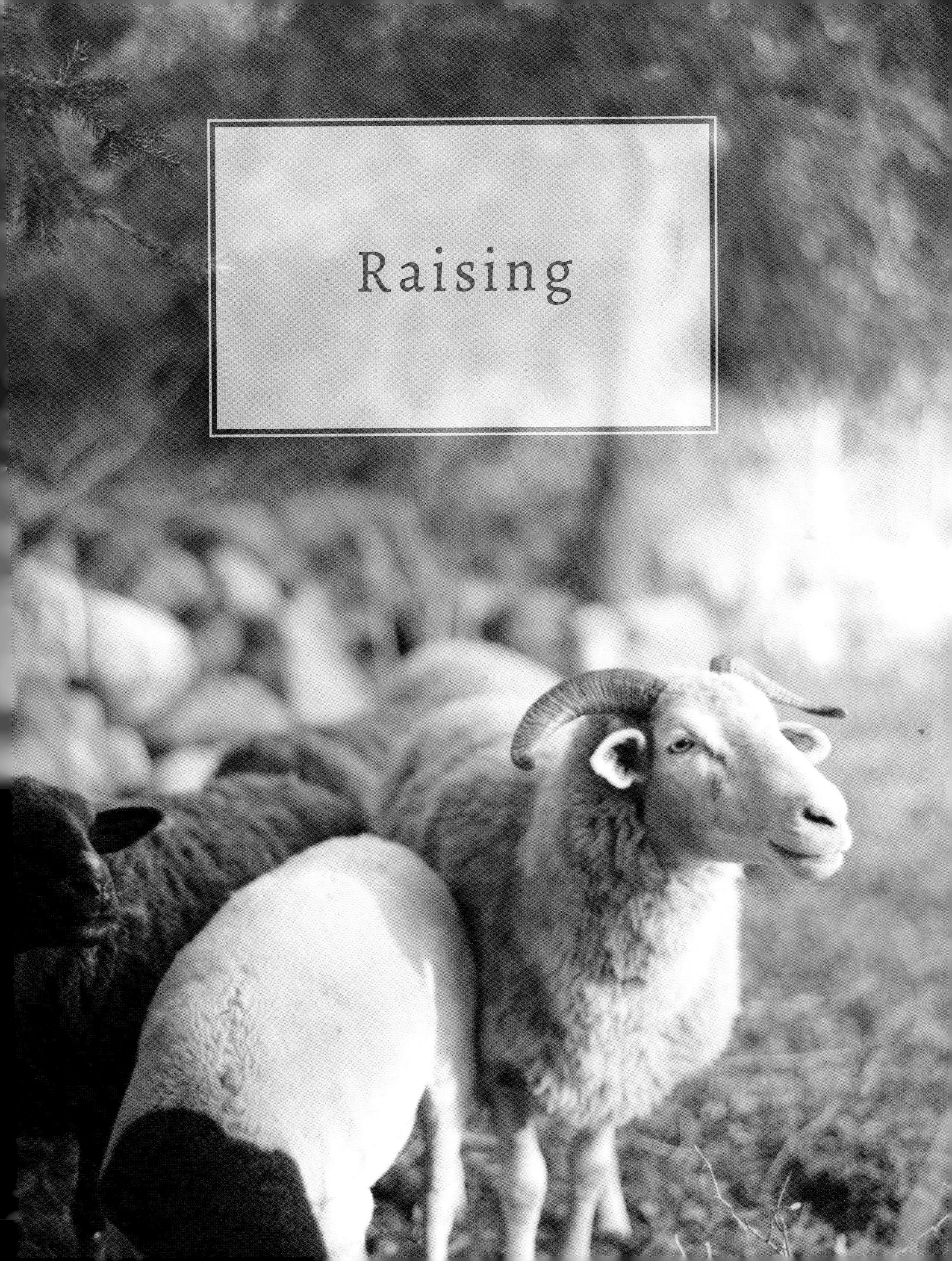

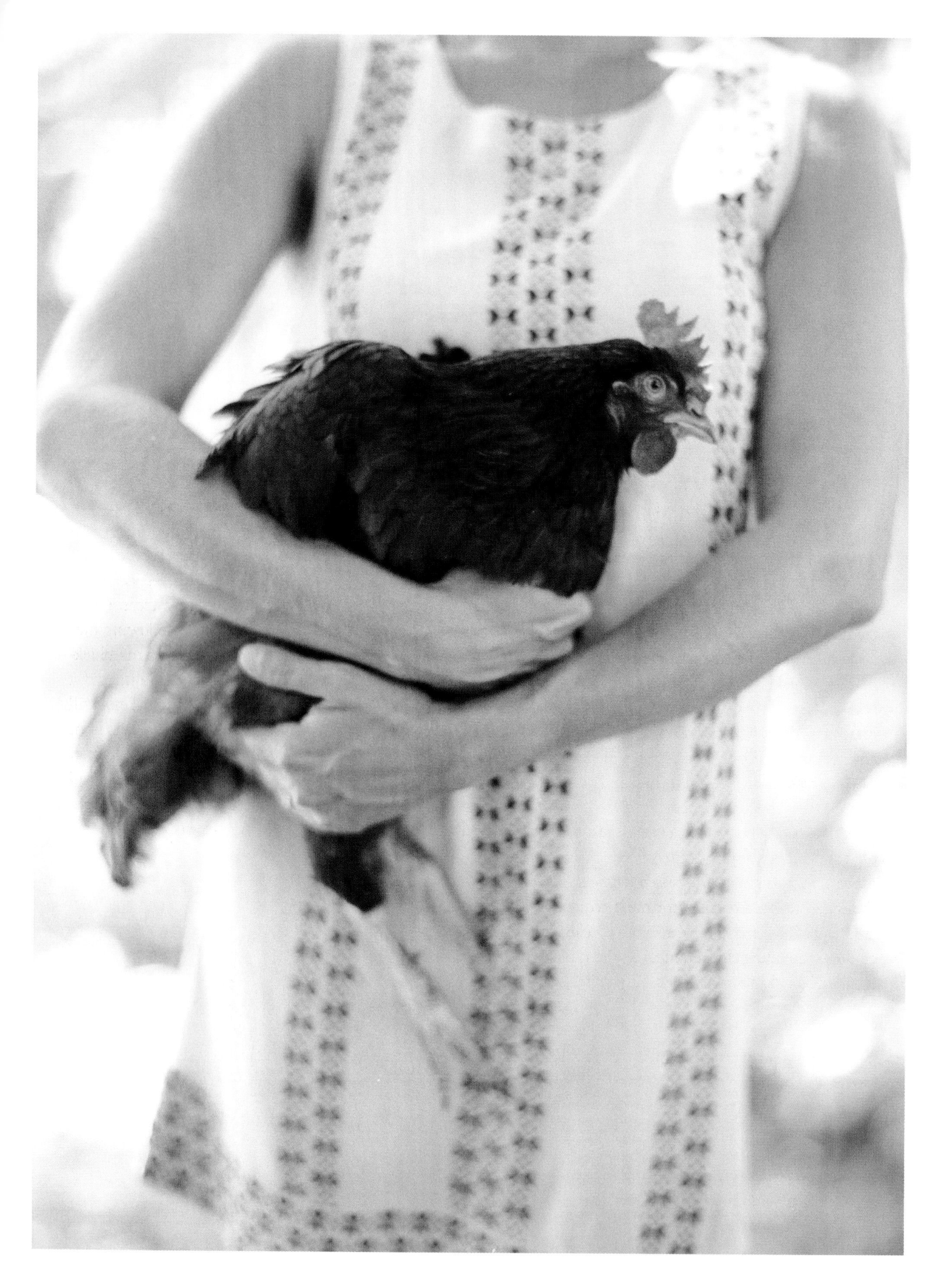

Chickens

NOTHING IS MORE IDYLLIC THAN A HOMESTEAD WITH A FLOCK OF CHICKENS RANGING AROUND A RUSTIC OUTBUILDING. THE BENEFITS OF RAISING CHICKENS ARE MANY: FRESH EGGS, INSECT CONTROL, WEED CONTROL, FERTILIZER, AND ENTERTAINMENT, TO NAME A HANDFUL. AND BECAUSE CHICKENS ARE SMALL, YOU CAN RAISE MANY ON A SMALL PIECE OF LAND.

History

Humans have been coexisting with chickens for a very long time. Mashed chicken brains were a delicacy in ancient Rome. However, after the fall of the Roman Empire, humans didn't raise chickens on a large scale for quite some time. What really propelled our modern mass consumption of chicken was the fortification of feed with antibiotics and vitamins, which lets us raise large numbers of chickens indoors. Industrial-scale, modern chicken houses contain 20,000 to 30,000 boilers crowded together. It only takes two pounds of grain to produce one pound of chicken flesh, making chickens economically efficient compared to feed lot cattle, which require seven to sixteen pounds of grain to produce one pound of beef.

That's not to say that chickens aren't still raised the old-fashioned way, on pasture where they get plenty of fresh air, sunshine, and insects. It's relatively rare, though. Raising a chicken for meat requires a lot of labor, and if I were to raise enough chickens that we could eat as much chicken meat as the typical American, I'd be living on a chicken-only farm.

U.S. BROILER PRODUCTION, 1934–99

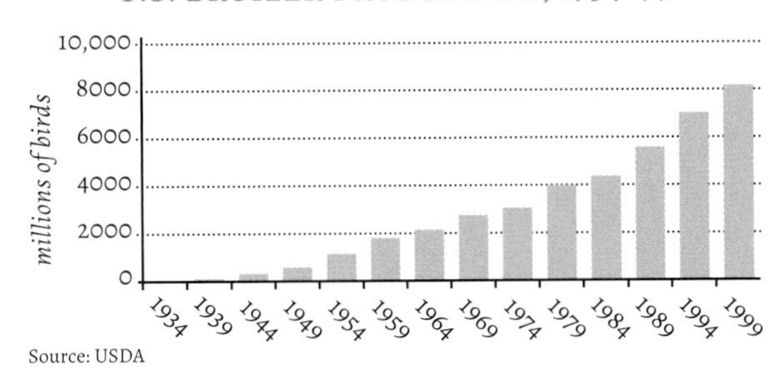

Source: USDA

Behavior

For my money, chickens are the most entertaining farm animals. Their constant movement, skittishness, aggressiveness, and one-eyed inquisitiveness are hilarious to watch. Chickens are very curious and will follow their owners around, especially if they think there's a chance of getting a treat. I'll often throw an insect at a chicken that's following me.

But while they're entertaining to us humans, chickens can be very aggressive towards each other. If a chicken has an injury or is sick, other chickens will quickly find it and peck at it. I'm not sure if this is an evolutionary mechanism to quickly rid the flock of weak members, but the speed at which chickens will cannibalize each other is shocking. Friendships and family ties are not strong among hens!

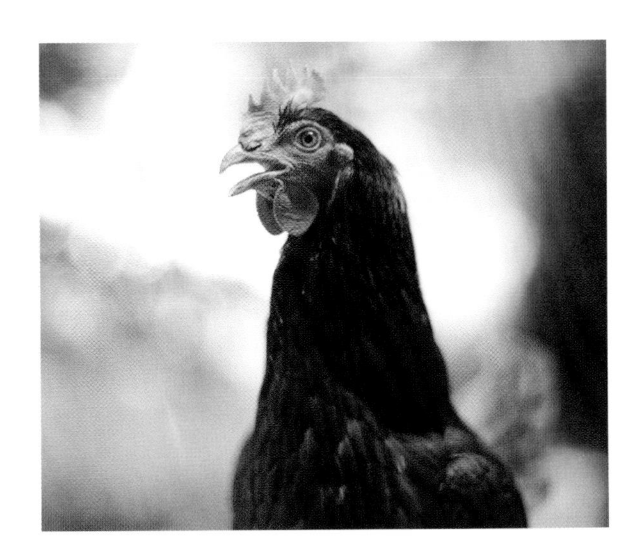

CHICKEN FAQS

DO YOU NEED A ROOSTER TO GET EGGS? Nope! Owning roosters has many benefits, but eggs (or more eggs) isn't one of them. Hens will absolutely produce eggs without a rooster around.

HOW MUCH SPACE DO MY LAYERS NEED? At the very minimum, each layer needs 4 square feet of floor space if it's spending the majority of its time inside a chicken coop. This means that if you have three birds, your coop needs to have 12 square feet of floor space. If your layers spend most of their time outdoors, 10 square feet of outdoor space plus 1 square foot of indoor space per bird is sufficient.

ARE ANY CHICKEN BREEDS MEAN? Chicken temperament varies greatly with breed. For friendliness, our favorite breed is Rhode Island Red.

ARE CHICKENS NOISY? Hens are not noisy. They often coo when curious about something and they squawk occasionally to alert each other to danger, but overall they are pretty quiet.

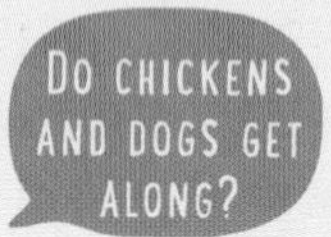

That depends on what you mean by "get along." Dogs love chickens—sometimes so much that they eat them.

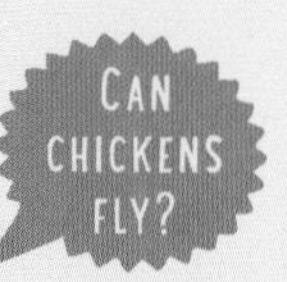

Sort of. Chickens aren't burning up the sky with their flying skills, but they can fly short distances.

DO CHICKENS BITE? Not really. Chickens are very curious animals and use their beaks to see if something is edible, but they aren't generally aggressive. I have a pair of polka dot rubber boots that the chickens love to peck at.

WHAT DO YOU DO IF A ROOSTER ATTACKS YOU? Roosters can become pretty mean over time, especially if kids have chased them around. If a rooster starts to get belligerent, don't run. Stand up to him. If all else fails, see the recipe for Big Bad Rooster Soup on page 262.

HOW MANY EGGS DOES A CHICKEN LAY EACH DAY? On average, a chicken lays one egg every day or two.

MY CHICKENS JUST LOST ALL OF THEIR FEATHERS—ARE THEY DYING? They're probably just molting, which is when they shed their old feathers and grow new ones. Chickens tend to molt when the days are shorter and the temperatures are cooler.

Nutrition

Eggs are one of the most nutrient-dense foods available. Most of this nutrition is located in the yolk, which is rich in B vitamins, iodine, phosphorus, many antioxidants, and vitamins A, E, and D. However, the health benefits of eating eggs are directly related to what the hens have been eating. Factory-raised chickens fed a diet of GMO corn and soy produce eggs that are much less nutritious than hens raised on pasture supplemented with organic grain. Eggs from pasture-raised chickens contain up to thirteen times more omega-3 fatty acids (the anti-inflammatory fatty acids that are beneficial for our health) than eggs from industrially raised chickens.

Chicken meat, on the other hand, is high in omega-6 fatty acids—which, unlike omega-3s, are pro-inflammatory; too much omega-6 and too little omega-3 is associated with all kinds of chronic disease. We don't eat a ton of chicken, but when we do, we roast an entire bird, eat the meat, and save the carcass for stock, which is incredibly nutritious (see the recipe on page 338). I have to say, though, we tend to eat a lot more lamb, pork, beef, and seafood than chicken. Wild seafood and herbivores raised on grass are far superior in their nutritional profile to poultry.

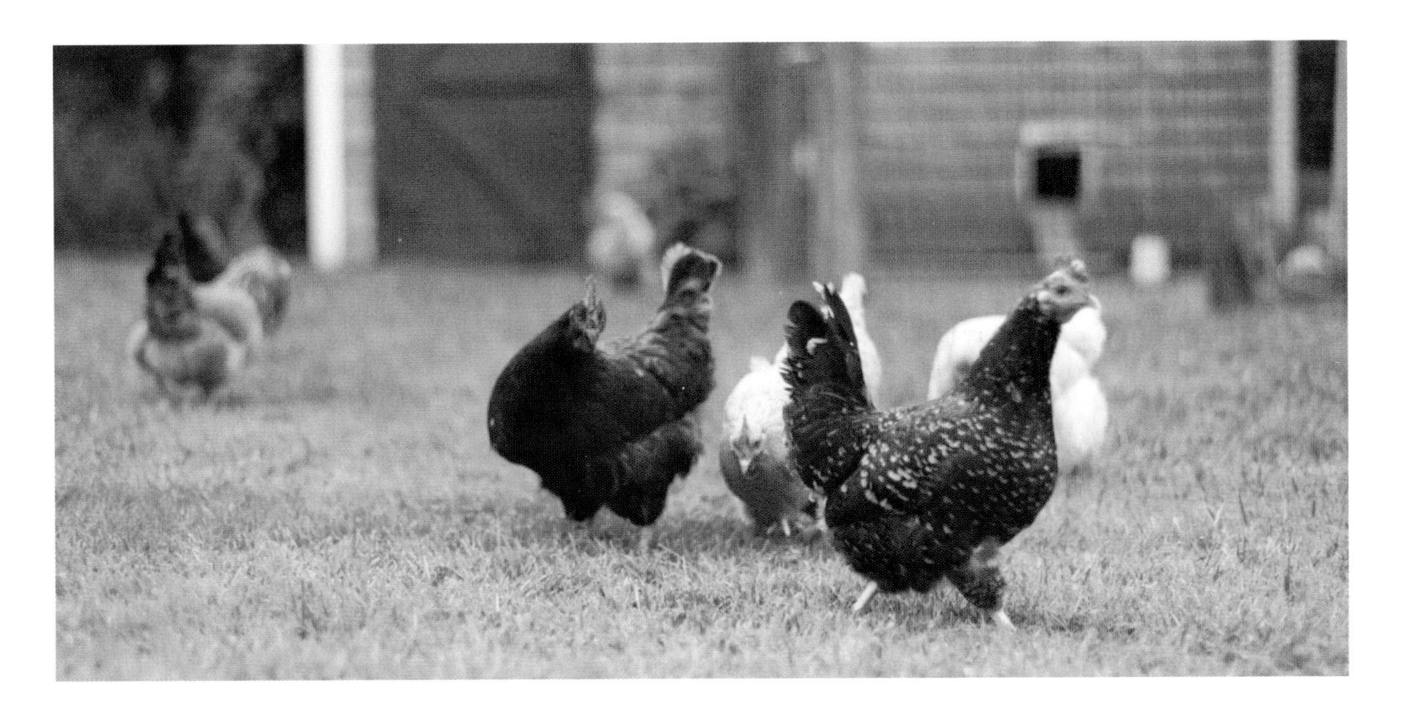

Selecting a Breed

Choosing a breed is essential to the success you will have with your flock. Chickens have been selectively bred for thousands of years, and each breed exhibits certain traits that are desirable for specific functions and locations.

Layers

Where I live in New England, heavy, brown egg-laying breeds like the New Hampshire Red, Rhode Island Red, and Barred Rock perform best with the rotational grazing system we use. The blue eggs of Aracuanas dazzle customers, but they do not lay as well in the chilly north, and their production significantly declines with the onset of winter. I like the hardiness of the Reds and the Barred Rocks—they thrive even in temperatures well below zero—and at the end of the season, they make nice roasters.

If you live in a hotter climate, go for a lighter breed that lays white eggs. Leghorns, Hamburgs, Andalusias, Minorcas, and Anconas are all well suited for warmer climates. You'll want to avoid heavily feathered birds like Orpingtons, as they can overheat easily. To cool down your coop, you might want to hose down the roof or put fans inside.

Broilers

Over the years, we have raised and slaughtered thousands of chickens. Our experience has been that the commercially popular, broad-breasted Cornish Cross is not a good breed for a natural, pasture-based system. Cornish Crosses are truly a marvelous example of the amazing success of the industrial agriculture machine. It worked feverishly for years to create a chicken that turns corn and soy feed into chicken protein as fast as possible, and it succeeded with the Cornish Cross, which develops into a full-sized, large-breasted chicken in six to eight weeks.

But while this is fantastic for the bottom line of a major poultry company, breeding hens that grow so fast meant sacrificing other aspects of their well-being. For example, Cornish Crosses grow so quickly and have such large breasts that their legs have trouble supporting their weight. By about eight weeks of age, many can no longer walk at all. And Cornish Crosses put on too much weight too fast for their internal organs to manage, and frequently die from pulmonary disease by about ten weeks. Plus, Cornish Crosses cannot reproduce naturally. But they're really efficient what they were bred for: converting corn and soy to protein.

Maybe there is some wisdom in the old saying "you are what you eat." Why would anyone want to consume animals that are dying from internal organ failure at ten weeks and can never reproduce? I believe we should be eating animals that are full of vigor and vitality.

For this reason, we recommend a category of breed called Red Broilers instead. When you call your hatchery, you can ask what breeds they have for Red Broilers. There are several variations on this breed on the market now, such as the Freedom Ranger, Red Ranger, and Pioneer, and in my experience they are all pretty good. They size up a lot slower than the Cornish Crosses, taking about twenty weeks to reach market weight, but they are much heartier, can escape predators, and will happily forage for food.

You can also do what we do: Instead of buying chickens specifically bred for meat, we slaughter our laying birds at the end of the growing season. Dual-purpose breeds, such as the New Hampshire Red, Rhode Island Red, and Barred Rock, are quite large by the time winter comes along.

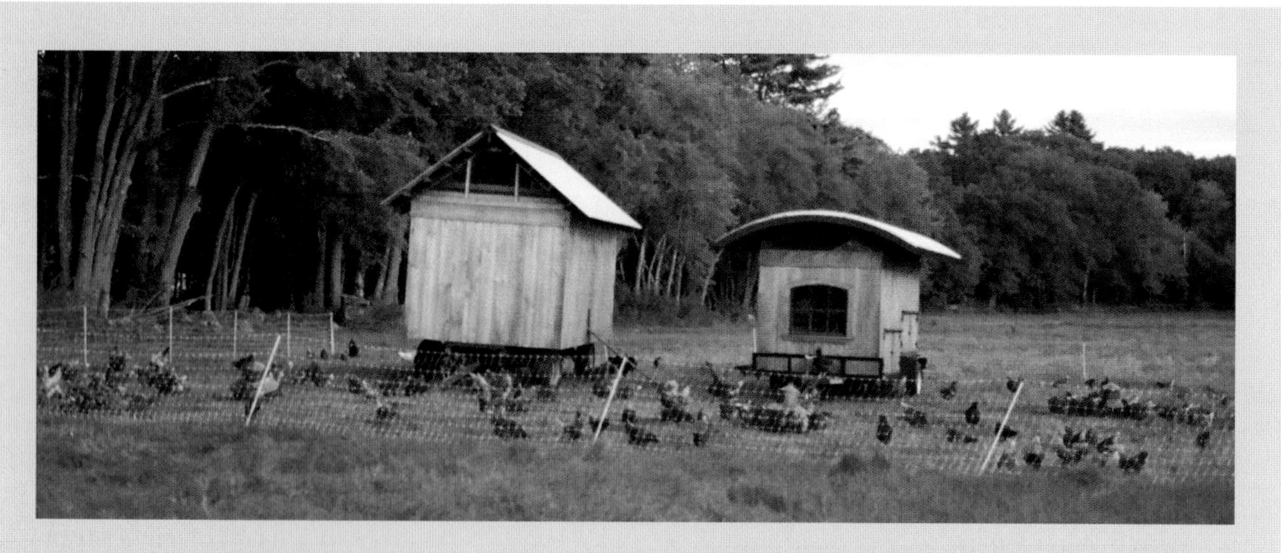

WHY CHICKENS ARE CRUCIAL FOR SUSTAINABILITY

At our farm, we always strive to be sustainable, and our chickens are critical in that effort. After harvesting vegetables from a field, we pull the mobile hen house onto the field and the hens feast on all the vegetative residue we've left behind. Not only are there literally tons of greens for them to eat, there are also thousands of insects and weed seeds, and there are minerals in the soil that the hens need. The birds concentrate all these calories, omega-3s, and minerals in the eggs they lay, making them a superfood. In fact, the eggs we get from pasturing the chickens on the field are more nutrient-dense than the field's primary crops (like lettuce, for example).

After about a week, it's time to move the hens to another harvested vegetable field. Weed seeds and insects have been consumed by the chickens, and hundreds of pounds of fertilizer have been left behind. The field is ready to be spaded and seeded with a cover crop, which will trap nutrients that would otherwise be leached away during the winter. After the cover crop has been established, it's time to bring the sheep and goats onto the field. The grasses grown on this soil are more nutritious, so the livestock grazing on it grow faster. The next season, the field is replenished and ready for a new vegetable crop to be planted.

This circular system is fundamental to a sustainable farm. After all, if a farm is constantly buying fertilizer, herbicides, pesticides, fungicides, and trace minerals, how sustainable is it? We strive to buy as little as possible, and we get better year after year at utilizing systems like this.

Roosters

Most towns do not allow backyard roosters, but if yours does, roosters can have a very beneficial effect on flock dynamics.

Roosters are concerned with only a few things: flock relations, flock protection, and reproduction. They quickly break up fights among hens and keep sick hens from being pecked to death. They are constantly vigilant against hawks and land-based predators; they have different warnings for different dangers, and the hens heed their warnings. As for reproduction, roosters (unsurprisingly) seem to have little concern for the hens' pleasure—they have all the fun here. The hens seem to tolerate it.

It's ideal to have one rooster for every twelve hens, and overall two roosters are better than one. If you only have one, it can develop a favorite hen, which can be very stressful for that hen. Two roosters will compete for all the hens and spread themselves evenly throughout the flock.

Deciding Whether to Hatch, Buy Chicks, or Buy Pullets

Hatching

Hatching eggs is a fantastic experience, especially for children. Watching the chicks struggle to break out of the eggs is nothing less than witnessing a miracle.

There are a few downsides, though. After the eggs arrive, they need to rest in an incubator for three weeks, and someone needs to keep watch to make sure the moisture levels are maintained and the incubator is performing correctly. More importantly, though, you will likely end up with 50 percent roosters and will have to figure out what to do with them all. Also, it is likely that some eggs won't hatch.

CHECKS IN THE MAIL

The phone rings. It's the postmaster: "Your checks have arrived. Would you like me to bring them by your place?" He waits for my response. Checks? What checks? Did I order checks? Maybe my husband did. Why would the postmaster be willing to bring my checks by? What great service. "Sure, bring them over!"

About twenty minutes later, a knock on the door signals the postmaster's arrival with my checks. To my amazement, the checks in the postmaster's hands are chirping. Oh yeah, my *chicks* were scheduled to arrive today!

Finally, if you don't already have an incubator, you'll need to take the cost of purchasing one into account. Basic models start at around $120, but those tend not to work very well. A good incubator costs about $200. You'll also need to buy an automatic egg turner. If the eggs aren't turned frequently, you won't get chicks.

Buying Chicks

Chicks can be purchased at a few days old through mail-order companies or at agriculture supply stores. The benefits of buying chicks are that the company you purchase them from guarantees that they'll live for a couple days, and the chicks have already been sexed—you'll know the gender of your birds. Accidents do happen, though, and poultry companies often sneak in some roosters with the hens.

Before your chicks arrive, you must have their brooder set up. Nothing is worse than getting the chicks home and keeping them in their shipping box, where they can get too cold or too hot.

For the first week of the chick's life, they must be kept at 90 degrees in a draft-free space. I recommend using a red heat lamp instead of a white heat lamp, since red is said to prevent pecking. You can reduce the heat by 5 degrees each week until they have "feathered out"—you'll see actual feathers instead of fuzz. You'll know if you have the proper temperature

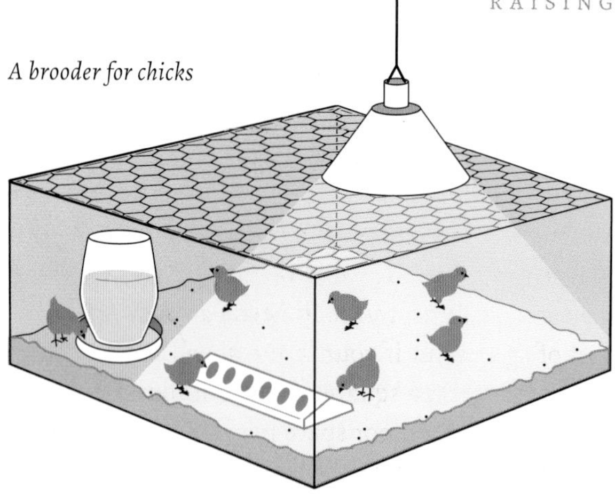
A brooder for chicks

in your little brooder when the chicks are evenly spread out. If they all flock to the edges, the light is too close and they are hot. If they are all directly under the light, they are too cold.

Chicks need a constant supply of water and feed—preferably an organic chick starter mash. When you move the chicks from the shipping box to the brooder, introduce them to the water and the mash by carefully dipping their beaks into the water and then into the mash. This will teach them where everything is and get them going.

The chicks should be happily walking around their enclosure with enough food and water until about four weeks, when they will have feathered out and become too large for the brooder.

When the birds have feathered out, it's time to move them into their permanent home. They're not ready to fend for themselves on pasture, though—keep them safe in their coop for another couple weeks. At around eight weeks, the young hens can be let outside. They're still quite young and small, so be vigilant against predators. An animal as small as a rat or kestrel can make a meal of these birds.

Buying Pullets

Buying pullets—teenage hens—is by far the most cost-effective, least stressful, most economical, least exciting, and most successful way to start your flock. Pullets are typically sold at around seventeen weeks. This means the birds have survived the most vulnerable days of their life, are fully feathered out, and are most likely thriving. They are also only a couple months away from starting to lay eggs! I've done the math several times, and you will save significantly by purchasing pullets instead of eggs or chicks.

Be aware that for the first week or so, you'll need to put your pullets to bed each night, until they understand where to go when the sun goes down. That means that you literally have to pick them up and place them in the house every night. Eventually they'll understand the drill and automatically walk into their house at dusk, so all you'll need to do is shut the door when it gets dark.

Housing

You can spend a lot of time and money creating the hen house of your dreams for your chickens. Some hen houses are nicer than most people houses. I've seen birds in these coops thriving and producing eggs at impressive rates—but I've also seen birds that live in a dilapidated doghouse laying at an ideal rate. However you decide to house your chickens, there are some basic criteria to keep in mind:

- The chicken coop should provide shelter from the elements and be draft-free (though it doesn't need to be heated).
- I highly recommend providing nesting boxes, which give chickens a safe, dark place to lay their eggs. They also keep you from having to do on a daily egg hunt in rock walls and other places hens love to lay eggs.
- The chicken coop should be near your house for convenience. Make taking care of them easy on yourself—nobody wants to trek through tons of snow every day to care for chickens.

- The coop should keep the birds safe from predators. That means no holes larger than 1 square inch. Anything larger will allow weasels to get in. Weasels, raccoons, fisher cats, and snakes are unbelievably great predators. Take them seriously. In fact, the most common reason that homesteaders get out of raising chickens is that predators are constantly killing their flocks.
- Chickens prefer to sleep on a roost, which is basically a branch. You can provide them with a few perches built from branches, sturdy pieces of wood, or wooden tomato stakes. They should look like wide ladders, set an angle.
- If you want a consistent egg supply during the winter months, try installing lights on a timer to ensure the hens are exposed to light twelve hours a day (the sun from 8 a.m. to 4 p.m., then the indoor lights from 4 p.m. to 8 p.m.).

Meat birds can be housed with your laying flock. Just be sure to band the birds so you can tell which are meat birds and which are layers. Leg bands—just what they sound like, a kind of bracelet that is placed around the leg—are available through chicken supply stores. If you are raising just meat birds, there is no need to build nesting boxes, as it's unlikely they will lay any eggs before you are ready to process them.

Make sure the chicken coop provides enough space that your birds will be comfortable. Each bird needs about 4 square feet of floor space, so if you have twelve birds, the coop needs at least 48 square feet of space. But if your layers spend most of their time outdoors, 10 square feet of outdoor space plus 1 square foot of indoor space per bird is sufficient.

Don't forget to make the housing work for you, too. Twice a day, every day, seven days a week, fifty-two weeks a year, for many years, you will likely need to visit your chicken coop. While the hens will be happy with the coop so long as it meets their basic needs (shelter from the elements and safety from predators), you will be complaining and resenting your flock if the coop isn't human-friendly. Make it easy to get in and out of, keep it clean, and make sure it's easy to gather eggs from. For example, our coop has a little door that gives us access to the nesting boxes from the outside, so we don't have to crawl inside the tiny coop to collect the eggs. Also, you and your neighbors will be looking at the coop for a long time to come, so consider making it aesthetically pleasing. (For suggestions on where to buy a chicken coop and places to buy plans for building your own, see page 398.)

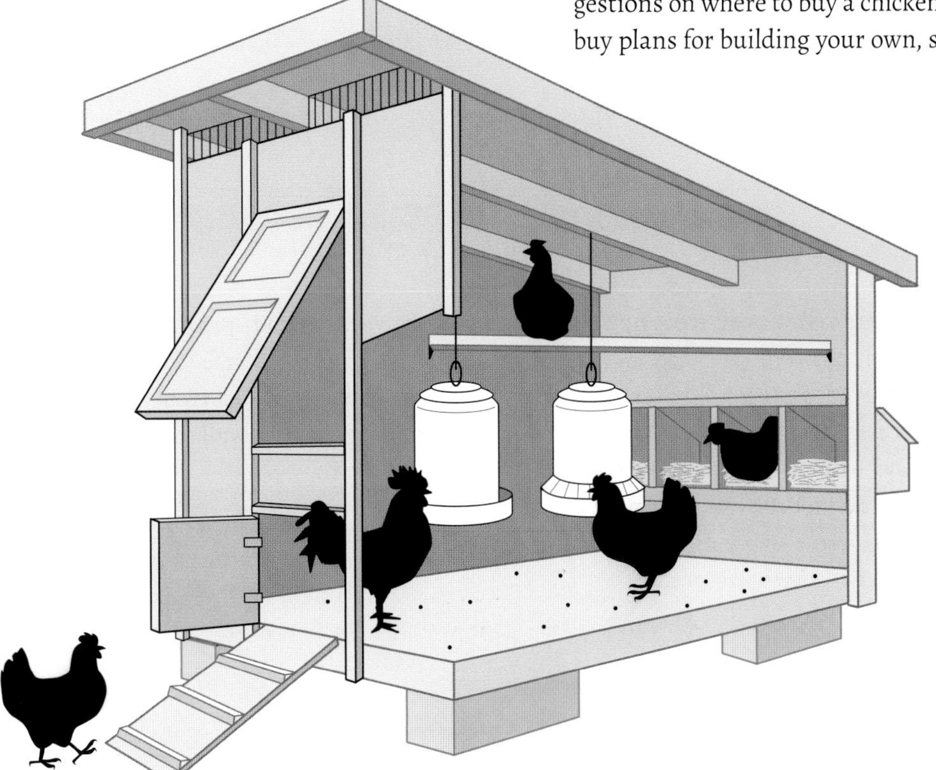

Example of a stationary hen house

Mobile or Stationary Chickens?

Part of establishing housing for your hens means deciding whether to let them roam your yard or keep them penned in one place. There are pros and cons to each.

Mobile Chickens

Benefits: Birds that are left free to roam take care of a lot of their own nutrition needs. They will hunt all around your property for insects, plants, seeds, and minerals that they need. That grazing can also get some of your chores done for you. If you allow them to enter your garden (after vegetables have been harvested!), they'll do some weeding, eat pests, and fertilize. Also, there's no mucking if your birds are free-range. Don't underestimate how nice it is to not have to muck. Mucking is time-consuming and heavy work.

Drawbacks: Stepping in chicken poop is pretty gross, and they poop all over the place. Chickens also like to eat your favorite, most beautiful flowers if they can get to them, and without fencing predators will have easy access to the birds.

Stationary Chickens

Benefits: Permanent hen houses with chicken yards keep your hens from wandering into areas you don't want them to be, like your vegetable garden or, worse, your neighbor's. Chicken yards can also be made predator-proof. Be sure to bury chicken wire 1 foot deep and angle the fence away from the yard to protect against predators that will try to dig under it.

For healthy chickens and to create fantastic compost for your garden, it is very important to provide organic material in your chicken yard. A layer of leaves several inches thick works wonderfully. The leaves sop up chicken manure and create a habitat for insects and worms, which the chickens love. In the process of scratching through the leaves to capture bugs, the chickens mix their manure with the organic matter and aerate the soil. Every season, clean out the yard and add this material to your compost pile, and in no time you'll have an amazing soil amendment. To make this even easier, follow the example of a friend of ours who keeps her compost pile in a tall cylinder of wire within her chicken yard. The chickens hop in, eat the chicken scraps and bugs, then hop out.

Drawbacks: With the birds permanently in one area, manure builds up, and the increase in manure and bedding also increases the population of flies and chicken parasites. If you aren't vigilant, rats can also become a problem—they're drawn to the chicken feed and kitchen scraps that can build up in the yard, and once they're entrenched, they're very hard to get rid of using organic techniques. Prevent rats from being attracted to the yard in the first place by not overfeeding your chickens, so the feeders are empty at night, and not allowing the hens to waste kitchen scraps. When you do see a rat, trap or kill it immediately. If rodents are a big problem, though, consider letting your chickens be mobile, or at least providing a mobile enclosure, so rodents have less of an chance to settle in. Finally, disease can be more prevalent in a stationary chicken yard. When chickens are constantly moving to new grass, there is less manure build-up, which means less incidence of disease.

Example of a permanent hen house with a fixed chicken yard

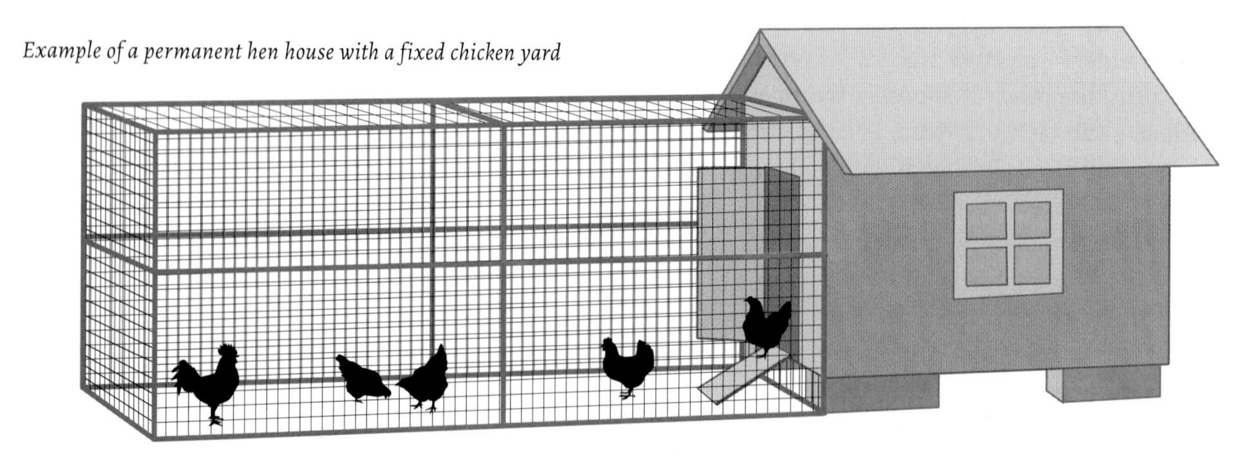

Mobile Enclosures: The Best of Both Worlds

One way to keep your chickens from roaming free all over your garden and still give them access to different parts of your yard, is to get a "chicken tractor" or other type of mobile enclosure for your birds. These can be easily built or purchased from a chicken supplier. This is what we have on our farm, and I recommend it—it gives you and your hens the best of both worlds. The chickens have a house on wheels that is moved to new grass regularly, and you can use mobile, solar-powered electric fencing (see page 56) to keep them safe from predators.

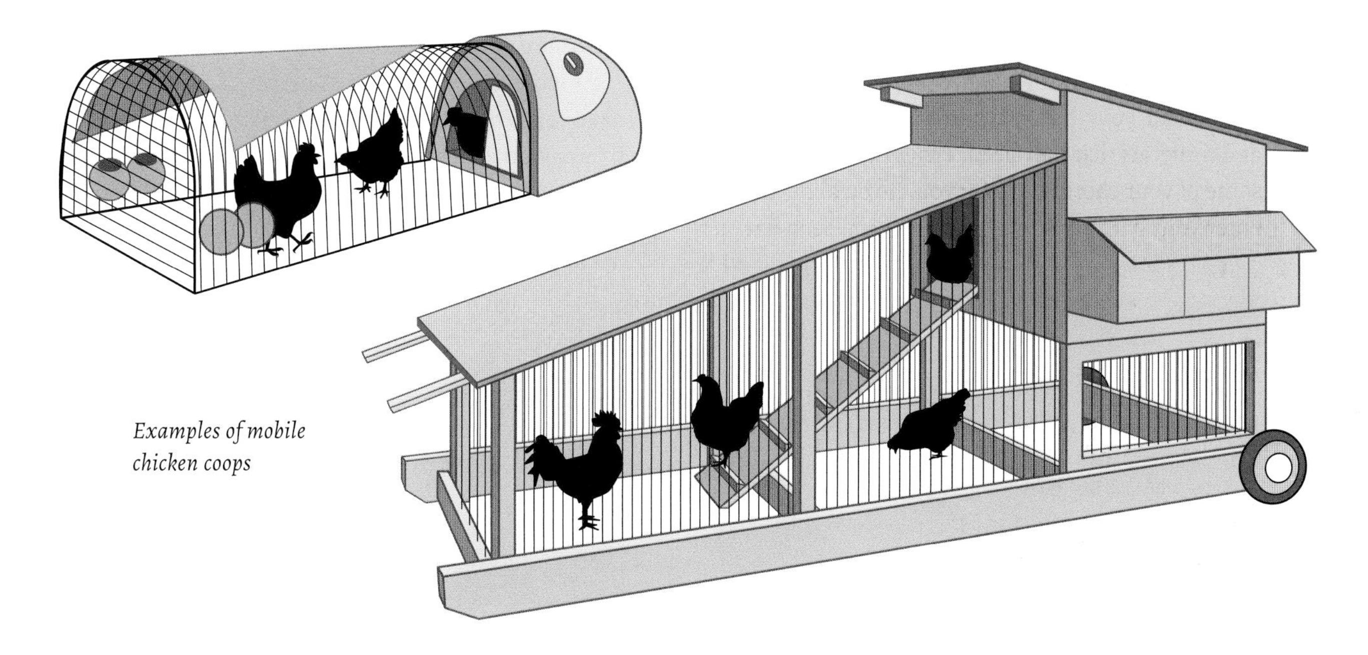

Examples of mobile chicken coops

Food and Water

Chickens are omnivores and prefer a good source of protein over any other food. Spend some time watching chickens on pasture and you'll see them range surprisingly far in the hunt for nice, juicy bugs. They'll also gladly eat any greens and seeds that they encounter, but their main goal is to find insects.

For the beginning homesteader, I recommend buying an organic, soy-free layer pellet to supplement your hens' nutrition. It is possible to raise chickens without grain on lush pasture and insects, but some grain supplementation tends to give better results. Organic, soy-free grain is gaining in popularity, and most agriculture supply stores will order it for you. Chickens can eat a quarter pound of grain a day.

Be careful when storing the grain for your chickens. It can attract many wild animals, particularly rats, so make sure you store it in a rodent-proof container. Metal garbage cans work well for small amounts of grain: one 30-gallon metal trash can easily holds 50 pounds of grain. Also, don't let your hens be messy eaters. You can train them to be thrifty with the grain by letting the feeder go empty at times. Hungry birds will seek out all the dropped grain on the ground, and as a bonus, they'll also put more effort into searching for food on their own.

While it's okay to let your hens go without food for several hours, don't let them go without water, especially in hot weather. A chicken waterer—basically, a bucket or plastic jar overturned on a saucer—works well. Keep the waterers clean and close to their shelter. Countless times I've observed poultry water containers in the middle of a field, without a place for hens to run to in order to escape predators. While you do want your birds to range, you don't want to set the dinner table for hungry hawks. I use one 5-gallon waterer for every forty birds.

Collecting and Storing Eggs

Your farm-fresh, pastured eggs should be collected daily from the nesting boxes in the chicken house. There's usually no need to wash the eggs—simply brush off any shavings or poop—but very dirty eggs can be washed with warm water. While they can be stored at room temperature, refrigerating eggs (even if you choose not to wash them) will extend their shelf life. Eggs held at room temperature will last about one week while refrigerated eggs will last six weeks or longer.

Health

Check your flock over regularly; the chickens should have bright eyes, upright postures, and an alert look. Especially during winter, when chickens are susceptible to respiratory illnesses, keep the hen house clean and make sure they have plenty of fresh water and food.

Any sick birds should be isolated immediately. Some symptoms to look for are not eating or drinking, coughing, mucus in the eyes, diarrhea, and lice. As professional farmers, we cull chickens that seem unwell. As a homesteader, you may want to do more to save your chicken. If your local vet is unfamiliar with chickens, there are some great books and websites listed in the Resources section that may be helpful (see page 396).

CARING FOR YOUR CHICKENS

Daily (about 20 to 30 minutes)	**Weekly** (1 to 2 hours)	**Monthly** (1 to 2 hours)
Let them out of the coop. Provide water and feed. Collect eggs. Shut the door of the coop at night.	Check fencing. Move a mobile flock. Clean out water containers.	Muck out the hen house.

Processing

"Processing" basically means "slaughtering." No one loves this part of keeping animals, but it's unavoidable for homesteaders, and everyone needs to know what to do when a chicken is sick or no longer laying eggs, or when an angry rooster is harassing the neighborhood kids. As professional farmers, we keep our chickens for one to two years while they are at their maximum egg-laying capacity, then process them for meat and start fresh with a new flock. Most backyard homesteaders, however, keep chickens much longer.

While larger animals need to go to a slaughterhouse, chickens and other fowl are usually processed at home. The best way to learn how to process poultry is to have someone with experience demonstrate the process for you. Keep in mind, killing and cleaning an animal is not for those with weak stomachs, and confidence and competence are necessary to do a good job and properly respect the animal. It's critical to be as calm as you can, which will keep the animal less stressed throughout the process. (See page 398 for links to videos on processing poultry.)

One tip for processing ducks: adding a tiny amount of detergent to the scalding tank will make the plucking easier.

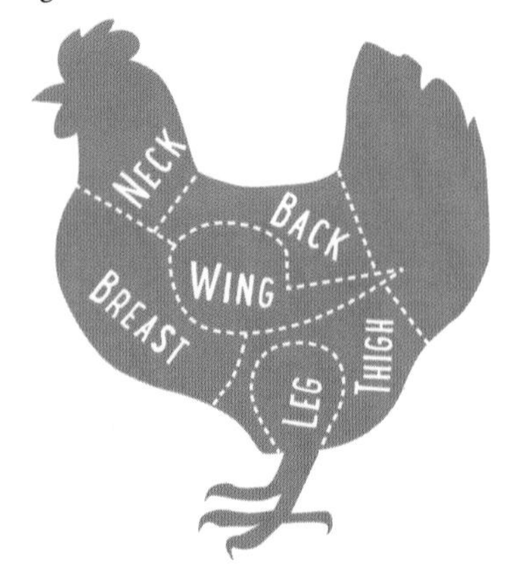

Turkeys and Ducks

Raising ducks and turkeys is similar to raising hens, but there are a few different housing needs to consider.

Our favorite breeds of ducks are Indian Runners and Khaki Campbells. Both lay very well and are a riot to watch running around. Indian Runners are excellent foragers and, given enough room, thrive without any grain supplements. Khaki Campbells are extremely hardy and have the added benefit of growing quickly. Both Runners and Campbells are great layers and produce enormous, golden-yolked eggs, which make a great substitute for chicken eggs. One duck egg is the equivalent of two chicken eggs.

Because of their short legs, ducks will not be able to jump up into hens' nesting boxes, so keep their nesting boxes on the floor of their house. We use scrap wood and construct three sides of a box up against the wall. Placing milk crates on their sides is also a great idea.

For several years we raised turkeys for the Thanksgiving market. For the best-tasting meat, our favorite breeds are the Bourbon Red and Narragansett. In the past, we have tried the traditional Broad Breasted White, the kind you'll find in a grocery store, but we found that they get too large, and their breasts are so heavy that the birds have a hard time walking. Turkeys can be an excellent source of income, and most of the work is processing, which occurs at a time of year when the farm isn't so busy.

Like chickens, turkeys like to sleep on roosting bars. However, there's no need for nesting boxes if you're raising them for Thanksgiving, since you won't see eggs before then. Turkeys can grow to 30 pounds. Given their enormous size, each bird needs 6 feet of space in the coop.

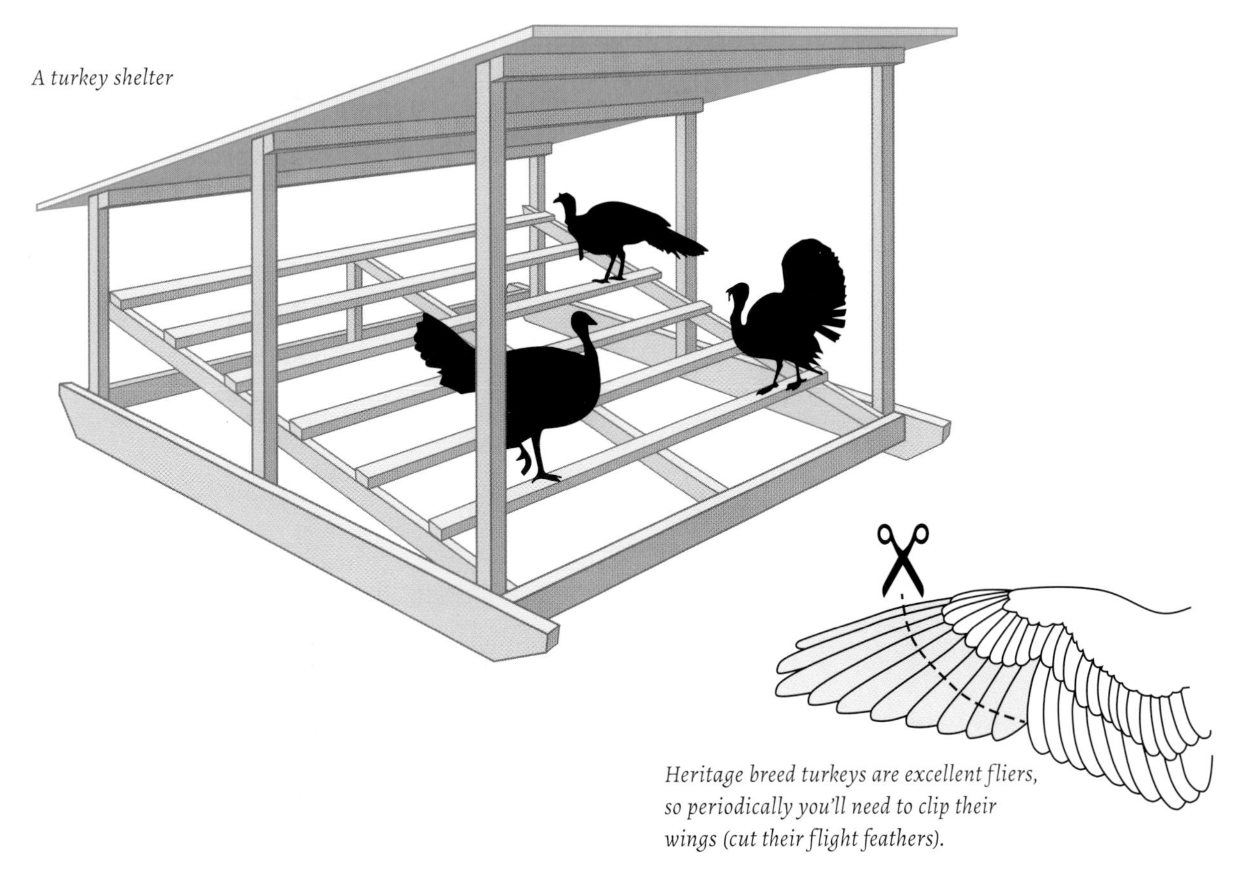

A turkey shelter

Heritage breed turkeys are excellent fliers, so periodically you'll need to clip their wings (cut their flight feathers).

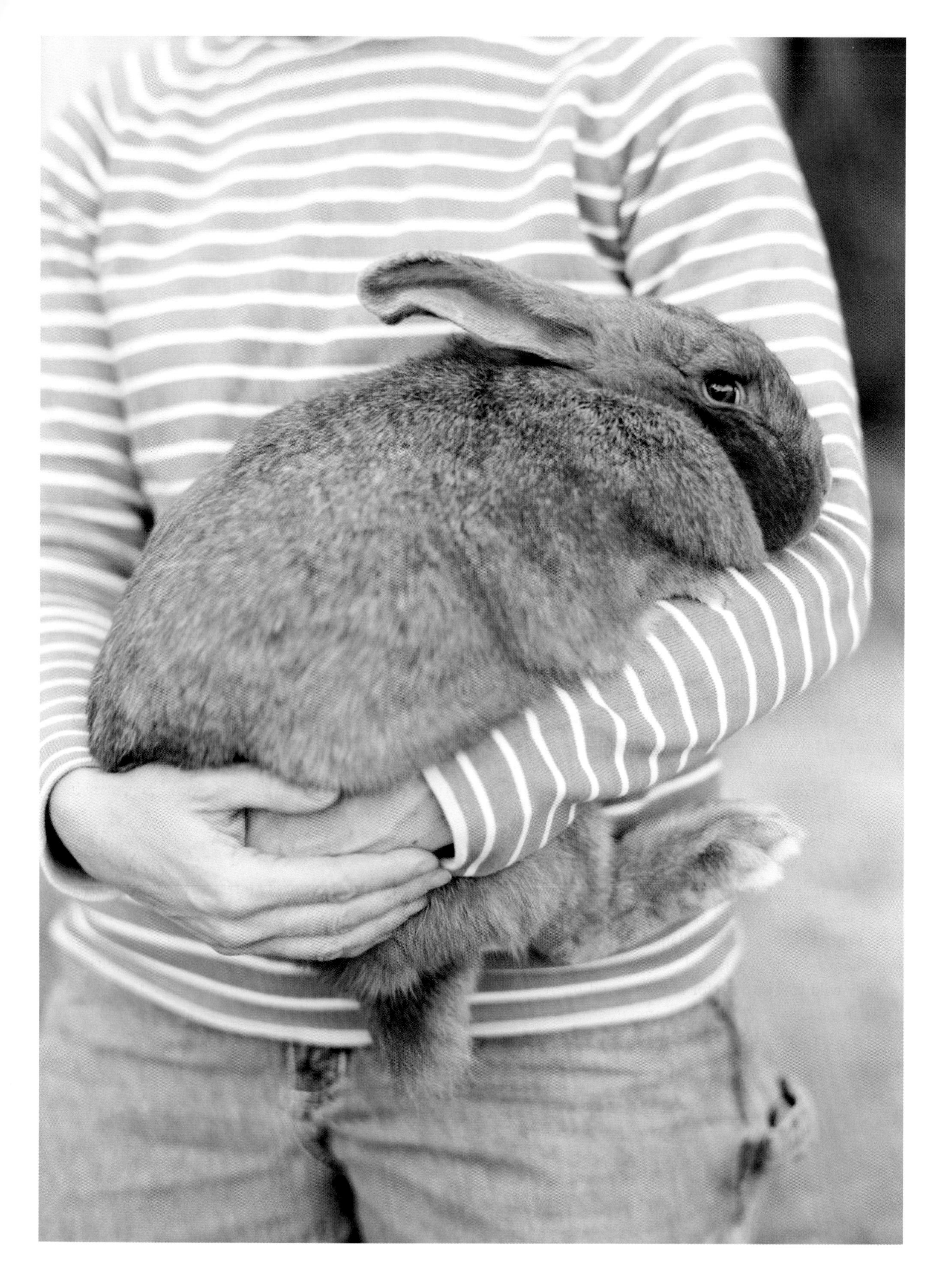

Rabbits

If you have limited space but still want to raise your own meat, rabbits can be a great solution. They are easy to care for, compared to other farm animals, and prolific. Rabbits are often raised for food in France, Italy, Malta, and Spain, although in the United States they're more often seen as pets. There are over one hundred breeds of domestic rabbits and they range in size from dwarf to giant, which can weigh over 20 pounds.

Although we do eat rabbit, Andrew and I have not yet raised them for profit on our farm, so for this chapter I picked the brain of my friend and rabbit expert Jennifer Hashley. She and her husband raise about 250 rabbits on pasture every year for profit, in addition to raising chickens, pigs, and sheep. Jen also runs a program called the New Entry Sustainable Farming Project at Tufts University, training new farmers and providing access to land, technical assistance, and market connections. She gave me the skinny on all you'll need to know to raise your own nutritious backyard bunnies.

History

Today's domestic rabbits are descended from the wild European rabbit. Although the early Romans kept wild rabbits in walled gardens called *leporia*, rabbits weren't domesticated until the Middle Ages, when monks began selectively breeding them for size and color. Medieval sailors released rabbits on islands to breed and flourish, then returned to catch and eat them—a neat way to avoid caring for rabbits on their ships while still getting fresh meat.

Like other invasive species, these rabbits thrived at the expense of native plants and animals. In 1859, Thomas Austin released twenty-four rabbits into the wild in Australia for hunting, and by the 1920s, these had given rise to an estimated 10 billion rabbits. Feral rabbits also became a serious problem in New Zealand, which, like Australia, offered a favorable environment, abundant feed, and an absence of predators. The exploding rabbit population in these countries is believed to be responsible for the extinction of many native species, and efforts to control it have had mixed results.

During the Victorian era, rabbits began to be raised as pets, and the popularity of rabbit meat declined in Britain and the United States. But that popularity often rose again during hard economic times, such as the Great Depression and World War II, since rabbits can survive on table scraps, reproduce quickly, and don't need much space. Today, rabbit meat is becoming trendy in the U.S., and it's still eaten widely throughout the rest of the world.

RABBIT FAQS

WHAT DOES RABBIT MEAT TASTE LIKE? It tastes sort of like sweet chicken breast.

DO RABBITS MAKE ANY NOISE? Most of the time, rabbits are very quiet. When they are frightened, however, their scream is bloodcurdling.

HOW QUICKLY DO RABBITS REPRODUCE? A doe can reproduce four to six times in one year. The gestation period is twenty-eight to thirty-four days.

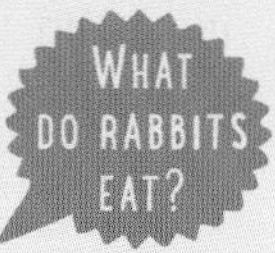

Rabbits do very well on a mix of grass, dry hay, and a supplement of rabbit pellets.

DO RABBITS SMELL? Generally, if their area is kept clean, there is very little scent from the does, though the bucks can have a strong odor at times.

CAN RABBITS BE AGGRESSIVE? Rabbits are known to bite and scratch when they're frightened. Be sure to wear old clothes when you handle them, as their powerful hind legs can rip a hole in your shirt and scratch your skin. Does also can be very protective of their babies, so use care when checking on them. The more rabbits are handled by humans when they are young, the more docile they tend to be. (A note of caution, however: If you impart too much of your scent on newborn bunnies, the mother may abandon them.)

HOW LONG DOES IT TAKE FOR A RABBIT TO BECOME FULL-GROWN? Rabbits are ready to breed at five months old. On average, rabbits that are bred for meat reach market weight in twelve to fourteen weeks.

IS THERE SOMEWHERE I CAN TAKE RABBITS TO BE PROCESSED? Unfortunately, it's unlikely that you'll find someone who can do the dirty work for you. If you're unprepared to slaughter them yourself, raising rabbits for meat probably isn't for you.

DO YOU NEED A LICENSE TO RAISE RABBITS? Check the zoning laws in your town; some do require an animal permit. But there's no need to announce to the town clerk that you are going to raise a ton of rabbits for meat—just read the ordinances. People raise rabbits all of the time as pets, and nobody needs to know what you intend to do with them.

CAN YOU RAISE RABBITS ALL OVER THE COUNTRY? Rabbits prefer cooler temperatures, and anything above 90°F is very stressful for them—males can even go sterile in high heat. So if you live in a hot climate, rabbits may not be for you.

RAISING RABBITS IN DEVELOPING COUNTRIES

Several factors make rabbits an ideal food source for developing countries: They do not compete with humans for food; the entire animal can be consumed at one meal, so there's no need for refrigeration; and they grow and reproduce quickly. Unfortunately, rabbits don't do well in tropical climates, although they're better able to handle the hot, dry climates of the Mediterranean and northern Africa. Some countries are also reluctant to introduce rabbits for fear of their prolific nature—no one wants the problems that Australia and New Zealand have faced with their rabbit populations—and then, too, the image of cute, warm, fuzzy bunnies discourages many from trying rabbits as meat.

Behavior

Rabbits are curious. They love to hop around and are more active at night than during the day. Rabbits can be trained to use a litter box and come when they are called. However, if you are raising them for meat, I suggest you don't treat them as pets—it's too easy to get attached. When your rabbits are around five months old and ready to breed, you'll need to put each rabbit in a separate cage to keep them from fighting.

Nutrition

Rabbit meat tastes a lot like a sweet version of chicken breast, but it's much higher in beneficial omega-3 fatty acids because rabbits consume less grain and more grass than chickens. Rabbit is also a good source of niacin, iron, phosphorus, and selenium, and a very good source of protein and vitamin B12. If you compare the vitamins and minerals in rabbit meat to those in chicken, rabbit wins by a landslide. It can be substituted for chicken in most recipes, and it's delicious broiled, roasted, barbecued, and of course stewed, as in Cajun Rabbit Stew with Andouille Sausage and Mushrooms (page 288).

Selecting a Breed and Purchasing

Some of the best breeds for meat are New Zealand, Florida White, and Californian. Pound for pound, these breeds are the best bet for the backyard homesteader looking for good meat production.

Be sure you seek out a reputable breeder. Ask for recommendations at your local agricultural supply store or look around online. (Yes, many rabbits are sold via mail-order!) If you find your rabbits through a show breeder, you may end up paying fifty dollars per rabbit, but it can be worth it to get quality rabbits to begin your own breeding herd. Be wary of anyone charging five dollars per rabbit: you get what you pay for. A good breeder should be able to show you a breeding record and detailed pedigree for each rabbit. Also, look around the farm. It should be clean and well organized. The rabbits should all look very healthy, and the breeder should guarantee your complete satisfaction, proudly standing behind their product.

To start out, get yourself a trio—one buck (male) and two does (females). Be sure they are not closely related. They will be the rabbits you breed to start your herd, which will later be separated into breeders and meat rabbits. Since you are looking for good breeding ability, ask the breeder if they come from productive lines. If the rabbits are young, ask to see their parents to make sure they look healthy and fit. Find out what they have been eating and how often they're being fed. If their food is very different from what you plan to feed them at home, be sure to make the change gradually to prevent digestive upset.

RABBIT TERMINOLOGY

Doe
Female rabbit

Buck
Male rabbit

Kit
Baby rabbit

Fryer
Young rabbit under twelve weeks old and about 4 to 5 pounds. Males tend to taste best at this stage.

Roaster
Rabbit that's between 5½ and 8 pounds

Stewer
A rabbit older than 6 months and weighing over 8 pounds. Stewing and braising are the best cooking methods for these.

Housing

All predators love rabbits, so keep them safe and don't allow them to roam free unless you intend to feed the neighborhood. Rabbits need a dry, durable hutch for shelter, but they don't really need a ton of room. An eight- to ten-pound rabbit needs a hutch that's 7½ to 10 square feet, and if you provide a nesting box for breeding does, a hutch that's 1½ feet by 3 feet by 2 feet is better. Rabbits can gnaw at a wood frame, so a wire hutch is best—it also lets their droppings fall through, so they don't accumulate on the floor of the hutch, and it's much easier to keep clean and dry. Rabbits do need protection from sun and elements, so be sure it has a sturdy roof. In the winter, you can wrap plastic sheeting around three sides of the cage for added protection from wind, rain, and snow. A hutch with 14-gauge wire is ideal for large meat breeds, and the floor should be a mesh of no larger than ½ inch by 1 inch. Be sure the door overlaps the cage on three sides. Rabbits are excellent escape artists!

If you live in a populated area, don't let your rabbit operation become an eyesore. You may want to shelter your rabbit hutches in some sort of pretty little shed with lots of ventilation (you shouldn't be overwhelmed by the smell of rabbits when you enter). Just don't put an open side of the shed right against your house, as your rabbits could urinate all over your home. Allow 3 feet between the hutches and walls of the shed.

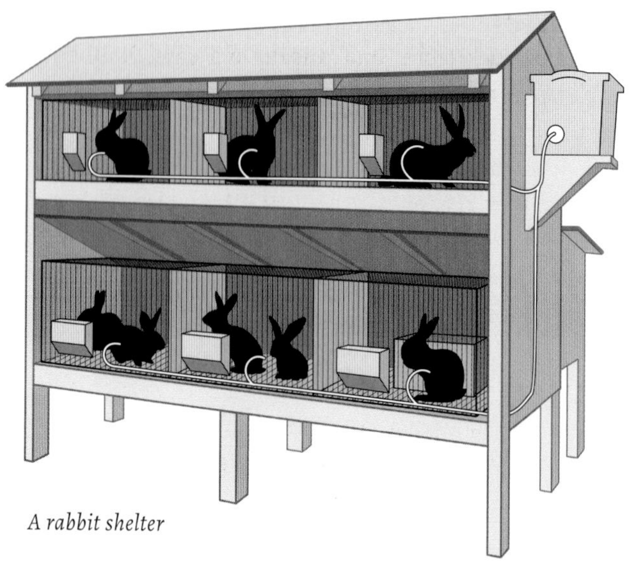

A rabbit shelter

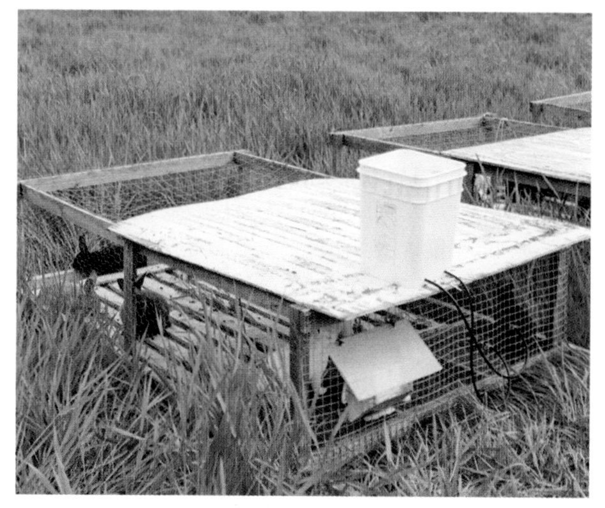

A mobile grazing pen for rabbits

A nesting box is necessary for your breeding does. These wire boxes are about 18 inches long, 10 inches wide, and 10 inches high. Fluff it up with some straw and it's the perfect place for the mama to have her babies. Add it to the hutch on day 27 or 28 after breeding day, just before she delivers on day 30 to 32. If you introduce it too soon, it will become a litter box.

Rabbits being raised solely for meat can be placed in an outdoor grazing pen or mobile rabbit hutch, which can be purchased online and look very similar to a mobile chicken coop. These allow the rabbits to graze on fresh grass but keep them safe from predators and prevent them from digging out of the box. A 6-by-10-foot box can hold about ten rabbits. Each day, move the cage to a new patch of grass that offers some shade. Keep an eye on the temperature in the summer; if it gets too hot, you can spray them with a hose, which they hate, but it will cool them off. In the winter, be sure their drinking water doesn't freeze. The grazing pen doesn't need to be heated, but rabbits do require protection from the wind. A simple tarp on windy days works well.

Bucks should always be separated from does. Does can live together, two to a hutch, until they are ready to be bred, then they should be separated.

Food and Water

In the wild, rabbits eat a mix of grass, seeds, bark, and other plant matter. In order to mimic this mix, it's ideal to feed your rabbits dry roughages like grass hay and alfalfa hay, greens like lettuce, and rabbit pellets, which contain a mix of grains and seeds. Non-GMO, soy-free pellets are best for the rabbit's health. Read the labels—rabbits are herbivores, so you don't want to purchase pellets that include beef or other animal by-products. Rabbits also love produce scraps from beets, carrots, lettuce, sunflower seeds, and turnips. Don't feed greens to baby rabbits as they can cause diarrhea. Store rabbit food in a galvanized can to keep it safe from rodents—if you leave the bag in the corner, you're inviting trouble.

Feed your rabbits every day, ideally in the late afternoon or early evening, when they are most active, but morning is also acceptable. Once a week, feel each rabbit's back and belly. If you can feel the knobs of its spine, it's too thin and could use more pellets in its ration. Rabbits need more feed in the winter than in the summer, and young, growing rabbits and pregnant and lactating does also need more. At the same time, you don't want to overfeed your rabbits. Their food is expensive, and an overweight rabbit will not breed well.

Rabbits drink about a quart of water a day. Watering systems with nipples or bite valves are cleaner than water dishes, which can collect bacteria, and can be found at any agricultural supply store. However, bottles can crack when frozen, so keep an eye on them in the winter.

Rabbit	Amount of pellets per day for average meat breed
Buck	3–8 oz
Doe	6–9 oz
Doe, 1–15 days after breeding	6–9 oz
Doe, 16–30 days after breeding	7–10 oz
Doe plus litter (6–8 kits) 1 week old	10–12 oz
Doe plus litter (6–8 kits) 1 month old	18–24 oz
Doe plus litter (6–8 kits) 6–8 weeks old	28–36 oz
Young rabbit, weaned, 2 months old	3–9 oz

Health

Your rabbits should be bright and mobile, with a glossy coat, and they should be eating well. If you suspect you have a sick rabbit, isolate it from the others. Common illnesses include parasite infections and ear cankers, but these usually occur only when there's a build-up of manure, so a wire hutch—which lets the droppings fall right through the cage—can help prevent them. Routinely look for any discharge from the eyes or a runny nose, and check their poop to make sure it's well formed. Also look for sore hocks (hind legs), which are often caused by a bacterial infection and can be treated with antibiotic ointment. Check each rabbit for deformities on the genitals, buck teeth, and misaligned ears. Rabbits with these traits are fine to eat but should not be bred—you don't want to pass on these traits in your breeding line.

Trimming the toenails of your breeders makes them easier to handle. This is best done with regular toenail clippers.

Rabbits don't handle heat well. During warm weather, make sure your rabbits have plenty of water, place grazing pens in a shady spot, and provide indoor rabbits with a fan. You can also fill a plastic jug with water, freeze it, and then place it in the rabbit hutch to help them stay cool.

Breeding Your Rabbits

Rabbits are ready to breed when they're about five months old. Before breeding your rabbits, make sure they are in good health and have healthy coats. Check the genitals of the doe: the vulva will be purple or bright red when she is ready to breed, while pale pink means she's not in the mood, so don't even try. A doe is fertile most of the time—they ovulate upon copulation—but it's possible that she may not get pregnant right away.

Here's how to breed your rabbits:

1. Weigh the doe and take her to the buck. If you take the buck to the doe, she will become territorial and fight with him.
2. Watch the mating. Don't leave them alone or turn away for a second—without supervision, they could fight.
3. When they're done, the male normally does a dramatic dismount and can even scream. It's pretty funny.
4. Take the doe back to her cage.
5. Repeat the mating the next day to ensure success. The doe usually ovulates within ten hours of copulation, so the repeat performance helps guarantee that she'll conceive.
6. Weigh your doe again in two weeks. If she's pregnant, she'll be about one pound heavier. You can also palpate her abdomen at that point and feel for little baby balls.

If the buck is uninterested, you can place him alone in the doe's hutch overnight while she stays in his. Her scent may stimulate him to get in the mood. If that doesn't work, try putting him on a diet. A fat buck won't do his job properly.

If the doe is uninterested even though her vulva is the right color for breeding, you can force the issue: holding the doe by her shoulders, place her rear end into the cage. The buck will mount the doe and do his business.

Rabbit gestation is twenty-eight to thirty-four days. On day 27, place the nesting box in her cage. Line the bottom with shavings, then add a layer of straw. In the winter, line the box with cardboard first to provide extra insulation.

When the doe has given birth, she will pull some fur from her belly and use it to cover up her babies. You do not need to assist this process; she knows what to do. Be sure to give the doe her space for the first few days so that she doesn't kill or abandon the kits. Newborns should be handled very little so that you don't impart too much of your scent on them, but after about three days, you can gently pull up the fur and check on the babies. Remove any dead ones and quickly replace the fur over the rest.

After about two weeks, the kits will start to come out of the nesting box, and you can remove the box after one month. Wean the litter starting at eight weeks, moving the breeders to hutches and the meat bunnies to grazing pens. Move a few at a time and spread the separation out over a few weeks so the doe's milk supply can dry up gradually. Give the doe two weeks to rest after the last kit is weaned before breeding her again. If you do not intend to breed the doe again, she can be left with the female babies for several months.

Record how many babies each doe has, and if you're keeping any for future breeding stock, record who their parents are to help prevent inbreeding. A hutch record card is useful for recordkeeping.

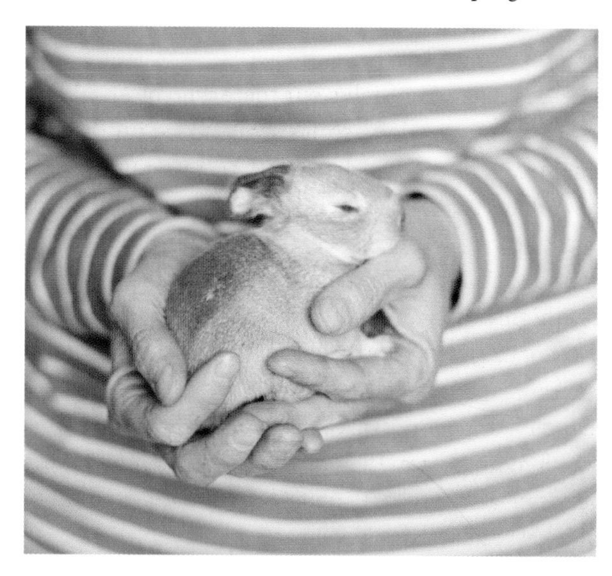

HUTCH RECORD CARD

Doe.................................. Ear Tattoo.................................. Breed.. 1 Yr. Weight........................

Nipples.............................. Born....../....../........... Fertile....../....../........... Sire............................ Dam.............................

Buck	Breed Date	Palpate Date	Nest Box Date	Due Date	Kindled Date	Number Kindled	Number Dead	Fostered Kids	Planned Rebreed Date	Weight Avg. at 5 Weeks	Grade A=Best F=Worst

CARING FOR YOUR RABBITS

Daily (10 to 20 minutes)	**Weekly** (about 1 hour)	**Monthly** (about 2 hours)
Provide fresh food and water. Move grazing pens to new pasture.	Clean hutches with a wire brush. You can use a butane torch (not when the rabbits are in there, of course!) to burn away fur that's stuck to the cage. Check on the rabbits' general health.	Breed, if desired. Wean any eight-week-old kits. Maintain records. Trim the nails of breeding does. Process any rabbits that have reached market weight.

Processing

There aren't tons of folks out there who offer rabbit-slaughtering services, so it's likely to be up to you. The best way to learn how to process a rabbit is to have someone with experience teach you. The next best alternative is to watch a video online so you can see how it's done. (See page 398 for a link.)

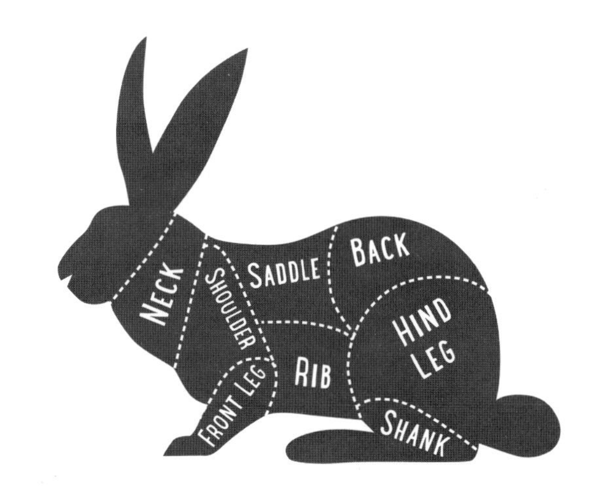

I highly recommend slaughtering your rabbits by shooting them with a pistol. You can break their necks instead, but it's tricky to do this fast and accurately, and until you're really good at it, a gun is much more humane. If you don't want to use a gun, you can also use a Rabbit Wringer, a device that quickly breaks the rabbit's neck.

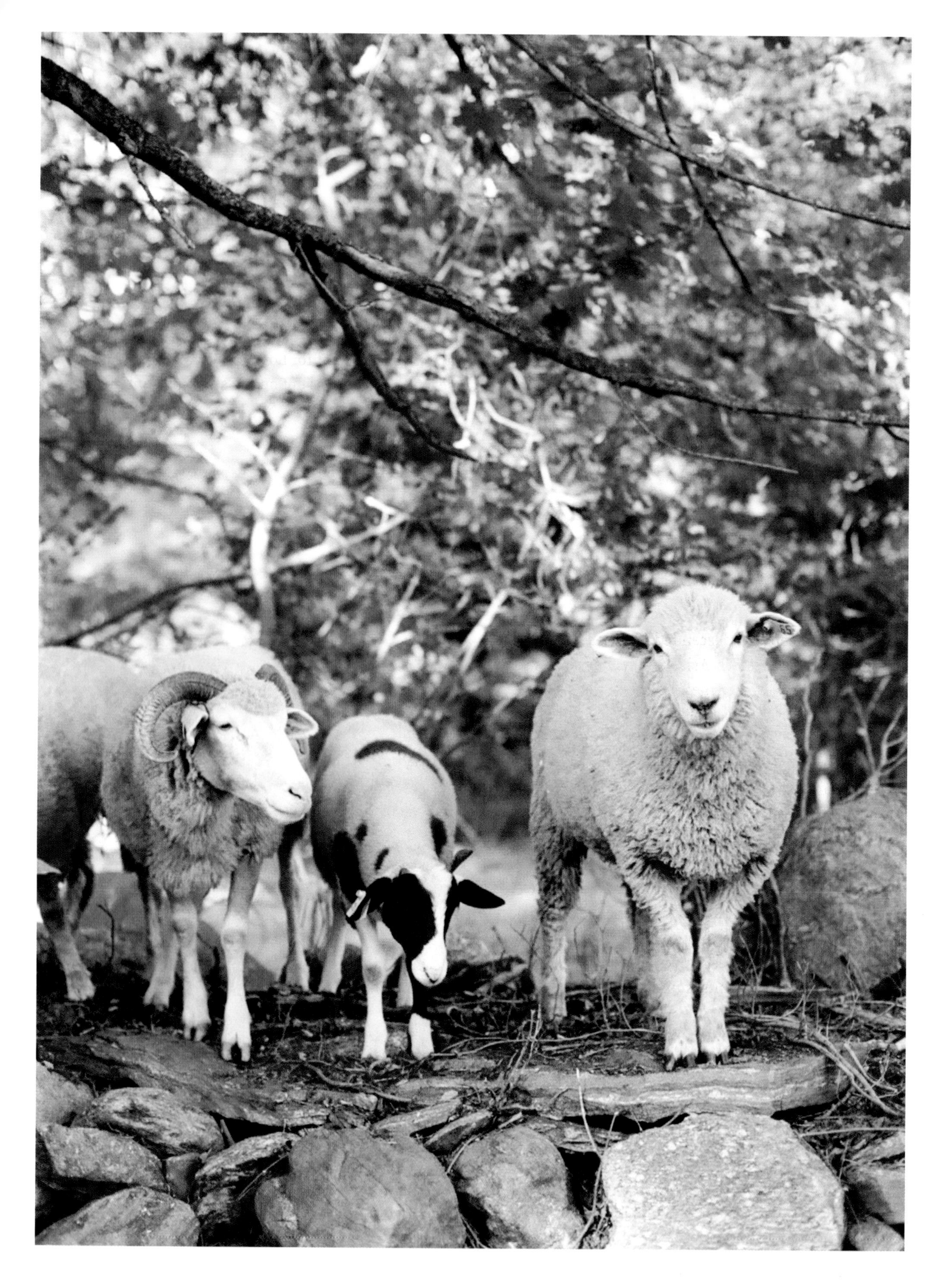

Sheep

Sheep have a special place in my heart. I've been breeding them for over ten years and am constantly learning more and gaining a deeper appreciation for them. Not many animals can instill the deep sense of calm that comes from watching a flock of sheep contently grazing a lush pasture.

Sheep have been selectively bred over thousands of years to provide us with many resources: meat, skins, wool, and milk. Their small size and abundant gifts make them ideal for a homestead with some pasture, and their docile nature and, again, relatively small size make them great for kids to work with. Sheep are especially great for homesteaders because five to seven sheep can be kept on the same amount of land needed for a single cow. Sheep are also more nimble than cows and can graze in ditches, woodlots, and orchards, not just pasture.

History

Modern sheep are descended from the wild mouflon sheep of western Asia. Because of several positive attributes—manageable size, early sexual maturity, docile nature, high reproduction rates, and valuable milk and meat—sheep were one of the first animals to be domesticated by humans. Interestingly, though, sheep were initially kept solely for their meat, milk, and skins, not wool. Woolly breeds developed much later.

Sheep farming reached its peak in the U.S. in 1884, and the number of sheep continues to fall today. Consumers only purchase about one-third the lamb that they purchased thirty years ago. On the positive side, because the sheep industry hasn't been taken over by corporate giants, small producers can still do quite well.

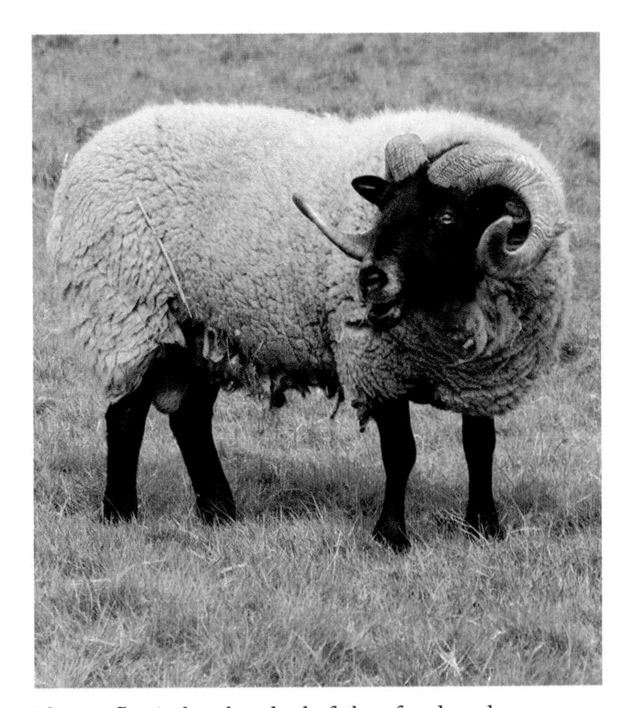

The mouflan is thought to be the father of modern sheep.

SHEEP FAQS

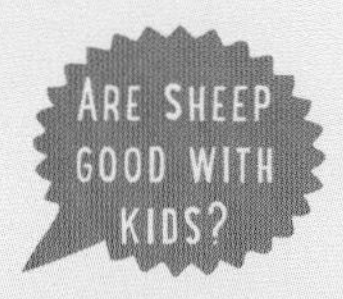

With their small size and calm disposition, sheep are ideal for kids who want to work with animals.

ARE SHEEP REALLY THE DUMBEST FARM ANIMAL?

Yes. There's only one farm animal dumber than a chicken and that's a sheep.

WHAT ARE THE LAWS ABOUT KEEPING SHEEP IN MY TOWN?

Towns have very different rules regarding keeping livestock. Be sure to check with your board of health before buying your flock.

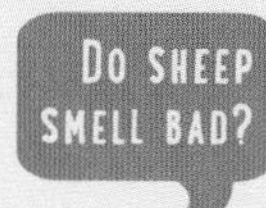

Every animal has a specific scent. Sheep have a pleasantly sweaty and oily smell, with a hint of grass and soil.

WHAT DO SHEEP EAT?

Sheep eat grass and leaves. You can also give them a small amount of grain to get them to follow you into the barn, then out to the pasture.

HOW MANY SHEEP DO I NEED?

Sheep are highly social and prefer to be kept in a group. I wouldn't keep any fewer than four sheep, but I have seen some backyard farmers with two.

HOW MUCH PASTURE DO FOUR SHEEP NEED?

In general, four sheep need at least 1 acre of pasture.

DO ONLY MALE SHEEP HAVE HORNS?

No. In some breeds, both the ewes and rams have horns.

ARE SHEEP HARD TO CONTAIN?

Sheep will definitely find the weaknesses in your fencing. While they're not as Houdini-like as goats, if they're underfed or have some need that's not being met, they will try to get out of their pen.

DO LAMBS NEED TO BE SHEARED?

No. Lambs are slaughtered while still young (less than a year old), and although their wool can get quite long, if you are raising them for meat you don't need to shear them.

WHAT DO I DO IF ONE OF MY LAMBS IS SICK?

The best thing to do is call a veterinarian. Unfortunately, there are not as many vets who are knowledgeable about sheep care as there used to be. Before you bring your flock home, do some research and find one that can help you.

DO I HAVE TO WORM MY LAMBS?

It is a good idea to make sure your lambs were wormed by the breeder before you take them home. If they weren't, do a preventative worming with a broad-spectrum wormer.

Behavior

Sheep are highly social animals with a strong flocking instinct. They're also generally fearful, especially when encountering something new, and their flocking behavior is a great adaptation against predators. By forming a tight group, they make it harder for a predator to target one sheep.

Their strong flocking instinct, combined with the clear hierarchy of power within the flock, can also get sheep into trouble. If a more dominant sheep decides it is time to move, the rest of the flock will follow, and if your fences are not strong, they may follow the leader right over them and out to greener pastures.

Take the flocking instinct in account when you need to work with one sheep and do not isolate it from the flock—a solitary sheep will be very stressed out. Instead, bring the entire flock into a small pen to do the job. If you do need to isolate a sheep (for example, after lambing), place the sheep in a pen where she can see the rest of the flock.

Nutrition

Lamb is by far the favorite meat in our house. It's tender and has a much nicer flavor than beef. Once we get our lamb in the freezer, it's the first to go, even before the bacon! Lamb is also very nutritious. It's a good source of niacin and zinc, and a very good source of protein and vitamin B12. Grass-fed lamb is also rich in omega-3 fatty acids, which reduce inflammation. Typically, the sheep meat you find in U.S. stores is lamb, though in many other countries, hogget—a young sheep between one and two years old—is considered even more desirable.

SHEEP TERMINOLOGY

Ewe
Adult female sheep

Wether
Adult castrated male sheep

Lamb
Young sheep, under 12 months old, that does not have any permanent incisor teeth

Hogget or hogg
Young sheep or maiden ewe that has no more than two permanent incisors

Mutton
Meat from an ewe or wether with more than two permanent incisors, or from a sheep over two years old

Selecting a Breed

Sheep have been selectively bred over thousands of years for specific traits and climates. If you are looking for an animal that will give you more than just one really great product, I recommend an all-around breed such as Border Leicester, Cheviot, Columbia, Dorset, East Friesian, Lincoln, Montadale, Polypay, Rambouillet, Romney, Shropshire, Southdown, or Targhee.

On our farm, we have found that the best sheep for our northeastern climate and on our pasture is a cross between a Horned Dorset and a Southdown. I often experiment with some other breeds to enhance our sheep genetics, but overall I'm very pleased with this mix. They can handle the harsh winters well, thrive on our pasture, and put on weight well. They're also very calm and passive, unlike other breeds, which can be skittish. They breed well and frequently have twins. In warmer climates, choose a breed that is well suited to handle heat, like a Dorper, which has hair instead of wool.

Try to find a reputable local breeder who can answer any questions you might have about breeds.

Meat Breeds

Best: Columbia, East Friesian, Hampshire, Oxford, Suffolk

Still Great: Border Leicester, Blue Leicester, Cheviot, Dorper, Dorset, Katahdin, Lincoln, Montadale, Panama, Polypay, Rambouillet, Romney, Shropshire, Southdown, Targhee, Texel, Tunis, Wiltshire

Wool Breeds

Best: American Cormo, Booroola Merino, Columbia, Corriedale, Debouillet, Delaine Merino, East Friesian, Panama, Ramouillet, Targhee

Dairy Breeds

Best: Assaf, British Milksheep, Clun Forest, East Friesian, Lacaune

Housing and Fencing

Sheep require some protection from the elements. During the summer, they need a roof to provide some shade and protection from a downpour. During the winter, they need shelter from frigid winds, rain, and snow. A three-sided horse run-in is usually sufficient, but if you have a lot of predators in your area, you may need to lock them in a barn at night.

At our farm, we use electric netting to fence off pasture for our sheep and goats. It's 4 feet tall and comes in rolls of 160 feet. It's powered by a 2 joule 52B battery energizer support box with a 20 watt solar panel and a 12 volt 4 amp solar regulator attached to a 12 volt battery. One person can easily set up a small pen in 15 minutes, which is important when you're moving sheep around for rotational grazing.

If you're looking for more permanent fencing, we suggest 5-foot-tall metal livestock fencing with 6-by-6-inch squares, held up by 6-foot metal T posts. This type of fencing comes in 330-foot rolls and is very heavy to maneuver, but once it's up, you'll sleep soundly knowing that your sheep are safely fenced in.

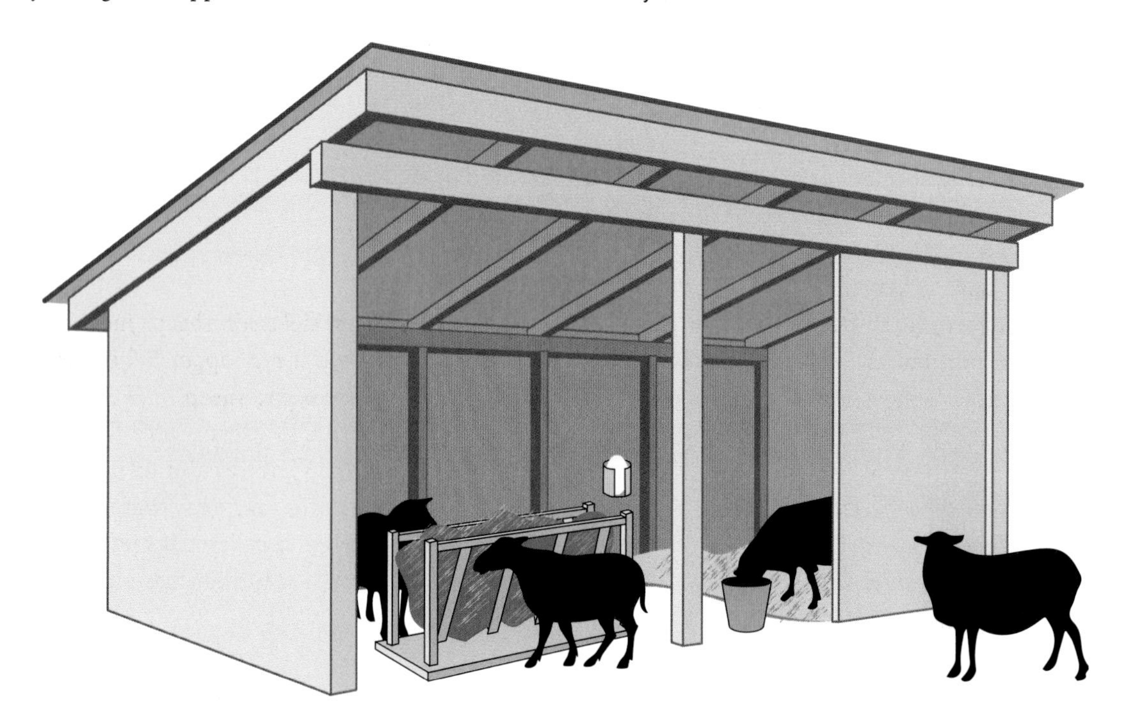

Food and Water

Sheep need pasture. A very general estimate is that 1 acre of pasture can support four sheep. If you live in an arid climate, though, that's way too many sheep for 1 acre. Likewise, if you live in a lush green area such as the Northeast, you can have more sheep on your land. If you do not have enough pasture and are planning to buy hay year-round, be prepared to spend a ton of money to feed your flock.

No matter your climate, rotational grazing—in which sheep graze in a small area for a limited time before being moved to another area—is key for maximizing your pasture and minimizing your hay bill. (See page 61 for more on rotational grazing.) After the sheep graze a piece of land, we move the chicken flock onto it. They eat worms, pick through the manure left by the sheep, scratch at the ground, and leave their own droppings. It all adds up to healthy, fertilized grass with few worms to infect the sheep the next time they graze there.

If you live in a region with cold winters, you'll need to provide hay during the winter months. Each sheep needs 4 pounds of hay per day when they aren't on pasture. So to calculate how much hay you'll need, multiply the number of sheep by 4 and then by the number of days your pasture is not growing. Most square hay bales weigh about 40 pounds, so then divide the number of pounds of hay you need by 40 to get the number of bales of hay you'll need to get through your pasture's off season.

Sheep can be wasteful with hay, so build or buy a hay crib to minimize spillage, and don't give them more hay until they've finished what they have.

Many farmers supplement lambs with some grain to help them reach market weight faster, but this is not necessarily good for the lambs' digestion, nor is it good for your wallet. Sheep do love grain, though, and it helps ewes put on weight in the fall, so they're more likely to have a successful twin birth in the spring. On our farm, each ewe gets about a half a pound of grain per day as the weather gets cooler. During the spring, the new lambs and their mothers are primarily grass-fed, but we use a touch of grain in a bucket to lead them out to the fields. It's much easier to get sheep to go in and out of the barn with the promise of a handful of grain.

Unlike grain supplements, mineral supplements are absolutely necessary. Most agricultural supply

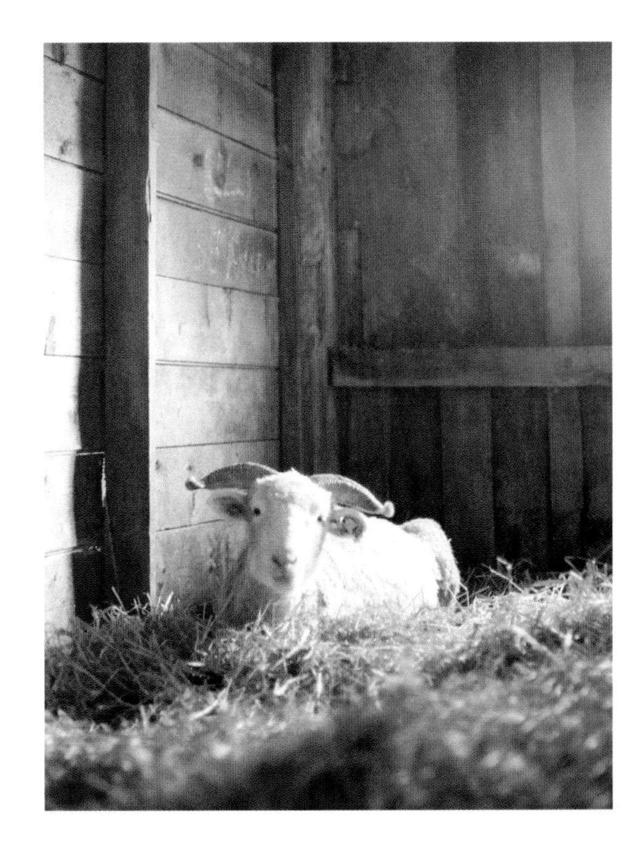

stores sell mineral licks for sheep. Just make sure that you do not give sheep copper. While goats tolerate it just fine, it's toxic to sheep.

You'll want to provide clean water for your sheep and make sure they have access to it at all times. They don't tend to tip over their water buckets too often. We use a few five gallon buckets for our flock. If you only have two sheep, they may only go through half a bucket a day.

Predators

Sheep have many predators: coyotes, bears, wolves, even domestic dogs. Lambs are also vulnerable to foxes, bobcats, and even fisher cats. If you plan to leave your sheep out on pasture at night, you will need to have a guard animal or bring them into a barn at night. I recommend you bring your sheep in at night, especially if, like us, you live in a highly populated area: Although guard dogs are ideal for protecting the farm against predators, they can be aggressive to other dogs and to people. For us, it's just too much of a liability. We have had great success with llamas guarding the sheep, though; they were kept in the field with the sheep, and they did a great job and were quite entertaining. Other people we know have used donkeys as guard animals.

Health

Keep an eye on your flock and watch for any sheep that are laying down a lot, aren't eating or drinking, or are separated from the flock—these are all signs of illness. When you find a sick sheep, it's a good idea to isolate it for a few days and give your vet a call. We've found that sheep are more susceptible than our other animals to a variety of issues, from parasites to poisoning from toxic plants to hoof problems (see page 59).

Parasites

Sheep are far more likely to die from a parasite infestation than from a predator attack. All sheep carry a parasite load, but a healthy sheep isn't adversely affected by the parasites. If a sheep is sick from parasites, it's necessary to cull it from your flock.

Rotational grazing plays a huge part in preventing parasite infestations. Most parasites live low down on the stem of the grass, so if the sheep don't overgraze, they won't come into contact with the parasites. Without a host, parasites eventually die, so over the years rotational grazing can drastically reduce the amount of parasites living on your pasture.

A sheep suffering from a heavy parasite load is often anemic, which shows up in gums and eyelids that are very pale instead of pink. Other signs of a parasite problem include diarrhea, lethargy, weight loss, and just generally sluggishness. Although we almost never have to treat our sheep for parasites, you can get a dewormer from an agriculture supply store if parasites become an issue.

Toxic plants

Sheep can be poisoned by the following plants:

- Trees in the rose family (cherry, serviceberry)
- Nightshades (potatoes, tomatoes, peppers)
- Beets
- Buckwheat
- Chard
- Goldenrod
- Lupine seeds
- Milkweed
- Mountain laurel
- Pigweed
- Rhododendron
- Rhubarb
- Skunk cabbage
- St. John's wort

These plants are very common in much of the United States. If you see any of them growing in your pasture, it is important that you remove them. It take only a tiny amount of these leaves to make your lambs sick or even kill them.

CARING FOR YOUR SHEEP

Daily (15 minutes)	**Weekly** (2 hours)	**Monthly** (5 to 10 minutes per animal)
Provide water and hay or pasture, depending on the time of year. Make sure droppings are well formed.	Rotate sheep to new pasture. Clean out water troughs. Spend some time looking at the flock to see if there are any unhealthy sheep.	Bring sheep into the barn and do a thorough check of each animal. Check gums and eyelids for paleness, which could be a sign of anemia. Check hooves to see if they need trimming.

Caring for Sheep and Goat Hooves

Unlike chickens, ducks, turkeys, and pigs, sheep and goats need some routine care to keep them healthy. On our farm, we trim their hooves every six weeks, but if you have more rocky terrain, you may need to trim them less often. It may be helpful to watch a video first to see how it's done (see page 398 for a suggestion), or better yet, have someone show you how to do it.

Before you begin to trim their hooves, it can be helpful to prop sheep up on their butts. It makes it easier to get to their hooves and keeps the animal immobilized. You can also trim goats' hooves this way, but sometimes it's easier to work on goats while they're standing up, working on one leg at a time.

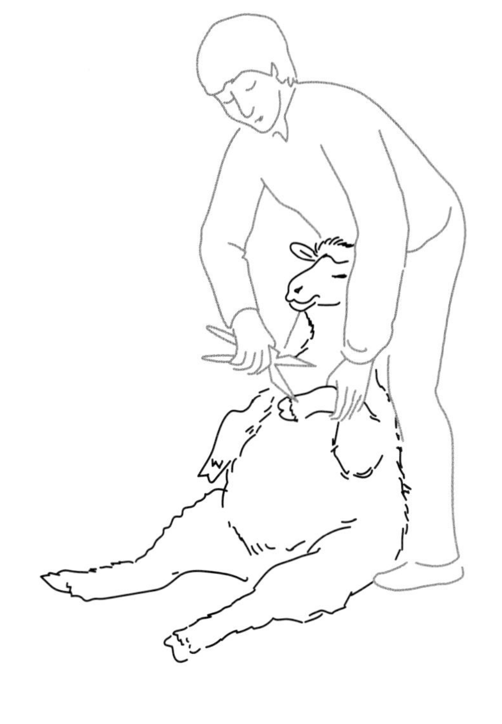

Bad: Note that one side of the hoof is longer than the other and the hoof tips up at the end.

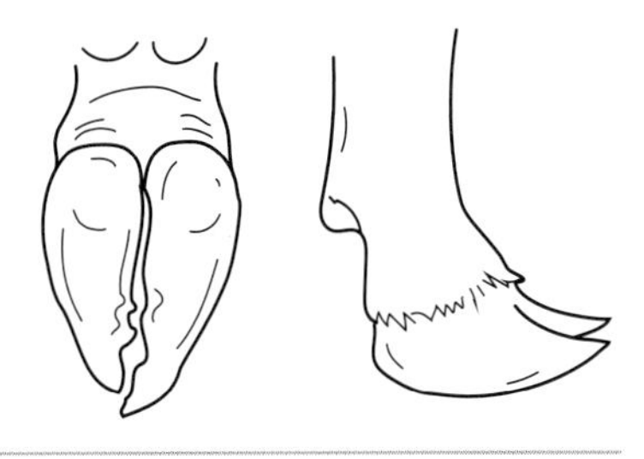

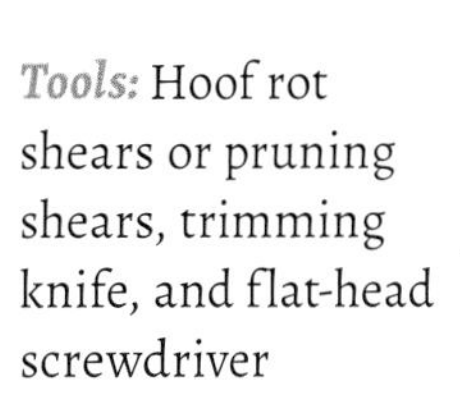

Good: Both sides of the hoof are even and neatly trimmed.

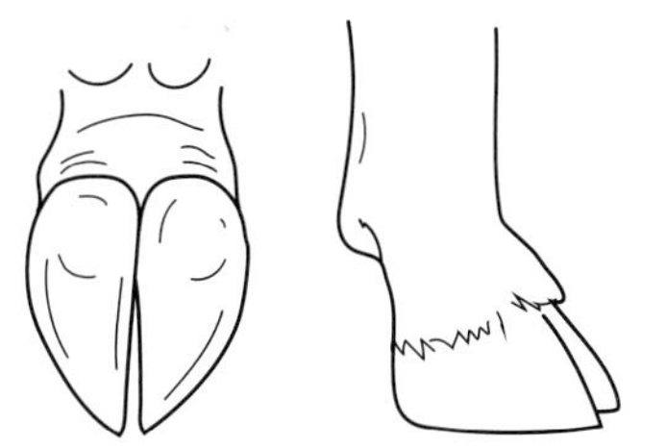

Tools: Hoof rot shears or pruning shears, trimming knife, and flat-head screwdriver

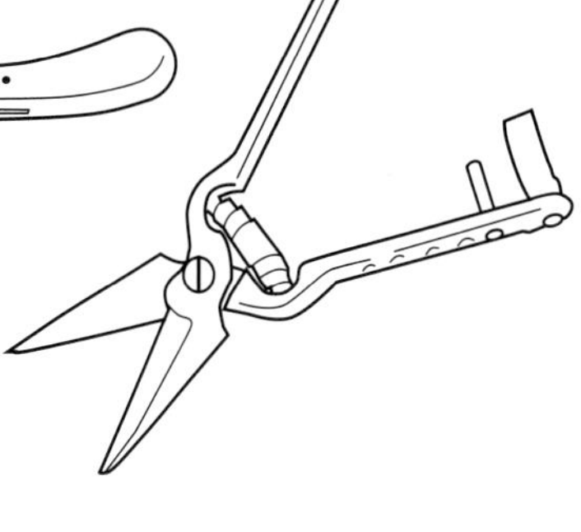

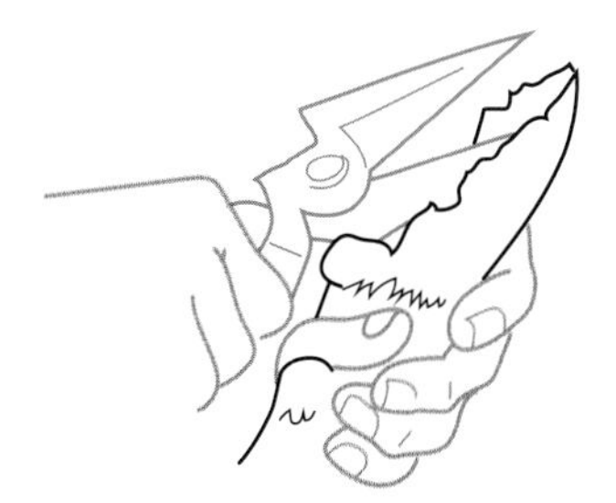

Step 1: Clean the hooves with the screwdriver or shears, digging out any dirt or stones.

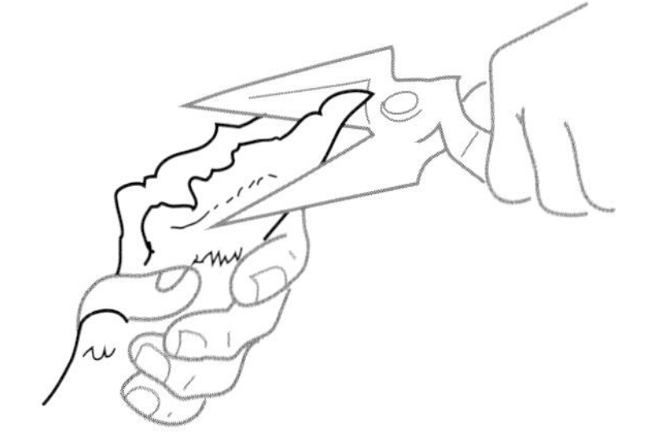

Step 2: Make the base of the hoof level by trimming it parallel to the hairline with the shears. Once properly trimmed, the pad (the center part of the hoof) will be even with the nail.

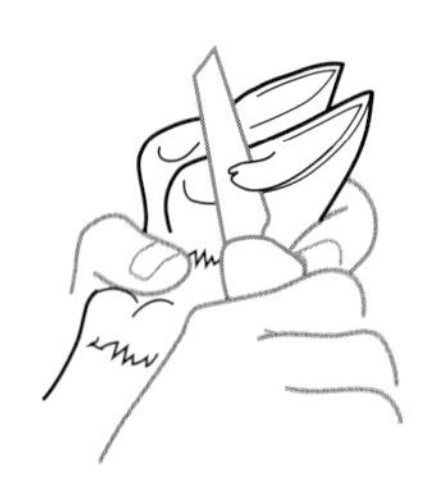

Step 3: Use the trimming knife to pare the nails until they are level and even.

Shearing Your Sheep

Sheep need to be shorn of their long woolly coats once or twice a year, depending on the breed and climate—if the breed has a particularly long coat or you live in a warm climate, you can shear them more often to keep them cool. Shear your sheep four to eight weeks before lambing, and if summers get hot where you live, you may want to shear again before the temperatures spike. While sheep don't enjoy the process of being shorn, they are a lot happier after it's done.

Shearing day is one of the most exciting days on a farm. It's an early sign that spring is coming, and that we'll soon have new lambs. We often schedule school groups to come watch, and the kids are pretty silent in awe as our shearer—Kevin Ford, who is one of the last to use old-fashioned hand shears, not electric shears—does his magic.

There are many uses for the fleece. You can card and spin the wool into yarn yourself, sell it to a local spinner, or use it as mulch for your tomato plants. There are also companies that you can pay to spin your raw wool into beautiful blankets.

Here are some tips to keep in mind for shearing day:

- If your sheep are out on pasture, bring them in the barn the day before shearing so they have time to dry. You do not want to shear a wet sheep.
- Don't allow your sheep any food or water for eight hours before shearing. A sheep with a full belly is very uncomfortable during the shearing process. They can eat and drink all they want right after.
- Keep the sheep in a cozy pen. Large, open pens are stressful for them; they prefer being snugged up next to other sheep.
- Have a clean, dedicated shearing area. You can use a sheet of plywood or a tarp to separate the area from the rest of the pen. Sweep off the shearing platform between sheep to keep it clean.
- Each time you collect a sheep to take to the shearing area, try not to make it into some sort of rodeo. Keep things calm.
- Make sure you have good lighting.
- Keep a first aid kit on hand in case the shearer gets cut.
- Have heavy-duty plastic bags on hand to put the fleeces in.
- Shearing is a great time to take a careful look at your sheep. Once their heavy fleece is shorn, you can get a good look at their udders and see if they're full of milk, ready for the new lambs.

Processing

Lambs are ready to be slaughtered when they're between twelve weeks and one year old. At our farm, we process the males and keep the females for breeding stock. I prefer to have our lamb processed when they are about seven months old, when they're still very tender and have a mild flavor. For more on processing, see "Dealing with a Slaughterhouse" on page 75.

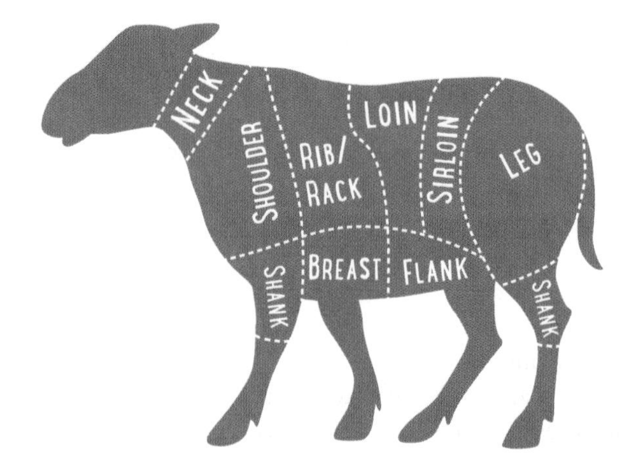

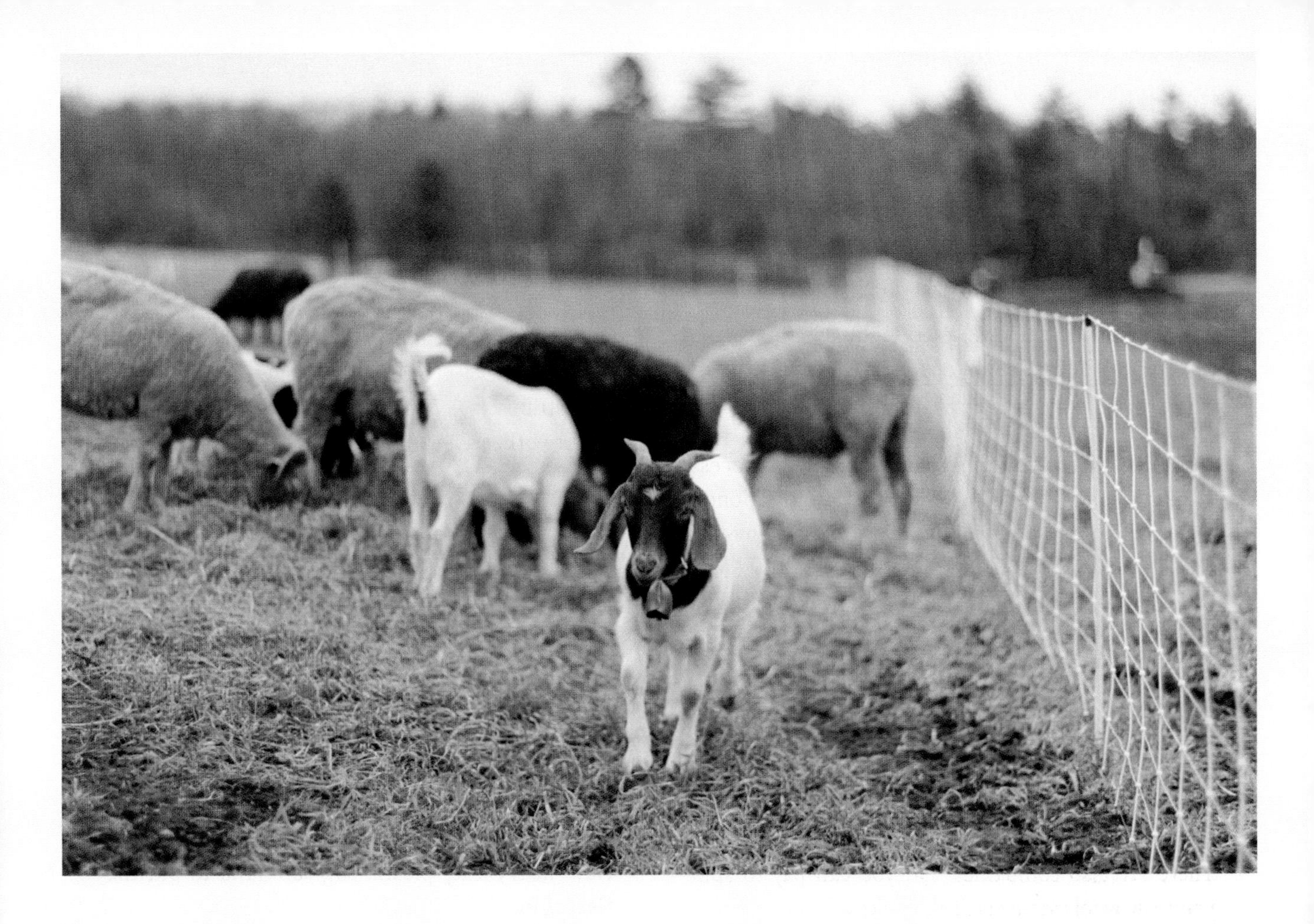

ROTATIONAL GRAZING

WHETHER YOU'RE RAISING SHEEP, GOATS, OR COWS, ROTATIONAL GRAZING IS KEY FOR MAXIMIZING YOUR PASTURE AND MINIMIZING YOUR HAY BILL. KEEPING YOUR ANIMALS IN ONE PATCH OF PASTURE AND THEN MOVING THEM TO ANOTHER IS EXCELLENT FOR THE GRASS AND SOIL, AND IT HELPS KEEP THE ANIMALS HEALTHY, TOO.

The process itself is pretty straightforward: Section off a piece of land with movable fencing and allow the animals to graze until the grass is down to about 4 inches, then move them to a new area of pasture. When you decide how much space to fence off for the animals, there are several factors to take into account. How lush and dense is the pasture? How long is the grass? Do your animals like this pasture? If you don't have great pasture yet, you can supplement with hay until your animals help you improve the land with their manure.

There are two benefits to keeping the grass above 4 inches: First, it lets the grass recover quickly. Second, most parasites live on the stem of the grass close to the ground, so when the grass is above 4 inches, the animals are less likely to ingest parasites. Over time, the parasites without a host will die off, so rotational grazing can help eliminate parasites from the pasture. Don't move the animals off the pasture too soon, though. If you do, they'll only eat their favorite grasses, and you don't want to encourage picky eaters.

If you have chickens, consider bringing them on to an area of pasture right after you move the grazing animals off. The chickens eat any worms and parasites, and their droppings and scratching at the ground help keep the soil healthy.

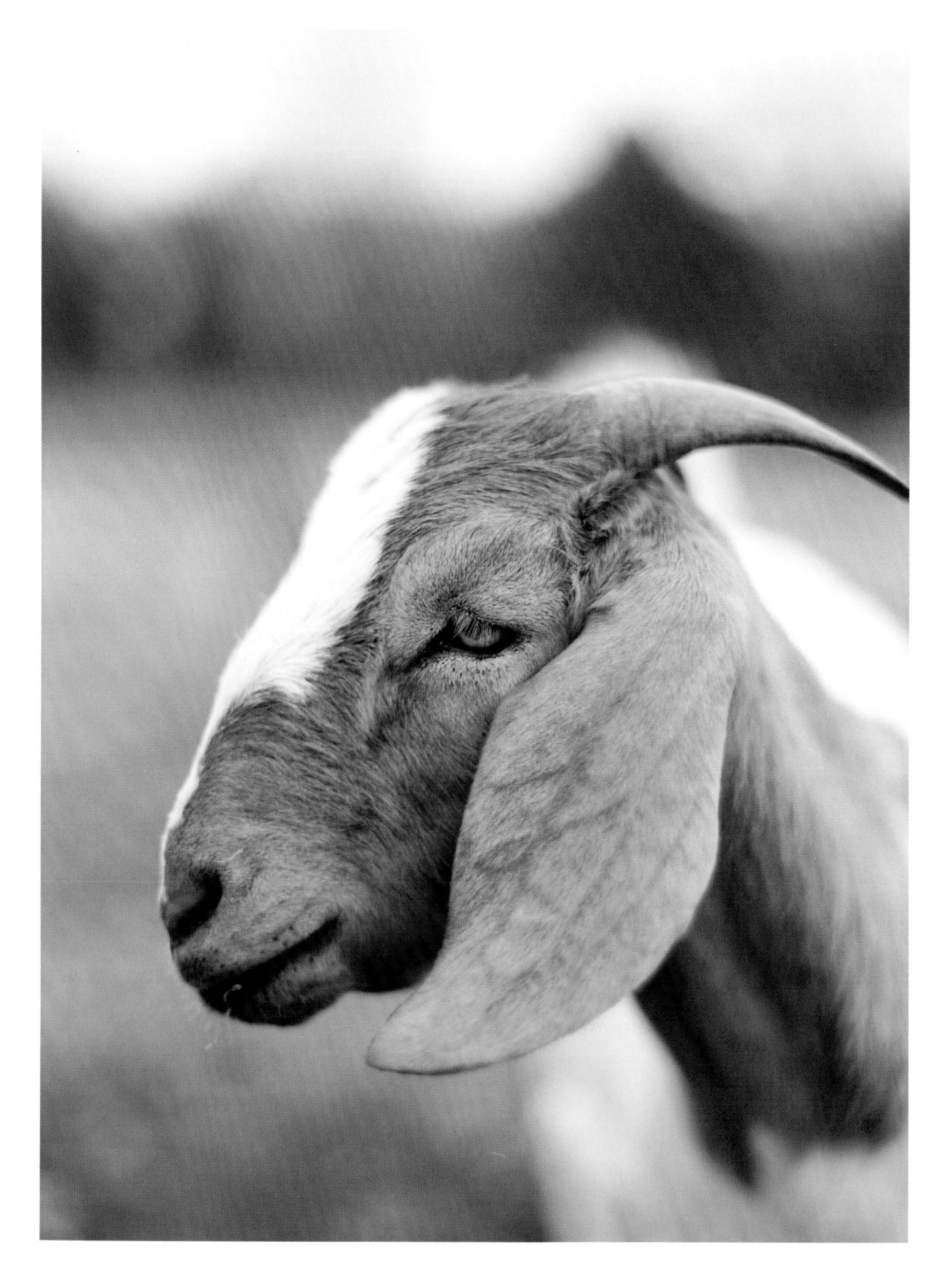

Goats

Goats are a great addition to any homestead. They efficiently keep brush under control and add a fantastic meat or cheese to your table. Goats are also cute, inquisitive, and incredibly entertaining. Goats are herd animals, so I suggest you keep at least two.

History

About 10,000 to 11,000 years ago, people in the Near East began keeping small herds of goats for their milk and meat. Goats also played several roles in ancient religions: depictions of many gods, such as the Greek god Pan, show them in goat forms; the Jewish practice of designating a goat to bear the sins of the people on Yom Kippur led to the term "scapegoat"; and goats were often used in religious sacrifice. Over time, goats have become smaller than their wild ancestors, and their horns have also shrunk. However, they have kept their natural curiosity, vitality, and gumption, which endear them to us humans.

Today, more than 80 percent of the world's goats live in Asia and Africa. They adapt well to a variety of terrain and climates, much better than cattle do, and they can largely fend for themselves without much human intervention. But although goat meat is a fundamental protein for many across the globe, Americans generally only keep goats for their milk—their meat is seen as too pungent, and with the wide availability of other meats here, goat is not considered a delicacy.

Behavior

Goats act like a cross between dogs and sheep: they are curious and playful, and they enjoy affection. They like human company, and when you're in the pasture, they'll follow you around as you do your chores. Bucks like to sneak up on you from behind—sort of funny, but also kind of dangerous! An aggressive buck will try to knock you over if you're not careful.

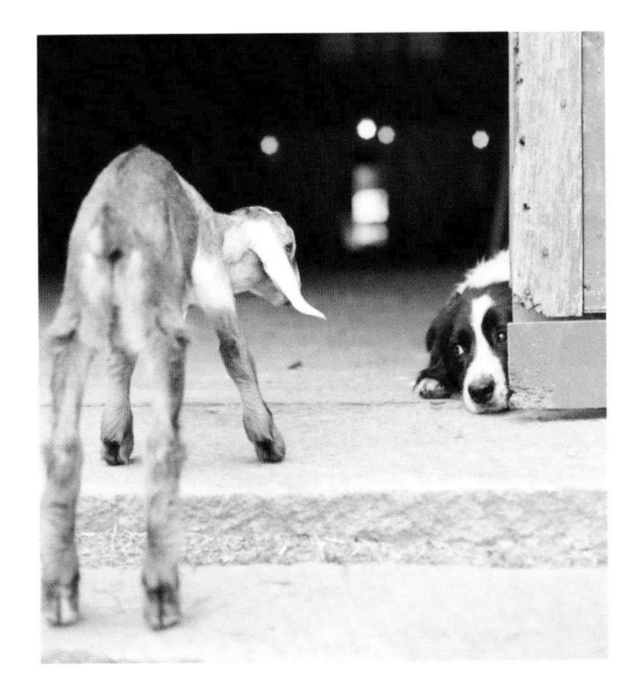

GOAT FAQS

Do goats really eat everything?

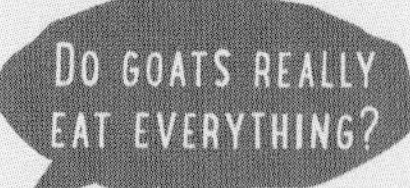

Contrary to what you've seen in cartoons, goats do not eat everything, but they are curious and will nibble at many things—including your jacket. Be careful not to allow plants that are toxic to goats on your property.

Do goats smell bad?

Female goats and young male goats have a very pleasant grassy, earthy smell. Some mature male goats can have a very strong odor that many people find very offensive, but we've also known some bucks that don't smell bad at all.

Are goats safe around children?

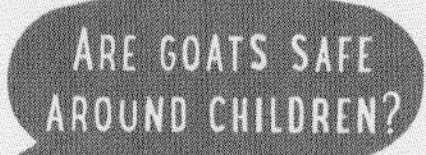

Yes, goats are generally kind animals. They are more rambunctious than sheep, though, particularly—as with most animals—the males. Males can range from annoying to very aggressive, so it's best to keep them away from children.

Can you milk all breeds of goats?

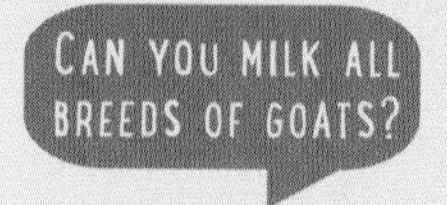

You could, but dairy breeds are far more productive than meat breeds.

Does goat meat have a strong taste?

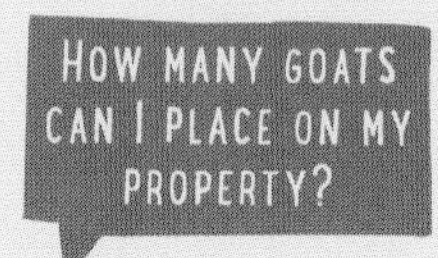

Young goat meat tastes a lot like lamb and is quite delicious. Older goat can be tough and strong-tasting, though. Curries and other slow-cooked dishes are great for meat from older goats.

How many goats can I place on my property?

It varies with the quantity and quality of the available plants, but in general, 1 acre of pasture can support four to eight goats.

Can you run goats with other livestock?

Yes, goats work well as companion grazers because they prefer plants that other livestock won't eat. Goats even prefer weeds over grass and clover, leaving those for sheep and cows.

Nutrition

The molecules in goat milk are similar in size to those in human milk, making goat milk easier for babies to digest and suitable for a range of dairy products. Unlike cows, goats convert carotene to vitamin A in their milk, making it bioavailable to humans. Goat milk is naturally homogenized because it does not contain agglutinin, the compound in cow milk that enables the fat globules to rise to the top—so goat milk won't separate. It also contains less lactose than cow milk, so those with problems digesting lactose may have an easier time digesting goat milk.

Goat milk tastes different from cow milk and is particularly good for making cheese. Some breeds produce a more musky-tasting milk, and if there is a buck around, the milk may have a stronger taste. In general, the fresher the milk, the sweeter the taste. We did a taste test with our kids, and they almost always preferred goat milk to cow milk.

Goat meat is low in calories and fat—it doesn't marble like beef does—and high in protein and iron. Meat from a relatively young goat is quite tasty, though the cuts can contain more bones than lamb cuts. I generally make stews and curries with goat meat, and I use the bones for added flavor. Smoked goat leg is also fantastic. I tend to avoid meat from bucks, as the flavor is quite strong. If you'd like to try goat meat and aren't ready to raise it yourself, try seeking out a butcher that caters to Middle Eastern or Caribbean customers.

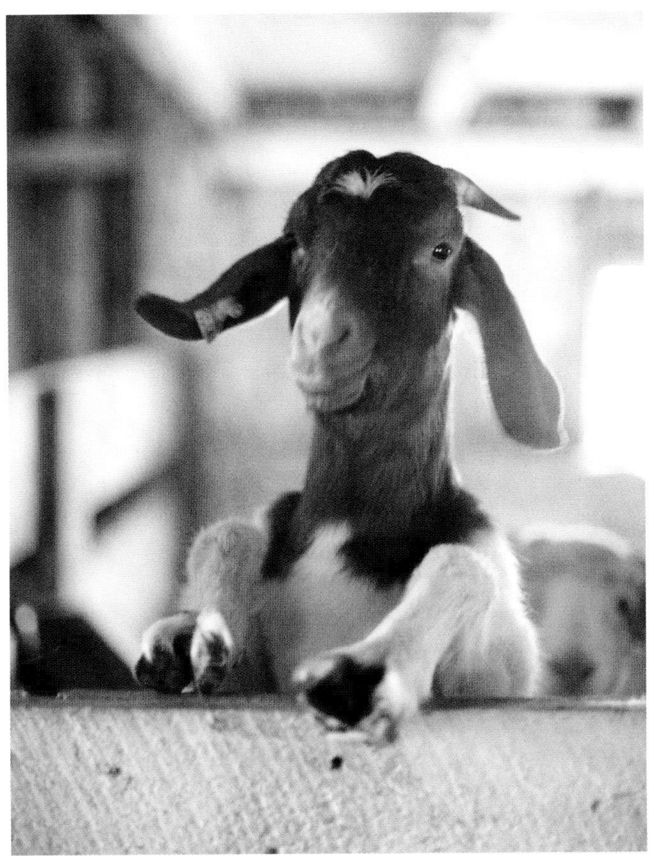

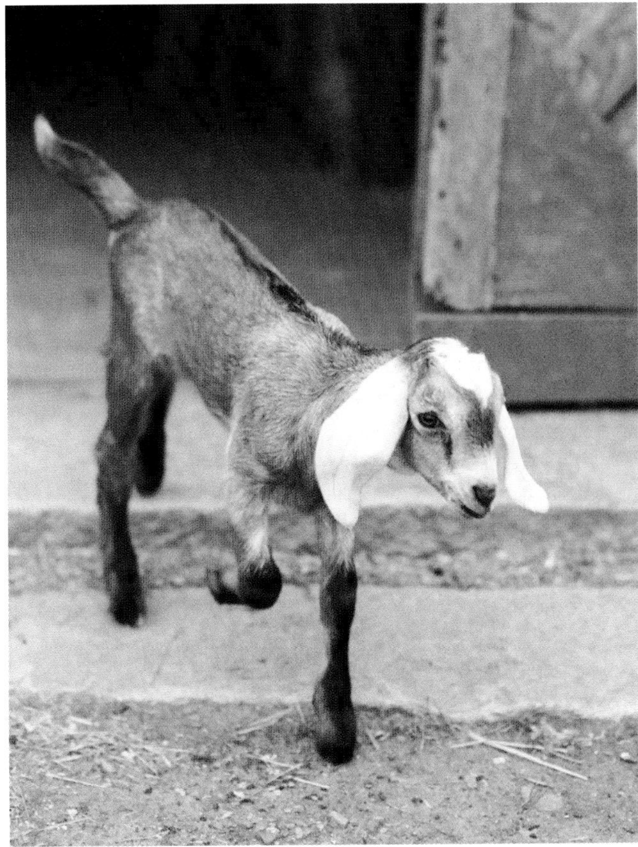

Selecting a Breed

Dairy goats are generally very hardy and live for over a decade. If you're looking for a dairy breed, Nubians are adorable and very friendly, and they produce milk that's high in butterfat, making it good for cheese and soap. Alpines are also a popular dairy breed. If you don't have much space, you might want to consider Nigerian Dwarf goats, which need half the space of standard-size goats, produce milk that's high in butterfat, and make very good pets.

Most meat breeds are short and stocky and aren't as friendly as the dairy breeds, but they're curious and playful nonetheless. At our farm we raise Boers for meat. Boers are considered one of the best breeds for meat because of the way they put on weight. We've been very happy with their temperament, size, and ease of care.

No matter what breed you choose, make sure you buy from a reputable breeder who has an established track record of disease-free goats.

GOAT TERMINOLOGY

Nanny
Female goat

Kid
Baby goat

Buck or billy
Male goat

Wether
Castrated male goat

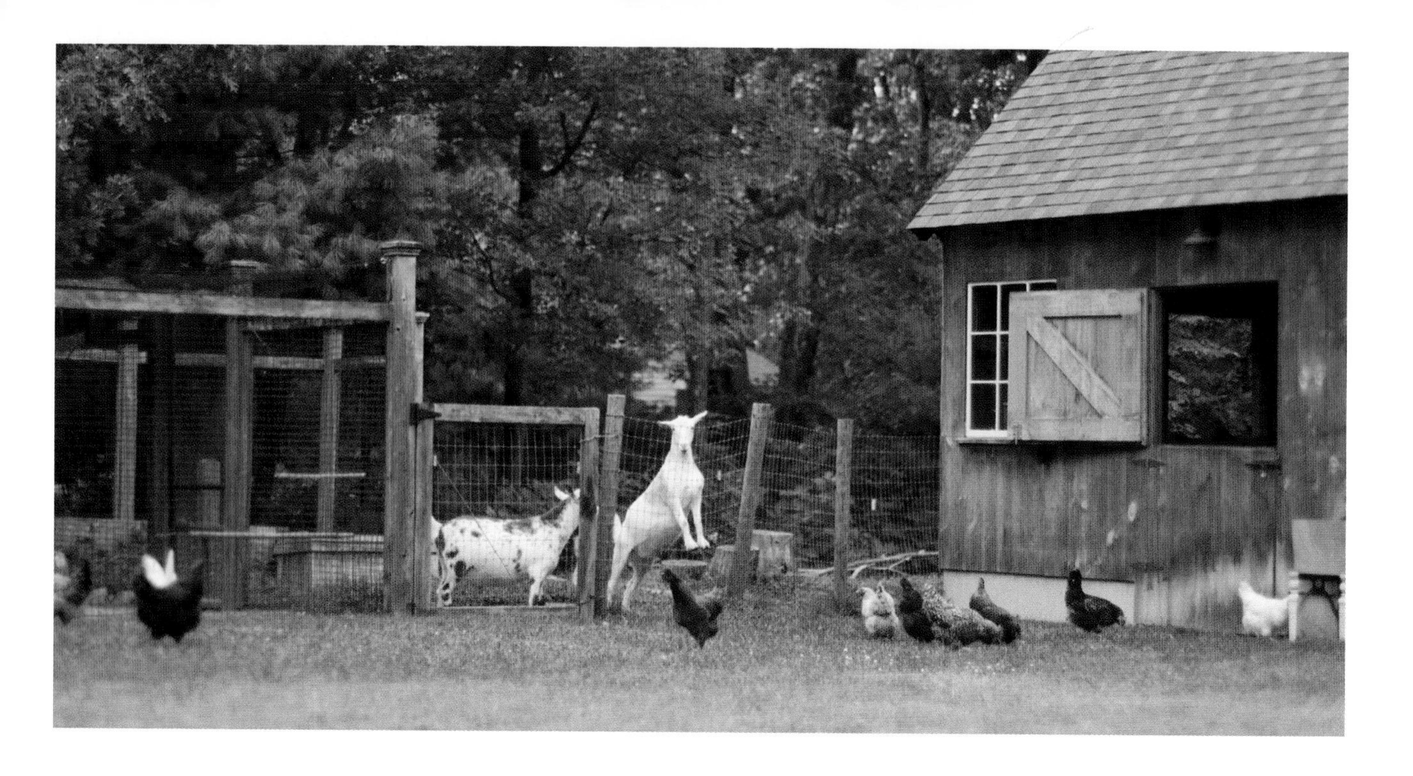

Housing and Fencing

Like sheep, goats need shade and protection from rain during the summer and shelter from wind, rain, and snow during the winter. A three-sided horse run-in (see page 56) works just as well for goats as for sheep, but if predators are a concern in your area, it's best to lock them in a barn at night.

Electric netting works well as temporary fencing on pasture. It's easy for one person to set up, which is important when you're moving animals to a new area. It's 4 feet tall, comes in rolls of 160 feet, and is powered by a 2 joule 52B battery energizer support box with a 20 watt solar panel and a 12 volt 4 amp solar regulator attached to a 12 volt battery. For permanent fencing, try 5-foot-tall metal livestock fencing with 6-by-6-inch squares, held up by 6-foot metal T posts.

Goats are much craftier than sheep when it comes to escaping from their field. They are curious and smart, and they can jump over fencing. The electric fencing is more of a psychological barrier: they can jump out if they really want to, but if their needs are being met—they have enough food and some goat friends—then they probably aren't going anywhere. That being said, we do have one goat that just loves to get out, constantly. She doesn't go far; usually she just hangs out on the other side of the fence and taunts the other goats that are still in the pasture.

CARING FOR YOUR GOATS

Daily (15 minutes)	**Weekly** (2 hours)	**Monthly** (5 to 10 minutes per animal)
Provide water and hay or pasture, depending on the time of year.	Rotate goats to new pasture. Clean out water troughs.	Bring goats into the barn and do a thorough check of each animal. Check hooves to see if they need trimming, and take a look at their gums and eyelids to see if they look pale, a sign of anemia from a possible parasite infection.

Food and Water

Although goats will eat grass, they prefer leaves, vines, weeds, and shrubs. In fact, they'll do a great job of cleaning up any weedy, brambly corners of your land.

In general, an acre of pasture can support four to eight goats, depending on the quality and quantity of plants available on your land. Rotational grazing, as always, is key for keeping the pasture and the goats healthy. (See page 61 for more on rotational grazing.)

During the winter months, you'll need to provide hay for your goats. Each goat needs 4 pounds of hay per day when they aren't on pasture, so to calculate how much hay you'll need, multiply the number of goats by 4 and then by the number of days your pasture is not growing. Divide that by 40 to get the number of hay bales (which weigh about 40 pounds) you'll need. Starting in the fall, we feed pregnant goats about 1 pound of grain per day to help them put on weight, which helps ensure a healthy delivery in the spring.

You'll need to provide mineral supplements year-round for your goats. Mineral licks can be found at most agricultural supply stores. And of course, be sure to provide your goats with a clean supply of water. Five-gallon buckets work just fine.

Health

Goats are very hardy and thrive when given proper care. However, they do tend to suffer from problems with their hooves, especially in lush pasture. Keep goats on dry land as much as possible. If there is standing water, you're asking for trouble. To keep their hooves neatly pared and healthy, see the instructions on page 59.

Like sheep, goats are susceptible to parasites, which are gradually becoming resistant to the drenches used to control them, posing a looming threat to goat farming. One alternative is to breed healthy animals that have a resistance to internal parasites. It also helps not to routinely deworm the entire flock if one goat is sick with parasites, and rotational grazing can minimize goats' ingestion of parasitic larvae—for more on that, see page 61.

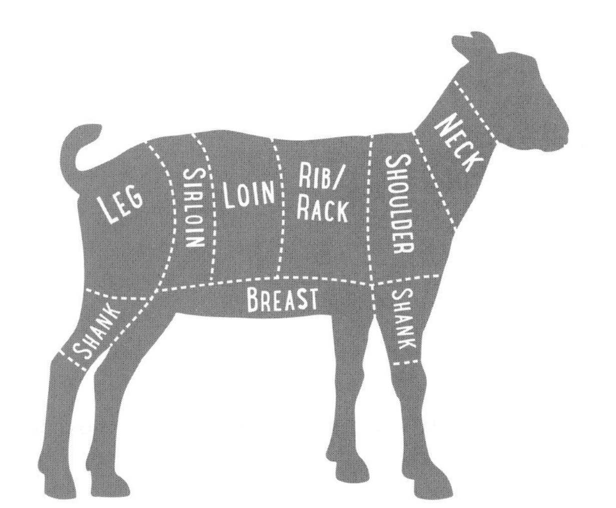

Processing

Meat goats are ready for processing at six or seven months old. For more on processing, see "Dealing with a Slaughterhouse" on page 75.

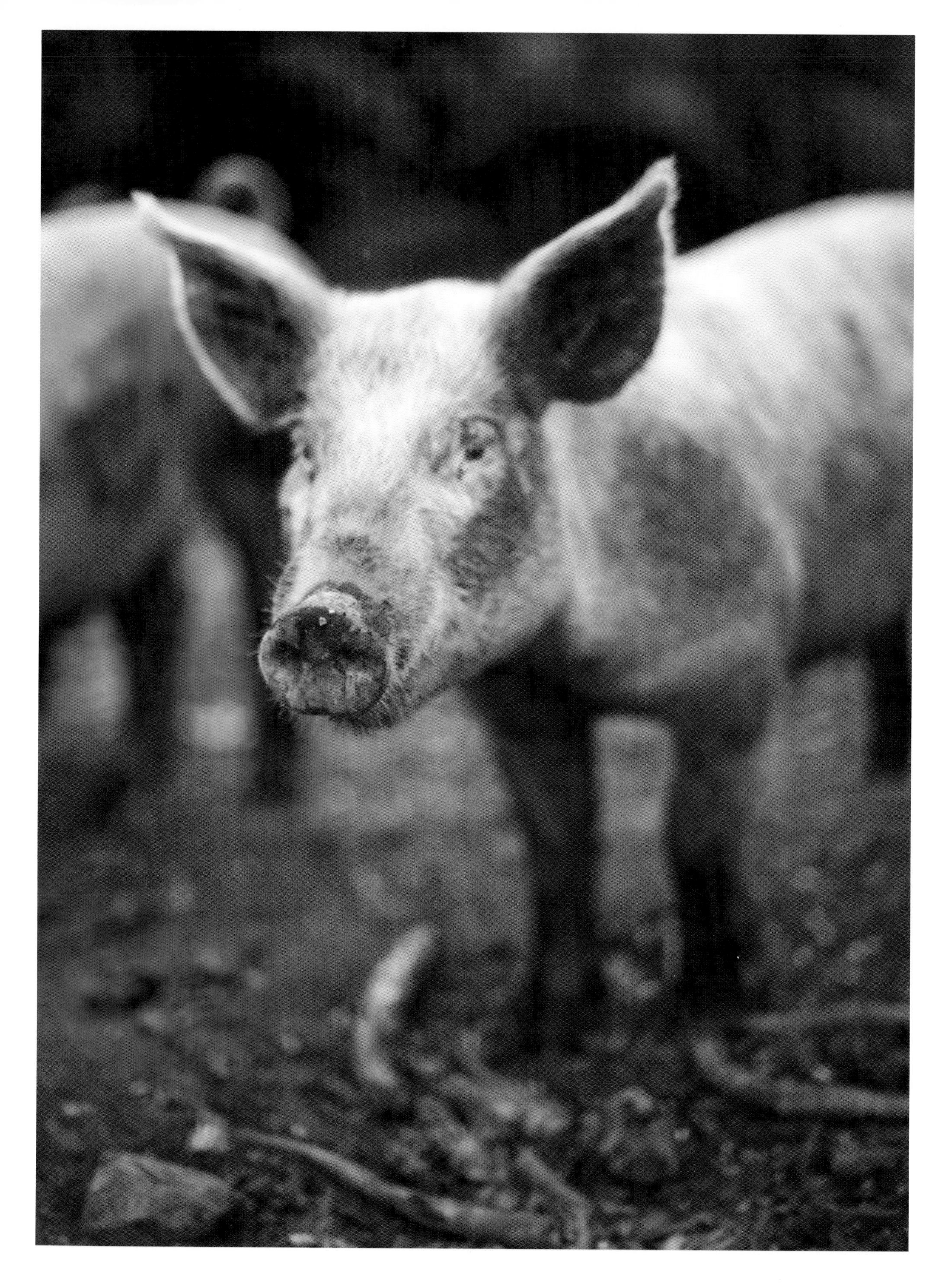

Pigs

If you have the space, enjoy amazing relationships with your neighbors, and live in a town that does not prohibit raising swine, consider adding some pigs to your homestead. They are incredibly efficient at converting kitchen scraps, garden waste, and grain into delicious bacon, ham, and pork—one or two pigs will yield hundreds of pounds of pork. That's a lot of bang for your buck. Our family consumes about two pigs per year, and the cost of raising these pigs is minimal compared to the return. In about six months they're ready to slaughter and you see a great return on your investment, and the labor only amounts to about fifteen minutes per day.

History

Pigs were domesticated in central Asia about 10,000 years ago. They've always been a good way to translate scraps and waste into tasty meat. In fact, in several cultures, "privy pigs" mostly consumed human excrement, and before sewage systems were in place, many cities used pigs for sanitation—gross but efficient, and it kept pork cheap and plentiful.

During colonial times in America, domesticated pigs freely roamed the woods foraging for food and were rounded up and slaughtered in the fall. According to New England lore, early settlers often left pigs to fend for themselves on small islands and then plucked them off to slaughter as needed. If you live in coastal New England, have you ever noticed how many islands are named "Hog"?

Today in America, pork is not as popular as beef or chicken, primarily because of the misplaced fear of fat and of *Trichinella spiralis,* the parasite that causes trichinosis, which has largely been eradicated in our meat supply. In modern pork production, pigs are injected with growth hormones, eat only grain, and spend their days in cramped, industrial-scale barns with no access to sunlight. It's a profitable industry, however: Pigs are prolific, giving birth to an average of ten piglets after a gestation period of only 4 months, and in the first six months of life, they can increase in weight by 5,000 percent. Plus, pigs thrive on a variety of cheap food. It all adds up to a high return for pork producers.

The variety of breeds of pigs has suffered from the trend toward a few commercial breeds (for more on this trend, see page 23). In the 1930 USDA Yearbook of Agriculture, there were more than fifteen breeds of pigs. Today, more than half have disappeared.

PIGS FAQs

ARE PIGS SMART?

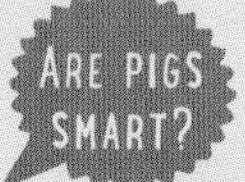

Pigs are generally considered the smartest of all farm animals. Some people even think pigs are as smart as dogs.

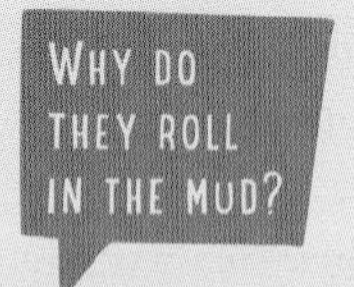

Pigs roll in the mud to cool their body and protect themselves from sunburn. Mud also works as an insect repellent.

DO THEY MAKE GOOD PETS?

Remember the big pot-bellied pig fad of the 1990s? That craze did not end well for all those pigs, many of which ended up abandoned when they grew larger than their owners expected. While pigs are smart and social and can be housebroken, they are not as socially accepted as cats and dogs, and they can get very large.

HOW MUCH BACON CAN YOU GET FROM ONE PIG?

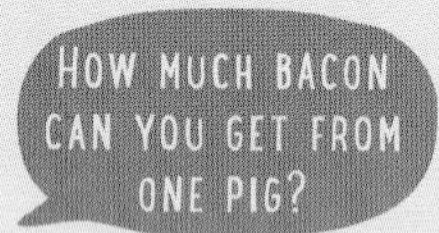

On average, a market-size hog yields about 10 pounds of bacon. Some breeds, such as the Tamworth and Large Black, have been bred especially for great bacon, so if that's a priority for you, go with one of these.

DO PIGS SMELL?

Pigs do not have much of an odor, but their droppings do. The more room you give your pigs, the less odor will develop. There are also some very well-designed pigpens that use the Korean natural farming method, which involves indigenous microorganisms, to almost completely eliminate pig odor.

CAN PIGS GET SUNBURNED?

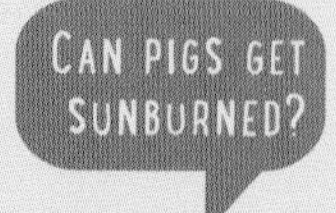

Yes, this is why pigs need to have shade and mud to protect their skin.

ARE PIGS NOISY?

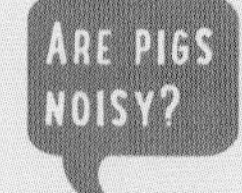

No, pigs are one of the quietest farm animals. They can get vocal when stressed, though.

DO PIGS BITE?

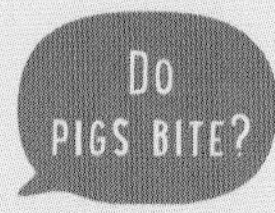

Pigs have a very powerful bite. Be careful with children and whenever you're in a pen with pigs, especially with larger pigs. We have found the bigger they are, the hungrier they are.

CAN YOU RAISE A PIG BY ITSELF OR DO YOU NEED MORE THAN ONE?

Pigs are playful, social animals, so raise at least two pigs at a time. They all need another pig to play with.

HOW LONG DOES IT TAKE TO RAISE A PIG TO SLAUGHTER?

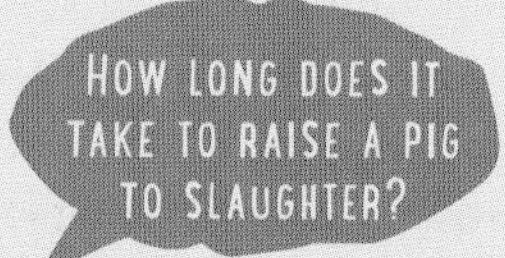

From weaning to slaughter, it takes about 5 months, depending on nutrition and breed. The pig should weigh about 250 pounds at 5 months old and will yield about 175 pounds of usable cuts.

WHAT DO I FEED A PIG?

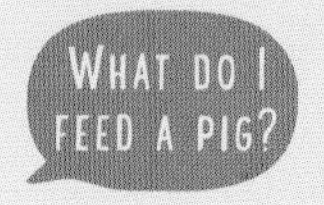

Pigs are omnivores. Their favorite foods are corn, cooked grains, fruits, and vegetables.

Behavior

Pigs are very social animals and have a herding instinct, not unlike sheep. They enjoy being in close proximity to each other at all times. When sleeping, they often form a "pig pile"for warmth and comfort. They're playful, too; I've often watched pigs playing some game whose rules I never quite figured out. Pigs are also curious, and their curiosity goes beyond the search for food. Whenever I need to check fencing or fix something in their yard, the pigs escort me and watch everything I do. I think they're trying to figure out the rules to the game I'm playing.

Despite their reputation, pigs are very clean animals. They devote one area of their yard for their bathroom, unlike all other farm animals, which go wherever they happen to be. It's nice to not have to muck out the entire pen.

Nutrition

Pork fat from pastured pigs is rich in omega-3 fatty acids and vitamins D and E. Pork is also a good source of potassium and a very good source of thiamin, niacin, vitamin B6, phosphorus, and selenium. On top of all this, it tastes fantastic! Pork is a winner with our family, for sure.

Although there's been some concern about nitrates in ham and bacon, there isn't really any good science supporting that fear. In the body, nitrates are converted to nitrite, which is reduced to nitric oxide, a potent vasodilator that's responsible for the blood pressure–lowering effects of vegetables. Yes, bacon does have more sodium than uncured pork products, but if you're consuming a Paleo diet and avoiding processed foods, the additional sodium isn't really enough to worry about.

Selecting a Breed and Purchasing

While raising purebred heritage breeds can be rewarding, I prefer pigs that are crosses of two different breeds. Hybrids grow faster and are healthier, and on our farm, we make choices based on health above all else. My favorites pig crosses are Berkshire/Hampshires, Yorkshire/Berkshires, and anything crossed with a Tamworth.

Whatever breed you select, if you buy a male, make sure that he has been castrated. I have raised intact boars, and they tend to be more aggressive. Their pork also seems to have a slightly stronger flavor, and while I personally liked it, most people are accustomed to pork that has a very mild flavor.

When selecting your piglets, insist on seeing their parents. Make sure the parents are healthy and strong. Look for bright eyes, a curly tail, perky ears, and large hams (think bubble butt). And avoid any runts; you want your pigs to grow large.

Housing and Fencing

There's no need to invest big bucks into your pigsty. After all, it's a pigsty! A thrown-together "A" frame, an old shed, and even a tarp tied to some trees are all suitable houses for pigs. They just need protection from the hot sun, rain, and snow. Make sure your pig yard also has sunny spots; pigs like to bask in the sun, especially on chilly days in the spring and fall.

They do need very strong fences, though. Pigs are rooting animals. They view the world through their nose, and when they're not sleeping or eating, they are digging. Over the course of a season, one pig can tear up an acre of ground. For this reason, your fencing must be extremely strong.

For backyard pigs, I recommend using 6-foot-long, heavy-gauge T posts pounded 18 inches into the ground and hog panels, which are made from thick metal with strong welds. They come in 16-foot-long panels and are easy for two people to install. Place posts every 8 feet to ensure the fence doesn't get bulldozed over. This will give you a secure fenced-in area that pigs will have a hard time escaping from.

If you have a lot of space, you could use our method of electric fencing. After a few years of piglets escaping from an electric fence enclosure, we found that it works best to first place them in a small fenced-in yard and gradually expose them to the electric fence, so they learn to avoid it.

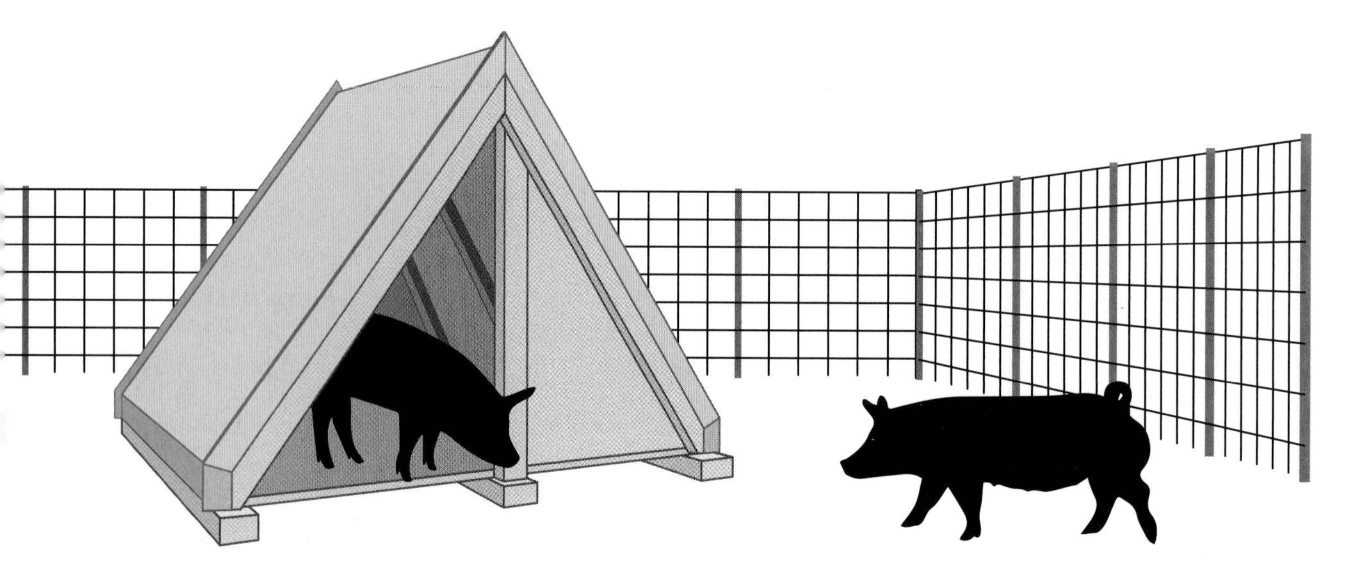

An "A" frame shelter for pigs and a hog panel

After purchasing the piglets, I place them in a small, 16-by-16-foot yard created by setting up four hog panels in a square and surrounding them with electric netting. As the pigs get comfortable in their new home, I expose a small opening in the panels so the pigs will be introduced to the electric netting.

Over the course of a few days, I increase the amount of electric fencing the pigs are exposed to. After hitting the fence just a few times, the piglets learn to stay away from it. But I do not recommend this system if you have neighbors nearby. While pigs have escaped through our fencing occasionally, we have enough space on our farm that they did not damage anyone else's property. If you live close to neighbors, I recommend that you use a permanent fence, as described above.

If you want to go with electric fencing, I recommend the following equipment:

- Strong charger, such as the Intelishock 52B, which runs about $500
- Multiple grounding rods
- Three lines of ½-inch heavy-duty poly tape —it's more portable and easier to use than wire, and it's more visible to the pigs

It's always important to inspect the fences daily to make sure they're strong and intact, but it's especially important if you're using electric fencing.

Space Requirements

In nature, pigs are forest-dwelling animals that live in large extended families, and they need to range far to forage for enough calories. At our farm I like to give pigs a lot of space to mimic, as much as possible, their natural environment. The more space pigs have, the more they can forage for food and the healthier they will be—and for you, more space means less odor. I typically provide between 6,000 and 20,000 square feet per pig. To a conventional farmer raising pigs with only 40 square feet per pig, that probably sounds ridiculous, but I think it's important to create an environment as close as possible to their natural habitat, and when you think about it, 6,000 square feet really isn't that much space—just an eighth of an acre per pig.

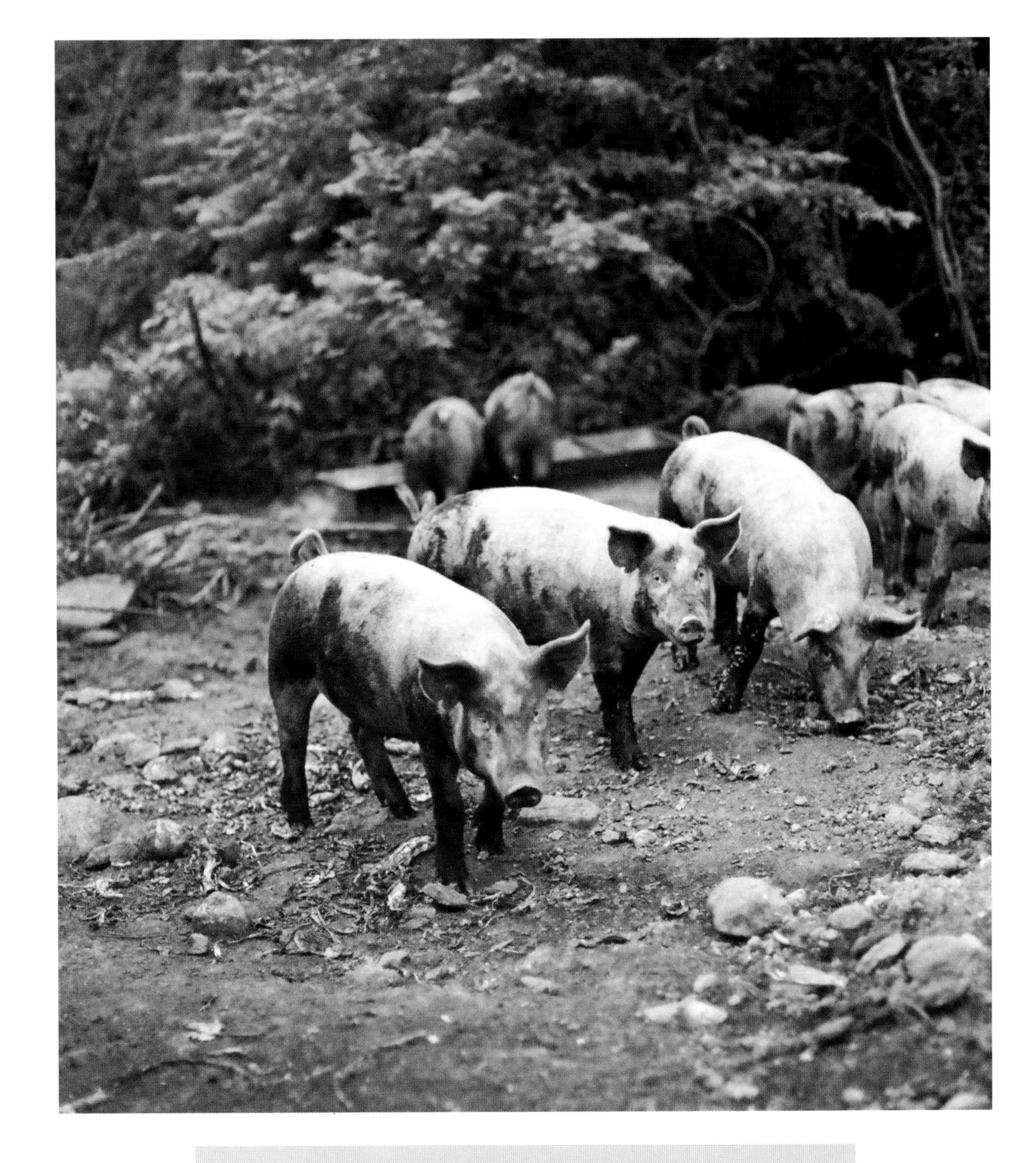

CARING FOR YOUR PIGS

Daily (15 minutes)	**Weekly** (30 minutes)
Check fencing. Feed and make sure they have clean water.	Thoroughly clean troughs with a stiff wire brush and a strong spraying hose.

Food and Water

Pigs are omnivores. Most farmers raise pigs primarily on a fortified grain ration supplemented with kitchen scraps, and those I know who decided not to feed their pigs grain have not had great results: their pigs were generally too thin and sometimes sickly. That being said, pigs would much rather eat vegetables, fruits, nuts, breads and wild edibles—they'll only eat grain when there is nothing else to eat. At our farm, I bring the pigs kitchen scraps, slightly too-old vegetables, and weeds. If you find a restaurant chef who is willing to barter their scraps in exchange for pork, try to make a deal. You can realize enormous savings if the pigs are getting enough scraps. Just make sure there is no garbage accidentally thrown in with outside scraps. One year I lost a pig to an intestinal obstruction that turned out to be a bunch of twist ties.

Pigs require lots of water to stay healthy. For the backyard homesteader, I suggest a 25-gallon water trough; each pig needs about 5 gallons per day. There are many great automatic waterers on the market that ensure the pigs have adequate water and keep water troughs clean longer, which is no small benefit. Keeping the water trough clean can be time-consuming—I rinse it once or twice a day, every day. An open water trough is a poor option for pigs unless you can check on it frequently throughout the day, because as temperatures climb, pigs like to climb into their water trough and go for a swim. Nice for the pigs, but not a good way to provide clean water.

Health

As a general rule, we've found pigs to be very hearty animals, requiring little medical attention compared to sheep. As with any animal, check pigs' poop to see if it's well formed, and keep an eye on their skin for any sign of disease. Good hygiene can help prevent gut infections, such as enteritis and diarrhea (scour), and parasites, such as lice and mange. If you suddenly notice raised, diamond-shaped patches on their skin, it's likely erysipelas, a bacterial infection: contact your vet immediately.

Processing

We process our pigs at about seven months old, and like all large animals that we sell, they need to go to a slaughterhouse rather than be processed on site like chickens and rabbits. (See page 75 for more about slaughterhouses.)

To get the pigs to go on the trailer to the slaughterhouse, it's best to park it right in their fenced-in area for about week and feed them in the trailer, so they get used to it. This will make their transport to the slaughterhouse much less stressful for them. The morning you're ready to go, feed them in the trailer, then close the doors and drive away.

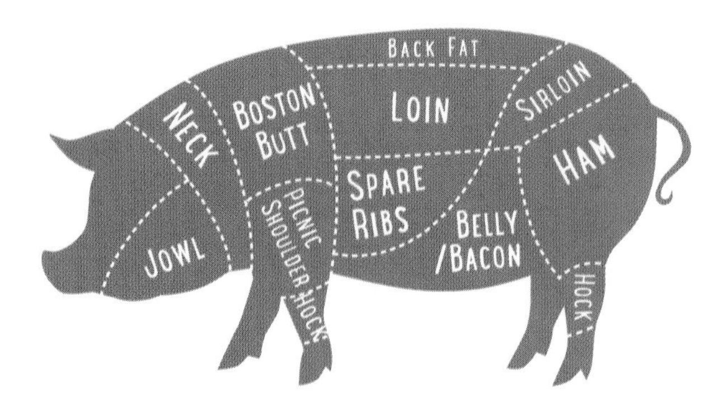

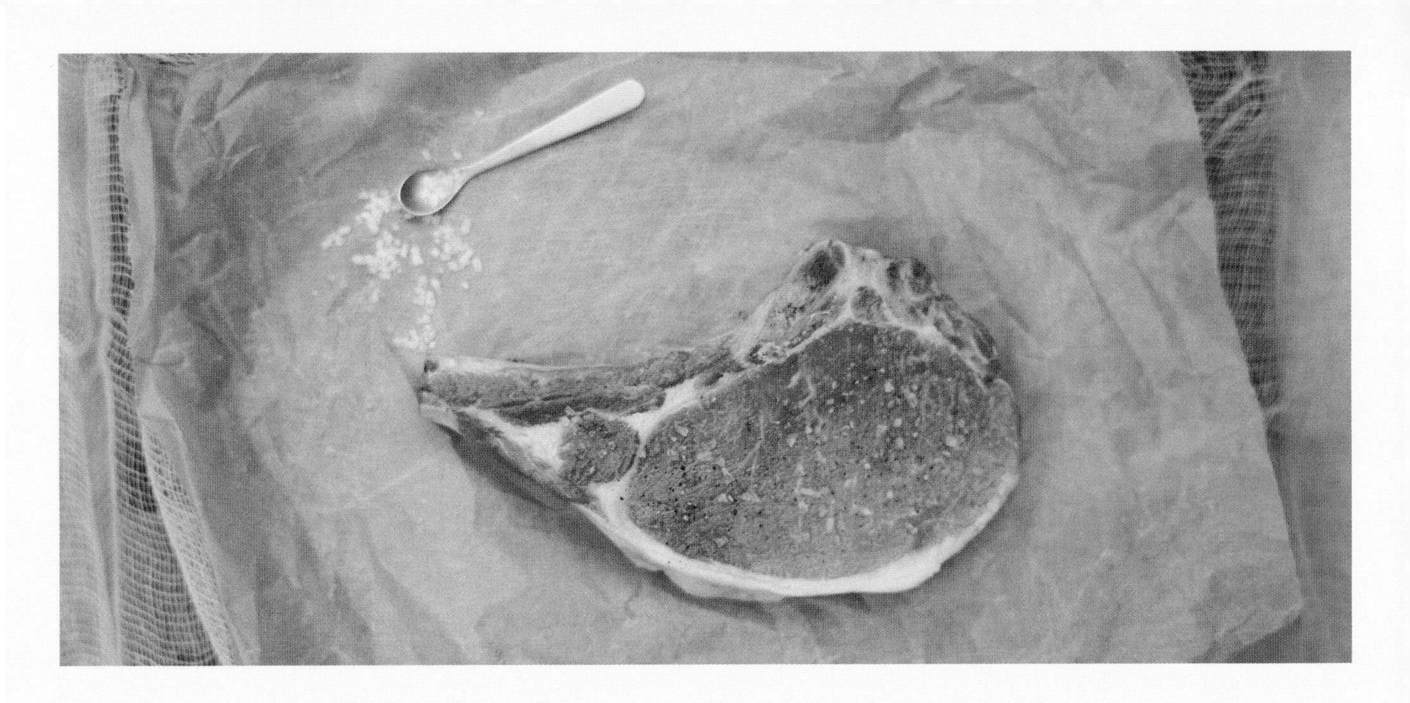

DEALING WITH A SLAUGHTERHOUSE

For the small-scale homesteader, it's usually easiest to process rabbits and poultry at home, but for all other animals, we recommend using a slaughterhouse.

Finding a Slaughterhouse

Although many people use the terms "slaughterhouse" and "butcher" interchangeably, they're not the same. A slaughterhouse kills the animal. A butcher cuts the carcass into pieces of meat. Most small-scale slaughterhouses have butchers who do their work at the end of the slaughtering process, but there are also stand-alone butchers who break down whole or partial pieces of animals for customers.

If you're planning to sell your meat, many states have an inspection program that allows you to sell state-inspected meat within state lines. However, if you plan on selling meat across state lines, you must use a USDA-certified slaughterhouse. If you won't be selling your meat, you can have a butcher custom-cut your animal without inspection, and they will mark it"not for sale."

If possible, try to find a slaughterhouse that uses humane techniques. Ask about their practices or view an actual slaughter (if they'll let you) before you commit to taking your animals there. The Animal Welfare Approved program (animalwelfareapproved.org) provides labels for meat and dairy products that meet certain criteria for humane treatment of animals, including humane slaughter. While other certification organizations, such as Certified Humane, may have slightly different standards, in general humane slaughter techniques include the following:

- Flooring must have good traction to prevent cattle from falling or slipping.
- Animals must be handled in a calm manner, with as little loud noise as possible.
- Animals must not be abused or maltreated.
- Clean water must be provided in the holding pen.
- Animals from different farms or transport groups must not be mixed in holding pens.
- Stunning must render animals immediately insensible to pain on the first attempt.

What to Expect in Return for Your Live Animals

Keep in mind that when you get your animal back, it will not be the same size as when you dropped it off. The hanging weight ("hangwt") is the weight of the animal on the rail, without the head, hooves, organs, or hide. Once the animal is butchered and more of the bones are removed to create steaks and other cuts, the weight of the meat you get back will be even lower. For pigs and lamb, you should expect to get about 70 percent of the hanging weight, and for cows you will get about 60 to 65 percent. If your cutting instructions include lots of bone-in cuts, your yield will be higher, and a skilled butcher can add about 5 percent to the yield. Keep in mind that you'll get about 30 to 40 percent of your cow in ground beef, depending on how you cut it—there is not very much tenderloin!

Animal	Live weight	Hanging weight	Finished cuts
Beef	1100–1200 lbs	550–650 lbs	350–400 lbs
Pork	300–350 lbs	175–225 lbs	110–150 lbs
Lamb/Goat	70–100 lbs	40–75 lbs	30–50 lbs

For all that meat, you may need a separate freezer. A whole lamb will fit into a standard-sized freezer above a refrigerator, but not much else will fit in there with it. Pork and beef require a separate chest freezer. The meat from two whole pigs or one cow will fit in a 20-cubic-foot chest freezer.

Before Processing Day

Be sure you schedule your processing date well in advance—I typically schedule my fall slaughter dates in early spring. Some slaughterhouses have a list of "haulers" you can hire to bring your animals to the slaughterhouse. Hiring an experienced hauler can mean less stress on the animals and on you.

If you're transporting your animals yourself, it's best to move them in a horse trailer, so if you don't have one, borrow one from a friend. Park the trailer in the yard for about a week before the processing date and allow your animals to explore it. Move their water, hay, and grain (if you offer grain) into the trailer so they will be more comfortable inside it. It may take a few days for them to even step onto it, but giving them time to acclimate to the trailer will make the animals much less stressed on processing day.

As the processing day approaches, there are a few things to think about:

- **The types of cuts you want:** Most slaughterhouses provide a "cut sheet," a menu of all the different cuts they offer. Keep in mind that choosing one cut may mean that you can't get another cut.
- **If you want the lard or organ meats from your animal:** If you do, make sure you request them specifically. Most places we've worked with don't include them unless you ask.
- **If you would like the meat vacuum-sealed or wrapped in wax paper:** I personally prefer vacuum-sealed because our farm's customers like to see the cuts rather than buy a mystery package of paper-wrapped meat. It's also quicker to thaw meat that is vacuum-sealed, and it's less likely to dry out. It does cost a little more than paper-wrapped meat, but it's worth it.
- **How many pounds of meat you should be getting back:** Do the math before you head to the slaughterhouse so you'll know what to expect. See the chart above for guidelines on how much meat you'll get from your animals.

If there's anything you're unsure about or that is unclear, don't be afraid to ask questions at the slaughterhouse! Once the animal is cut up, there's no putting it back together.

On Processing Day

The morning of your drop-off date with the slaughterhouse, feed the animals only a very small amount in order to lure them onto the trailer, and then shut the door. Don't fill them up with a "last meal." When the animals have fasted, there is less material in their intestines, which makes the slaughtering process cleaner and helps prevent fecal matter from getting on the carcass and contaminating the meat. Animals are also often more relaxed in a fasted state.

Getting the animals into the trailer isn't always as easy as it sounds, and you may want to have another set of hands helping to encourage them. If you kept the trailer in the field and fed the animals there during the week before, they'll be accustomed to it and it will be easier to get them inside. The slaughterhouse usually wants you there early in the morning, so plan on being organized for an early arrival.

Going to a slaughterhouse can be overwhelming. We've found that basic customer service and normal pleasantries are often forgotten in the culture of the slaughterhouse, but knowing what to expect can make it easier. Every slaughterhouse is a little different, but in general, here's what happens when you drop your animals off at a small-scale, certified-humane, USDA-approved operation:

1. When you arrive at the slaughterhouse, you're greeted by the employees, who tell you where to back up your trailer. Your animals are placed either in a short-term holding area, to be processed right away, or in a barn, to be processed within a few days. If this is your first time sending animals to processing, mentally prepare yourself for the separation, especially if you have an emotional bond with them.
2. Some slaughterhouses allow farmers to watch the slaughtering process. It can be difficult, but I believe that observing the slaughter is an important part of fully understanding and appreciating the entire process.
3. When the staff are ready, the animals are led in a line toward the kill floor. One at a time, they are led into a special chute, separated from the other animals by a door so those behind can not see what is happening. Once in the chute, each animal is shot in the head with a stun gun, which is called "knocking" and renders them unconscious. Quickly after, the animal's throat is slit, and it's hung upside down to bleed out. When done correctly, this process is fast and causes as little stress to the animal as possible.
4. After it's bled out, the animal is skinned and the internal organs are removed.
5. The animal carcass is then inspected by an official and moved into a cooler to wait to be butchered.
6. The butchers break down the animal carcass into the specified cuts, which are usually quickly frozen and boxed for you to pick up, though some slaughterhouses provide you with fresh, not frozen, meat.

After Processing

It usually takes a couple weeks before you get the call to pick up your frozen, unsmoked meats from the slaughterhouse. If you want smoked pork, it can take quite a bit longer. However, I'd advise against getting smoked meats from most slaughterhouses. It's often a liquid chemical smoke, not a wood-based smoke, and I've found that they generally don't taste good. Do some research and find a traditional smokehouse instead. It costs more, you might have to travel a bit to get to the smokehouse, and you get less meat back because real smoking removes water from the meat, but amazing ham and bacon are worth it.

Small slaughterhouses that deal primarily with family farmers can often dry-age grass-fed beef, pastured pork, and lamb for you, allowing it to hang for at least ten days. This process allows the muscles to relax and enzymes to begin to break down the meat, resulting in tenderization. There is also a slight loss of moisture, which decreases your effective yield but concentrates the flavor.

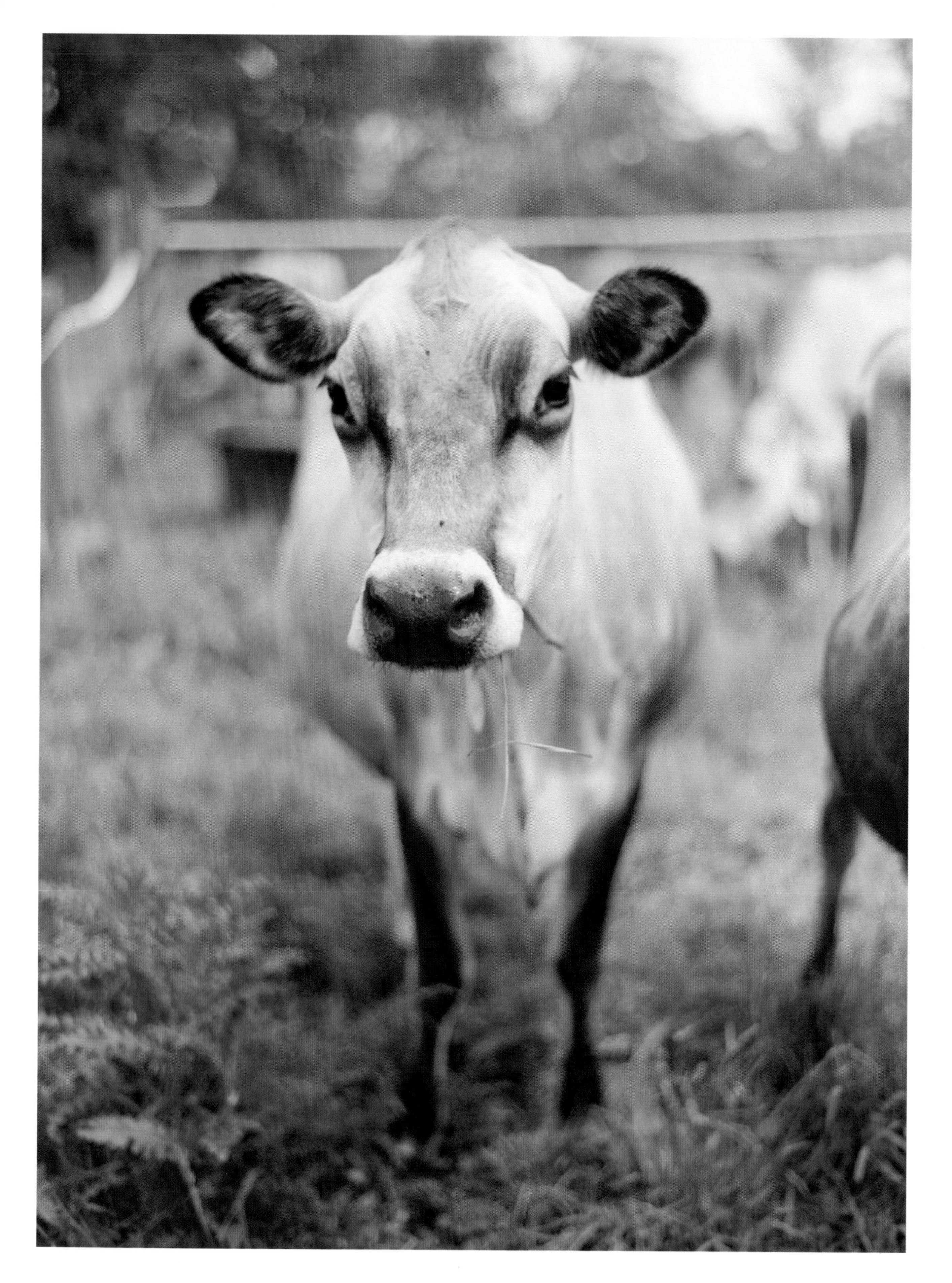

The Family Cow

If you want a great lawnmower in addition to some delicious milk and/or meat, a cow could be an excellent addition to your homestead. Even if you don't have a lot of pasture space, there are some fantastic miniature breeds out there that can graze marginal land that is too poor for crops.

History

Cattle have been domesticated for less than 10,000 years, compared to about 12,000 years for sheep and goats. But they've been one of the most valuable animals for humans because of the many benefits they provide: milk, meat, hides, dung (for fertilizer and fuel), and draft power. (Although, interestingly, cow milk wasn't an important component of the European diet until the 1600s, making it one of the latest animal products to be used by humans.) In fact, the term "livestock" literally means "living wealth," an indication of just how prized the animals were in centuries past.

In addition to the products they provide, the labor of cattle made them invaluable. It is thought that cows made it possible for humans to settle new lands throughout history by carrying heavy weights over mountain passes and providing fresh food along the way. During the colonial era in America, dairy cows often worked the land for four or five hours, then were parked in the barn, milked for the dinner table, and refueled for the next day's work, all while producing just as much milk as if they'd stayed in the barn all day. Oxen were valuable for logging because they were more patient and less skittish than horses.

Cows even played a key role in the invention of the smallpox vaccine. In the late 1700s, English physician and scientist Edward Jenner noticed that milkmaids were immune to smallpox, which he suspected was because they'd been exposed to cowpox, a similar but milder version of the disease. He collected the pus from milkmaids' cowpox lesions and used it to develop a successful smallpox vaccine.

Behavior

Cows can be domineering, loving, mischievous, and friendly (sometimes overly so). They like to be part of a herd and will stick together—when one gets a drink, they all do—but they do all right on their own, too. Like other farm animals, cows sometimes have a pecking order. You may have read that certain breeds are more docile than others, but there is generally more difference among individual cows than among breeds. Be sure to buy one with a mild temperament and that has been handled and doesn't tend to kick. Cows will always come to you if you have food, which is the best time to make friends with them.

COWS FAQs

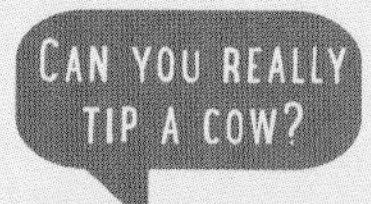

Yes, they sleep standing up and you can tip them over. But it's not a very nice thing to do.

DO COWS GET MAD WHEN THEY SEE THE COLOR RED?

No. However, it's no joke that bulls can be aggressive if provoked. I don't recommend keeping a bull on a homestead farm.

HOW MUCH LAND DO I NEED PER COW?

It depends on the cow's purpose. A milking cow with a calf needs more room than a steer that you intend to butcher. A miniature breed needs less space than a standard-sized cow. Some farmers keep one cow per acre. Others raise one or two standard-sized cows on five acres, or eight to ten miniature cows on the same piece of land. If your land doesn't have great pasture, though, you may need much more space per cow.

CAN ALL COWS PRODUCE MILK?

Yes, any breed can produce milk, though some produce more milk than others. Cows need to have a calf before they can produce milk. I wouldn't suggest milking a bull.

HOW MUCH WATER DOES A COW NEED WHEN PRODUCING MILK?

To make one gallon of milk, a cow needs to drink 2 gallons of water.

HOW MUCH MILK DOES A COW PRODUCE?

A dairy cow can produce upwards of about 6 gallons a day, though most family cows produce about 3 gallons per day.

HOW OFTEN DO YOU NEED TO MILK A COW?

Cows need to be milked twice a day, every twelve hours. However, if you are keeping the calf with the cow, milk her just once a day.

DO COWS HAVE FOUR STOMACHS?

Not exactly. Cows have just one stomach with four chambers: the rumen, reticulum, omasum, and abomasum. The four chambers allow cows to consume tough plant matter that would otherwise be indigestible.

RAW MILK

The consumption of raw milk—milk that hasn't been pasteurized or homogenized—is something of a controversial topic today. When cows were kept on small farms and their milk used by people on the farm, there was very little risk of illness from fresh milk, provided it was consumed quickly. Butter and cheese were generally safer because they were more easily stored and transported. Today, though, fewer of us live on farms and dairy cows are not as healthy as they once were, and milk from industrial-scale dairy farms must be pasteurized to be safe to drink.

I do believe that raw milk from small, organic, pasture-based farms, consumed in moderation, can be beneficial for those who tolerate it, since it retains the vitamins and minerals that are lost during pasteurization. However, I've also seen heavy milk consumption impede weight loss, aggravate autoimmune conditions, and cause acne. Milk is great at putting weight on young mammals. That's what it's for. So, for kids, milk can be a fantastic food in moderation. For adults not looking to put on more pounds, it's not so great. (For more on milk and its nutrients, please see page 18.)

If you are interested in drinking raw milk, I suggest you do your research well. Don't assume that raw milk from the dairy up the street is safe to drink just because the cows there look happy. I only consume raw milk products from a trusted source, and I make sure that bacteria levels are monitored, the herd is small and on pasture, and only one person milks the cows, to minimize unsafe handling practices. If you're planning to drink raw milk from your own cow, you need to be sure to use extremely clean methods, and the cow should be on grass, not grain. If the cow looks sick, don't drink her milk.

Nutrition

Grass-fed beef is higher in anti-inflammatory omega-3s than feedlot beef. It's important to clarify that there is a difference between grass-fed and grass-finished cows. Be sure the meat you're buying was not finished on grains, which can dramatically affect the fatty acid profile of the meat. A producer may claim that grain-finishing improves the flavor, due to the marbling of the meat. While it is true that grass-finished beef has a different flavor than grain-finished beef, it's also much healthier for you. Beef from grass-fed cows is also good source of protein, vitamin B12, and phosphorus, and a very good source of niacin, vitamin B6, zinc, and selenium. Grass-fed beef and milk also contains more conjugated linoleic acid (CLA), which helps support healthy cell structure and has been shown to reduce risk for cancer. Grass-fed beef is lower in total fat and calories than grain-fed.

In addition, because cows are such large animals and grazing requires minimal input from the farmer, grass-fed beef is an excellent choice for environmental sustainability.

Selecting a Breed and Purchasing

With hobby farmers on the rise, smaller versions of standard breeds, such as a miniature Jersey or lowline Angus, are becoming more and more common. You can even find miniature Texas Longhorns. For smaller farms and homesteads, we like Dexters, a small, dual-purpose breed that's generally mild-tempered and thrives on average pasture. Jersey and Guernsey cows are excellent dairy cows: they produce milk much higher in butterfat than other breeds, which really makes a difference in nutritional value and taste. But don't discount the value of a crossbreed cow. The benefits of hybrid vigor can make one a fantastic choice.

When you're ready to purchase a dairy cow, contact local dairies or search Craigslist instead of rushing to a local livestock auction, where you'd be buying a cow from an unknown source. If you're new to raising cows, I suggest that you try to acquire a middle-aged, good-natured, lactating cow, instead of a dairy heifer that needs to be bred. Find out if she's currently pregnant. A pregnant cow isn't necessarily more expensive, and once her calf is weaned, you can sell it to help pay for the upkeep of your cow, or you can keep it and raise it for beef.

Before you purchase your cow, find out important information: Has she been machine- or hand-milked? (If she's only been machine-milked, you'll need to get her accustomed to hand-milking.) Has she had any problems calving? How many times has she calved, and were they all successful births? Is she a good mother? You'll also want to milk her yourself or watch her being milked to ensure you have a friendly cow, and be sure to get proof that she is free of tuberculosis and brucellosis.

COW TERMINOLOGY

Cow
Female over two years old that has given birth

Steer or ox
Castrated male

Heifer
Unbred female under two years old

Bull
Intact male

Housing and Fencing

At the minimum, cows need some sort of shelter from the elements, like a large, open-front shed—although a barn is ideal, especially for harsh winters. For milking, it's best to have a clean area with a concrete floor and running water, but it is also possible to milk a cow right in the middle of a field, though you risk getting more contaminants in the milk.

As with sheep and goats, rotational grazing is key for the health of both cattle and the pasture (see page 61 for more on rotational grazing). The amount of pasture required depends on the quality of the grass, but generally each cow needs about 1 to 2½ acres. Strong electric fencing can be moved easily and works well for rotational grazing. With cattle, make sure the bottom wire is no more than 3½ feet from the ground, though it's best to have a second one about 18 inches from the ground, especially if you have calves. With all our electric fencing, we use a 2 joule 52B battery energizer support box with a 20 watt solar panel and a 12 volt 4 amp solar regulator attached to a 12 volt battery.

Food and Water

It is far more economical to raise a cow on pasture than on grain—not to mention healthier for the cow. (For more on that, see pages 14 and 18.) It also gives you the highest-quality milk. When fresh green grass isn't available, you can supplement with hay. It's also important to supplement a lactating cow with alfalfa hay or have her on a grass-legume pasture, in order to meet her protein requirements and ensure healthy milk production. Cows also love to eat garden scraps, such as cabbage and root vegetables.

You'll need to provide your cows with a salt lick, mineral block, and plenty of clean water. The soil in certain parts of the country is deficient in various minerals. In the Northeast you'll see less cobalt, and then there is the "goiter belt"—the northern Midwest and Great Lakes region, where a lack of iodine in the soil led to thyroid problems before the introduction of iodized salt. A mineral block for cows fills in any gaps in the cow's nutrition. Find out what is a specific concern in your neck of the woods—you can have your soil tested to be sure (see page 107).

Milking Your Cow

You don't have to have a dairy breed to milk your cow, though dairy breeds are generally a bit more inclined to cooperate if you're looking for milk on a regular basis. The average family dairy cow produces 3 gallons of milk a day, depending on the breed.

Most farmers breed their cows yearly in order to keep up their milk production. You can get away with every other year, but the quantity of milk will decline. If your cow goes longer than two years between calves, it's just not worth it to milk her. The quantity of milk will begin to decline around six months after she gives birth, and it's best to allow the cow to go dry for about two months before she is bred again. When you're ready to breed your cow, get a good book that covers it in depth and learn all about it—*The Family Cow*, by Dirk van Loon, is a great resource.

A happy cow is a one that is milked on a regular schedule. A cow with full udders is uncomfortable and wants you to milk her, so pick a milking schedule and stick to it. It's not a good idea to milk a cow at 8 a.m. and 8 p.m. one day, then 5 a.m. and 5 p.m. the next.

A calf needs to drink about half of the milk that the cow produces, so until the calf is weaned, keep it with the cow during the daytime and separate them at night, then milk the cow in the morning before turning them both out on pasture for the day.

Although some cows are calm enough to be milked right out in the pasture, most farmers tether their cows indoors before milking them. Getting the cow to follow you into the barn is much easier if you offer her a bit of grain. Give her a little treat for coming to you, and depending on her temperament, you may not even need to tie her up to milk her.

Before you try milking a cow on your own, you may want to have someone show you how, or look up a how-to video online (one suggestion is in the Resources section on page 398). Take a deep breath; you got this! Here are the basic steps.

You'll need:

- A stool
- A spray bottle filled with warm water and a splash of disinfectant, such as bleach
- A milking bucket

1. Sit down on the stool. Don't place the bucket under the udder just yet.
2. Spray the teats with the mix of water and disinfectant to help prevent mastitis. Leave the disinfectant on the teats for approximately 30 seconds.
3. Take two teats firmly in your hands.
4. Press the teat between your thumb and index finger, then close your fingers on it while gently pulling down. Alternate between your hands.
5. Keep this up and the milk will flow. Allow the first few squirts to fall on the ground just in case your cow has any extra dirt or an infection, so it won't end up in your milk bucket.
6. Wipe off the udders with a towel after the initial stripping squirts.
7. Now position the milking bucket under the udder and begin milking. If your cow doesn't have a calf, work all the teats until the udder is empty. If she does have a calf, stop milking before the udder is completely empty.
8. If your cow doesn't have a calf, spray the disinfectant on the udders once more to prevent mastitis. If she does have a calf, you can skip this step, as the calf will disinfect the udders when it nurses (always spray on the disinfectant before milking, though, even if she has a calf).
9. After milking, bring the milk inside and strain it through a strainer and a few layers of cheesecloth to remove any specks of dirt or hair. Wash the strainer well after you're done.

If you'd like to use just the cream, allow the milk to sit in the fridge for day. The cream rises to the top and is about 22 percent fat. The rest of the milk is less than 1 percent fat. Milk that low in fat is fantastic to feed to your pigs, who will be so excited to have it. With the cream, you can make butter (see page 348) or experiment with simple cheeses. One of the best things I've ever tasted is raw, cultured butter from a grassfed cow. There's just nothing like it. If you notice the flavor of the milk or cream seems a bit off, that can sometimes be caused by weeds or plants with strong flavors, such as garlic, cabbage, and wild onions.

CARING FOR YOUR COW

Daily (30–45 minutes)	**Weekly** (1 hour)	**Monthly** (1 hour)	**Yearly**
Milk the cow and care for the udder. Provide clean water. Check fencing.	Muck out the stall if needed. Set up new fencing and rotate the cow to new pasture.	Monitor the mineral block and salt lick and replace as needed. Check hooves, eyes, and teeth and keep an eye on the cow's overall health.	Breed your cow and wean the calf at between 3 and 8 months old (older is generally better). Process if desired.

Health

A healthy cow has a good appetite and appears bright and alert. Your cow should also have relatively firm manure, not too dry and definitely not watery. If your cow seems anxious, is breathing heavily, lays down a lot, or has a temperature above 102.5°F, it's a sign that something is wrong. (A quick note on taking a cow's temperature: It needs to be done rectally, and it's best to have someone show you how. Be sure to tie a string to the thermometer so you don't lose it!) Any abnormal posture can be a sign that the animal might be in pain. Get yourself a good vet and a book outlining common cow diseases so you know what to look for.

Mastitis

Mastitis is a bacterial infection of one or more teats. It can be caused by a few things:

- When an udder is bumped or bruised, infection can set in.
- If a teat is dirty because the cow lay down in mud or manure, her calf may not nurse from it, allowing the udder to become swollen and full of milk. If she's not milked completely and in good time, the teat can become infected.
- A milker can carry bacteria on his or her hand and infect the teats.

Mastitis can be dangerous and even life-threatening if the infection enters the bloodstream. If you suspect your cow has mastitis, call your vet immediately. The best way to avoid mastitis is to select a cow with average, not high, milk production and to be sure to take care of her udders. Keep them clean and dry, and protect them from frostbite and becoming chapped.

Milk fever

Milk fever is associated mainly with dairy cattle, but it can affect beef cows as well. It is a result of low calcium and occurs when the cow is producing colostrum, the first milk produced right after giving birth, which is high in calcium. Be on the lookout for milk fever right after your cow gives birth. Early symptoms include lack of muscle coordination and twitching. Call your vet right away if you notice these symptoms.

Processing

Most farmers wait until the calf is two years old before they slaughter it, though this depends on the breed and the type of feed it's given (grain-fed animals fatten up much sooner). On an industrial-scale dairy farm, cows often only live for about four or five years, but a happy family cow can make it to twenty.

As with sheep, goats, and pigs, it's best to take your cow to a slaughterhouse to be processed (see page 75 for more on slaughterhouses). It may be worthwhile to take a class in butchering, though, just so that you are familiar with the cuts of beef.

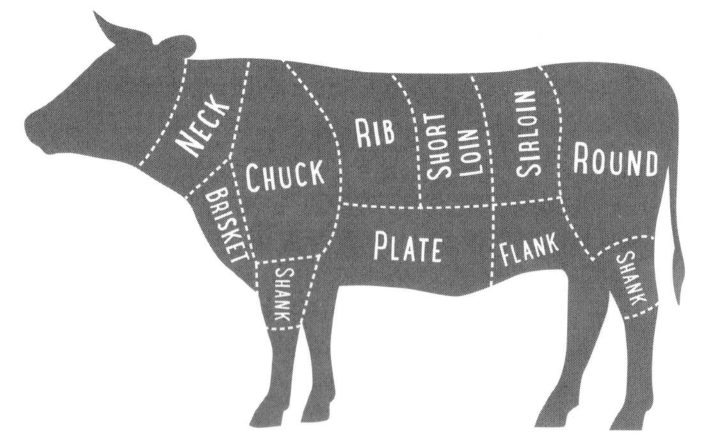

SUSTAINABLE SEAFOOD

ALTHOUGH FEW HOMESTEADERS FARM THEIR OWN FISH, IT'S IMPORTANT TO KEEP SUSTAINABLE SEAFOOD PRACTICES IN MIND WHEN WE SHOP, AND TO THAT END, IT'S HELPFUL TO HAVE A GENERAL UNDERSTANDING OF THE SEAFOOD INDUSTRY. HOWEVER, IF YOU LIVE IN A COASTAL AREA OR NEAR A CLEAN RIVER OR LAKE, PLEASE CONSIDER LEARNING HOW TO FISH FOR YOURSELF, OR GET OUT THERE AND COLLECT SHELLFISH (WITH A PROPER LICENSE, OF COURSE). FISHING AND GATHERING CLAMS AND MUSSELS IS ESPECIALLY FUN TO DO WITH KIDS, SO IT CAN BE A FAMILY OUTING INSTEAD OF A CHORE.

Wild Fish

The commercial fishing industry has had a devastating impact on our oceans. Overfishing is depleting them, and it doesn't affect just the species that are overfished; it also has serious effects up and down the food chain. In addition, the fishing of certain species leads to a phenomenon called "bycatch," in which another species, like turtles, is caught and often dies during the pursuit of the marketable fish. Making it worse is the fact that there are few property rights in the ocean, which makes it vulnerable to exploitation. And many countries actually subsidize unprofitable fishing fleets, which encourages overfishing.

Although there are still some species of fish that are relatively sustainable to consume, the Food and Aquaculture Organization (FAO), which monitors 600 marine fish stocks worldwide, estimates that nearly 30 percent of all fish stocks are being overfished. We need to choose species of wild fish that have healthy ocean populations and that are sustainably fished. Helpful guides are available online (see page 86).

Farmed Fish

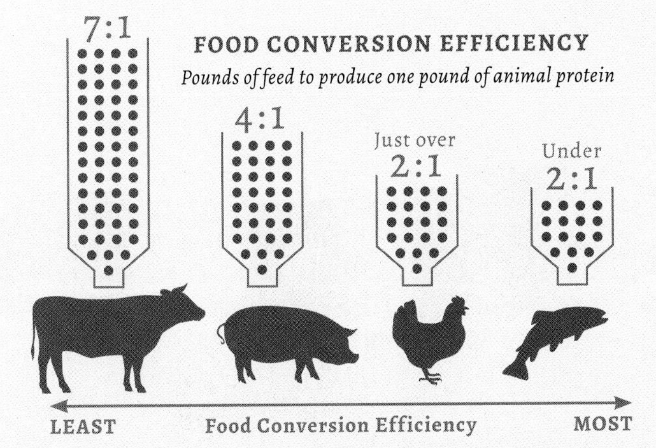

Source: http://www.earth-policy.org/books/pb2/pb2ch9_ss4

Note: *This information applies to conventionally raised animals, not pastured animals, which have different food conversion ratios.*

When it comes to converting animal feed to protein, fish are incredibly efficient, especially compared to conventionally raised meat. The chart at left shows food conversion rates for conventionally raised animals and farmed fish, all of which are fed grain. Hands down, fish need the least amount of grain to create protein. That alone makes farmed fish a better choice than conventionally raised meat. There are some concerns about farmed fish, however:

- Farmed fish can get loose and interbreed with wild fish, weakening the species and spreading disease.
- When non-native species escape offshore fish farms, they can overtake wild species of fish and cause problems in the local ecosystem.

- Farming carnivorous fish is unsustainable and highly inefficient. It means either raising other fish on grain first or catching and grinding up wild fish—so it requires many more resources to get a single pound of fish to the table.
- Farmed fish may contain higher amounts of toxins than wild fish.
- Even though they do eat less grain for each pound of animal protein they create, farmed fish are still fed grain, and it's usually GMO grain, which isn't good for the environment, the fish, or our health.
- Although there are some small-scale, sustainable fish farms, most are large, industrial operations, and putting huge groups of animals in a confined space is not only stressful and unnatural for the animals, it's also bad for the environment because of the concentrated amounts of waste produced by these operations.

WORLD FARMED FISH AND BEEF PRODUCTION, 1950–2012

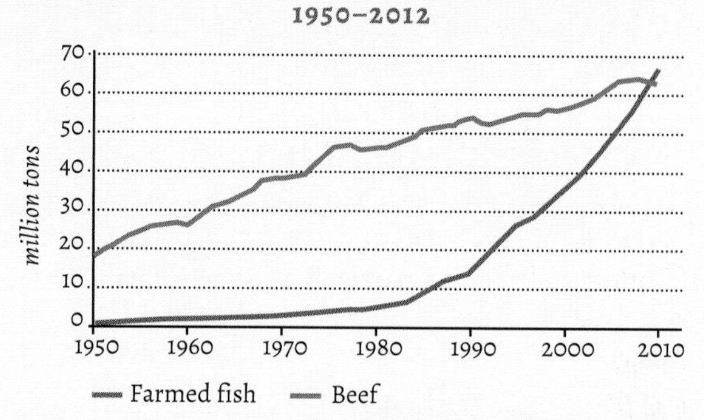

Source: Earth Policy Institute (www.earth-policy.org)

Despite these concerns, the aquaculture industry is growing at an unprecedented rate. More farmed fish is now being raised than beef. And with many species of wild fish in peril from overfishing, sometimes farmed fish is a better choice. We just need to make sure we buy fish that is farmed as responsibly and sustainably as possible.

Choosing Which Fish and Shellfish to Buy

One easy way to support sustainability is to try a "trash fish"—one that's local to your region, so it doesn't travel far, and is of little value in today's fish market. Despite the name, trash fish doesn't have to taste bad or be unhealthy. Lobster, for example, used to be considered trash fish in New England. Sometimes a fish is considered a trash fish in one location but not elsewhere—carp is a trash fish in the U.S. but is highly desirable in Asia. Broaden your horizons beyond salmon and tuna.

All the labels and verifications found on seafood in the grocery store can be confusing; sometimes they even seem to contradict each other. Fortunately, several guides can make choosing which fish to buy much easier.

Seafood Watch from the Monterey Bay Aquarium: The Monterey Bay Aquarium's Seafood Watch website (seafoodwatch.org) and mobile app provide three lists of seafood: those that are sustainable and ideal for purchasing, those that are okay to buy but have some sustainability issues, and those that should be avoided because they're caught or farmed in damaging, unsustainable ways. The lists are updated monthly and take into account where you live and the most recent data available on wild fish as well as fish farms. Seafood Watch also supplies a "Super Green" list of seafood that's particularly healthy for humans, with high levels of omega-3s and low levels of mercury, as well as sustainable.

Seafood Decision Guide from National Geographic: National Geographic's Seafood Decision Guide (nationalgeographic.com/foodfeatures/seafood-decision-guide/) is an interactive tool that helps you decide what fish and shellfish is best for your needs. It takes into account sustainability, omega-3 levels, mercury content, and whether the fish is good for heart health and pregnant women.

Seafood Selector from the Environmental Defense Fund: The EDF's Seafood Selector website (seafood.edf.org) rates fish choices according to how their fishing or farming methods affect the environment. It also allows you to search for fish that's both sustainable and particularly healthy, and a separate list provides the best choices for sushi.

Based on all of these guides, the smartest choices for wild fish and shellfish from the United States at the time of printing are listed below. (You can find up-to-date lists online at the websites discussed above.) This list doesn't include farmed fish because there are so many producers (mostly unsustainable, unfortunately) for every farmed species, and in a market it can be difficult to tell where a particular fish was farmed.

- *Clams*
- *Cod (Pacific and Alaskan)*
- *Crab (dungeness, snow, stone)*
- *Crayfish*
- *Halibut (Pacific)*
- *Mackerel (king and Atlantic)*
- *Mahimahi, troll- or pole-caught*
- *Mussels*
- *Oysters*
- *Salmon (Alaskan)*
- *Squid (longfin)*
- *Sardines (Pacific)*
- *Stripped bass/rockfish*
- *Tuna (albacore, yellowfin, skipjack/light), troll- or pole-caught*

Don't be afraid to try a new species of fish, and if you live near the coast, please don't forget to support your local fish market or join a Community Supported Fishery (CSF). A CSF is very much like a Community Supported Agriculture (CSA) program, except instead of investing in a farmer, you invest in a fishery. The details vary greatly among organizations, but the basic idea is that you pay upfront for a membership and receive a regular package of locally caught fish. You end up with a variety of sustainable choices, help support your local fishery, and get to eat lots of incredibly fresh fish—a win-win!

Also, keep in mind that frozen and canned seafood is often a more sustainable choice than fresh fish. Seafood is very perishable, and retailers often end up throwing out about 30 percent of the fresh fish on display. By purchasing frozen or canned fish, you eliminate that waste. Plus, much of the seafood on display was once frozen and is now thawed, which isn't a big deal if it was thawed that day, but if it has been thawed and on display for more than one day, it's likely to have a strong fishy taste and I don't recommend buying it.

What About Mercury and Other Harmful Toxins in Fish?

There's been a lot of worry about mercury in the fish we eat, but in truth, the trace amounts of mercury in most fish aren't high enough to pose a serious health risk for most people, although it's more of a concern for pregnant women, nursing mothers, and children. The FDA recommends that pregnant and breastfeeding women and young children eat two to three servings each week of fish lower in mercury, such as salmon, tilapia, cod, and catfish.

And here's some good news: Selenium binds to mercury in the body, making it harder for us to digest. If a fish contains more selenium than mercury, which is fairly common, the selenium has a protective effect, making it safe to eat. Mahi mahi, yellowfin and skipjack tuna, and swordfish all have higher levels of selenium than mercury.

There are also concerns about polychlorinated biphenyls (PCBs) in fish. PCBs cause cancer, harm fetal neurological development, suppress the immune system, and disrupt thyroid hormone levels. Like mercury, PCBs are found in higher levels in larger fish, but the highest levels of PCBs are actually found in beef, chicken, pork, and dairy products, according to a study in the *Journal of the American Medical Association.*

The benefits of eating fish—which are a great source of protein and can also be rich in omega-3s and many vitamins and minerals—far outweigh any risks posed by contaminants.

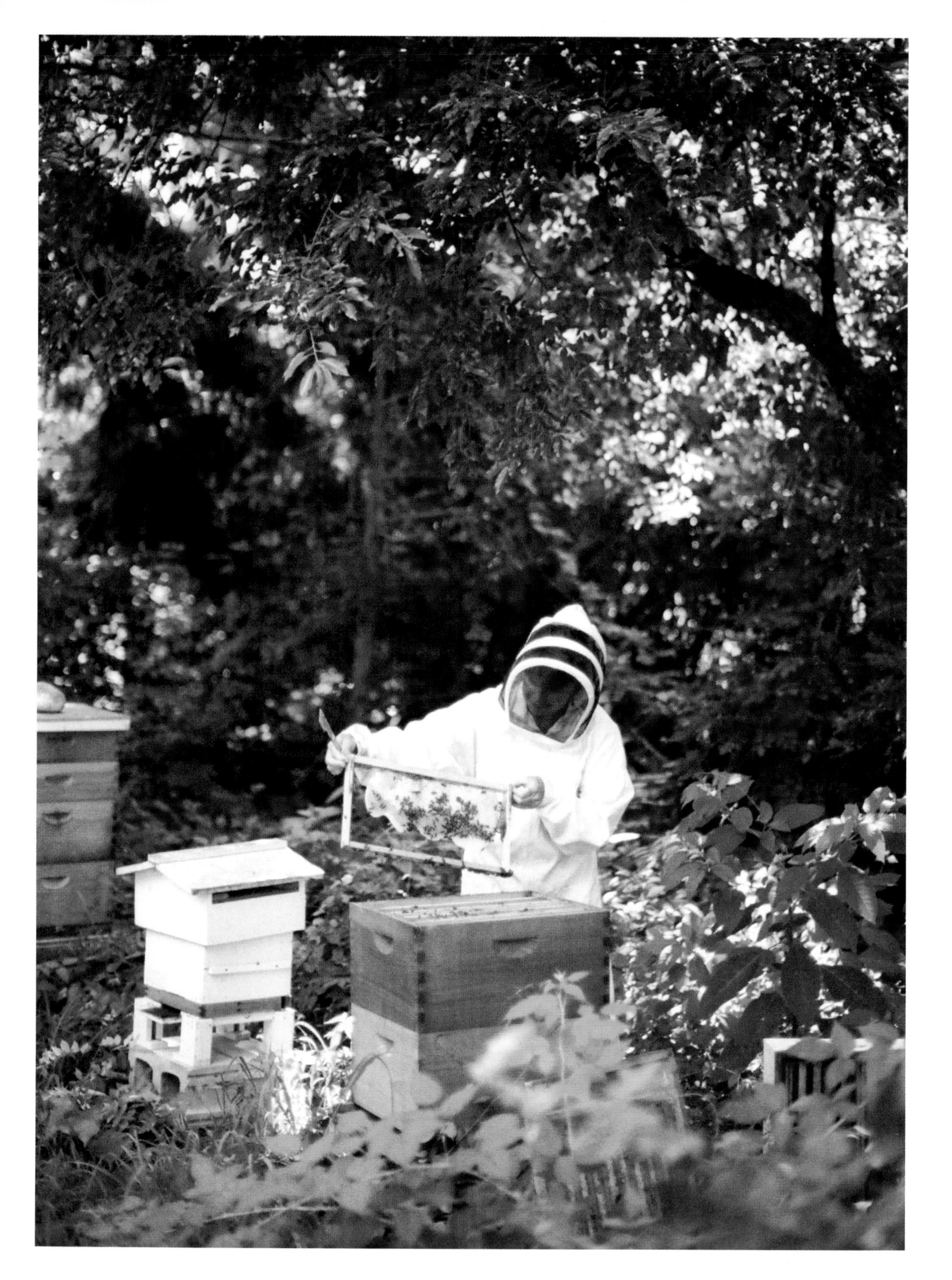

Bees

Adding a couple of beehives to your homestead will help improve your produce yield, but let's face it, I'll bet you're really interested in the liquid gold reward. And I certainly understand the draw: honey is delicious on its own or as a sweetener in recipes; it has less fructose and glucose than granulated sugar and contains vitamins and minerals, so it's better for you; and it's more sustainably harvested, especially if you can find a local source.

There are other benefits that come from keeping bees, too. There are dozens of uses for beeswax, from candles to skin creams to furniture polish and much, much more. Local honey, from local pollinating plants, can help curb seasonal allergies. And with wild bees being decimated by mites, pesticides, and urban sprawl, keeping a backyard hive can play an important part in restoring the honeybee population. That's especially crucial because bees not only pollinate plants, they also help keep the soil healthy by secreting formic acid.

Like most farmers, we hire a professional beekeeper to keep the hives on our farm. So in order to better understand the intricacies of beekeeping, I interviewed my friend Mary Mansur, a professional beekeeper who also runs a thriving business selling honey, candles, and other bee products.

History

Humans have been collecting wild honey and keeping bees for thousands of years. Cave paintings of honey gathering have been dated to 8,000 years ago, and archaeologists have found pots of honey in ancient Egyptian tombs. (It was still edible!) Many cultures used honey medicinally—it has antibacterial properties—and ancient Romans prized honey so highly that they even used it to pay their taxes.

Up until the nineteenth century, harvesting honey meant destroying the hive, since the honeycomb was fixed to the sides of the hive and needed to be cut out. Reverend Lorenzo Langstroth's 1851 invention of the movable-comb hive changed that. Frames in these hives are separated by one centimeter, which is exactly the right amount of space needed to prevent bees from building comb or using propolis, also known as "bee glue," to fill the space. Bees build comb in each frame without gluing the frames together, so it's easy for the beekeeper to remove the frames and get at the honeycomb without destroying the hive.

Royal Jelly

Royal jelly is a substance secreted by a worker nurse bee. All honeybees are fed a small amount of royal jelly, but the queen bee is fed only royal jelly—in fact, that's part of what makes a larva develop into a queen. Royal jelly is harvested by scooping out the contents of the queen cell. It is sold as a nutritional supplement and is said to have a number of health benefits, from lowering cholesterol to fighting cancer.

BEES FAQs

HOW FAR DO BEES FLY?

Bees forage in a two- to three-mile radius from the hive.

HOW MANY HIVES SHOULD I GET?

Start with two. There will be losses every year, and having two increases the chance of at least one hive making it through the winter. Also, if one hive is low on honey, the second can help make up the deficiency.

HOW MUCH HONEY WILL I GET?

You can get up to about 100 pounds of honey from one hive, not including what you need to leave for the bees, but in the first year it's likely to be less.

HOW MUCH DO BEES COST?

For about $120, you can get a package of bees that includes a queen and about 15,000 workers. The protective gear, hive, and other tools together cost about $400.

DO I NEED A LICENSE OR PERMIT TO KEEP BEES?

It completely depends on where you live. Contact your local town hall.

DO I NEED TO JOIN A LOCAL ASSOCIATION OR CLUB TO KEEP BEES?

You don't have to, but you'll learn a lot and meet some really interesting people. Beekeepers love to talk about bees, and your local bee club can help you find a mentor. I also highly suggest attending workshops and meetings to learn more about beekeeping—it has a steep learning curve.

DO I NEED TO START A NEW HIVE AT A CERTAIN TIME OF THE YEAR?

Yes, hives are started in the spring, but order your bees in January. Most bee farms sell out by the end of the winter.

HOW OFTEN DO BEEKEEPERS GET STUNG?

Every hive has its own personality; some are more passive or aggressive than others. The hive's aggressiveness also depends on the weather and the state of the hive. If a hive is healthy, it's a sunny day, and the bees are busy foraging, then the beekeeper may not need any protection from stings at all.

I WAS STUNG BY A BEE. WHAT DO I DO?

Remove the stinger as soon as possible by scraping it out with a fingernail or credit card. Don't squeeze it! That may release more venom into the skin.

DO BEES REALLY DIE AFTER STINGING A PERSON?

Yes, if a worker bee stings you, it will die shortly after. A queen bee may survive after stinging, but it's extremely uncommon to be stung by a queen.

AREN'T ALL THE BEES DYING?

In the past several years, many bee populations have been decimated by pesticides known as "neonicotinoids." Additionally, the toxins in mosquito sprays are responsible for killing an alarming number of beehives each year. Many beekeepers feel that mosquito spraying is overdone, and its effectiveness in preventing West Nile virus is being questioned.

Nutrition

Honey is a sweetener whose molecular profile is similar to high-fructose corn syrup. However, it has a few health benefits. It has been shown to increase the level of antioxidants in the blood and reduce inflammation. It also has antibacterial, antitumor, and antimutagenic properties, and it can help treat *H. pylori* infections—which can cause ulcers—and ease diarrhea in children. Raw honey, which has active natural enzymes, is best, and most honey sold at small farms is raw.

Be careful not to overconsume honey, though. I've found that my nutrition clients who have a hard time giving up sweets need to completely avoid honey during their initial thirty-day Paleo challenge to help break the cycle of cravings.

Snapshot of a Bee Colony

On average, there are 60,000 bees in a healthy hive. They are divided into three types: the queen, the workers, and the drones.

There is only one queen, and she is longer and more slender than the other bees. Her job is to produce pheromones that help regulate the colony and to lay up to 1500 eggs a day. Once in her lifetime, a virgin queen goes on a nuptial flight, flying high into the sky towards the sun. She is pursued by many drones and mates with the five or six that fly the highest. Upon her return to the hive, she immediately begins laying eggs. A fertilized egg becomes a worker bee, and an unfertilized egg becomes a drone. Queens can live for two years or more, but some beekeepers replace them as their egg production decreases.

Worker bees are much smaller than queens and have pollen baskets on their hind legs. They're responsible for gathering pollen, building honeycomb, repairing the hive, and pretty much everything else involved in keeping the hive healthy, aside from laying eggs and mating. Worker bees live about six weeks during the active season, when they are doing a lot of flying, and may live about four months in the winter. The younger ones are "house bees," which handle duties in the hive, and as they mature they become "field bees"and venture out to collect pollen.

The drones are larger than workers, although they're not as large as queens, and their eyes are much larger than those of queens and workers. They exist solely to mate with new queens and die soon after. Drones can't care for themselves and need to be fed by the worker bees, and as the mating season ends in the fall, the workers toss the drones out of the hive so that they won't be a drain on hive resources over the winter.

Purchasing Bees and Equipment

Before you buy any bees or equipment, make sure you have any licenses your town requires, and chat with your neighbors first to tell them about your plans to keep bees.

The Bees

There are several types of bees, all with different characteristics. If you're new to beekeeping, I suggest starting with Italian, Carolina, or Russian bees. They are all gentle, productive, and hearty.

Just like chicks, bees arrive in the mail. Place your order in January so that you'll have them by the time you're ready to start the hive in the spring. Your initial order of bees will be about three pounds, or 15,000 bees, which is just right for a new hive, and will come in a package that's about the size of a large shoe box. Be sure to order a marked queen—the dot on her back will help you easily identify her when you check on your hive.

There are many online bee suppliers, but I've found that the best way to find one is to ask at your local bee club, which probably has a "new beekeeper" program. Let your post office know that you're expecting a package of bees about a week before they're due to arrive, and give them your phone number so that they can call you to pick them up. Make sure you have your hive fully put together before you get the call from the post office.

The Equipment

The most important piece of equipment, of course, is the hive. I suggest you start with the most common beehive, the ten-frame Langstroth, which sort of looks like a chest of drawers. You can put it together yourself or buy it preassembled. Look for the higher-quality wood versions instead of the ones made from plastic or other materials; they're built better and will last longer.

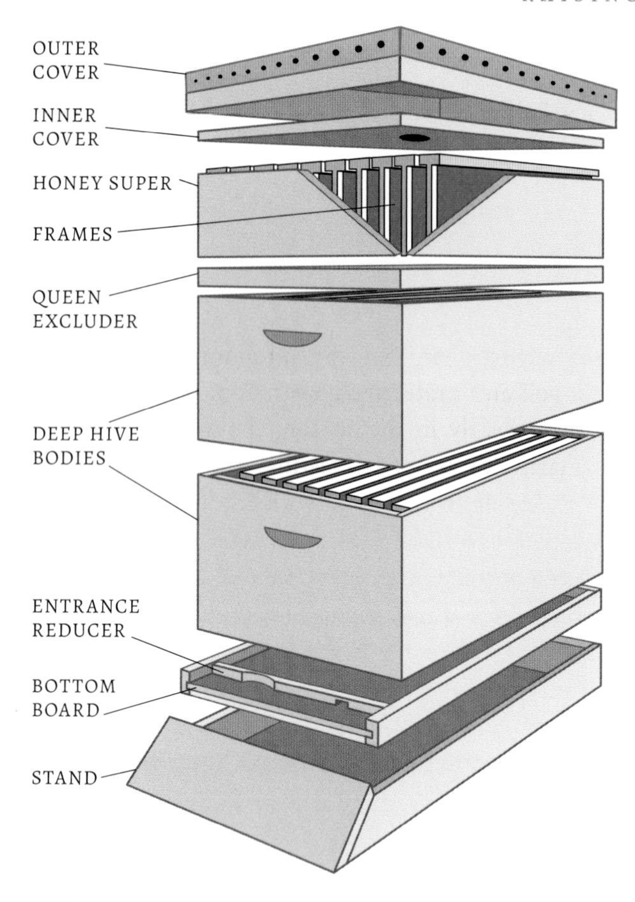

A hive is made of the following parts:

- **Screened bottom board:** The bottom board is the floor of the beehive. A screened bottom board, rather than a standard one, helps control mites: when the mites fall off the bees, they can't crawl back up into the hive.
- **Deep hive bodies:** Each contains ten frames of honeycomb. The lower deep is the nursery and the upper deep, which is added later, is the food chamber, where the bees store honey and pollen. Inside the hive bodies sit frames.
- **Frames:** The bees build their comb onto the frames, which usually come with a sheet of beeswax foundation to help the bees build uniform honeycomb. Despite the name, beeswax foundation is also available in plastic. Bees are slow to accept a plastic foundation, though, so if you really want uniform comb, use natural beeswax instead. But bees will also create their own beautiful honeycomb without foundation, and the process supports a healthier, stronger hive, so consider buying frames without it.
- **Honey super:** This looks like a shallower version of the deep hive bodies and is where the bees store surplus honey. You won't need it at first; add it to the hive around the end of the second month. You can purchase medium or shallow supers, but keep their weight in mind: when full of honey, a medium super weighs about 50 pounds and a shallow super weighs about 40 pounds. As the bees produce more and more honey, you can add more and more supers to the hive, stacking them on top like Legos.
- **Inner cover:** This cover sits directly on top of the super and has a ventilation notch on the front. It's optional, but it can help insulate the hive.
- **Outer cover:** This sits on the inner cover. It is often reinforced with galvanized steel, which protects it from the elements.

You'll also need to have some other equipment on hand before your bees arrive:

- **Entrance reducer:** This is placed between the bottom board and the lower hive body to limit movement in and out of the hive and control hive temperature and ventilation. It can also help bees defend against yellow jackets and robbing bees, since it reduces the size of the entrance. Use the entrance reducer in a new hive and during cold months, to keep the hive warm while allowing bees to come and go. Once the hive is established and when the weather is warm, you can remove it.
- **Queen excluder:** Used only during the honey season, this keeps the queen from laying eggs in the honey super.
- **Hive-top feeder:** This small box sits directly on top of the upper hive body, under the outer cover—no inner cover is used with a hive-top feeder. Adding sugar syrup to the feeder is an easy way to keep your bees fed.

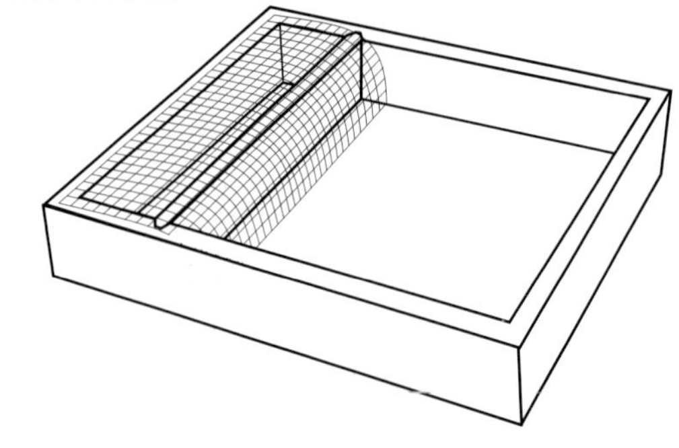

- **Smoker:** Produces cool smoke that helps calm the bees, so it's easier for you to inspect the hive.

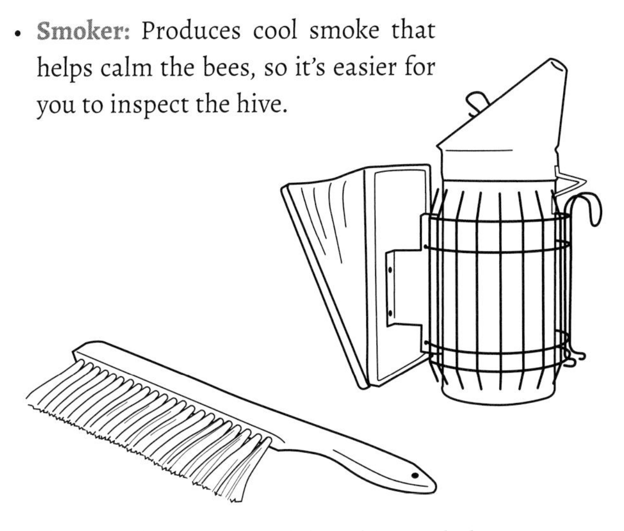

- **Bee brush:** It's optional, but this can help you gently brush bees off the hive in order to access the frames.
- **Hive tool:** Use this tool to scrape beeswax off the hive and loosen the parts of the hive, so they're easier to pry apart.

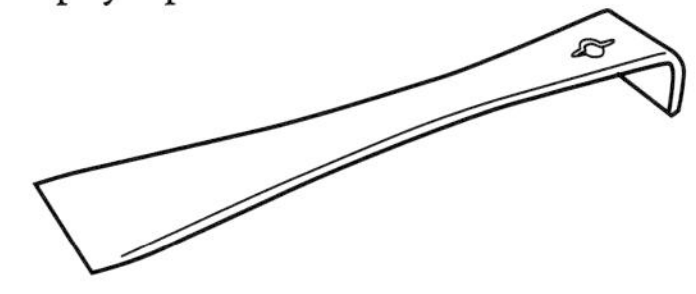

- **Protective gear:** At the minimum, you'll need a veil and protective gloves. You won't need the gloves early in the season, though; they're primarily for honey harvesting, and without them it's easier to be gentle with the bees. Coveralls are optional and range in price and thickness. If you opt not to wear coveralls, make sure you wear light-colored clothing and tuck it in, so bees don't crawl inside.

Setting Up a Hive

The ideal place for a hive is a dappled sunny place with a little afternoon shade, out of the way and relatively near a water source. It should be easy for you to access, but it should also be in a place where there isn't a lot of human or animal traffic to upset the bees. Be sure to place the hives at least 6 feet from your neighbors' property, and provide a water source so your bees aren't drinking from your neighbor's swimming pool or koi pond (see page 95 for more on providing food and water). Help keep your neighbors happy by giving them some honey once your hive is set up and productive. Also, consider elevating the hive on cinder blocks to help protect it from raccoons and skunks and make it easier to work with.

Once your hive is set up and your bees have arrived, it's time to add them to the hive. Install the bees in the hive within twenty-four hours of their arrival. It's best to introduce them to the hive on a cool morning, before they are too active, or in the evening, when they're more likely to settle than fly right away.

Your bees will arrive in a small package with 15,000 bees, the queen, and a feeding can. The queen will be in a separate, 1-by-3-inch cage whose entrance is plugged by a piece of candy or a marshmallow, called a "sugar plug." The bees the queen arrives with are not necessarily the bees she has been living with, and separating her like this protects her until her pheromones have a chance to spread throughout the hive and the workers accept her. The worker bees will eventually eat through the candy to set the queen free.

You'll need:

- An entrance reducer
- Two spray bottles, one filled with cool water and one with sugar syrup
- A veil
- A smoker
- A hive tool
- A nail
- Pliers
- A pushpin
- A hive-top feeder

1. Pick a nice sunny day to introduce your bees to the hive. They will be less defensive on a sunny day than if it's very cold or raining.
2. Place an entrance reducer on the front of your hive.
3. Remove the outer and inner cover. Take five of the frames from the deep body and set aside.
4. Spray the package of bees with cool water and put it in a cool place, such as a basement, for an hour. After the bees have had an hour to cool, spray them with nonmedicated sugar syrup (see page 95) to keep them from flying too much and give them a little extra food to start with.
5. Put on your veil and set up your smoker (see page 95).
6. Bring the bees to your hive and gently tap the top of the package so the bees fall to the bottom of the box. Now it's time to get the queen.
7. Use the hive tool to remove the feeding can and the queen cage from the package, taking care that the queen cage doesn't fall to the bottom of the box. Remove the cork from the queen's cage to expose the sugar plug and allow her pheromones will spread throughout the hive.
8. After removing the cork, use a nail to poke a small hole through the sugar plug. This gives the bees a head start in eating their way through the plug to release the queen.
9. Use your pliers to bend the metal around the queen cage to create a hanger from which to suspend the queen cage. Hang the queen cage in the middle of the hive, between the middle two frames, making sure that the wire front of the cage is parallel to the front of the hive. You can use a pushpin to hang it by its metal tab.
10. Gently pour the rest of the bees into the body of the hive. If there are bees left in the box, just place the box in front of the hive and they'll find their way in.
11. Give the bees a few puffs of smoke to keep them calm. (This is optional, and many experienced beekeepers will not smoke new bees, but I recommend it for new beekeepers.)
12. Replace the frames in the hive very slowly, taking care not to squish the bees below.
13. Place the hive-top feeder on the hive body, fill it with sugar syrup, and replace the outer cover.
14. After a few hours, watch at the entrance of the hive for bees fanning their wings. They are moving the pheromone scent outward so that the rest of the bees can find the hive.
15. After two days, check that the bees are continuing to eat through the sugar plug to release the queen. If the bees haven't eaten completely through the sugar plug after five days, you can enlarge the hole. If the plug is still there after seven days, you can safely remove it. Remove the queen cage from the vicinity of the hive as soon as the queen is released—if it's left near the hive, the queen's pheromones on the cage could be confusing to the bees.
16. While you're at the hive to check on the sugar plug, make sure the bees have enough sugar syrup. You'll want to feed them until there are five or six frames filled with comb and then let them feed themselves.

Completing the Setup

Three weeks after introducing the bees to the hive, it's time to open the entrance reducer to its largest opening, to provide more ventilation.

When your hive is a month old, you'll likely need to add the second deep hive body to provide more space, so the bees do not become overcrowded and swarm to create a new hive. The second deep hive body should be added when there is some comb in three-quarters of the frames (if you have ten frames, seven should have comb on them). Simply remove the outer cover, the hive-top feeder, and the top of the original hive body, place the second hive body directly upon the original, and fill the second hive body with frames. It will serve as a nursery for the next month or so, and after that the colony will use it to store honey for the winter.

By the end of the second month, remove the entrance reducer entirely. It's also a good time to see if the upper deep frames are drawn out—completely full of honeycomb. When this happens, it's time to place the honey super on top of your hive (called "supering"). Place the queen excluder above the upper deep chamber to allow the smaller bees to pass through but keep the queen out. Then add the honey super above the queen excluder and replace the outer cover.

Food and Water

You should provide water for your bees. A chicken waterer (see page 41) or a birdbath is great. Add some pebbles so they don't drown when they are drinking. Place the water source relatively close to the hive.

Bees don't necessarily need to be fed, but keep an eye on their honey stores to make sure they have enough. If the stores are low, it's best to feed your bees honey from another apiary (not simply store-bought honey). Sugar syrup should be used only as a last resort—and be aware that it won't be converted to honey. Only nectar from flowers results in honey.

To make sugar syrup, dissolve 5 pounds of white sugar in 2½ quarts of boiled water. Cool to room temperature before feeding your bees. In the winter, make a concentrated form of sugar water by dissolving 10 pounds of white sugar in 2½ quarts of water. Add any medication after the water is at room temperature.

Visiting with Your Bees

As a new beekeeper, you'll want to check on the hive about once a week. Visit between 10 a.m. and 5 p.m., and pick a sunny day. Don't wear wool or leather—bees dislike the smell—and avoid strong scents on your body, like garlic or perfume. Wear your veil at the very least, but if you have more protective gear, such as coveralls and gloves, put them on. If a bee gets into your veil, she is unlikely to sting you unless provoked. Don't scream, run, swat, or freak out. Just walk slowly away and slip off your veil to let the bee out, then replace the veil and return to the hive.

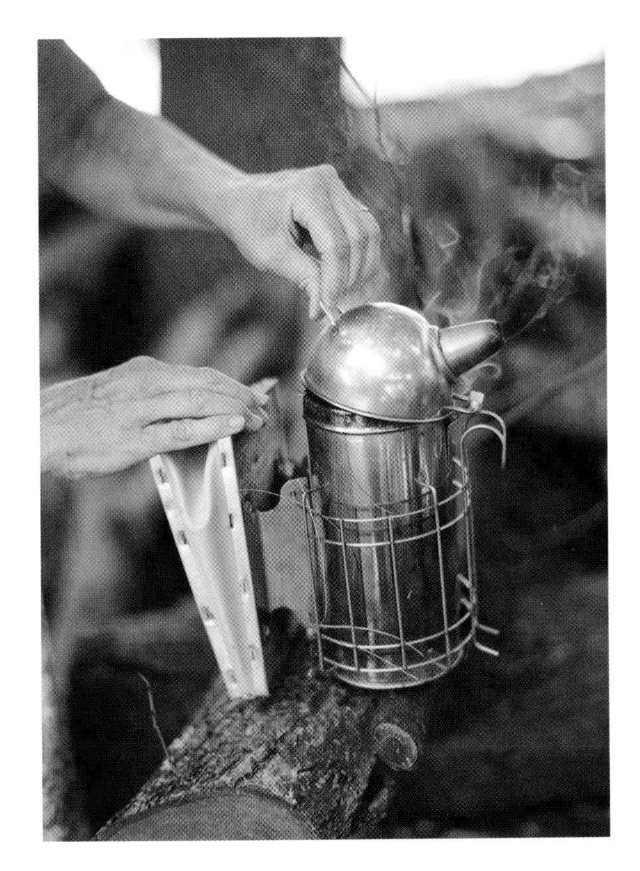

The smoker is a "knock on the door" to let your bees know you're coming, and the smoke calms the bees. Light your smoker with dried leaves or dried herbs from your garden. Once it's lit, pack it with small wood chips, then close the lid. If the fire goes out, shake everything and light the smoker again. It takes some practice. It's good to keep a box of wood chips near the hive for easy access. To use the smoker, stand about 2 feet away from the hive and send a couple of puffs of smoke toward the entrance. Walk a bit closer and smoke the top of the hive.

In the beginning, the frames won't be stuck together, but later in the season, you'll need to use a hive tool to pry up the feeder and outer cover. To avoid rattling the bees by making a loud cracking noise, use one hand to hold down the cover and the other to pry it up. Wait thirty seconds, then carefully lift one edge of the outer cover and smoke a bit more on top of the frames. Now put your smoker down and slowly remove the cover. Set the cover aside on the ground. Remove the inner cover as well.

Pick up one of the frames next to the wall by the ends. Be very careful not to crush any bees; just brush them aside if they're in the way. Gently rest the frame up against the hive. Loosen the next frame, pick it up and inspect it, then replace it and move on to the next one. Only the first frame should be taken out and laid on the ground.

To inspect a frame, stand with your back to the sun, so the wax cells are illuminated and you can get a better look at the eggs and larvae. Carefully rotate the frame to the right, then to the left, and finally upside down. Once you're done checking every frame, gently slide the frames all back and give the hive a puff of smoke, then shake the bees off the outside frame and replace it in the hive. Carefully replace the inner and outer covers.

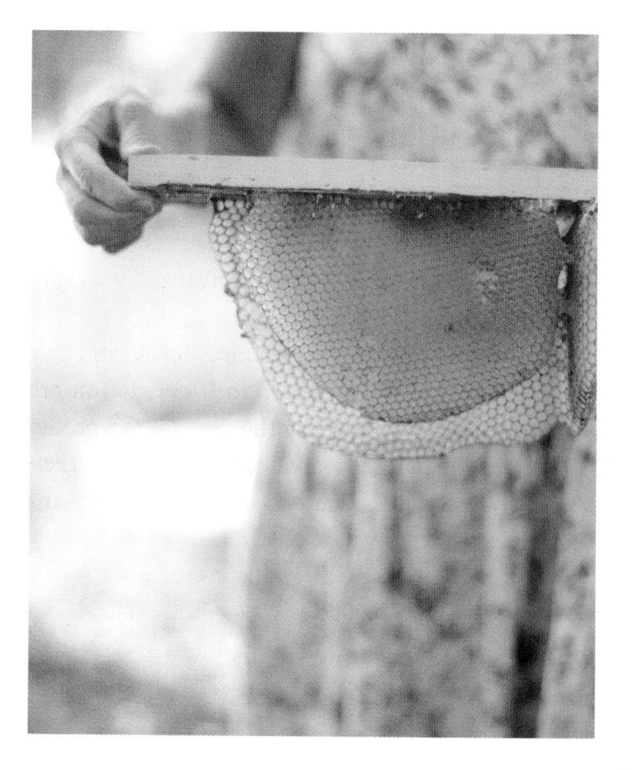

What to Look For

The queen: The main thing you're checking for is that the queen is alive and well. (If she's not, you may need to replace the queen—see page 97.) It will take a couple of weeks for the honeycomb to build up so that the queen has somewhere to lay the eggs, but once it does, you won't need to actually see the queen to know she is active. If she is there and doing her job, there will be eggs in the cells. This is your signal that you have a thriving colony of bees.

Eggs and larvae: Look for the tiny, translucent, rice-like eggs in the cells. You may need a pair of reading glasses (even if you don't normally need them) to get a better look. It takes three days for the egg to hatch and become a larva. Nurse bees feed the larvae and seal them in the cells with beeswax. After twelve days, the adult bee chews its way out of the cell and joins the colony. To see where adults have emerged, look for wax that seems broken and thin. There should be a tight pattern of active larvae cells; if they're intermittently dispersed, it could indicate an unhealthy queen.

Filled cells: By the end of one month, the bees should have drawn comb on nearly every frame (about seven out of ten), so that you need to add a second deep hive body to avoid overcrowding (see page 94).

Supersedure cells: When a queen becomes old or ill, the workers take an egg that's a few days old and place it in a supersedure cell—not a cell within the honeycomb but a structure that looks like a little peanut and hangs from the comb on the upper two-thirds of the frame. The larva in a supersedure cell is exclusively fed royal jelly so that it will become a queen. If you see more than three supersedure cells, it's pretty clear that your colony is looking to replace its queen.

Swarm cells: Though you're unlikely to see these in a new hive, they're something to be aware of. When a hive is overcrowded, the workers build swarm cells to raise up a second queen in anticipation of swarming to create a second hive. Like supersedure cells, swarm cells also look like peanuts, but they tend to form toward the bottom third of the frame.

Eight or more of these structures is a good indication that the colony will soon swarm. Most beekeepers remove swarm cells, but that doesn't solve the problem of an overcrowded hive or lack of ventilation, which can also lead to swarm cells. Anticipate problems before they arise and make plans to expand your hive or provide more ventilation.

REPLACING THE QUEEN

If your new colony loses its queen, you'll need to buy a replacement. However, if you have an established colony, you can also allow the colony to replace the queen on its own. A naturally raised queen may be more hearty than a purchased test-tube queen, whose immune system won't be as strong. In most cases, it's best just to keep an eye on things and, as long as all goes smoothly, leave the bees alone to manage their hive.

Winter Hive Maintenance

After the weather gets cold, don't open the hive. The bees have used propolis, a sticky substance made from tree sap and resin, to seal it up. If the beekeeper cracks these seals in late fall, the bees don't have time to seal the hive again. Place a cinder block on top of the outer cover to keep it in place in the wind and winter storms, and consider wrapping the hive with roofing paper to insulate it, but be careful not to cover the entrance. If it snows, visit your bees and make sure the snow is not covering the hive entrance.

During the winter, the bees curl up in a tight ball around the queen, which is called "clustering." They vibrate their flight muscles but keep their wings still, creating a kind of shiver. When the bees on the outside of the cluster get cold, they move to the center, so every bee gets a turn staying warm. They'll keep the hive at about 92 degrees through the winter.

Health and Predators

It's a good idea to familiarize yourself with common bee diseases so you can watch for them. There are so many variables that it's best to get a good book that covers the topic in detail and attend local beekeepers meetings to learn more. One common problem is dark brown cells with larvae inside, which indicates the larvae are dead. Also, if you see yellow streaks of bee feces down the side of the hive, it's often a sign of nosema, a common fungal infection.

Although many beekeepers are concerned about the mites that honeybees carry, the truth is, there have always been and will always be mites on bees. In fact, most beekeepers nowadays think of beehives as housing two kinds of creatures: the bee and the mite. The solution is not to try to kill off the mites with chemicals but to make the bees strong enough that they can coexist. Antibiotics and other chemicals used by some beekeepers can actually weaken the bee's immune system.

Raccoons, skunks, bears, mouse, birds, and other insects all are as interested in honey as you are. Elevating your hive is really the best way to protect against most four-legged honey thieves, but there are other techniques you can use for different animals. You can purchase metal mouse guards for your hives through beekeeping supply companies. If ants are a problem, try dusting the ground around your hive with cinnamon, which ants hate. Bears can be held back by an electric fence.

CARING FOR YOUR BEES

Bees require much less maintenance than other farm animals, which makes beekeeping a great hobby for someone who works full-time. Here's what to expect each season.

Spring and summer (March through October)	**Winter** (November through February)	**Throughout the year**
Visit the bees once a week and make sure the queen is there and the hive is healthy. Look for signs of swarming. By midsummer, add additional honey supers if your bees are producing a surplus. Harvest honey in mid to late summer.	Every three weeks, and every time there's a big snowfall, make sure the hive entrance is clear.	Clean supplies. Order new bees if needed. Attend beekeeping meetings and read up on bees.

Harvesting the Honey

Bees store their surplus honey in the super. That's honey that you can harvest at the end of the honey-making season, which can be any time between June and September, depending on your region. If you're not certain when exactly you should be harvesting the honey, check with other local beekeepers.

When you harvest honey, be sure to leave enough to feed the bees. They need about 50 to 60 pounds of honey to make it through the winter—up to 80 or 90 pounds if you live in an area with long, snowy winters. As always, if in doubt, check with your local beekeepers association and find out what other successful beekeepers are doing.

When the bees determine that the honey in a comb cell has the right moisture content, they cap the cell with wax. Before you begin harvesting honey, make sure the bees have filled eight out of ten frames with capped honey. If liquid spills out when you shake the frame, the honey has too much moisture and will spoil your honey harvest, so put the frame back and wait. But you don't want to wait so long that the honey under the wax cap has hardened, so harvest when the weather is still warm.

If you can, help a friend harvest honey before you attempt to do it on your own. That way, you'll be more comfortable when it's your turn. Don't try to bottle honey outdoors—it attracts all kinds of bees and will be a huge mess. Pick a good indoor space for your honey production center, such as a garage or basement, cover the floor with newspaper, and have everything set up before you begin.

You'll need:

- **Bee escape:** Lets bees out but doesn't let them back in. Placing one under the super you'll be harvesting is an easy way to clear bees from the frames.
- **Uncapping fork:** Removes the wax cap from the cells.

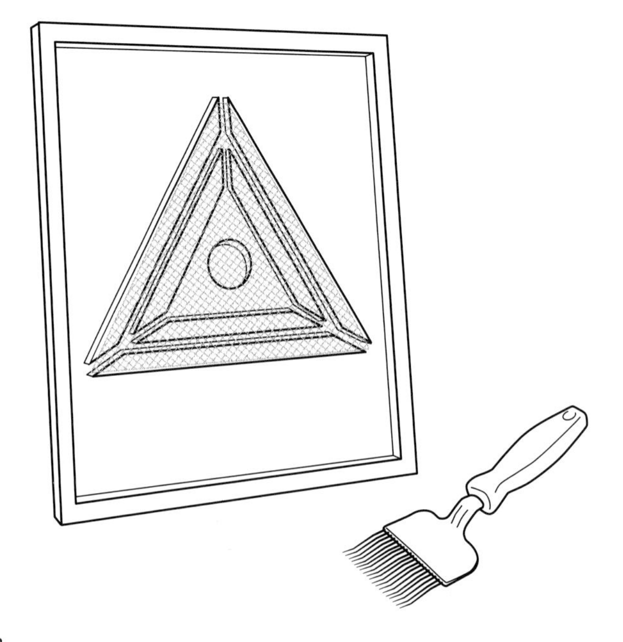

- **Extractor:** Spins to extract the honey from the comb. Extractors can be hand-cranked or electric, and a good one can cost $250 to $400. Before you make the investment, see if you can rent one from your local beekeepers association or borrow one from a friend to help you decide which kind you'd like to buy.
- **Honey strainer:** Ensures no bee heads end up in your honey. You can use a fine-mesh kitchen strainer or one specifically made for straining honey.
- **Bottling bucket:** Five-gallon bucket with a gate valve, which makes it easy to bottle your honey.
- **Jars:** Any clean glass or plastic jars will work to store your honey. One full super yields about 30 pounds of honey, so you'll probably need around twenty pint jars.
- **Helping hands:** Harvesting honey is a fun activity for a group of people, and the extra help will be welcome. Invite your friends and neighbors to help you in exchange for a bottle of liquid gold at the end!

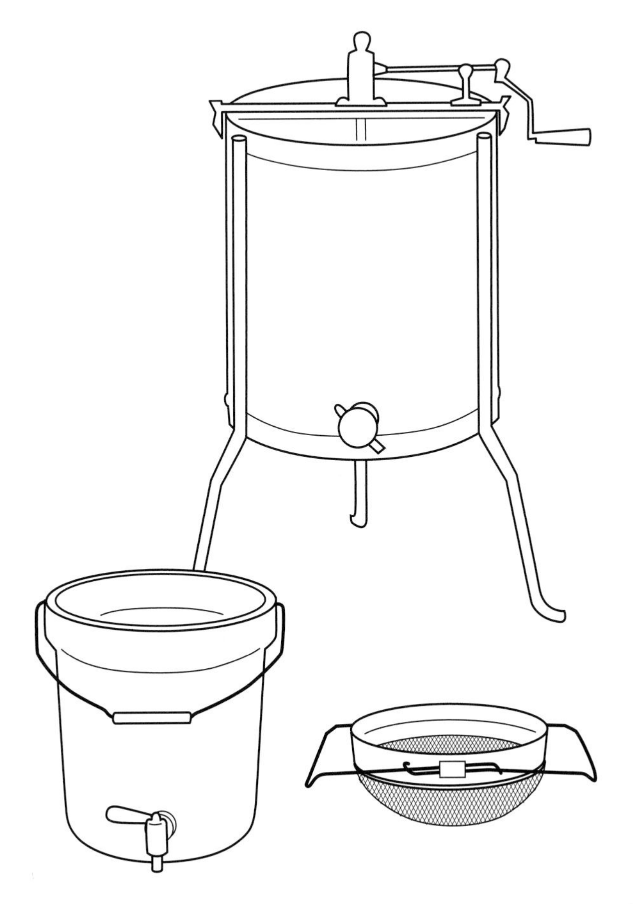

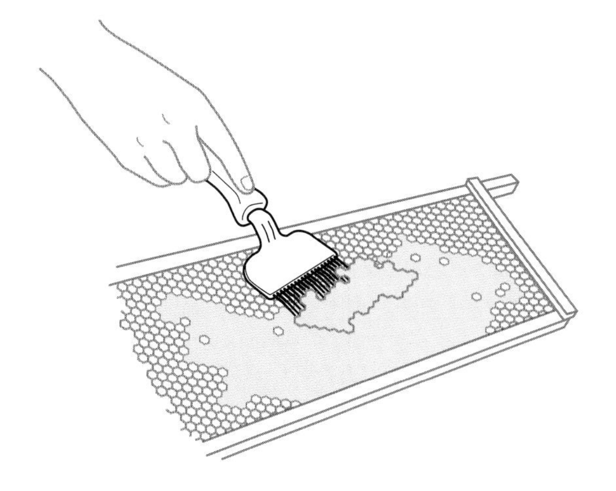

Removing wax caps with an uncapping fork

First, you need to get all the bees off your frames. The day before the harvest, place a bee escape under the super you'll be harvesting. Bees will leave the super and not be able to get back in, so the day of the harvest, nearly all the bees will be off the super's frames.

Remove the super and all the frames and take them to your honey production space. Use the uncapping fork to remove the wax caps, revealing the honey. Place the frame in your extractor and spin to extract the honey. Drain the honey through the strainer and into your bottling bucket, and then use the bucket's valve to fill the jars.

Cleaning the frames after extraction couldn't be easier. At dusk, place the sticky super on top of the hive. The bees will eat all the honey remaining on the super. Before storing the super and frames for the winter, coat them with wax moth control to prevent wax moths from infesting the hive.

Sometimes if honey gets cold, it crystallizes and turns hazy instead of clear. No big deal—just place the jar of honey in warm water and it will liquefy again. However, if honey crystallizes in the frames, it's near impossible to extract, so be sure not to wait until cold months to harvest your honey.

When you are done harvesting your honey, the super goes into storage until the next year's honey season. If you live in a cold climate, however, leave one super full of honey on the hive to feed the bees during the winter.

HUNTING

FOR SOME, HUNTING IS A DEEPLY SPIRITUAL ACTIVITY; FOR OTHERS, IT'S ABOUT GETTING OUT WITH FRIENDS; AND FOR STILL OTHERS, IT'S A WAY TO PRACTICE AND HONE THE SKILLS OF TRACKING AND SHOOTING. BUT NO MATTER THE MOTIVATION, HUNTING, LIKE FARMING, IS HELPS YOU CONNECT WITH NATURE AND YOUR FOOD.

One reason for hunting that I find particularly compelling is that, in many parts of the country, it's an important part of conservation efforts. As habitat loss causes a decrease in the number of predators, the population of prey species can reach unnaturally high levels. For example, in much of the Northeast there are way too many deer. That has led to a sharp decrease in certain plant species, which in turn has led to a shift in the forest ecology. For one, the disappearance of low-growing shrubs harms the native songbirds that nest in them.

Also, eating wild game, especially herbivores and fish, has many health benefits. Because the animals are moving freely and aren't eating factory-farmed grains, wild game is leaner and has more anti-inflammatory omega-3s.

And let's not forget that it's free! Well, after you pay for your gear, license, travel, processing, and so on. But seriously, my buddy Charles Mayfield got four deer this past season. That's about 350 pounds of meat, and even with all the associated costs, it's a pretty good deal.

I'm fortunate to receive a steady stream of venison and other wild game from hunter friends, most of whom learned to hunt as kids. I polled several of them to find out how I could learn to hunt as an adult. If you've never done it before and think hunting is something you'd like to pursue, here are some tips from folks who are regulars:

- **Take a gun safety course and a hunting safety course.** Gun safety courses are usually offered through local police departments, and your state wildlife agency will have information about hunting courses.
- **Try a few different types of hunting.** You may like hunting quail much more than hunting elk. Maybe you like being still in a duck blind, or maybe you prefer being more mobile. Or maybe fishing is your thing. Try a bunch of different styles out until you find the one that suits you. If you have a friend who can take you, you can usually tag along and observe without a hunting license, and some states offer apprentice hunting licenses. Testing the waters is also a good way to figure out what type of gear you'll need before you make the investment.
- **Look up the "Unlimiteds."** Conservation organizations such as Ducks Unlimited, White Tail Unlimited, and Trout Unlimited can teach you everything you need to know about the animal you'll be hunting. Most of them have outings and other opportunities to expose you to hunting, and they're great ways for those who didn't grow up hunting to get acquainted with it. Many also have social media outlets where you can post that you're looking to tag along on a hunting trip. It's a great way to connect with other hunters.
- **Decide how much money you'd like to spend.** There are two main approaches to hunting: with little time and a lot of money, or with a lot of time and little money. For a hefty price tag, a big game ranch will take you out to shoot at anything from elk and buffalo to gazelles and wildebeests. They'll teach you everything, including how to load a gun and where to point it. The more economical option is to borrow some guns to figure out which you really like before you buy, to test out some local hunting options with friends or a local unlimited chapter, and to accumulate your gear slowly.

- **Learn how to process.** When we were in our early twenties, Andrew once brought me a whole trout, assuming I knew how to clean it. I had no idea what I was doing and made a huge mess in the sink, and we ended up with no meat. Knowing what to do with your game is critical. Plus, if you can field dress a deer, you'll spend a lot less energy hauling it back to your vehicle, and examining the liver and other organs can also give you a clue about the health of the animal. It's ideal to learn field dressing from a fellow hunter. It's also a good idea to take a basic butchering class. While in some areas there are places that will butcher your animal for you, it's a great skill to have yourself.
- **Own your bullet.** At the end of the day, great hunters understand that once the bullet leaves their gun, they're responsible for it. You own your shot. Before you pull the trigger, be sure you have properly identified your target so that you don't shoot something you don't intend to eat. You are holding the life of another being in your hands, and that's no small thing. Taking another life should be done with respect, humility, and a mindful understanding that the animal is giving its life so that you can eat. It's also critical to leave the environment better than you found it. Pack up your trash and respect the land you are using.

"ONE DOES NOT HUNT IN
ORDER TO KILL; ON THE
CONTRARY, ONE KILLS IN
ORDER TO HAVE HUNTED."
—Jose Ortega y Gasset

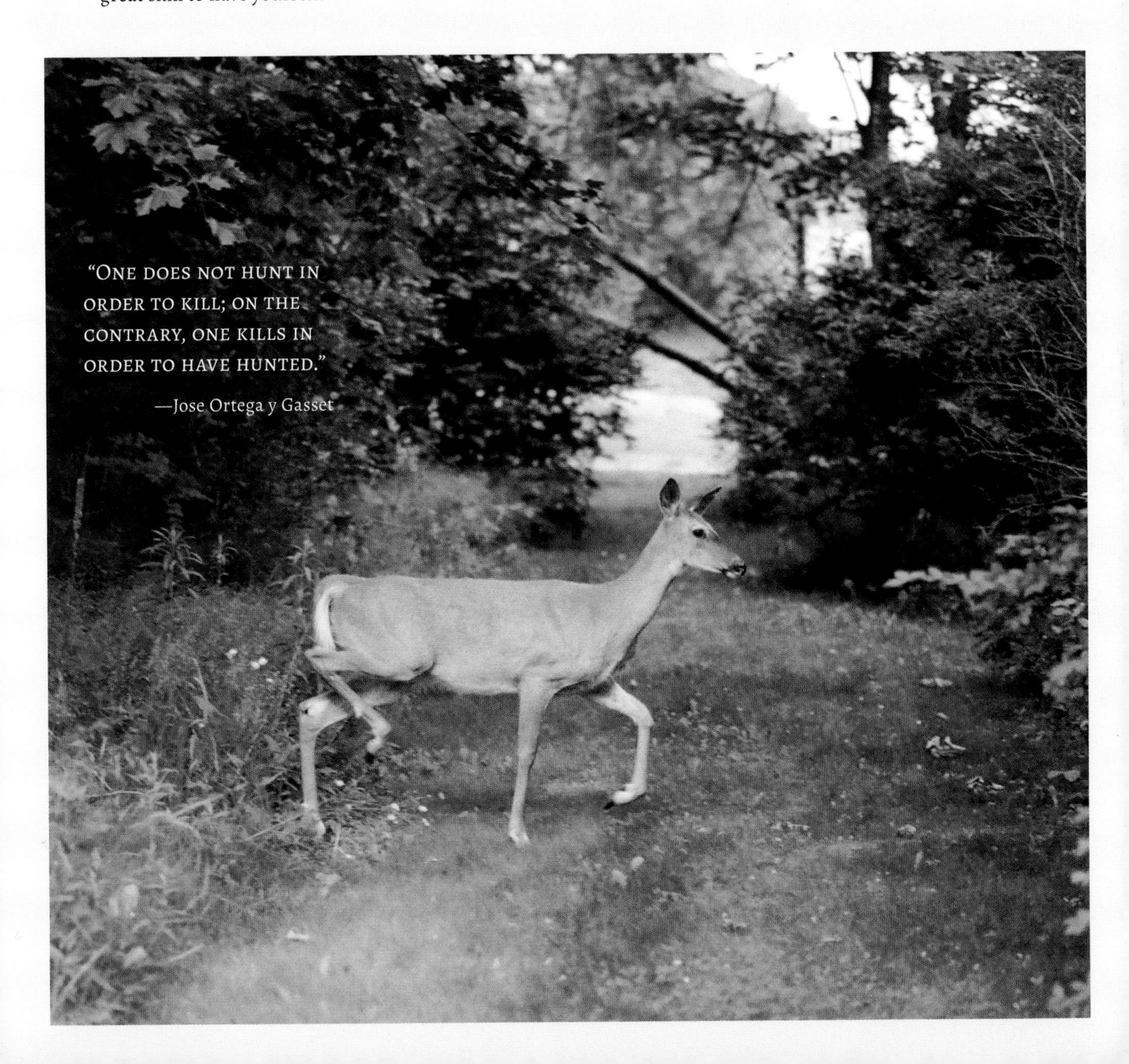

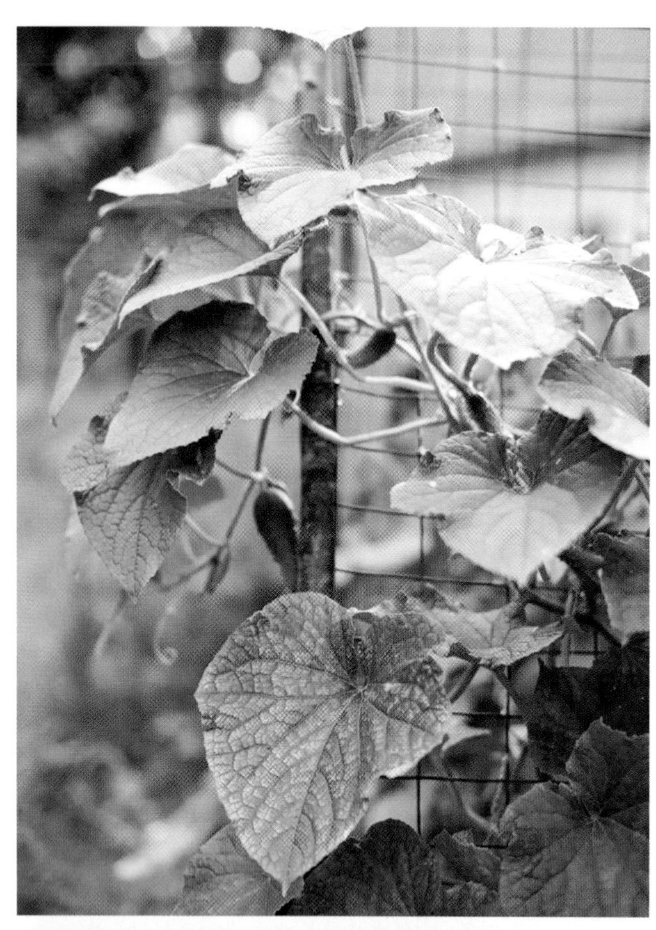

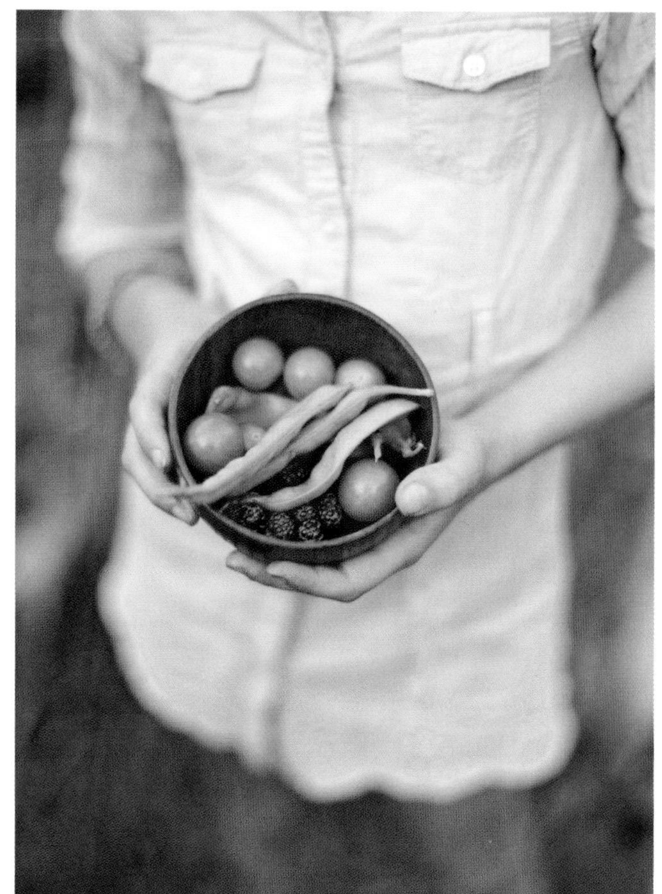

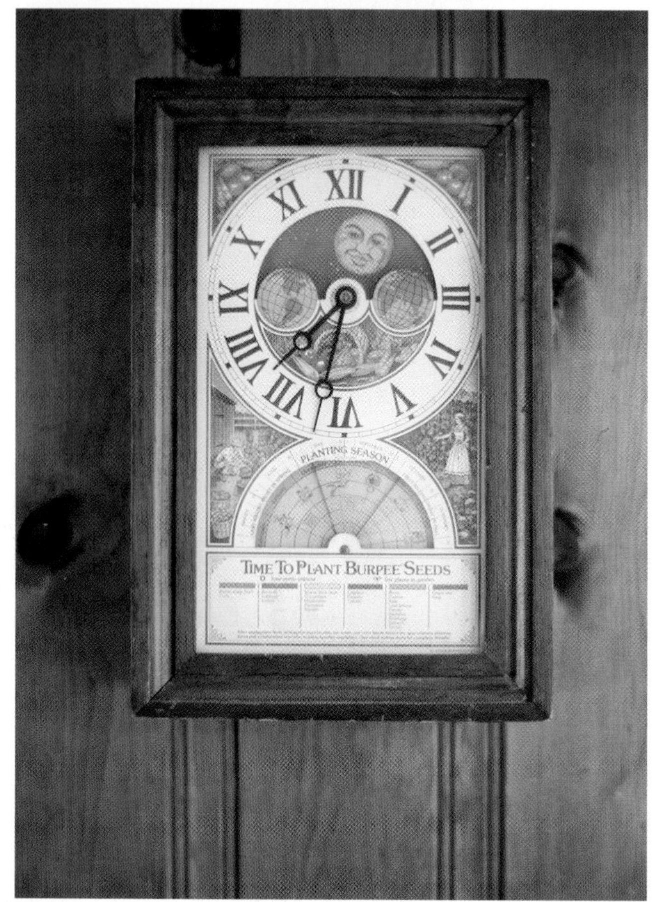
PLANTING SEASON
TIME TO PLANT BURPEE SEEDS

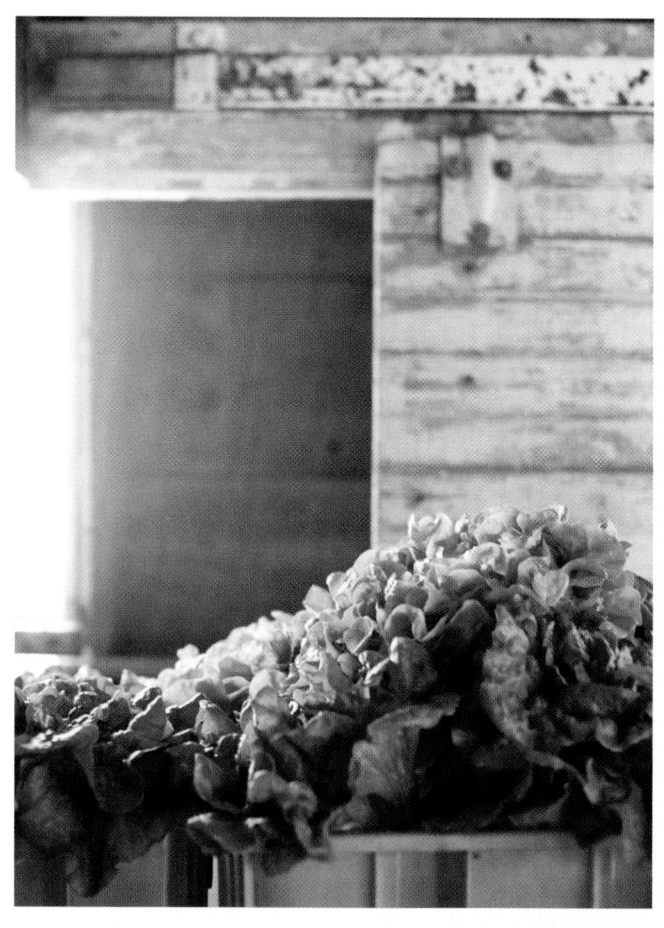

Growing

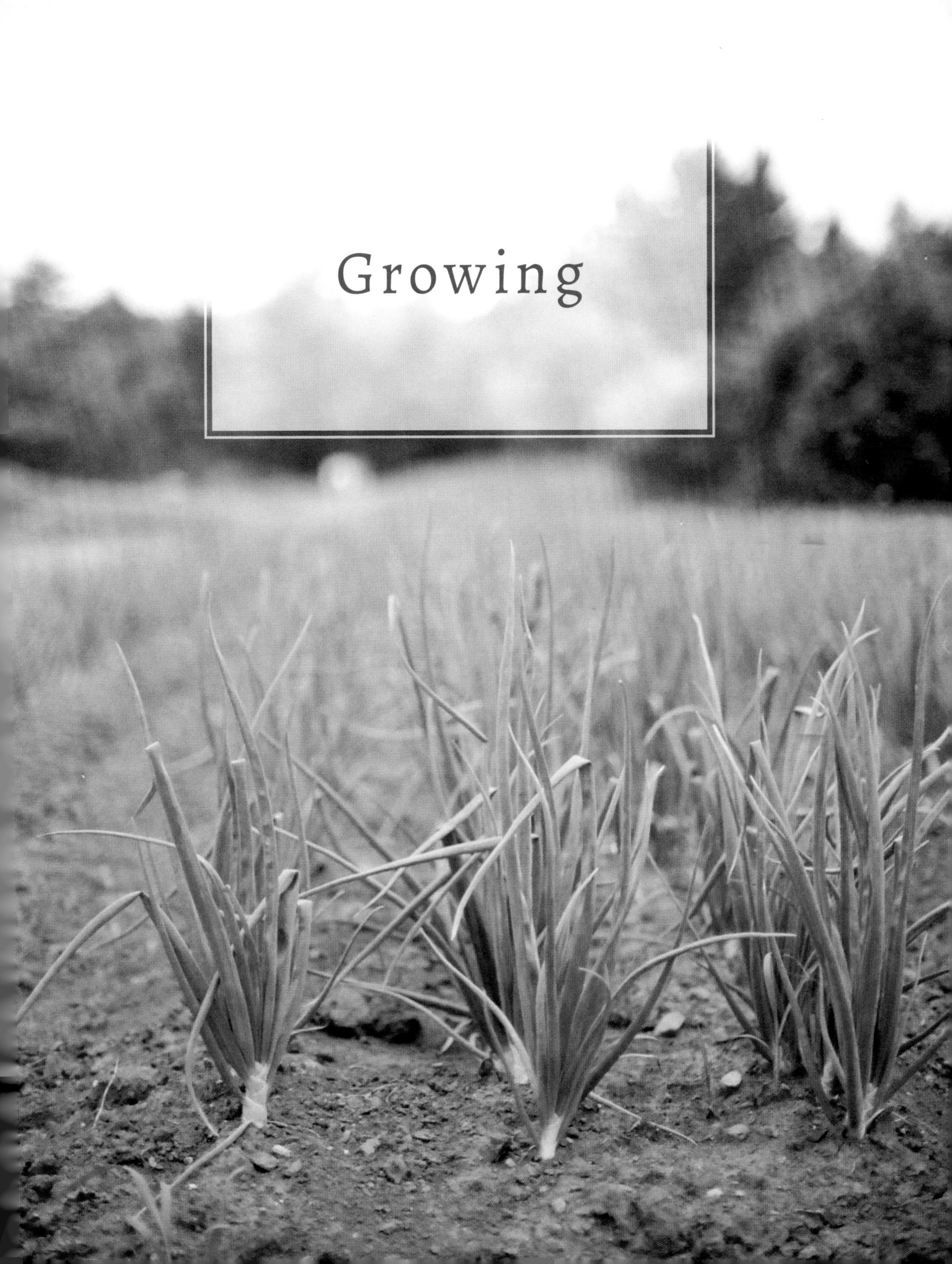

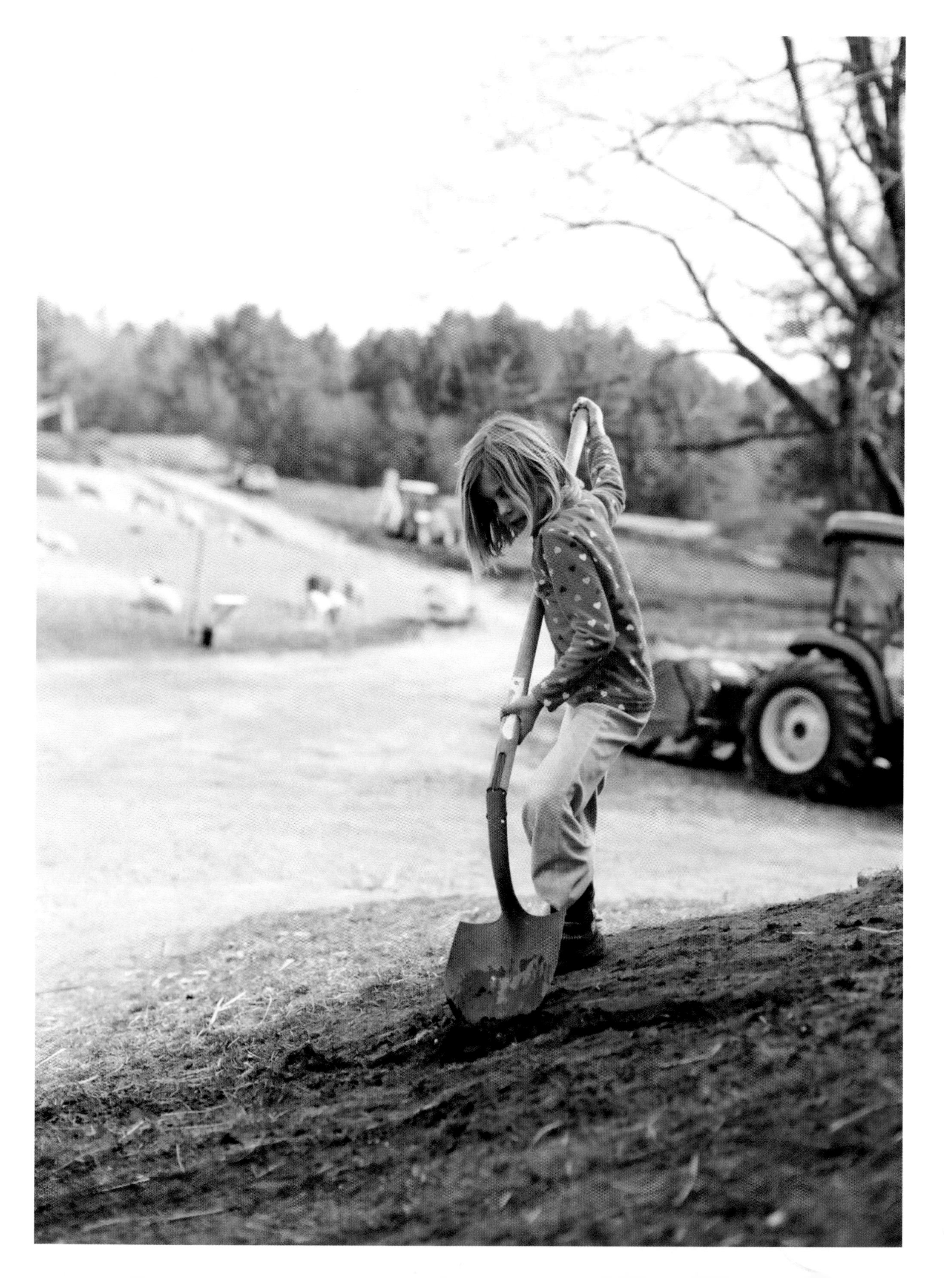

Getting Started with Your Garden

I'm not sure who originally said it, but it's true that growing your own vegetables is like printing money. There are some upfront costs, and of course you'll need to put in some time and labor, but you'll save money by growing your own organic produce, which can be expensive at the grocery store—plus, produce fresh from your own garden is simply more delicious!

Try starting small, so that it's not overwhelming; make your own fertilizer with homemade compost; and focus on growing vegetables that you know your family will eat. Gardening is a great way to spend your time outdoors, a good workout, a stress reducer, and you'll actually learn a ton—about food production, insects, weeds, pests, and more. Gardening is also simply fun, especially with kids, and they're much more likely to try a new food if it comes from a garden they helped to take care of. I can't think of a better family hobby than growing and cooking healthy food.

Planning

When you're planting your first garden, it's best to start simple and plant the very easiest-to-grow vegetables. Even so, gardening is a learning process, and your first attempt will be just grist for changes and refinements based on your microclimate. Planning exactly what you're going to plant and where, finding the best spot for your garden, and testing the soil can all increase your chances for success.

Some of the easiest vegetables to start with include:

- Cucumbers
- Zucchini
- Tomatoes
- Herbs
- Peppers
- Kale
- Potatoes
- Green beans
- Peas

Make a Plan

Plan your garden down to the last foot of space, and then stick to the plan. I know how easy it can be to impulsively buy twenty more tomato plants at the garden center, but trust me, it won't work out. If you can't fill your garden space with the plants you want to grow, then just cover the extra space with a mix of a perennial grass and a legume to fix nitrogen in the soil (more on that on page 112). If it really breaks your heart to not use every last inch of space, then plant some potatoes or sweet potatoes.

Find a Spot

Pick a sunny location—you'll have the best luck if the sun shines as much as possible on your garden. If you have a shady plot of land, try thinning the trees to let more light in. Your location also determines how quickly you can start planting your garden. If you're creating a brand new garden out of a grassy space, it's best to start the process of creating your garden at least a year before you start planting, to give the soil time to transition to a different use (see pages 107 to 109). If you are working with an established pasture or lawn, it will be a relatively quick one-year transition. If you are taking down an established forest, though, it will take several years for the soil to be ready to grow an annual vegetable. While you're working on making great soil (more on that starting on page 107), you can grow some vegetables in containers (see page 136).

GARDENING FAQs

HOW MUCH TIME DOES IT TAKE EACH WEEK TO CARE FOR A GARDEN?

It takes about three to four hours a week to maintain a typical home veggie patch that's about 20 by 20 feet.

HOW OFTEN DO I HAVE TO WATER THE GARDEN?

This is a hard question to answer. Depending on the weather and time of year, a vegetable garden in New England needs about 1 inch of water a week. If you live in a more arid climate, your garden will need more water. Also, certain crops, such as celeriac, like to keep their feet wet, and container plants in sunny locations need a lot more water. In general, plan on spending at least 15 minutes a week watering.

HOW MANY ACRES DO I NEED TO PLANT TO JUSTIFY BUYING A TRACTOR?

Guys always want to know this. You really don't need a tractor for less than 2 acres of crops.

WHAT'S THE BEST WAY TO FERTILIZE MY GARDEN?

Bagged organic granular fertilizer is great for a vegetable garden. Apply it when you sow seeds or transfer seedlings and again when the vegetables begin to fruit.

MY PLANTS ALWAYS DIE. CAN I DEVELOP A GREEN THUMB?

Yes, you really can. Keep at it and you will have success.

HOW MANY TOMATO PLANTS ARE NEEDED TO FEED A FAMILY OF FOUR?

You will need about two slicer plants (as opposed to cherry tomatoes or plum tomatoes) for a family of four. To make enough preserved tomato sauce to last the winter, you will need about ten to twenty plants.

HOW LARGE SHOULD MY GARDEN BE?

A 20-by-20-foot garden will go a long way toward satisfying your vegetable needs during the growing season.

HOW DO I KEEP DEER OUT?

Deer fencing is the only way to go. Good deer fencing is 7 feet tall and made of a durable material, like livestock fencing. I've had success excluding deer for a year or two using shorter, temporary fencing.

WHAT ARE THE FIVE BEST VEGETABLES TO GROW IN CONTAINERS?

I recommend tomatoes, herbs, bell peppers, eggplant, and strawberries. (For more on container gardening, see page 136.)

WHAT VEGETABLES DO WELL IN PARTIAL SHADE?

Vegetables won't grow in full shade, but you can have some success with partial shade, about six hours of sunlight a day. Lettuce, spinach, kale, Swiss chard, and arugula can all thrive in partial shade.

WHY IS MY LETTUCE BITTER DURING THE SUMMER?

Lettuce prefers cooler temperatures. As it matures and the weather gets warmer, it gets more bitter. While there are heat-tolerant varieties of lettuce that are less bitter, even they will get bitter if they don't get enough water.

CAN I USE TREATED WOOD TO MAKE MY RAISED BED?

No. Pressure-treated wood has had pesticides infused into it. In other words, the wood lasts a long time because it is poisonous. The pesticides will leach into the soil and end up in your food.

WHAT IS THE BEST MANURE TO USE FOR MY GARDEN?

The best manure for a garden is sheep and goat manure. Chicken manure is loaded with great nutrients as well, but it must be aged or composted in order to "cool it off"—otherwise, it has too much nitrogen and can burn the roots of your plants. Whatever manure you use, don't spread it within ninety days of harvesting the crop.

Test the Soil

It's always a good idea to know what is in your soil so that you can either remove and replace it or remediate it. The levels of lead, arsenic, and cadmium in your soil are of particular concern for health reasons. At our farm, we test our soil twice a year, so we have up-to-date information about what amendments we need to add. Your state's agriculture extension service will test samples of your soil for little or no cost, although they don't always test for heavy metals. If your state does not, the University of Massachusetts Extension Service does offer this service and will also help you interpret the results. Instructions on how to correct any deficiencies or excess minerals will be included with your test results.

Preparing

The work of gardening actually begins a year before you plant anything. That's when you start preparing the soil, so it's ready to nourish vegetable plants, and create raised beds for your crops. For the new grower, I suggest starting with a plot no larger than about 20 by 20 feet.

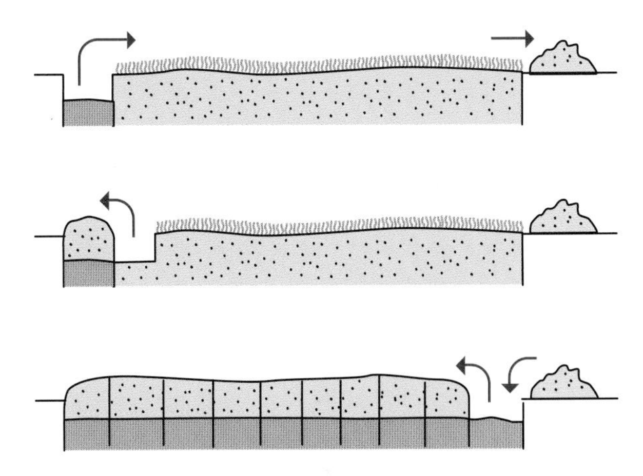

Double digging

Remove Grass and Weeds

In the early summer, the year before you want to grow vegetables, turn the grass over to kill the roots and seeds of any weeds or grass in the soil. The best way to do this is to plow your field or, if you have a small space and don't have a plow, "double dig." Double digging loosens the soil more than 1 foot down to create a more favorable environment where plant roots can thrive.

Mark out your bed and, starting at one end, dig a small trench 1 foot wide by 1 foot deep, placing the removed dirt in a wheelbarrow. Next, use a spading fork to loosen the soil in the bottom of the trench, going down another 10 inches or so. When you're done, make a second trench next to the first, only this time, you can take the dirt removed from trench #2 and place it in trench #1. Loosen the soil at the bottom of the second trench with the spading fork. Continue making trenches and moving the soil to the previous trench until you have completed the entire plot. At the end, use the soil from trench #1 that you placed in the wheelbarrow to fill the final trench. This is a fantastic workout as well!

After you turn over the grass, I suggest you try "stale bedding," which is simply running through the garden with a tiller every couple weeks until the fall. Depending on the size of the garden, this can be done by hand with a spading fork or stirrup hoe, or by machine with a rototiller. (A rototiller will save you time, but if you don't have one and your plot is relatively small, consider stale bedding to be your workout of the day). Stale bedding kills grass as well as any broadleaf weeds, and it gets rid of grubs that thrived in the pastured environment and would love to eat the roots of your vegetables.

Stirring up your garden plot through double digging and stale bedding introduces oxygen to your soil. The next step is to add compost.

Add Compost

In the spring about a year after you started turning over the soil, it's time to add compost. Apply about ½ to 1 inch of compost throughout the garden and mix it into your soil. This is the year you're going to plant!

It is imperative that the compost you use in your garden has been well managed. I cannot stress how important this is. In 2011, dozens of farms near ours were devastated by compost that contained not only glass, syringes, and other garbage in it, but also herbicides that prevented vegetables from growing. Do not buy compost from anywhere but an organic composting facility, which should happily provide you with a third-party analysis of their compost. Generally, though, the best option is to use your own compost, so you always know exactly what's in it. For that reason, it's best to start a compost pile when you start turning over the soil, about a year before you plant.

Form Your Beds

Raised beds are by far the best way for the home gardener to grow vegetables. Despite the name, raised beds aren't really lifted off the ground. It simply means that the area you've been working is surrounded by an edging and the soil is built up within the growing area. Compared to in-ground gardens, raised beds warm up earlier in the spring, are easier to weed, and have fewer problems with diseases and pests. You can use rocks, bricks, or wood to edge your beds, or you can use low-lying plants like creeping thyme. Avoid using pressure-treated wood, tires, concrete, or any other material that has chemicals that can leach into the soil.

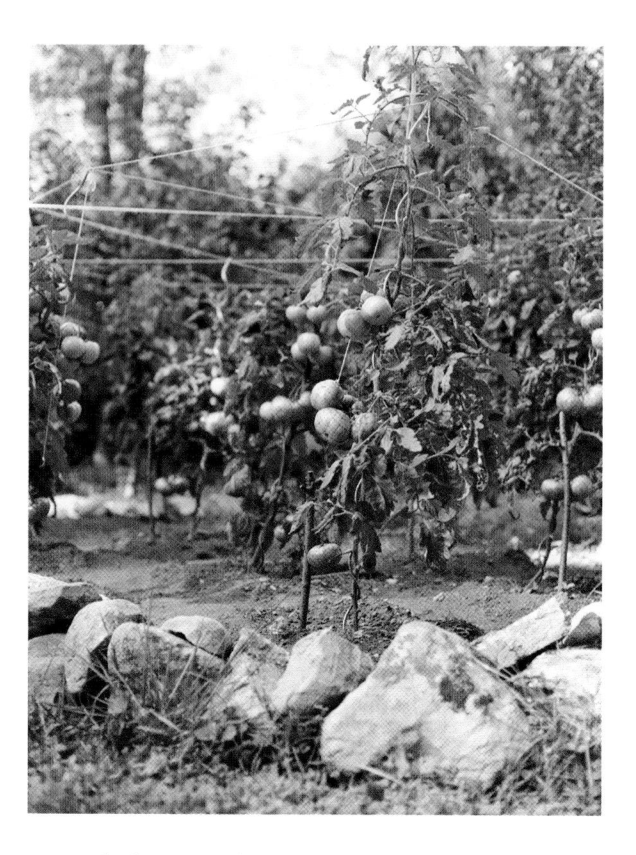

Weed the Garden

I know what you're thinking: *Why weed now, when I haven't planted anything?* But it's much easier to weed now than when vegetables are growing in the bed. Your newly formed raised beds are an ideal growing space for all plants, including weeds, and they'll be germinating beneath the soil in response to the tilled soil and compost. Drag a hoe through the soil, or pull the weeds out by hand and feed them to your chickens. It only takes a few minutes now and saves hours of backbreaking work later.

Planting

Plant

Some crops can be "direct seeded"—the seeds are sown right in the soil—while others do best when seedlings are transplanted. In the chapter on planting (page 117) we'll cover the most common crops for home gardeners and tell you which to direct seed and which to transplant.

Remember to space vegetables appropriately. Less is always more with gardening. Providing enough space between plants isn't just about how far apart you plant them; it's also about how well you prune them. One tomato plant spaced appropriately yields more tomatoes than two plants crowded together, it has less disease and insect pressure, and as long as it's pruned properly (see page 129), it puts its energy into a select few fruits instead of lots of little fruits. Proper spacing also allows more sunlight to hit the leaves so they stay drier, leading to healthier plants with less fungal disease. If you're not sure how much space a plant needs, just follow the directions on the seed packet.

Fertilize

Fertilize at the same time you plant. I recommend using a certified organic granular fertilizer. Conventional fertilizers are tremendous at making plants prolific, but they're terrible for the soil. Chemical fertilizers are prepared from inorganic materials and contain harmful acids, which stunt the growth of microorganisms and leach into rivers and streams, poisoning fish and wildlife. Conventionally fertilized gardens have much greater problems with disease and insect pressure, and the leaves of conventionally fertilized plants grow too quickly—you want your vegetables to grow sturdy and strong, not leggy and weak. Organic fertilizers, on the other hand, simply feed the soil, which in turn feeds the plants.

Water

Right after planting, give the plants a drink. Unless you're planting in the rain, don't wait for nature to take care of watering your plants.

Mulch

Covering the exposed soil between the crops helps hold in moisture, prevents weeds, and keeps soil temperatures cooler during a hot summer. There are lots of natural options for mulch, such as straw, or you can plant "living mulch," such as New Zealand white clover or creeping thyme. If you're using hay or straw, be very careful of seeds, which will become weeds in your garden. I also highly suggest avoiding bark mulch. The minute you put down a ground cover, the microbes in the soil begin to try to break it down. Straw is easy to break down and doesn't require much energy. Bark mulch, however, takes tons of energy from your microbes and drains the nitrogen stores in the soil very quickly, leaving few nutrients for your plants. (Acid- loving blueberries are the only crop for which this doesn't apply, and we mulch our blueberry plants thickly with bark chips.)

Maintaining

Set up a weekly maintenance program for the garden and build the time it needs into your schedule. The bigger your garden, the more time you need to devote to it. It takes about fifteen minutes to weed a vegetable garden that is 1,000 square feet. That's only if there is not a weed to be seen in the garden, however—you need to weed before any weeds are really visible, when they are the size of microgreens. This is where mulching helps; it prevents weeds from growing and saves you lots of labor. If a 1,000-square-foot garden has been neglected and weeds have taken over (which can happen very quickly), it can take you days to reclaim it from the weeds.

CARING FOR YOUR GARDEN: WEEKLY TASKS

Weeding: 15 to 20 minutes once or twice a week for a 20-by-20-foot garden

Watering: 15 minutes or as needed

Harvesting: 30 minutes to 1 hour, depending on the season

Scouting (looking for pests and disease): 15 minutes. You can do this while you weed to save time. Keep in mind, though, that if you have kids weeding your garden, they might not notice an emerging pest or disease problem.

Total: 1 hour, 15 minutes to 1 hour, 50 minutes each week

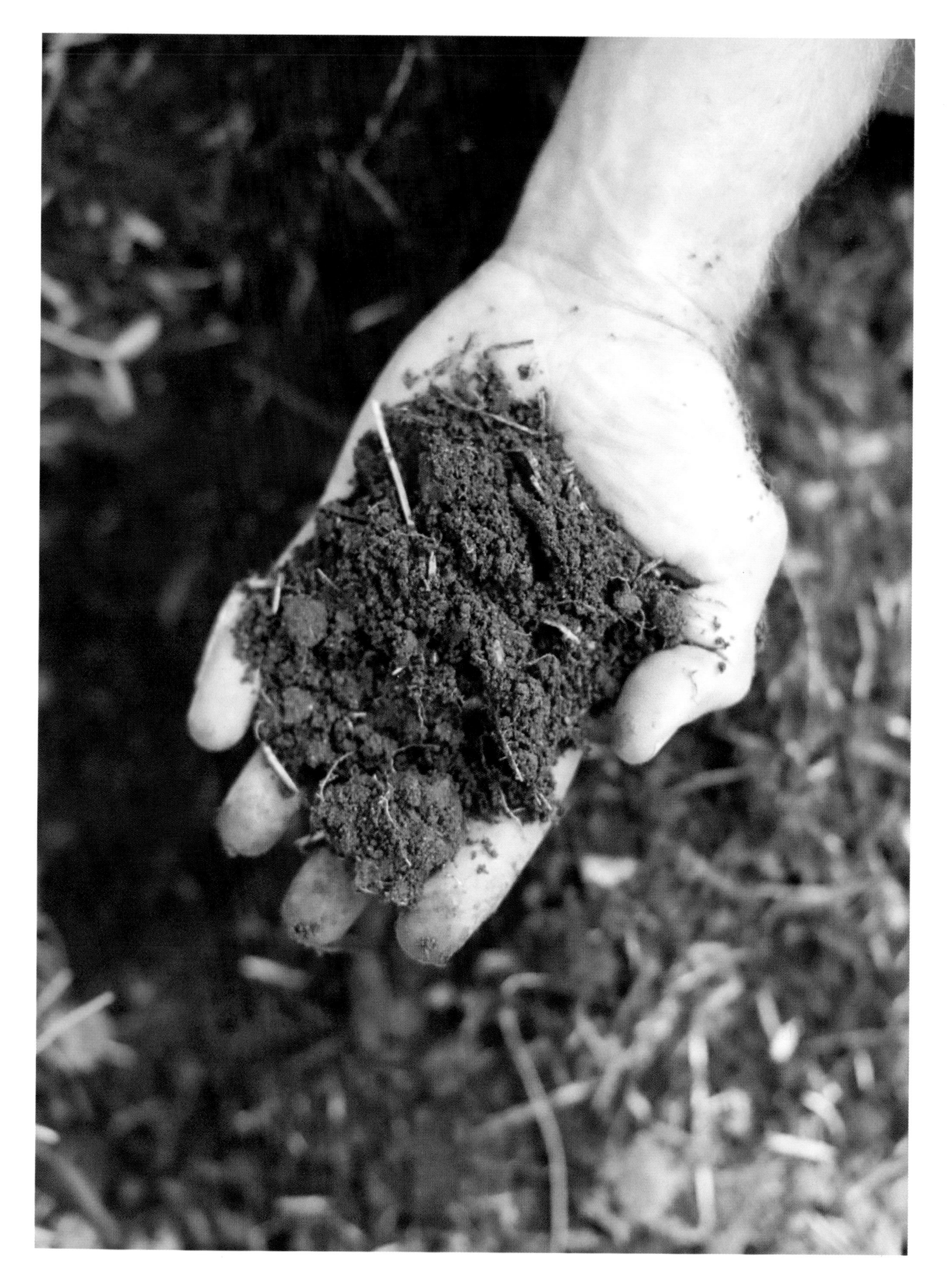

Building Healthy Soil

Soil is the foundation of an organic gardener's success. You cannot grow good crops unless you have good soil, end of story. Chemical fertilizers give conventional farmers a much better chance of success growing in poor soil, while organic crops grown in poorly managed soil tend to be small, misshapen, diseased, and riddled with insect damage.

Soil is an incredibly interesting, endlessly complex subject. Scientists are far from understanding all the complex interactions that occur in it. One thing that is understood, though, is that without soil, there is no human life.

There's still no agreed-upon scientific definition of "soil," but for our purposes, we can think of it as a growing medium that is required in order to grow crops. This growing medium is composed of:

- **The parent material,** made of sand, silt, and/or clay. This is the anchor for the plant roots and a magnet that nutrients cling to.
- **Organic matter,** living organisms as well as dead ones. This material holds onto water like a sponge, houses beneficial microbes, and sops up fertilizer.
- **Air space,** which allows roots to breathe.

When it comes to soil, growing crops can be thought of as a really slow, inefficient mining operation. A farmer comes along, digs up the grass or clears the forest, and then sows seeds. The seeds germinate and grow into plants. As the plants grow, they use their roots to find the minerals and water they need within the soil. Once the plants are mature, the farmer removes them from the field. All the minerals, metals, nutrients, and organic matter that the harvested plants drew from the soil are now gone—they've been mined out of the soil. While the amount of material each plant takes from the soil is minute, as this process is repeated year after year, generation after generation, the soil becomes depleted. As responsible growers, it's our job to return those mined nutrients to the soil.

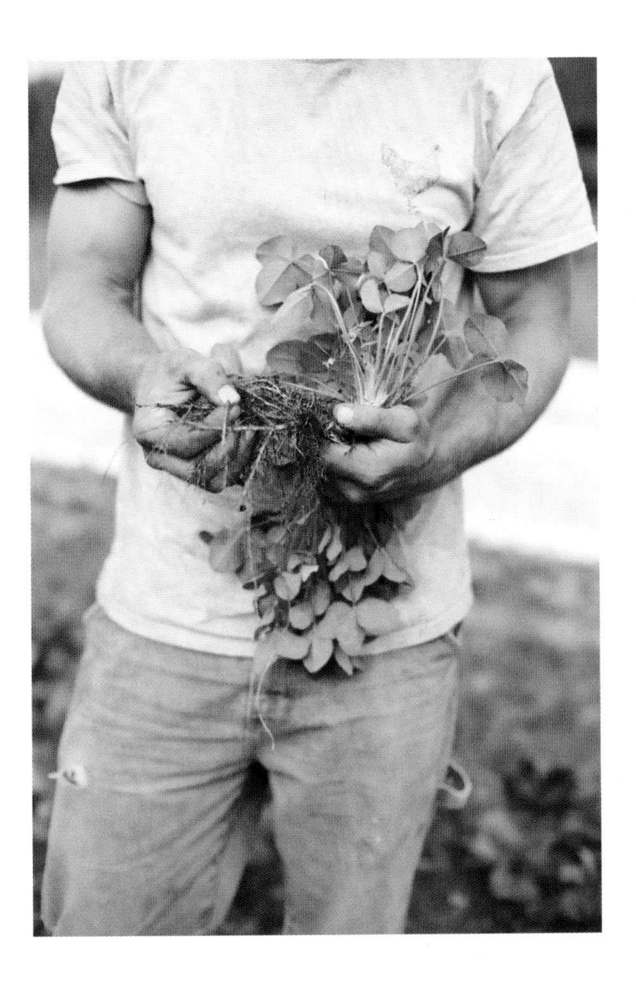

Think of your soil as a massive bank account. You cannot keep withdrawing from this account year after year without making deposits. Our withdrawals are crops, and our deposits are minerals and organic matter in the form of animal inputs and compost. Every year, our goal should be to deposit more than we withdraw.

Animal Inputs: Blood, Bones, and Poop

The composition of the parent material that dominates your soil depends on where you live. Chances are, if you live in the South, you have a clay soil. If you live near a river, you probably have a silty soil. On our farm in the Northeast, we have a lot of sandy loam. Some parent material is more beneficial for plants than others, but while you can't change the parent material of your soil, you can improve your soil's fertility by adding organic material.

By far, the best organic material to add to your soil is derived from animals, whether it's composted manure, dried blood, bone meal, or best of all, the manure left by living animals rotating through your garden. Consider the soil of the Midwest, one of the most fertile soils in the world. Americans did not invent this soil. It is not a product of our work ethic or ingenuity. It developed over thousands of years through symbiosis with herds of large herbivores, which migrated through the plains of the Midwest, grazing on the wild grasses, leaving their droppings behind, and ultimately dying on the plains. This symbiosis between herbivore, grass, and soil provided the soil of the Midwest with a fertility that has lasted many generations.

On our farm, we plant a cover crop such as oats on our vegetable beds in the fall and allow the animals to graze through, which fertilizes the soil. After the animals eat down the crop, the cover crop's roots help keep the dirt in place over the winter, cutting down on soil erosion. If you are not able to have animals such as chickens, sheep, or goats rotate through your vegetable garden, use composted manure and bagged organic fertilizers that contain blood meal—dried blood, which contains vital nitrogen for your soil—and bone meal—steamed, ground bones, which provide phosphorus and calcium.

Compost

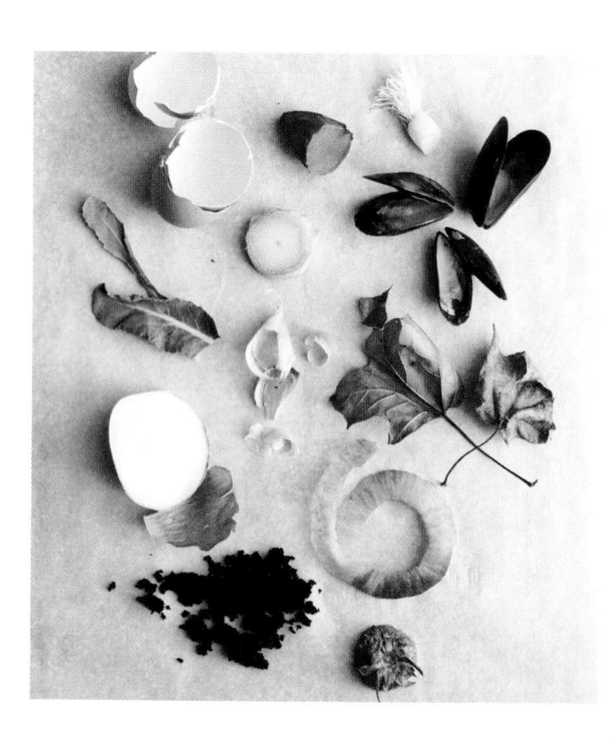

Compost is a very effective way of returning nutrients to the land, and on our farm, it's critical to the way we manage our soil fertility. While we do use fish emulsion and bagged organic fertilizer early in the spring, as we are preparing the soil for planting, compost provides the overwhelming majority of our soil input. We typically apply about 1 to 2 inches of compost throughout our vegetable fields early in the spring. The rest of the year we build compost piles and turn them, getting them ready to apply to the fields the next spring.

Compost has several advantages over conventional fertilizers and even bagged organic fertilizers. Well-made compost supplies your garden with lots of organic matter, billions upon billions of beneficial bacteria, many different micronutrients, and all the essential macronutrients for healthy plant growth.

Building Your Own Compost System

The compost system you use really depends on where you live, although in all compost systems, the ratio should be about thirty parts brown (dead leaves, straw, old hay) to one part green (kitchen scraps, manure, grass clippings). Many resources say the ratio should be three parts brown material to one part green, but in most situations, this will create an anaerobic environment—which means a stinky mess for the backyard homesteader. The ratio doesn't have to be exactly thirty to one, but the closer you get to that, the more oxygen your compost pile will have, creating a healthier environment for proper breakdown.

Here are some composting tips to help you get started.

Urban: Some cities make composting easy by offering curbside pickup of compostable materials; you can then purchase the finished compost, which supports the municipal composting system. If your city doesn't offer this, or you want to compost behind your building, consider buying a compost tumbler—it's basically a barrel with air holes on the sides and a screw-top lid, and it rotates on a frame. We have tested a bunch, and while they aren't optimal, the fact that they're small and have a lid that keeps out large animals may make them the best option in a big city. Be sure to not add animal products to a compost tumbler, as this will attract animals, some of which, like rats and mice, can fit through a compost tumbler's air holes.

Suburban: The three-pile system is a great way to produce compost without creating a mess. Build a container with three bays: the first bay is for new material, the second bay is for material in the cooking phase (nothing should be added to it), and the third bay is for finished compost. Be careful about adding animal products to this system; it can draw raccoons, rats, and other pests. Because the volume of material is small, it's difficult to keep food scraps buried in each pile. Covering the bays with chicken wire can help keep pests out.

To start your three-pile compost system, make sure you have enough material to get the compost cooking quickly—about 90 gallons of brown material (a pile about the size of a kitchen island) and about 3 gallons of green material. Sprinkle a dusting of high-calcium lime on the ground in the first bay; worms will bring this up into the compost from underneath, which helps adjust the pH and gets things really rocking in the compost pile.

Next, spread several inches of brown material, then add about 1 inch of green material on top of the brown. Continue to layer brown and green material in this fashion until you have used up your green material. The final layer should be a thick layer of brown material. Sprinkle water over your finished compost pile to get it wet. Depending on the time of year, the pile will shrink.

In about four weeks (depending on the temperature and how active your compost pile is), the pile will be about one-third the size of the original pile or smaller. This is when it's time to move it to the second bay. With a pitchfork, transfer the "cooked" compost from bay 1 to bay 2. Mix up the contents of bay 2 well. The compost in bay 2 can stay there until a new batch of compost is ready to be moved from bay 1 to bay 2; at that point, move the pile from bay 2 to bay 3.

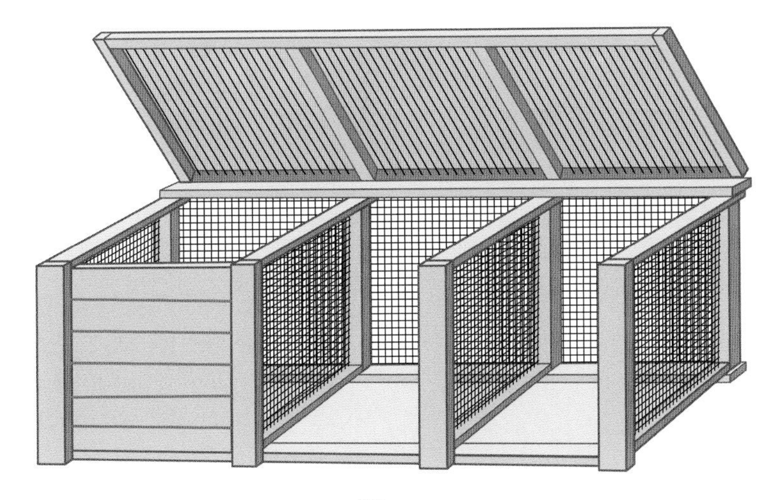

Compost container for a three-pile system

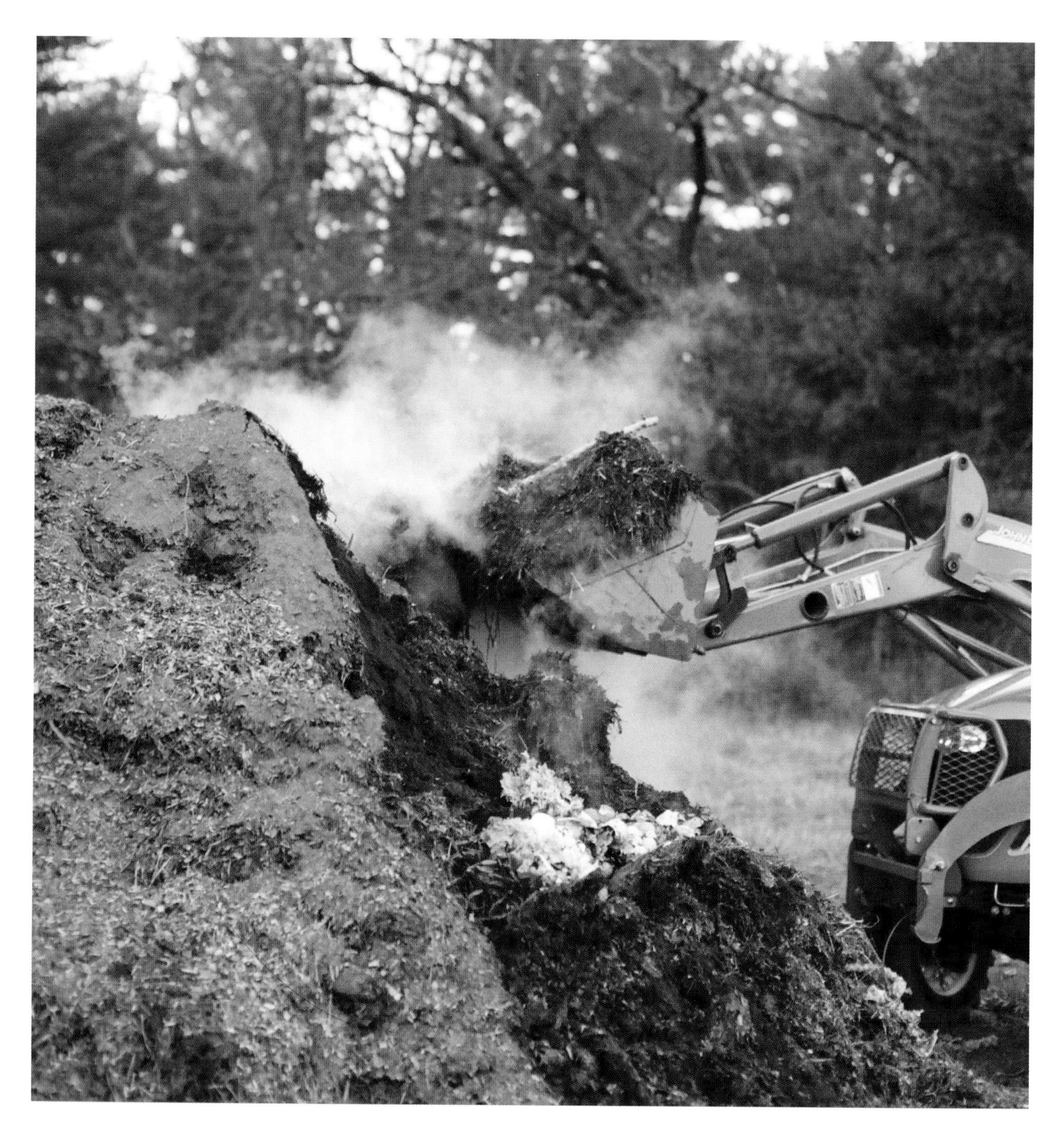

Rural: If you live in a rural area and have a lot of space—at least 70 by 70 feet—we like windrow composting, in which compost is heaped into very long, narrow piles called windrows. The shape and surface area of the windrows create the ideal conditions for decomposition. Start by accumulating compostable materials in a holding area. When you have enough material, mix it all together and pile it in a windrow that's about 8 feet high and 12 feet wide; that provides the optimal surface area while still allowing the pile to heat up. The windrow can be hundreds of feet long. The pile should be turned at least once a month (we use a bucket loader for this job). All compostable materials can be added to this system, even animal products—when we find a dead chicken on the farm, we add it to the compost pile. The bones and blood from the animal add precious nutrients to the compost.

Crop Rotation

Rotating crops in and out of fields reduces the occurrence of serious soilborne plant diseases and slows the depletion of certain minerals in the soil. Industrial agriculture has shown that monocropping year after year causes parasites, worms, bacteria, and fungus to build up in the soil. With a constant supply of a specific food (your tomato plants, for example) year after year, their populations continue to grow until you can no longer produce a marketable or economically sustainable crop. If you do not rotate your crops and they develop a soilborne disease, you may not be able to grow certain types of vegetables on that soil for decades, if ever.

Although you may think of crop rotation as something that's done on large farms, you can practice it on a smaller scale in the homestead garden. Divide your garden space into designated sections for each kind of crop you're growing. Ideally each section would be one raised bed, to reduce the chances of disease spreading from one section to another. Crops can then be divided into six categories: cucurbits (such as squash, cucumbers, melons, and zucchini), nightshades (such as tomatoes, potatoes, peppers, eggplant, and okra), alliums (such as onions, garlic, leeks, and chives), legumes (such as string beans and peas), brassicas (such as arugula, broccoli, kale, cabbage, and turnips), and, in the last category, lettuce, beets, and carrots. (Yes, I know they're from different families, but for crop rotation it's easier to treat them as one.)

The diagram here is just an example of how crop rotation might work; you don't have to rotate the categories in this specific order. Just plant a different category of crop in each section of the garden each year, and try to rotate them in such a way that a category isn't repeated in a section for at least four years.

DON'T EXHAUST THE SOIL!

Throughout my growing career I have advised homesteaders and gardeners on how to have healthy soil. The biggest problem I commonly see is exhausted soil: it's been worked intensively for thirty years and is simply depleted of minerals and nutrients. In response to dwindling vegetable yields, the gardener adds more and more fertilizer, but yields continue to decrease and disease continues to increase. The solution? Let the exhausted soil rest!

Since biblical times, farmers have been preaching the importance of a fallow period that lasts one or two seasons. While the land is resting, though, it can still be productive. At our farm, we seed fields that will lie fallow with a pasture mix of grasses and legumes, and we allow the animals graze on them during the growing season. This has three benefits: it keeps the fields generating income, it feeds our sheep and goats, and it fertilizes the soil with the animals' manure.

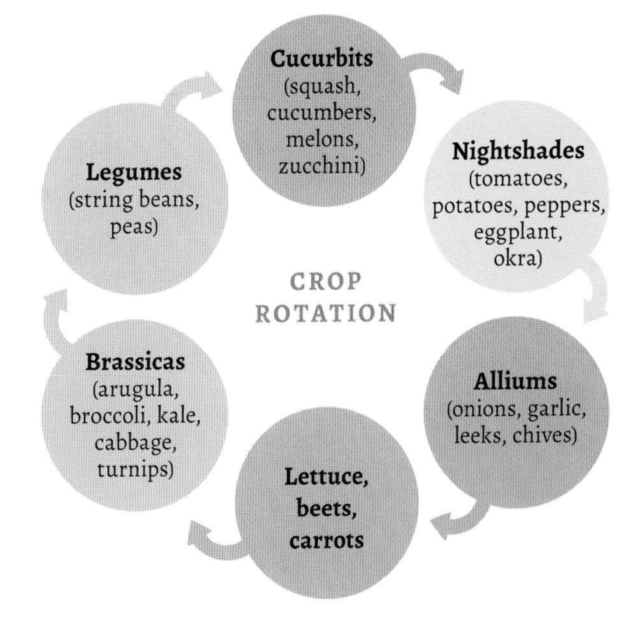

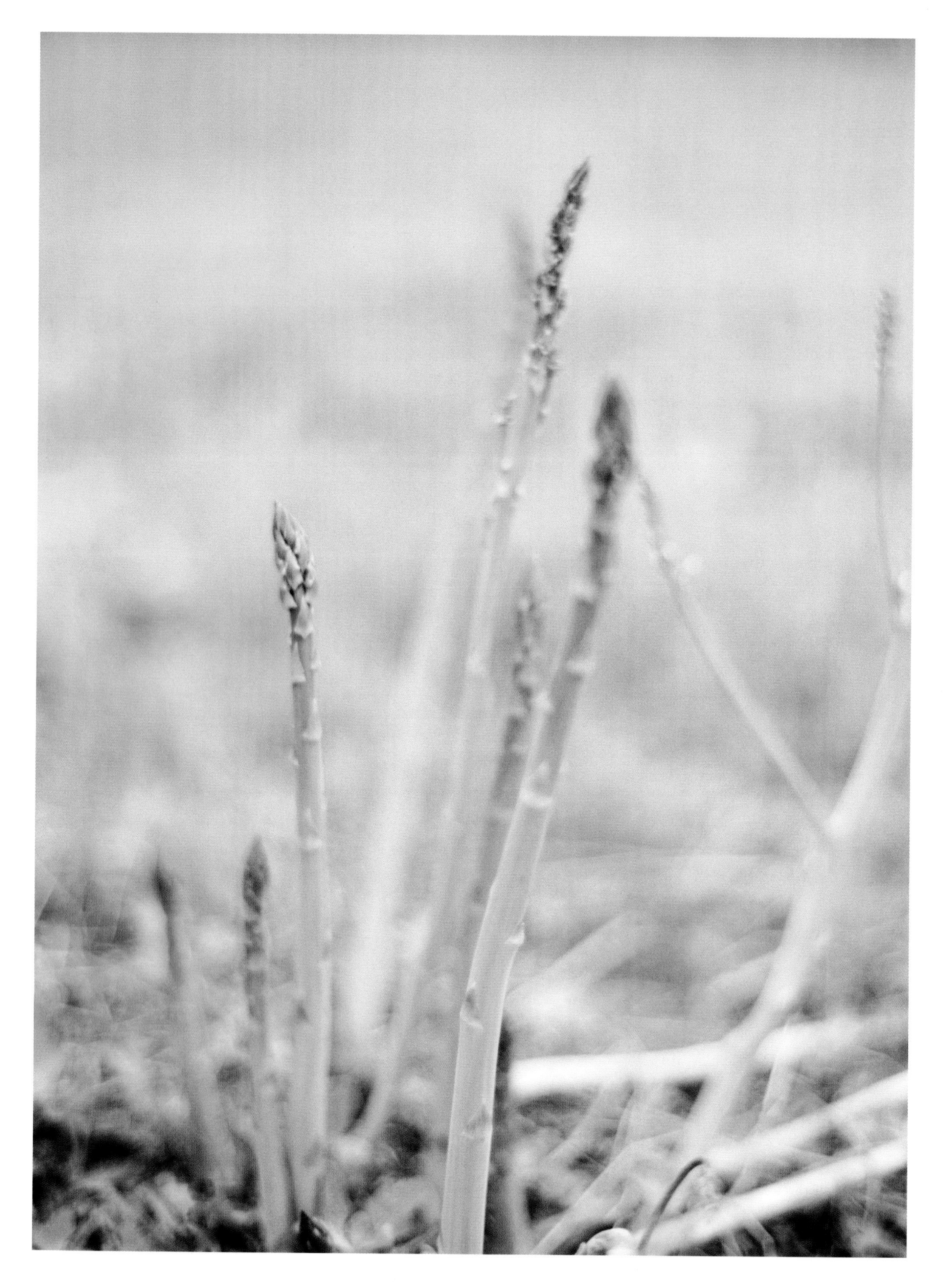

Planting

LIFE ON EARTH WOULD BE IMPOSSIBLE WITHOUT PLANTS. THROUGH PHOTOSYNTHESIS, THE PROCESS BY WHICH THEY USE SUNLIGHT TO SYNTHESIZE FOOD FROM CARBON DIOXIDE AND WATER, PLANTS MAINTAIN ATMOSPHERIC OXYGEN LEVELS AND SUPPLY ALL THE ORGANIC COMPOUNDS AND MOST OF THE ENERGY NECESSARY FOR LIFE ON EARTH.

With your garden plot set up, the grass turned over, and the soil prepared, it's time to plant your vegetables and make your own contribution to the life and health of the planet—not to mention, a very tasty, healthy contribution to your dinner table!

Plant Hardiness Zones

Average Annual Low Temperature

2. -40°F through -50°F
3. -30°F through -40°F
4. -20°F through -30°F
5. -10°F through -20°F
6. 0°F through -10°F
7. 10°F through 0°F
8. 20°F through 10°F
9. 30°F through 20°F
10. 40°F through 30°F

The U.S. Department of Agriculture provides a map outlining the zones where different plants thrive, based on average minimum winter temperatures. Figure out the zone you're in and when your last frost is. This will guide you in deciding when to sow your seeds or start your seedlings.

Seeds and Seedlings

Whether you sow seeds directly in the ground or transplant seedlings depends largely on the plant—we'll cover that later in the chapter.

It's absolutely worth seeking out organic seeds for your home garden, for many of the same reasons it's worth seeking out organic produce. Chemical pesticides and fungicides are used on the plant sources of nonorganic seeds, and they can affect the seeds and offspring. In addition, nonorganic seeds are often specifically treated with fungicides. Even herbicides can be a problem with nonorganic seeds: a chemical commonly used by commercial farmers to kill weeds is unsafe for our intestinal bacteria, which play a role not just in our digestive system but also in our immune, endocrine, and neurological systems. Chemical herbicides have also been linked to sterility, birth defects, and cancer in humans, and in animals such as birds, butterflies, and amphibians, major damage has already been documented. Unless you're buying organic seeds, you may be getting seeds that have been sprayed with all these chemicals, and the resulting plants may be affected.

Make sure the seeds you buy are also not genetically modified organisms (GMO). Contrary to common perception, GMOs aren't like hybrid plants, which have been around for thousands of years and often occur in nature. Hybrid plants are created by cross-pollinating two different plant species that are usually closely related—grapefruit, for instance, is a cross between a pomelo and a sweet orange. GMOs, on the other hand, are created by splicing genes from bacteria, viruses, animals, or other plants into crops—for example, a gene found in fish can be spliced into tomatoes, and rice can end up with daffodil and bacteria genes. Although GMO companies claim that their seeds are completely safe for human consumption, the jury is still out, and in fact, more than sixty countries have outlawed or restricted the use of GMOs. (For a list of companies that sell organic, non-GMO seeds, see page 398.)

Unless you have a hoop house or a large sunny spot in your home, it's usually better to purchase seedlings from a reputable organic farmer or garden center than to grow them yourself. But make sure you buy from the one who actually propagates the seedlings—otherwise, you may be buying seedlings that were grown at a disease-laden, out-of-state factory.

However, if you are dead set on starting your own seedlings from scratch and you don't have a hoop house, you can buy a setup or hack a DIY grow light shelving unit.

For this kind of setup, you'll need:

- A five-tier shelving unit (74 by 48 inches)
- Four 48-inch, full-spectrum fluorescent shop lights
- Eight S-hooks
- A power strip with timer
- Potting soil
- Germination trays with water liners
- Labels
- A spray bottle
- Twelve to fourteen hours of sunlight each day

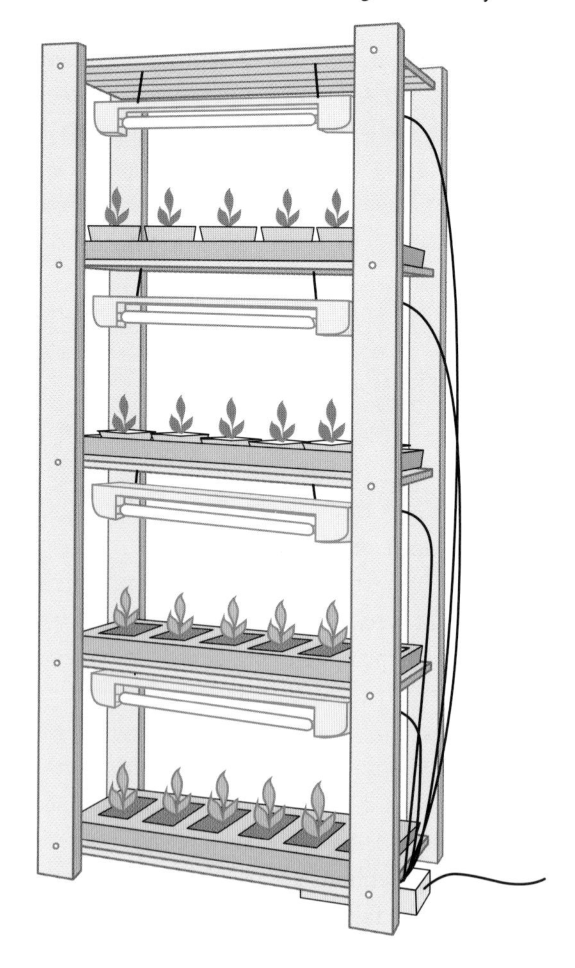

WEED MANAGEMENT

Here's a big secret that can give you unparalleled happiness and make your homestead into a nirvana: Keep your garden neat and the weeds under control. It's easy to get behind in weeding in the daily rush of work and cooking and chores, but weeds grow quickly from harmless, tiny things that can be wiped out of existence in a second with an effortless pass of a hoe, to towering monsters anchored to the ground with massive fibrous roots. And once that happens, weeds begin dropping their seeds, hundreds of thousands of them, which live in the soil for years and become even bigger problems. Plus, a weed-ridden garden is stressful to look at and doesn't produce much food, and what it does produce is small and blemished.

Whenever you walk by a weed, pull it out. If it's edible, eat it. If not, lay it out to let the sun destroy its roots. If it already has seeds on it, get it out of your garden—don't put it in your compost pile. Feed it to your chickens or pigs instead, or simply throw it out. On our farm, as soon as we have finished harvesting a crop and the animals have gone through the fields to eat any vegetative matter, I plant a cover crop so that weeds can't get established.

If you find that the weeds have gotten away from you—if you feel completely overwhelmed by the weed situation, or if they have gone to seed and more baby weeds are on their way—my advice is to start over: plow your garden under and begin again.At some point, no matter how heroic your efforts, you just can't save a garden. If it's not too late in the growing season, you can always reseed (though only if you have time to stay on top of weeding!). If it is late in the season, plow the garden under and sow a cover crop like oats, rye, clover, or hairy vetch to keep the weeds from returning before you reseed next year. You'll feel so much better about your homestead if you're looking at a lush, cover-cropped garden instead of a jungle of weeds.

After germination, use a liquid fish-based emulsion fertilizer on the seedlings every week until they are ready for transplanting. Don't wait too long to transplant the seedlings or they may get root-bound, with their roots growing so thick that they are coming out of the cell. If the seedling's leaves are yellow, it has run out of nitrogen and needs to be transplanted.

For each plant family, different signs will tell you when it's time to transplant. We'll cover those signs later in this chapter, along with the kind of care each plant family needs.

Vegetables

Alliums (garlic, leeks, onions, scallions)

Alliums prefer a rich, cool soil that's slightly alkaline, and they need lots of moisture.

Planting: Start onions, leeks, and scallions indoors about eight weeks before transplanting to your garden in early spring. During germination, keep temperatures around 70°F and water frequently. Direct seeding is also an option, depending on your climate, but you will have larger and better-quality onions with less disease if you grow or buy seedlings to transplant. Here in the Northeast, we always start them in a greenhouse. Garlic is planted directly into the soil in the fall.

Transplant leeks when they are about 6 inches high, right around the time of the last frost. Young leeks can handle a light frost.

Spacing: Space garlic and scallions 6 inches apart. Onions and leeks should be spaced 3 to 6 inches apart. Onions should be in rows 12 inches apart, but leeks require hilling (see page 120), so make sure you leave about 24 inches between rows of leeks.

Days to maturity: Onions and leeks mature about 100 days after transplanting, although some varieties of fresh onions are ready in about sixty days. Scallions mature after about seventy days. Garlic is harvested midsummer the year after it's planted.

When is it ready to harvest? I start harvesting scallions in the early summer and green onions (onions that don't have skins) in early July. Garlic scapes (the curly top shoot of a hardneck garlic plant) must be picked in early summer, before they become too fibrous; garlic itself should be harvested when a third of its leaves are brown. The flavor of leeks improves with frosts.

Onions are harvested when the bulb reaches the desired size—depending on the variety, that could be as small as a golf ball or as large as softball. Only certain onions can be stored. Storage onions contain less moisture than fresh onions and develop layers of protective, dry skins. Although it's possible to harvest and eat them early, if you'd like to store them, wait until their tops begin to dry. Check the variety to know whether your onions are storage onions or are meant to be eaten fresh.

Pests and diseases: Alliums are relatively hardy crops, but insects called onion thrips can be a problem. If thrips are common in your area, using a floating row cover (see page 123) can save your crop.

Special considerations: Onions grow best in warm, moist conditions. Some of the best soils for producing great yields are "muck soils," which are very wet and have a high organic matter content. Onions and leeks can tolerate relatively colder temperatures, and leeks can even handle freezes. Because alliums do not create a canopy over the soil, weeds are frequently a problem, so take extra care to keep your allium beds well-tended.

Our favorite varieties

- Fresh onions: Purplette
- Storage onions: Red Wing (red) and Cortland (yellow)
- Leeks: Lincoln
- Scallions: Evergreen
- Garlic: Depends on your location. Here in the Northeast, we love German Extra Hardy, but if you live in the South, you'll want a softneck variety. Check with your local garden center for a garlic variety that works in your climate.

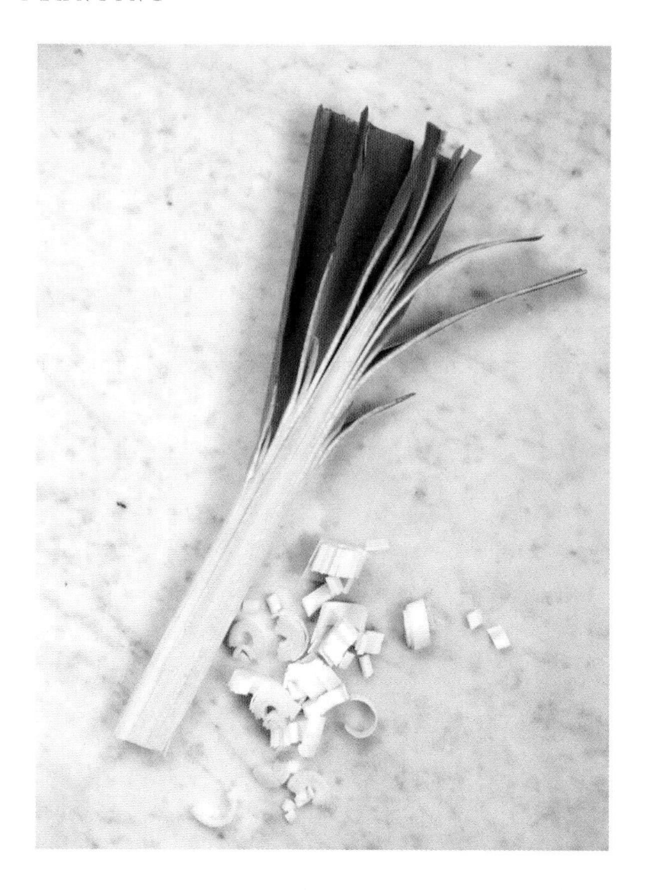

HILLING

Leeks, asparagus, and potatoes all require hilling. All that means, in practice, is that you need to occasionally build up the soil around the base of the plant. Once a week, as you weed your garden, just add some dirt around the bottom of the plants. For leeks, cover the stem with soil but keep the green tops exposed—this is what produces the white bottom part of the leek.

CURING

Before storing, onions and garlic need to be cured, which simply means drying out the excess moisture so they don't rot. Lay them out or hang them in a well-ventilated, shaded spot. Onions take about three weeks to cure and garlic can take a little longer, about one month. Do not wash the dirt off before curing, as this just adds extra moisture. Once the onions and garlic are dried, you can brush off any dirt or peel off the outer skin.

Asparagus

Asparagus is a perennial vegetable that prefers well-drained, fertile soil with a pH around 7. Unlike most vegetable crops, asparagus can tolerate partial shade, although yields are better with full sun.

Planting: Asparagus can be started from seeds or crowns. If they're started from crowns, they will have a greater yield, sooner. Begin to establish your asparagus in the early spring, as soon as the soil can be worked.

Spacing: Plant asparagus crowns 12 inches apart, with at least 4 feet between rows.

Days to maturity: Three years! Do not harvest any asparagus spears the first year. The second year, you can harvest for one week, but then you should not harvest any more. The third year, you can harvest for four weeks. After the third year, six weeks of harvest can be done. It is critical to follow this schedule to allow the plants' root structure time to develop.

When is it ready to harvest? Harvest spears when they are about 12 inches long.

Pests and diseases: In order to minimize damage from pests and diseases, keep your asparagus bed well weeded. Also, at the end of the year, be sure to cut dried ferns from the plant and remove them from the garden. Many pests and diseases can overwinter in the debris.

Special considerations: It takes a few years for asparagus roots to establish themselves, but if given proper care, a single bed will provide your house with a harvest for decades. When asparagus fails, weeds are usually the cause, so be vigilant about keeping the bed maintained. Asparagus does not grow as well in southern states.

Our favorite variety

- Jersey Knight

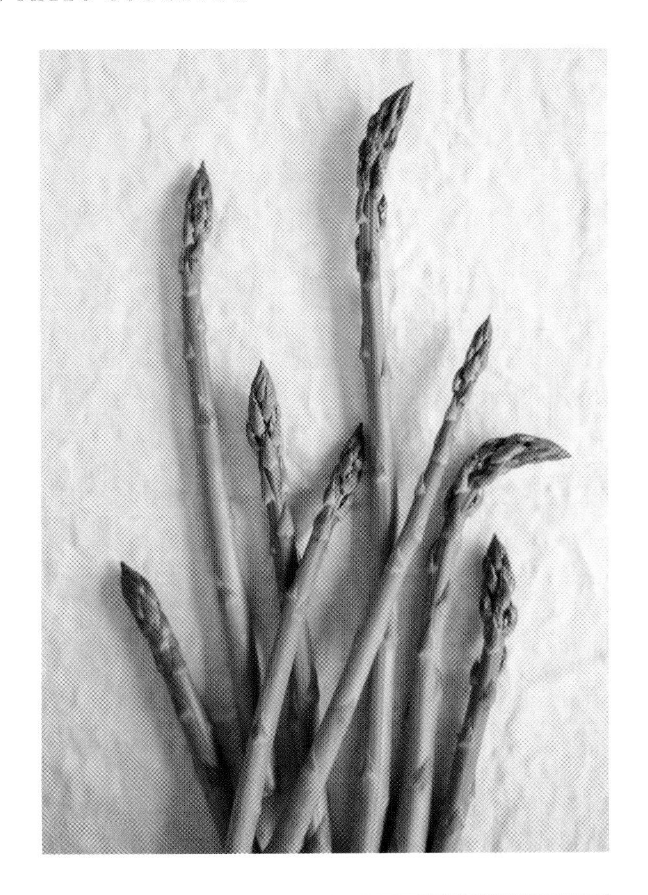

PLANTING ASPARAGUS

Planting asparagus is slightly different from planting other vegetables, but as with any garden, begin preparing your asparagus plot a year in advance. Apply aged manure to the area and weed thoroughly and repeatedly until no weeds germinate. When you are ready to plant your asparagus, dig a furrow. Space the crowns 12 inches apart in the furrow and spread out the roots. Cover the roots with 2 to 3 feet of soil. As the plants grow throughout the summer, add about 1 inch of soil per month to hill the plants, taking care not to damage the roots.

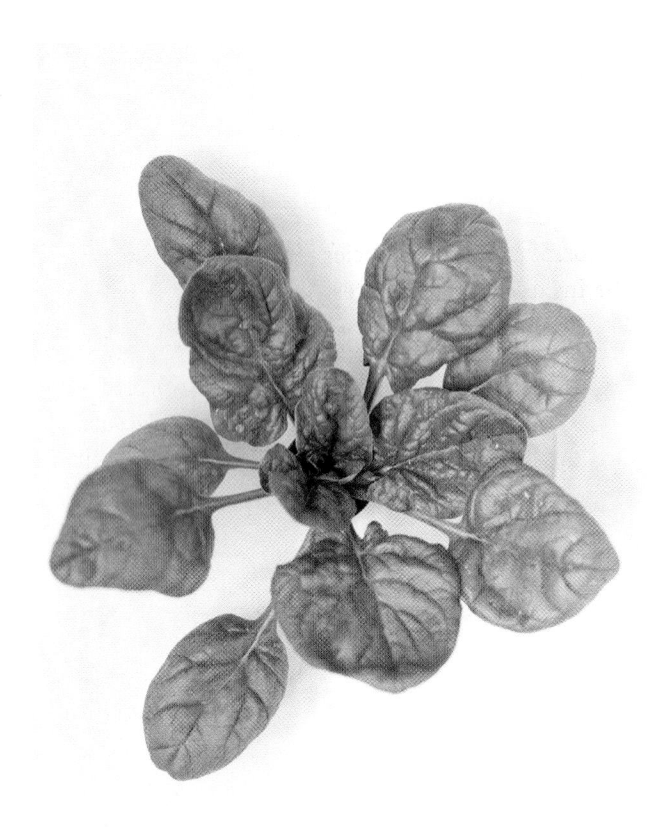

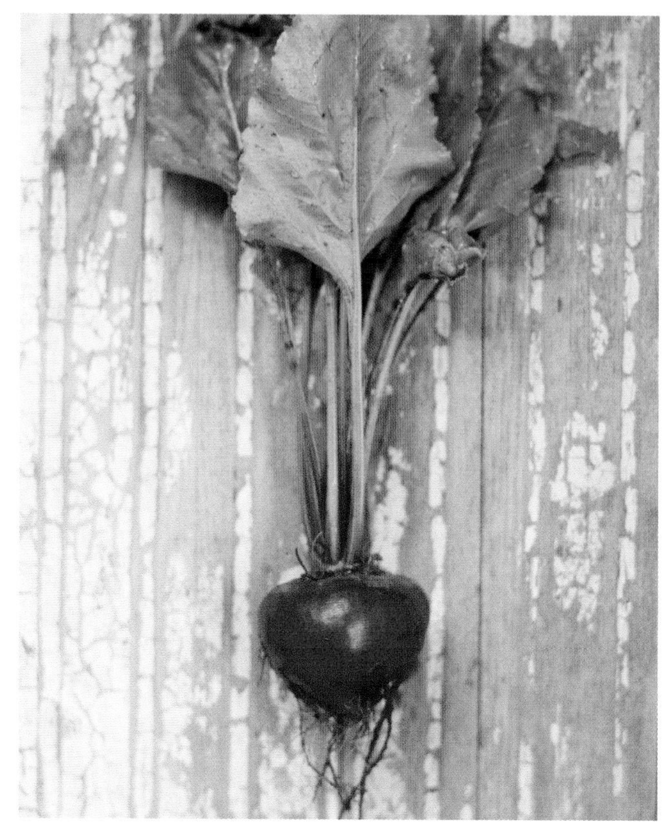

Beets, Chard, and Spinach

Beets, chard, and spinach prefer cooler temperatures and wet, pH-neutral soil with lots of organic matter.

Planting: Beets and chard can be direct seeded in the garden in the spring, once the soil has thawed enough to be worked. However, we always start them in greenhouses so that they reach harvest size faster. Freezes will stunt the growth of seedlings; do not plant until the danger of freezes has passed. Growing spinach is very difficult in hot temperatures, so plan to grow it in the spring and late fall. Beets, chard, and spinach should be transplanted before they are root-bound (have roots so thick that they come out of the cell).

Spacing: Space beet and spinach transplants every 6 inches, or thin seedlings from direct seeding to every 6 inches. While beets and spinach will grow if planted closer together, they will grow slower, they'll have less flavor, and they'll be more likely to experience disease. Space chard transplants 12 inches apart, or thin seedlings from direct seeding to 12 inches apart.

Days to maturity: Beets and chard mature about fifty days after transplanting. Spinach matures about thirty-five days after transplanting. If you direct seed, they'll need about two more weeks.

When is it ready to harvest? Beets, chard, and spinach are ready to harvest at any point after they mature, including as microgreens.

Pests and diseases: The fungus *Cercospora* is a major threat to these crops. Be sure to practice crop rotation, and don't allow standing water in the garden. If you see a puddle consistently forming in one part of the garden, work on your drainage system to get rid of it.

Our favorite varieties

- Beets: Merlin and Chioggia
- Chard: Bright Lights
- Spinach: Space

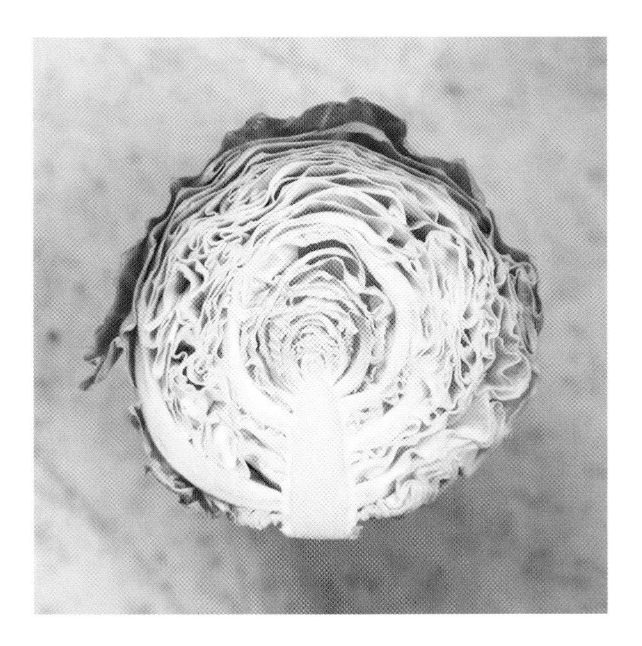

Brassicas (arugula, broccoli, Brussels sprouts, cabbage, cauliflower, kale, mustard, radishes, turnips)

Brassicas are a cool-season vegetable that prefers soil with a slightly alkaline pH and a lot of organic matter. Brassicas require consistent irrigation and thrive in a fertile soil.

Planting: Plant brassicas after any danger of a hard freeze has passed. Brassicas can handle temperatures below 32°F, although when the temperatures drop down to the mid-20s, damage is done. Radishes, turnips, and brassica greens, such as arugula, mustard, and cress, do best when direct seeded in the ground.

Broccoli, cabbage, Brussels sprouts, and cauliflower should be started indoors, or you can buy seedlings from a farm or garden center. The first two little leaves that sprout on a brassica are called cotyledons, after which the plant's "true leaves" appear. The plant will then put its energy into its true leaves and roots, and the cotyledons will die. This is the point at which you want to transplant the seedlings.

Spacing: For brassica greens, turnips, and radishes, sow one or two seeds per inch, about ¼ inch deep. Broccoli, cauliflower, and cabbage require more space. Plant one seedling every 12 inches in a row, and leave 2 feet between rows. Brussels sprouts require even more space than broccoli and cabbage. Plant one seedling every 18 inches to 2 feet, with 2 feet between rows.

Days to maturity: Brassica greens grow very quickly and are mature three weeks after seeding. Broccoli, cauliflower, and cabbage take about sixty days to mature after transplanting outside. Brussels sprouts take as many as 100 days to mature. Radishes and turnips mature within two months.

When is it ready to harvest? Brassica greens are ready pretty much as soon as you want to harvest them. Brassica microgreens are very tasty and are ready 1 week after seeding. Harvest broccoli and cauliflower as soon as florets have formed, and make sure you don't wait too long once they form. Broccoli will flower very quickly if it gets too hot. Cabbage is ready as soon as the heads are firm. Brussels sprouts are ready once the small heads have formed. Radishes are ready to be harvested at any size, although if you wait too long, they can become pithy. Turnips also can be harvested at any size, but they can stay in the field longer than radishes without danger of becoming pithy.

Pests and diseases: With brassicas, the most common pests are flea beetles and several types of moth larvae. Floating row covers are very effective at keeping brassicas free from pests. There are also several organic pesticides, such as Entrust and PyGanic, that can help control pests.

Our favorite varieties

- Arugula: Sylvetta
- Broccoli: Gypsy
- Brussels sprouts: Oliver
- Cabbage: Savoy
- Kale: Lacinato
- Mustard: Green Wave
- Radishes: D'Avignon and daikon
- Turnips: Hakurei

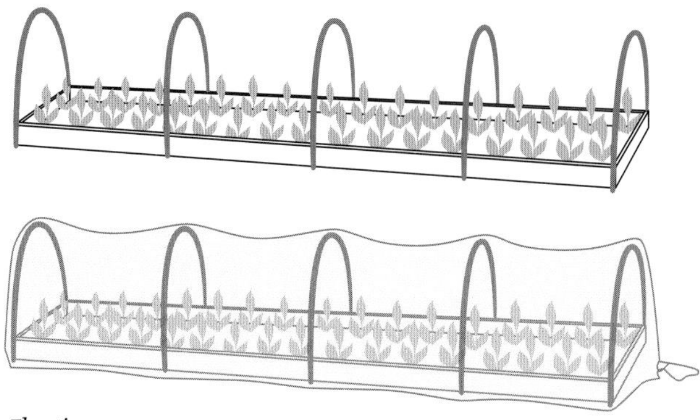

Floating row cover

Carrots and Parsnips

Carrots and parsnips thrive in a pH-neutral soil, and a loose, rock-free soil lets them grow straight. Carrots are not great at competing with weeds and do not transplant, so you have to really baby them in the early days. They don't like very warm soil, so it's best to sow carrots in the cooler months.

Planting: Carrots cannot be transplanted. Direct seed them in a row, ¼ inch deep, after the last deep freeze—in the Northeast, we seed our first planting of carrots in mid-April and continue to seed carrots until early August. Parsnips should be direct seeded in midspring, once the soil has warmed up (in New England, this means mid-May). Parsnip seeds need about three weeks to germinate and should be watered frequently. Make sure their area is kept weed-free during this germination time.

Spacing: Plant carrots in rows 12 inches apart, and once they sprout, thin them to 1 inch apart in the row. While it's possible to pack carrots closer together, overcrowded carrots take longer to mature, and their flavor can be more bitter. Parsnips need 18 inches between rows; once they sprout, thin parsnip seedlings to 1 inch apart in the row.

Days to maturity: It takes carrots about seventy-five days from direct seeding to mature. Storage varieties tend to take longer. Parsnips take a long time to grow. Most varieties don't mature until about 120 days after planting.

When is it ready to harvest? Carrots are ready to harvest anytime after they mature. Younger carrots tend to be sweeter than carrots that have been in the ground for a long time. Old, "horse carrots" also tend to be more fibrous. Carrots seeded in late summer and harvested after a frost are a special treat because they are extra sweet; our favorite variety for this is Bolero. Parsnips can be harvested at any size, but the flavor is better in older, larger parsnips. For sweeter flavor, harvest them after a frost.

Pests and diseases: Carrots and parsnips are pretty hardy overall, but wireworms, which love to eat most roots, can be a problem and are difficult to control organically. When we find wireworms in a field, we try to starve them out by not planting anything in the field for a full season, if possible.

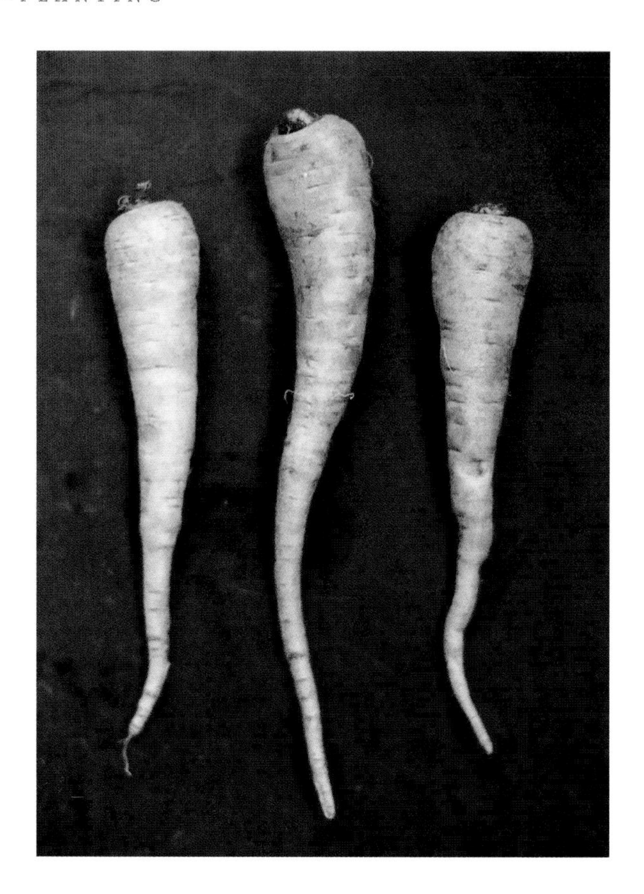

Carrots are also susceptible to some fungi, such as *Alternaria* and *Cercospora*. Crop rotation can help prevent fungi.

Special considerations: The best-tasting carrots are grown quickly. Be sure the soil is fertile and water them regularly. You can also speed up their growth by placing a floating row cover over them. Carrots are not good at competing with weeds, so be sure to stay on top of weeding. Once carrots have large tops, though, weed pressure isn't a problem. Do not weed or harvest parsnips on a hot, sunny day—a chemical in parsnip greens can cause a skin rash or blistering in direct sunlight.

Our favorite varieties

Carrots

- Sugarsnax
- Nelson
- Rainbow

Parsnips

- Javelin

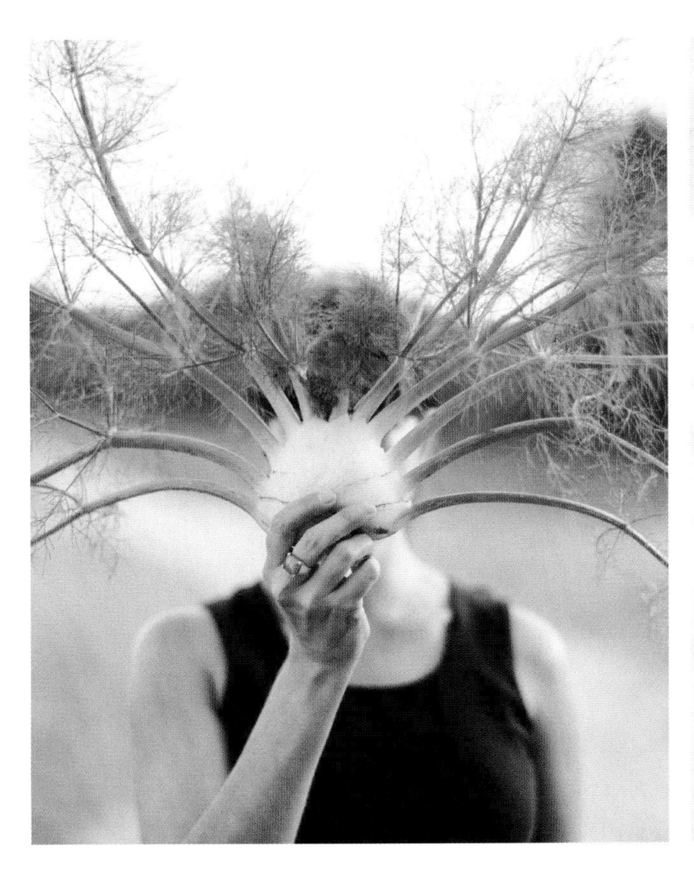

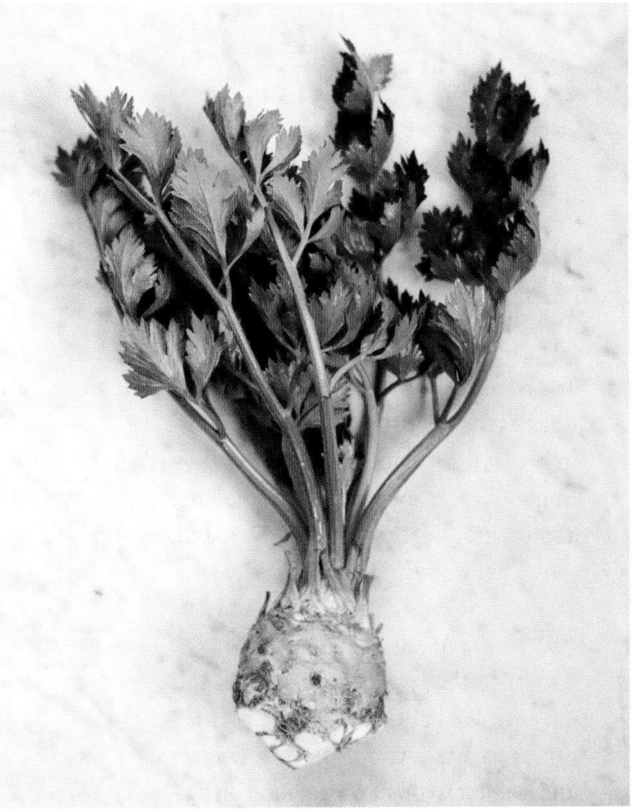

Celeriac, Celery, Fennel

Celeriac, celery, and fennel all enjoy similar growing conditions: a fertile soil with lots of organic matter and a pH between 6.0 and 7.0. Be sure you keep these plants wet and do not allow the soil to dry out; if it does, the plants become bitter.

Planting: Start seedlings about eight weeks before the last frost and transplant them outside once the danger of frost has passed.

Spacing: Plant seedlings 12 inches apart, with 12 inches between rows.

Days to maturity: Celery and fennel mature eighty days after transplanting; celeriac, about 100 days.

When is it ready to harvest? These crops can be eaten at any stage in their growth, including as microgreens.

Pests and diseases: Not many pests will bother these crops. Make sure there are adequate calcium levels in the soil to prevent blackheart disease.

Special considerations: Celery and fennel take a while to put on sizable growth. Keep beds well-watered and weeded at all times. Fennel cannot tolerate a freeze or frost. Celeriac is hardier than celery.

Our favorite varieties

- Celeriac: Mars
- Celery: Tango
- Fennel: Orion

Cucurbits (cucumbers, melons, summer squash, winter squash, zucchini)

Cucurbits prefer warm, well-drained soil with neutral pH, and they do best when the soil is rich and full of nutrients. They like full sun and do not like standing water.

Planting: Start seeds indoors four weeks before transplanting. Wait until transplants have four true leaves to ensure a good yield even if there is heavy disease and insect pressure. Alternatively, buy seedlings from a local farm or garden center.

Spacing: Space cucumbers, zucchini, and summer squash 1 foot apart, with 3 feet between rows. Plant melons and winter squash 2 to 3 feet apart, with 5 feet between rows.

Days to maturity: Cucumbers, summer squash, and zucchini mature about fifty days after transplanting. Winter squash mature about ninety to a hundred days after transplanting. Melons mature between seventy-five and ninety days from transplanting.

When is it ready to harvest? Summer squash and zucchini can be harvested at any size. The larger they get, though, the bigger the seeds in the fruit of the plant. To tell when winter squash is ready, keep an eye on its skin color. There are many different techniques for judging when a melon is ready; I wait until it's easily pulled off the vine and has a sweet scent. For watermelons, wait until the tendril opposite the fruit dries up.

Pests and diseases: The three major pests for cucurbits are striped cucumber beetles, squash bugs, and squash vine borers. To control these pests, delay transplanting seedlings until four true leaves have developed, use a floating row cover, and dust plants with kaolin clay. As a last resort, PyGanic can be an effective organic pesticide. Powdery mildew is also a major threat to cucurbits. We handle it through multiple plantings: older plants are the most affected, so by planting in succession, we have new plants bearing fruit when the older ones are most susceptible to powdery mildew.

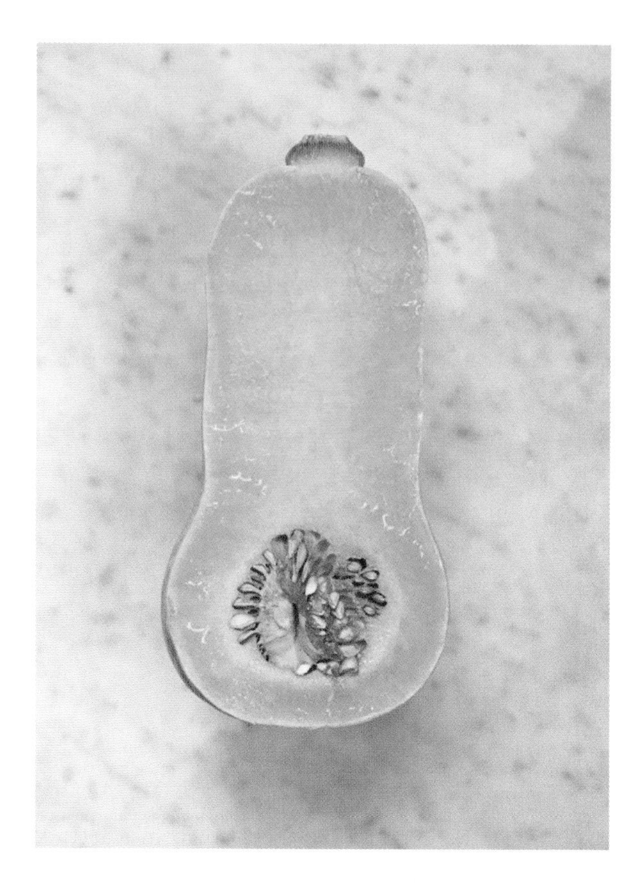

Special considerations: There are two tricks for a successful cucumber-growing season. One, transplant seedlings in batches every three weeks. Two, trellis—see the instructions for tomatoes on page 129.

Our favorite varieties

Cucumbers

- Slicing: Corinto
- Pickling: Little Leaf

Summer squash

- Magda
- Zephyr
- Pickling: Little Leaf

Zucchini

- Costata Romensco

Winter squash

- Butternut: Waltham
- Acorn: Tiptor PMR

Melons

- Watermelon: Sugar Baby
- Cantaloupe: Athena

Lettuce

Lettuce likes cooler temperatures and soil that's very wet, has a neutral pH, and has lots of organic matter. Avoid excess nitrogen in the soil or you'll have brown edges on the leaves.

Planting: Start lettuce seedlings indoors four weeks before transplanting them outside, or buy seedlings from a local farm or garden center. Transplant them into the ground after the danger of freezes has passed and the air temperature stays above 32°F. Lettuce is able to handle a frost as long as it occurs when the temperature is higher than that. Lettuce can also be direct seeded; just be sure to thin it to 12 inches apart for full-size heads. Lettuce can be planted continually throughout the growing season until about six weeks before the first killing freeze in the fall.

Spacing: For full-size heads, space transplants 12 inches apart and leave 12 inches between rows. For smaller heads, plant up to 8 inches apart.

Days to maturity: After transplanting, lettuce seedlings take about thirty days to form a lettuce head. Direct-seeded lettuce is ready in about sixty days.

When is it ready to harvest? Lettuce is ready to harvest anytime after it matures. Young, small heads tend to be sweeter than larger heads.

BOLTING

During a heat wave, many plants, especially lettuce, cilantro, basil, cabbage, and broccoli, can "bolt"—they quickly go into survival mode and send all of their energy into seed production. After bolting, the plant tastes very bitter and is basically inedible. It's not possible to prevent bolting in most plants, but to help stop basil from bolting, snap off the little flower heads—the plant will then put its energy back into leaf production. In general, keep plants well-watered when there is a lot of heat stress. If you want to enjoy salad in the summer, seek out a heat-tolerant variety of lettuce and water it frequently.

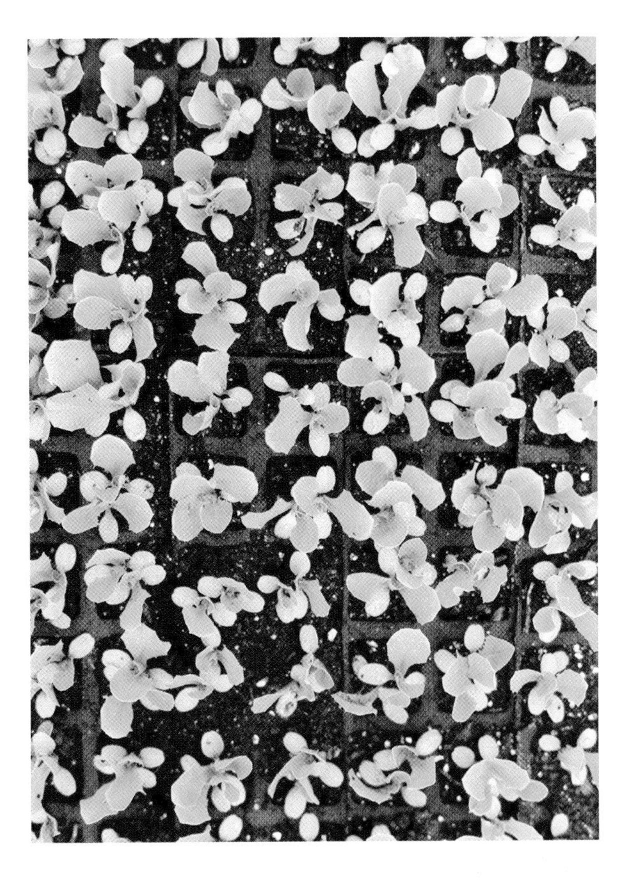

Pests and diseases: The most common pests for lettuce are slugs and cutworms. You can manage cutworms by being vigilant during weeding: whenever you notice a plant looking wilted, gently pull the soil away from the base of the plant and look for the grub, then remove it and squish it. Slugs can be removed from the leaves during the early morning, or try filling a jar lid with beer—slugs can't resist a good buzz and will drown.

Special considerations: Lettuce is very sensitive to high temperatures, so look for varieties that can tolerate high heat during the summer, and during hot weather, keep lettuce well-watered. Heat-stressed lettuce has a very bitter taste.

Our favorite varieties

- Romaine: Jericho
- Leaf: Panisse
- Heat-tolerant: Panisse and Skyphos
- Cold-tolerant: Winter Density

Nightshades (eggplants, peppers, tomatoes)

Nightshades prefer a warm, well-drained, acidic soil, with a pH between 5.5 and 6.0.

Planting: Tomatoes can be direct seeded or started as seedlings, but peppers and eggplants should be started indoors and transplanted after eight to ten weeks, when the first set of flowers appears. All three should be planted outdoors after any danger of frost has passed. In the Northeast, it is safe to plant after Memorial Day. If you are starting tomatoes from seeds, it's critical that you do not start too early! Tomatoes grow very quickly, and leggy tomato plants are more disease-prone and have lower yields.

Spacing: Nightshades require lots of space—plant seedlings 18 to 24 inches apart.

Days to maturity: Tomatoes begin to yield fruit about seventy days after transplanting. Peppers and eggplants yield fruit after about sixty-five days.

When is it ready to harvest? For tomatoes, firmness is often a safer indicator of maturity than color. An unripe tomato is very firm, while an overripe tomato is very soft. A perfectly ripe tomato should have just a little "give" when you press it. Tomatoes can be harvested early to mature off the vine, which is particularly helpful if there is a danger of frost in your area. With peppers, on the other hand, color is a good gauge of ripeness. Many people don't know this, but all green peppers are simply immature—most turn red as they ripen (though some turn orange or yellow). Bell peppers can be harvested when they're green or red (or yellow or orange, depending on the variety). Even jalapeños will turn red, but it takes a long time. Eggplants can be harvested at any time, as soon as they reach the size you want. We like to harvest them when they are relatively small and taste less bitter. Many cultures eat eggplants when they are no larger than a finger.

Pests and diseases: Common tomato pests are whiteflies, tomato hornworms, and tobacco hornworms. All three can be controlled if you're vigilant about maintenance. Colorado potato beetles love eggplant, and although they're generally manageable, if left unchecked, they can lead to a complete crop disaster. Squishing bugs is a very effective method of controlling outbreaks.

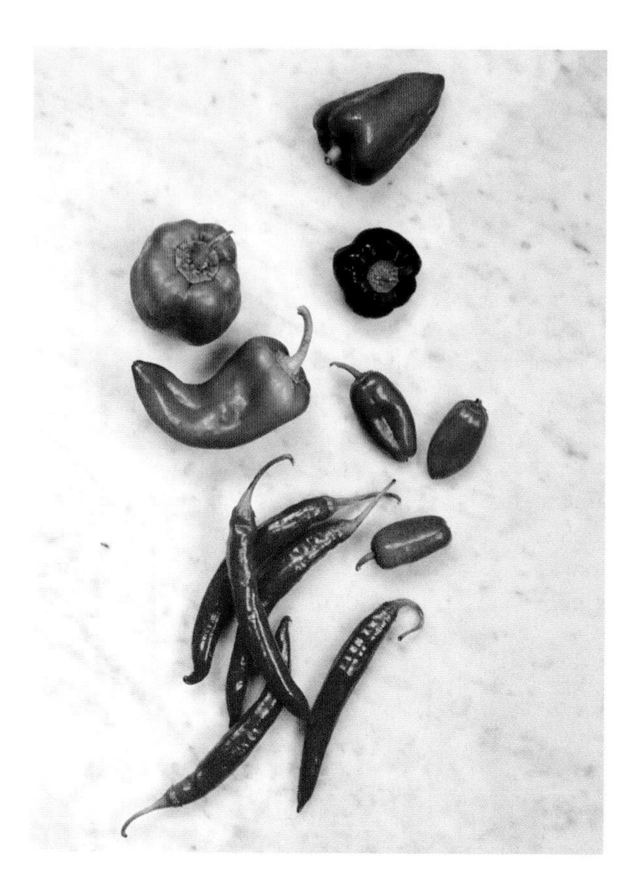

Special considerations: Peppers have a higher yield if they are given a cold treatment early in their development. Once a seedling has two sets of true leaves, subject it to temperatures around 50°F for several hours by placing it outside on a cool day. Repeat this daily for one week, and the plant will bear more fruit.

Our favorite varieties

Tomatoes

- Cherry tomatoes: Sun Gold
- Slicers: Striped German
- Plum tomatoes: San Marzano

Peppers

- Bell peppers: Lipstick and Lunchbox
- Hot peppers: Joe's Long Cayenne

Eggplant

- Orient Express
- Calliope

GROWING HEALTHY, THRIVING TOMATOES

Tomatoes are one of the most popular vegetables for home gardeners. While they're relatively easy to grow, a few practices can increase their yield and help your tomato plants thrive.

- **Trellising:** Disease is by far the greatest threat to your tomato crop. Most diseases thrive under dark, moist conditions, and the easiest way to prevent a disease outbreak is to provide plenty of light and airflow around your tomato plants and limit the amount of contact between the soil and tomato leaves. Trellising meets all these requirements. You can use a tomato cage, available at a garden center, or set up any number of different kinds of trellises ways with string or wood—you just need to provide a structure for the tomatoes to climb.

On our farm, we use the "Florida weave" method, sometimes called the "cat's cradle." Set up tomato stakes 10 feet apart between the plants. Then stretch several lengths of tomato twine between the stakes on both sides of the plant, close to the stem so that the plant is fully supported. As the plant grows, add twine higher on the stakes, so that the plant is always upright and supported.

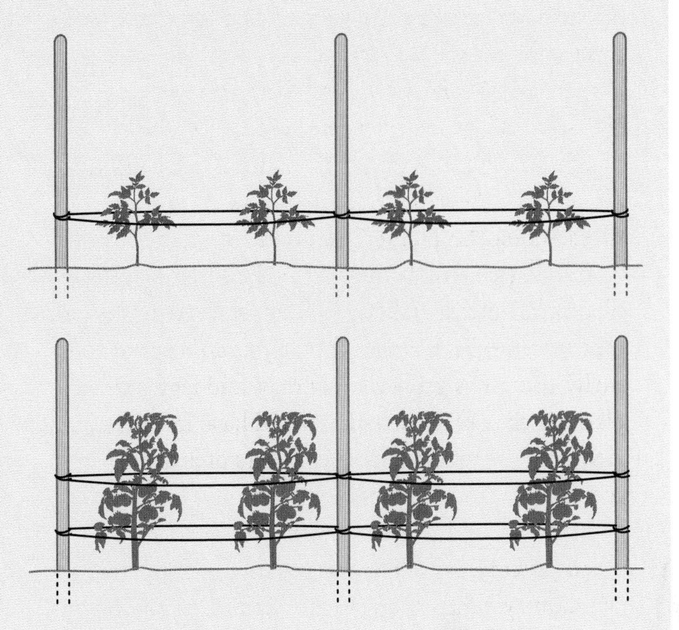

Florida weave trellising method

- **Suckering:** Removing newly formed growth tips from a tomato plant has several benefits: it channels energy into the growth of one or two main vines, cuts down on the plant's total biomass, increases air circulation around the plant, and produces higher-quality fruits. Just pinch off these "suckers," which appear between the main leader (the vine) and a branch or leaf.

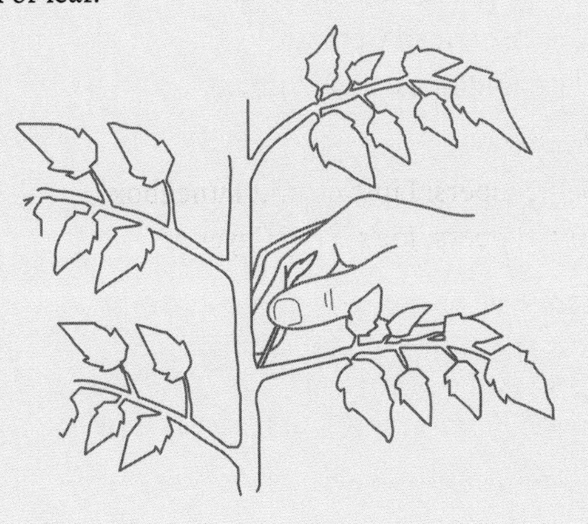

- **Pruning:** Under optimal conditions, tomatoes produce hundreds of flowers, and most of these flowers are pollinated and yield fruit. However, some of that fruit is tiny and misshapen. The best tomatoes are well-formed, large, and uniform in size and shape, and this can be achieved by pruning the flower clusters soon after pollination.

The illustration here shows a tomato plant that has been properly pruned—three flowers were removed from this cluster. Notice that the existing three tomatoes are evenly sized, and they grew faster than they otherwise would have.

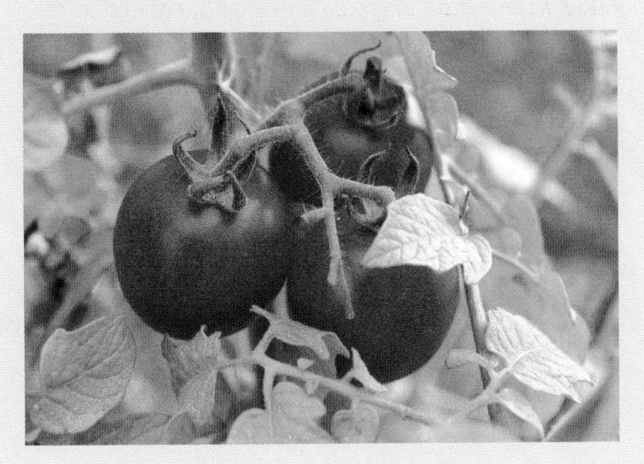

Potatoes

Potatoes prefer a well-drained soil with a pH around 6.5. Keep your potato crop well-watered to ensure large spuds.

Planting: Potato "seeds" are actually small potatoes. Plant them as soon as the chance of a freeze has passed. You can plant potato seeds from your previous year's crop, but be sure the seeds are disease-free. We recommend buying seeds to minimize the risk of disease.

Spacing: Space potato seeds 12 inches apart, leaving 36 inches between rows.

Days to maturity: Depending on the variety, potatoes mature between 60 and 120 days after planting.

When is it ready to harvest? You can usually tell that potatoes are ready to harvest when the leaves begin to die.

Pests and diseases: Watch out for late blight! Once the spots appear, copper sprays can help keep blight at bay, but they'll only buy you a few more weeks—hopefully that's enough time to get your harvest in. Another common pest is the Colorado potato beetle, which can decimate your crop. Squishing the bugs early on, before they mature and develop their hard shell, is the best control. The organic pesticide Entrust is effective if they get to the beetle stage.

Special considerations: The edible tubers of the potato plant grow off the main roots. As the potato plants grow, hill them up with soil to keep the sun from scorching the tubers (see page 120). By the end of the growing season, your potatoes should be hilled 14 to 20 inches above the ground.

Our favorite varieties

- Purple Peruvian
- Kenebec
- Dark Red Norland

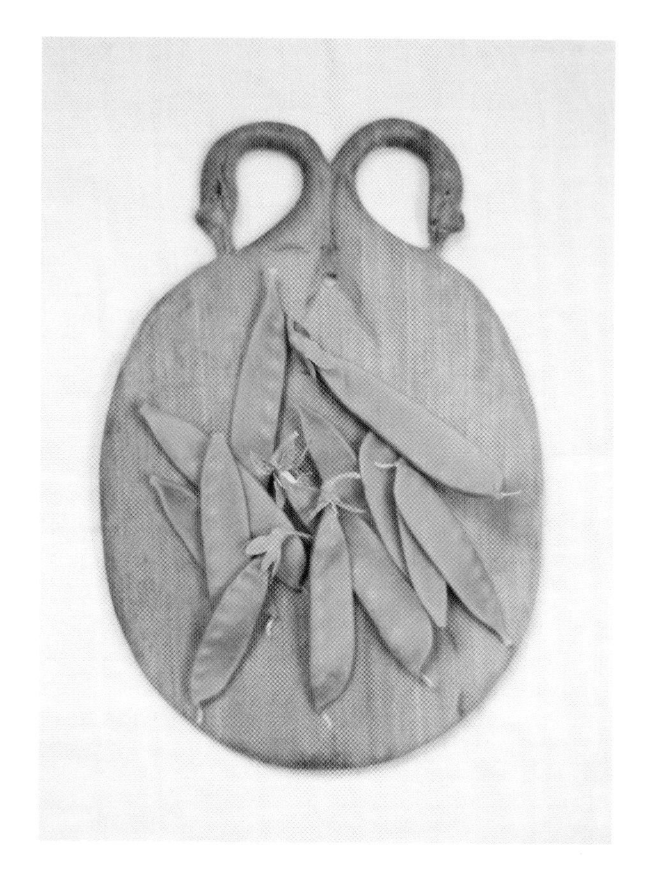

String Beans and Peas (shelling peas, snow peas, sugar snap peas)

String beans like soil that's rich and has a neutral to slightly acidic pH.

Planting: Direct seed peas early in the spring, as soon as the soil has thawed enough to be worked. Frosts and light freezes will not harm peas. String beans cannot be planted until the temperatures are staying above 65°F—if they're planted in cold soil, they tend to rot.

Spacing: Plant peas 4 inches apart in rows at least 2 feet apart, to allow space for harvesting. String beans require more space: plant them 6 inches apart and leave 2 feet between rows.

Days to maturity: Peas and string beans both mature about fifty days after planting.

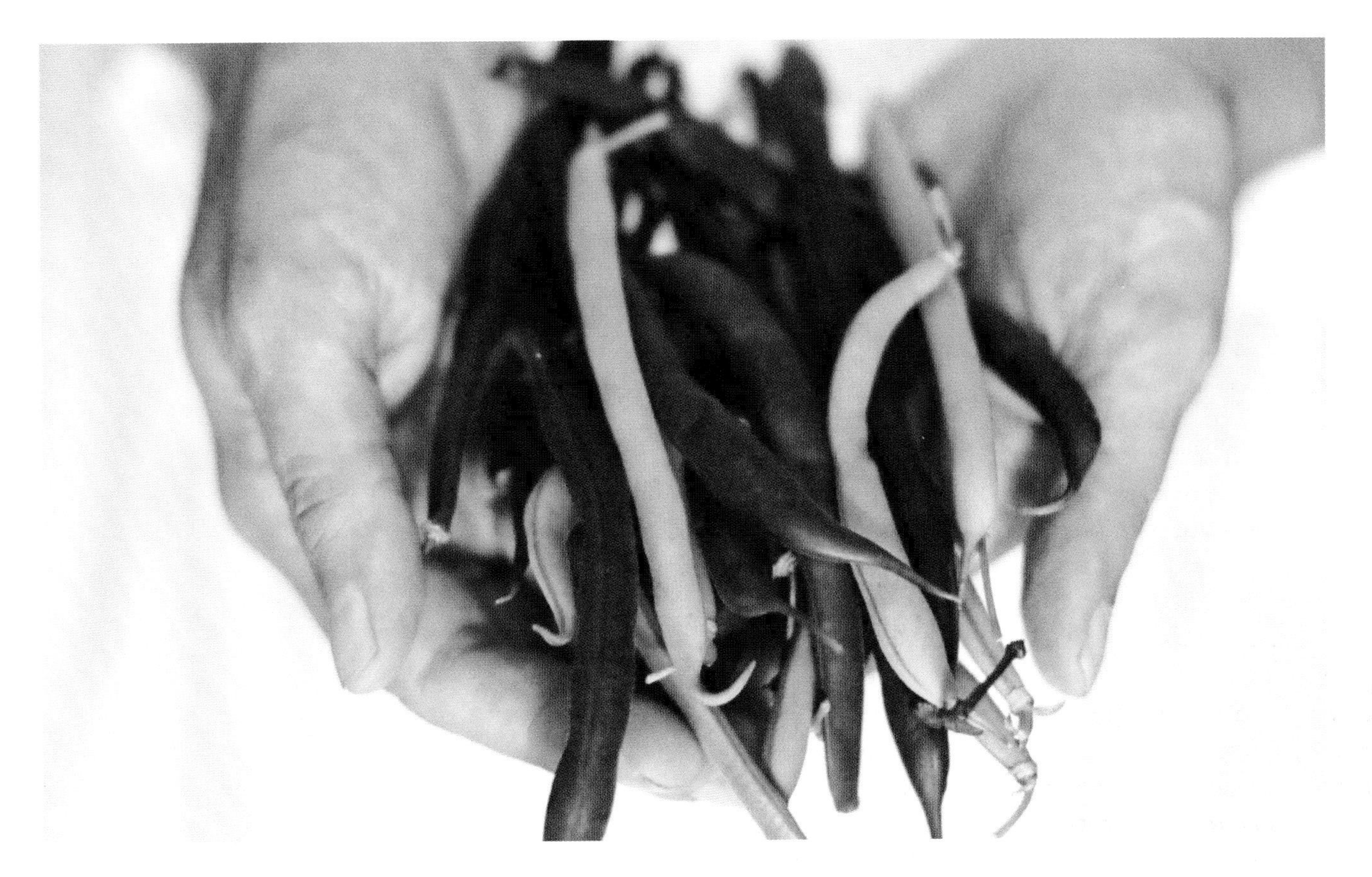

When is it ready to harvest? Sugar snap peas are ready whenever you want to harvest them. As they get larger, though, the pod gets more fibrous and the seed gets larger, less sweet, and starchier. Snow peas are perfect when they're not too large. We prefer to eat shelling peas when they are swollen but the pod hasn't yet turned yellow (at which point it becomes starchy), though some cultures prefer them much larger and starchier. String beans are ready at any size. Like peas, the larger they get, the tougher the skin and the larger the seed.

Pests and diseases: Pea root rot is the most common disease for peas. Well-drained soil is essential, and avoid overwatering. Powdery mildew can also be a big problem, so select mildew-resistant varieties. For string beans, the Mexican bean beetle is a common pest. The best way to control them is scouting and squishing, but beneficial nematodes—roundworms—can help control larvae.

Special considerations: By far, the best-flavored peas and green beans are the pole varieties. Peas and pole beans may require trellising (see page 129), but the great thing about them is that they send out tendrils and climb the trellis all by themselves—unlike tomato plants, they don't need clipping. Building a trellis does take a little time, but the yields, reduced disease, and flavor are worth the effort.

Our favorite varieties

Peas

- Sugar snap: Super Sugar Snap
- Shelling: Maxigolt
- Snow: Oregon Giant

String beans

- Fortex
- Marvel of Venice
- Red Noodle

Sweet Potatoes

Sweet potatoes are a warm-season vegetable that grows best in a well-drained, sandy loam with a pH around 6.5.

Planting: Sweet potatoes are started from "slips," shoots that are grown from a mature sweet potato. You can order slips online or purchase them at a garden center, or you can start your own slips, although it's an involved process (for a link to instructions, see Resources, page 398). Sweet potatoes cannot tolerate cold temperatures, so wait to plant slips until the soil is over 60°F and nights are warm. In the Northeast, this means no planting until mid-June.

Spacing: Plant sweet potato slips 4 inches deep and 12 inches apart, leaving 4 feet between rows.

Days to maturity: Sweet potatoes mature about 100 days after planting.

When is it ready to harvest? Harvest before the first killing frost. If a frost does occur before you are able to dig up your sweet potatoes, harvest them right away: rot will immediately start to spread from the vines down to the tuber.

Special considerations: Sweet potato slips can appear almost dead when you buy them. Wrap them in wet paper towels and keep at room temperature until you are ready to plant them. After harvesting, you'll need to cure sweet potatoes to trigger the development of sugar-creating enzymes—just store them in a warm, humid room for five to ten days. After curing, it's ideal to store them between 55°F and 60°F.

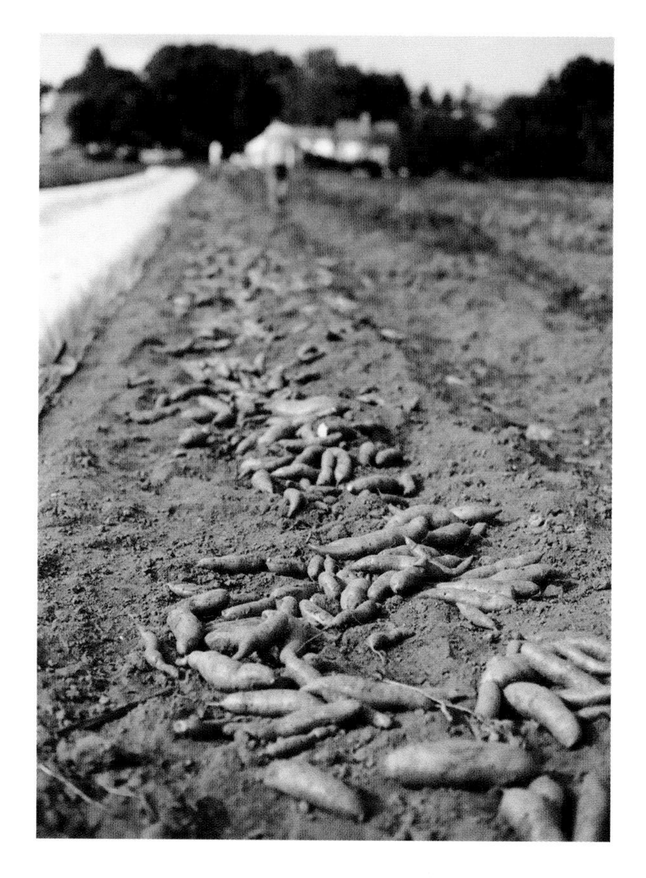

Pests and diseases: Sweet potatoes are remarkably pest-free, although Japanese beetles can be a problem. Deer also love to eat sweet potato vines—if they are an issue, deer fencing is really the best solution.

Our favorite varieties

- Beauregard

Herbs

While there's a lot of minutiae to know about growing specific herbs, it's easiest to just start with the basics of growing perennial and annual herbs.

Perennial herbs include:

- Chives
- Lemon balm
- Mint
- Oregano
- Parsley
- Rosemary
- Sage
- Thyme

Annual herbs include:

- Basil
- Cilantro
- Dill
- Savory
- Stevia
- Tarragon

When to plant: Perennial herbs are generally hardy and can be planted early in the spring, when there is still a danger of frost. Annuals, however,are more delicate; they cannot tolerate frosts and should not be planted until the temperatures are warm.

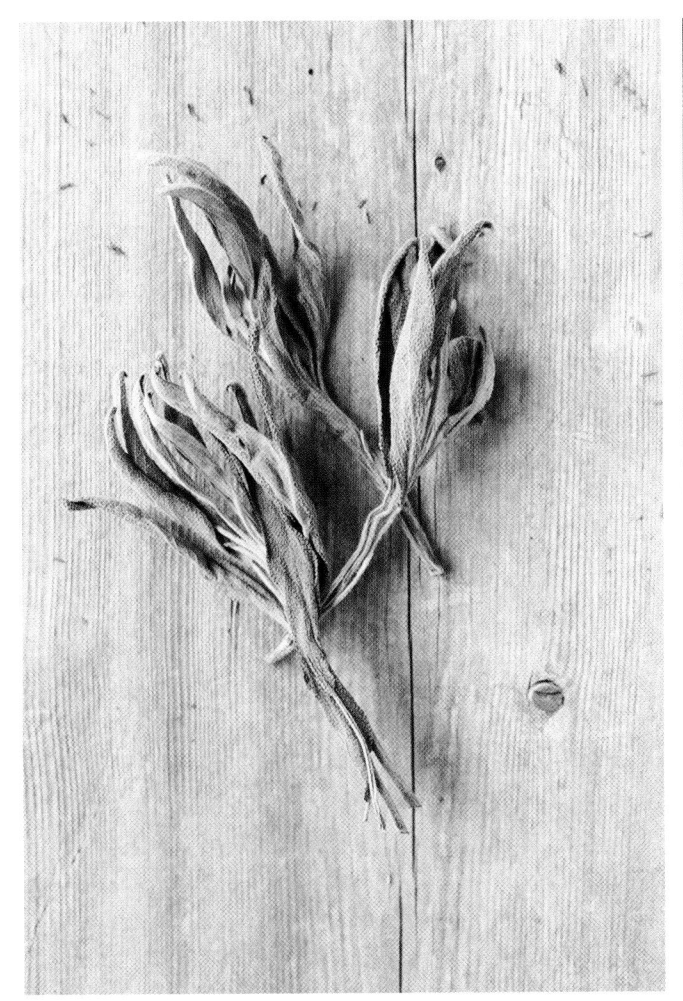

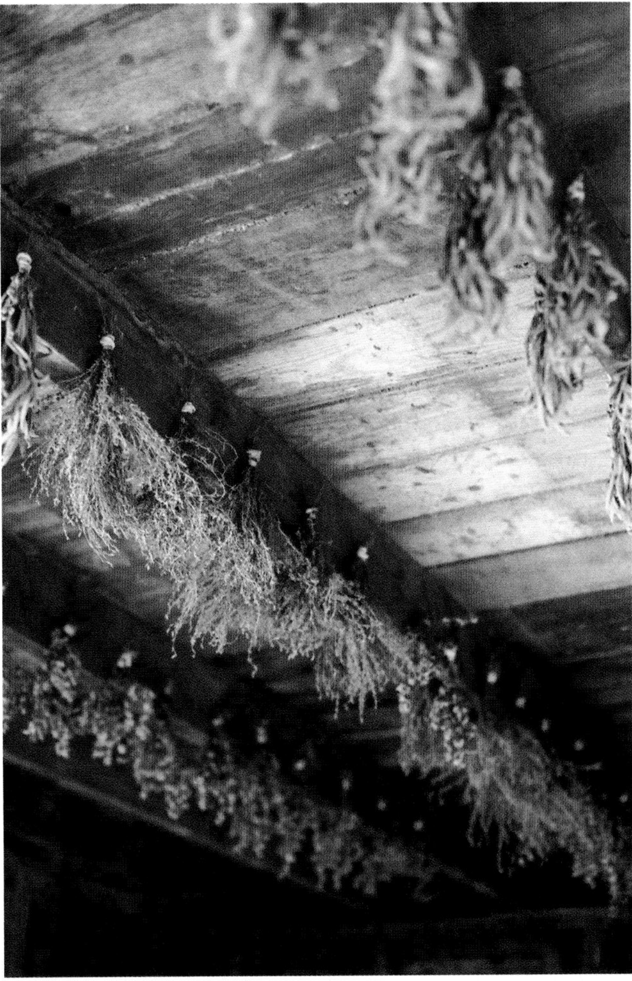

Spacing: Perennial herbs should be planted about 12 inches apart, with 18 inches between rows. Remember, they'll grow significantly over years, so less is more. Annual herbs can be spaced closer together: leave 6 inches between plants and 12 inches between rows. Basil can get very large and bushy over the course of the summer.

When is it ready to harvest? Herbs are ready to harvest at any time, though it's a good idea to wait for newly planted perennials to gain some size first. When you'd like to use an herb, snip off a few branches or leaves with scissors. Avoid trying to pull them off—you could end up accidentally ripping out the entire plant—and be careful not to overharvest, so the plant stays healthy. Be sure to harvest before the herbs bolt or flower (see page 127).

If you'd like to dry your herbs, tie them in bunches and hang them upside down in a dark space that has lots of air circulation. To avoid mold, try quickly drying moist herbs like chives and basil in a food dehydrator.

Pests and diseases: In general, herbs are pest-free. Basil is very susceptible to powdery mildew. Japanese beetles can also be a problem for basil. Putting out a beetle trap tends to just attract more beetles, so we suggest picking them off by hand. You can also try beneficial nematodes, which work on all grubs, including beetle larvae.

Special considerations: Perennial herbs require weed-free conditions to thrive. Be sure to stay on top of weeds so you don't lose your crop.

Berries

Blueberries

Blueberries are a long-lived perennial that will bear fruit for decades if taken care of properly. Blueberries require soil with a pH around 5, and they need full sun.

Planting: Plant blueberries in the early spring to allow them to take root before temperatures get cold again in the fall. Dig a hole about twice the width of the plant's root ball. Add peat moss and an organic fertilizer to the bottom of the hole. Place the root ball in the center of the hole and cover it with soil.

Blueberries can also be grown in containers. Be sure to use a container that's four times larger than the root ball, so the plant has room to grow.

Spacing: Plant blueberries 5 to 6 feet apart in beds 12 feet apart.

Days to maturity: Blueberries take several years to reach maturity. They should not be allowed to bear fruit for the first three years.

When is it ready to harvest? Blueberries are ripe when they are entirely blue. Even slightly unripe blueberries are tart, so wait for them to ripen.

Pests and diseases: The winter moth is a major pest in the Northeast. To control it, begin spraying an organic pesticide weekly before buds swell in early spring. Continue to spray once a week for four weeks. PyGanic and Entrust are both effective organic pesticides for winter moths. Birds can also become a significant pest; covering your bushes with bird netting can help.

Special considerations: Because blueberries are a long-lived perennial, it's important to keep the beds free of weeds. Although wood chips are too acidic to be a good mulch for other plants, blueberries thrive in an acidic soil, so add about 1 to 2 inches of wood chips every other year to keep weeds down. When a blueberry patch fails, the problem is often the soil pH. Before planting, apply sulfur to the bed, and test the soil annually to ensure the pH is in the desired range.

Our favorite varieties

- Rekka
- Blue Crop
- Blue Ray

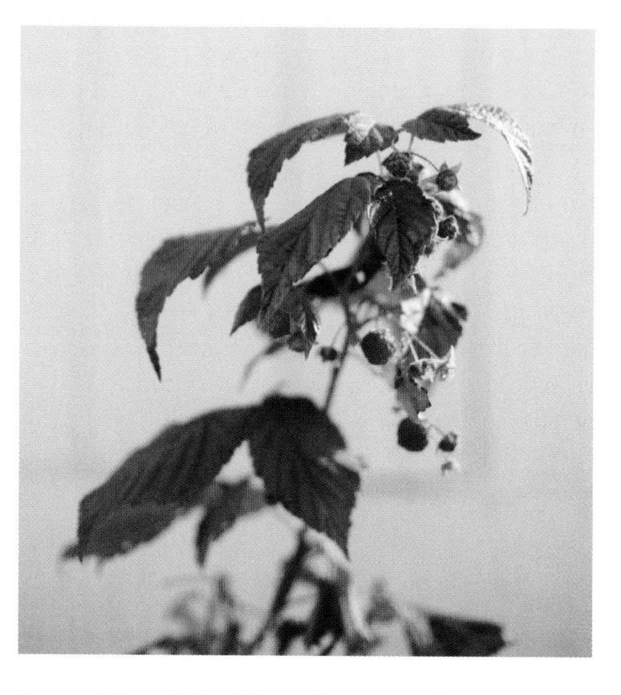

Brambles (blackberries, raspberries)

Brambles such as raspberries and blackberries, as well as several other varieties, tend to be hardy and can grow in partial shade. They prefer a slightly acidic soil, with lots of organic matter and consistent irrigation.

When to plant: Plant brambles any time throughout the spring and summer. Planting earlier in the year gives the plants more time to get established before the winter.

Spacing: Brambles have a tendency to spread . . . everywhere. Allow 2 feet between plants and 10 feet between rows. (The plants will eventually cover the entire area if you allow them to.) It's far easier to harvest berries if the beds are no more than 18 inches wide, so you can pick berries from either side of the bed. A narrow bed also allows for adequate airflow, which lowers the risk of disease and mold.

Days to maturity: Brambles take a year to get established. During the first year, prune the fruits to allow the plants to develop their root systems. Bramble seasons tend to be short, so plant multiple varieties to ensure a full summer of berry production.

When is it ready to harvest? Brambles are ready when the berries pull easily from the plant.

Pests and diseases: There are several pests common to brambles, including raspberry cane borers, raspberry fruit worms, spotted wing drosophila, and Japanese beetles. Organic pesticides like PyGanic can be effective in controlling many of these pests. In addition, larger animals like birds can steal your crop quickly. Nets can be helpful to keep birds off your plants.

Special considerations: Brambles spread aggressively, so make sure you have room for them before planting, and stay on top of them. Different bramble varieties bear fruit at different times, but if you choose varieties that fruit in the late summer and early fall, you can have berries all through the growing season: strawberries in June, blueberries in July, and raspberries or blackberries in August and September.

Our favorite varieties

Raspberries

- Anne
- Autumn Britten
- Caroline

Blackberries

- Chester

Strawberries

Strawberries are a low-growing perennial plant that prefers fertile soil with a neutral pH. For a good yield, it's extremely important to keep the strawberry bed free of weeds, and keep strawberries well watered throughout the fruiting period.

When to plant: Plant strawberry plants in the early spring, soon after the danger of freezes has passed.

Spacing: Plant strawberries 12 inches apart, in rows 18 inches apart.

Days to maturity: Although strawberries will form fruit in their first year, prune the flowers to allow the plant to focus more energy on developing its root structure. Harvest a year after planting instead. Most varieties bear fruit in the early summer.

When is it ready to harvest? Strawberries are ripe when they're fully red. Do not delay harvesting, as many insects enjoy eating the fruit and wet ripe strawberries grow moldy quickly.

Pests and diseases: From birds to deer to insects and slugs, there are many pests that love the sweet taste of strawberries. For bugs and aphids, PyGanic

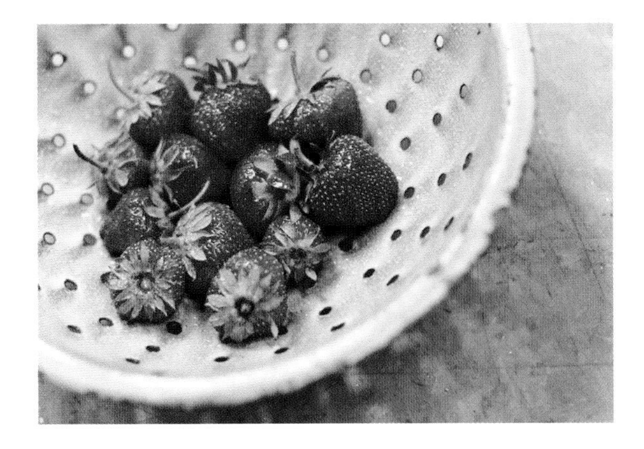

is an effective organic pesticide. Disease can also be an issue with strawberries, but keeping the beds weed-free lowers the risk of many diseases.

Special considerations: Weeds are a chronic problem in strawberry fields, so weed them frequently. In the fall, after a freeze, cover strawberries with several inches of straw and leave it in place through the winter. Strawberries often produce flowers very early in the spring, but flowers that undergo a frost will not produce fruit. To avoid crop loss, don't remove the straw until one month after the last frost and use floating row covers to keep your plants warmer on cold nights. Once the danger of frost has passed, uncover the plants so the flowers can be pollinated. Strawberries are often turned under after one year of harvest to avoid the build-up of weeds and because the berries get smaller as the plant gets older, but I have had strawberry plants that stayed productive for several years.

Our favorite varieties

- Jewel
- Cavendish

WAIT! WHY DIDN'T YOU INCLUDE FRUIT AND NUT TREES?

Fruit and nut trees and how to grow them vary widely depending on location, and we simply didn't have the space here to explore all the details. However, this doesn't mean that fruit trees shouldn't be part of your homestead. Please research what trees thrive in your area and consider incorporating them in your landscape. (For more, see Resources, page 398.)

CONTAINER GARDENING

If you're tight on space, or if you just want to try out growing on a very small scale, containers are a great option. Containers can grace stairs or balconies, and you can take advantage of vertical space by creating a trellis for plants like cucumbers, tomatoes, and squash. It's especially helpful to have a container of assorted herbs near your kitchen.

Choosing the Container

Picking the right container is really important, especially when you plan to eat what you are growing in it. First, a too-small container can stunt a plant's growth, so be sure to choose one that gives your plant enough room. Second, many chemicals from containers can leach into the soil and contaminate your plants. So even though you may see folks growing vegetables and herbs in all kinds of objects, from bathtubs to cinder blocks to wheelbarrows, it's important to be safe. Avoid all of the following:

- Pressure-treated wood
- Railroad ties
- Recycled wood that has been exposed to chemicals
- Galvanized steel
- Plastic
- Rubber (including old tires)
- Concrete containers

There are a lot of plastic containers on the market, including self-watering ones, which are very appealing. The problem is, even food-safe plastics are only safe up to certain temperatures, and a plastic container baking in the sun during the summer can exceed those temperatures—and when it breaks down, it'll leach chemicals into the soil and the roots of your vegetables. For this reason, we highly recommend wooden containers for growing edibles.

Getting the Soil

If you can harvest some rich, fertile soil from your own property, it will save you a lot of money. If you need to buy soil, make sure it's certified organic. Potting soil isn't quite what you want; a mix of soil and potting soil is better. Potting soil is mostly peat moss, and while it's a great medium for allowing seeds to sprout, it doesn't have the necessary nutrients for a mature plant to thrive. Sometimes you can find bagged soil labeled "container mix," but be sure it doesn't already contain chemical fertilizers.

Watering

Container plants need to be watered frequently. If you water them by hand, it can be time-consuming, but it's easy to turn any container into a self-watering one with a simple contraption. First, get a hose that's long enough to stretch along all of your containers. Then, for each container, punch an emitter into the hose. Emitters are little hose extensions that bring water directly to the container. Place each emitter into a container. Then just place your hose on a timer—we have ours set to water every morning from 8 to 8:30. This is really a fantastic system to keep your containers watered, without any effort on your part.

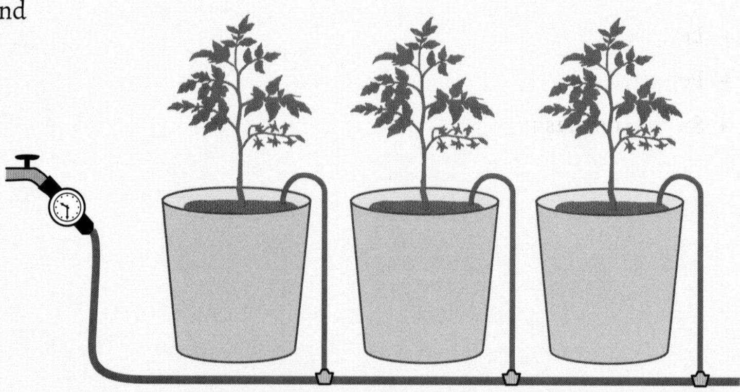

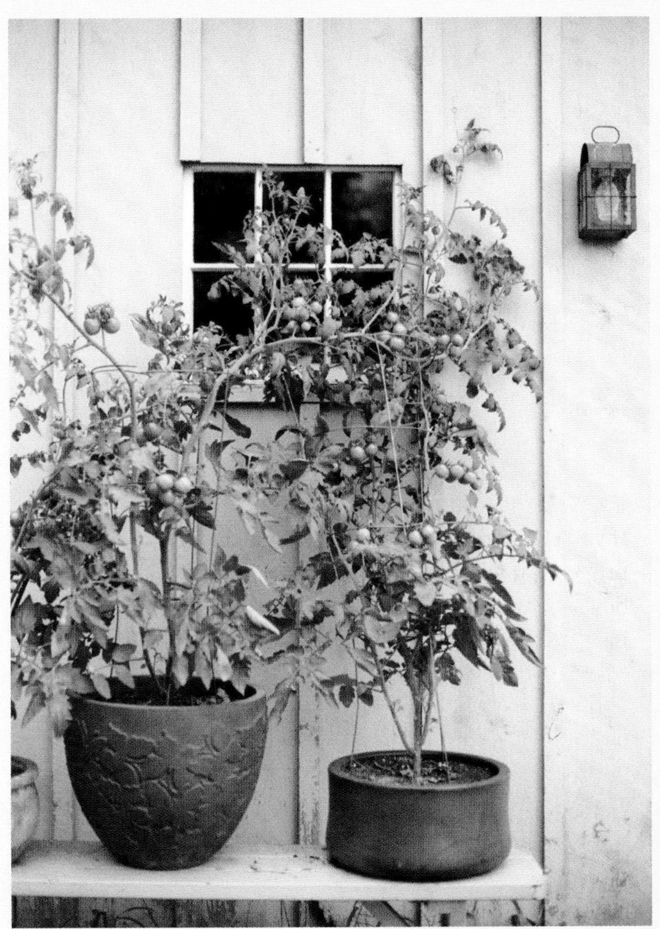

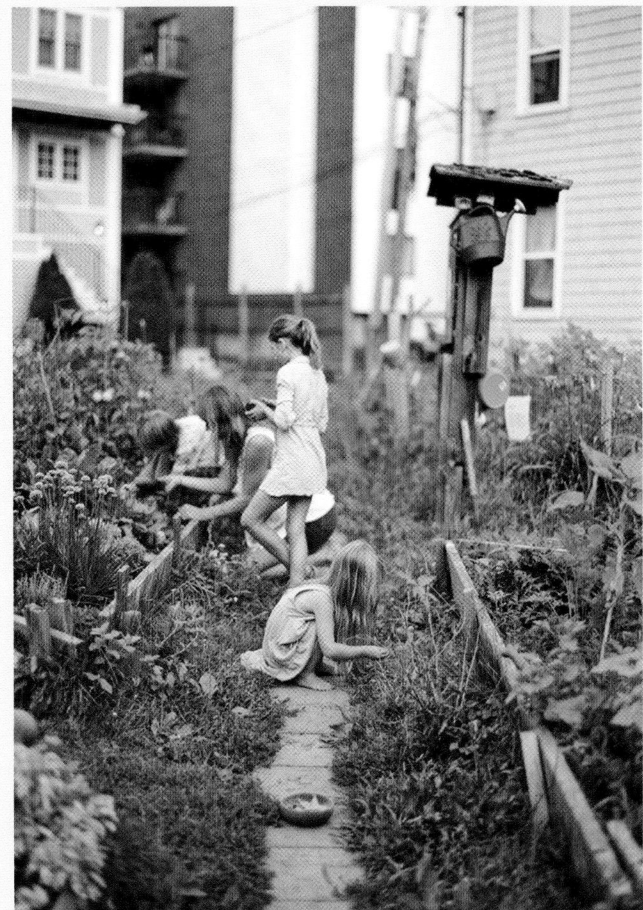

Fertilizing

Once a month, fertilize your container plants with an organic, liquid fertilizer, such as fish emulsion.

Our Favorite Plants for Containers

- Most herbs (basil, chives, mint, oregano, parsley, rosemary, thyme, etc.)
- Chard
- Cherry tomatoes
- Eggplant
- Lettuce
- Peppers
- Summer squash

Community Gardens

I get a big smile when I'm driving through a city and come across a vacant lot that has been transformed into a community garden. They're fantastic for bringing people together and beautifying neighborhoods. If you live in a city and don't have much room even for container plants, a community garden is a wonderful way to get your fresh vegetables and spend some time outdoors. And even if you do have space for vegetables at your home, it could be worth it to have a community garden plot for a few seasons—it's a great way to try out gardening before you decide to dig up your own backyard. Some of the larger community garden organizations have group compost deliveries, making it really easy to get compost right to your plot.

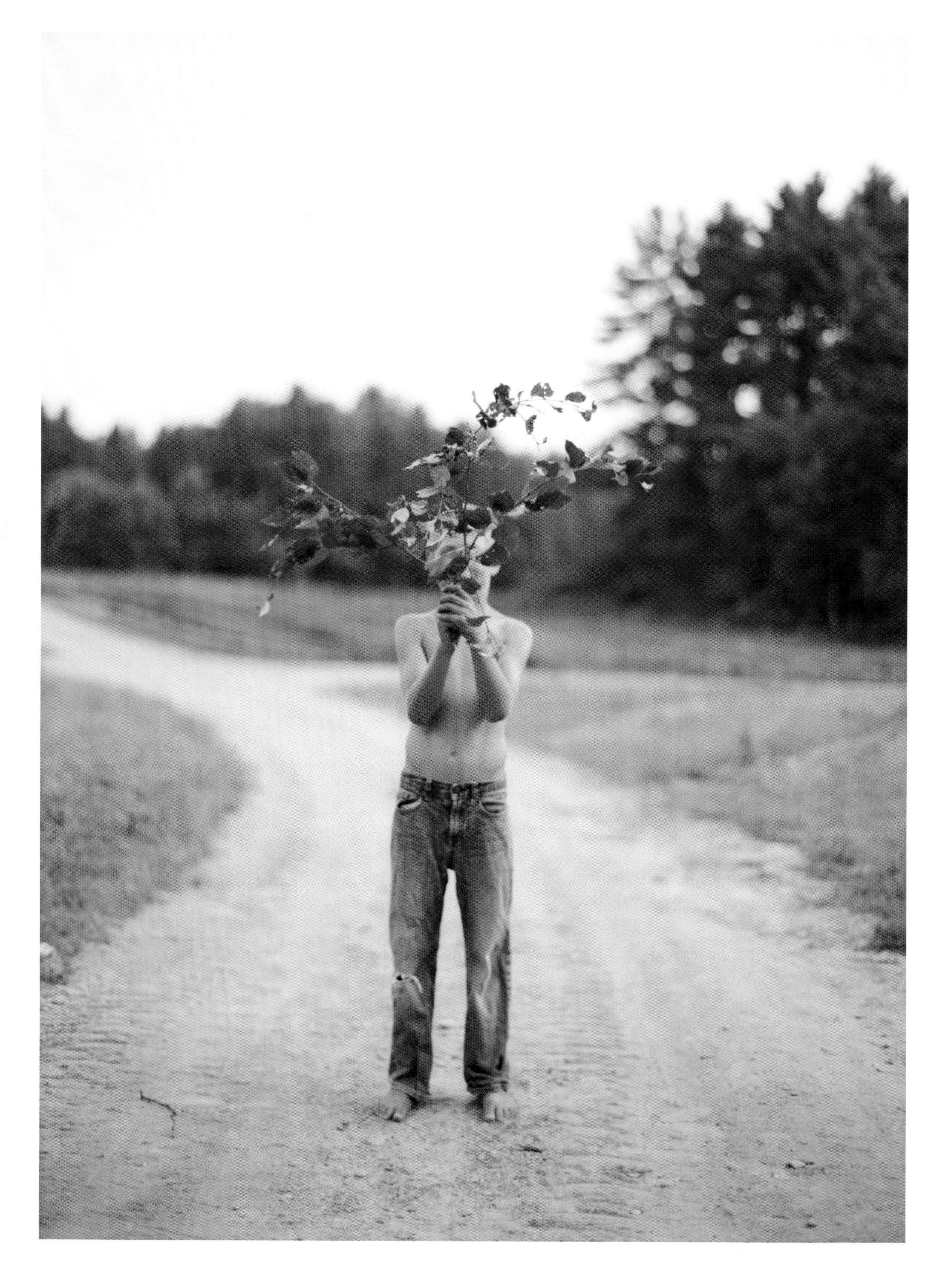

Get Wild: Foraging for Edible Plants

We all know it's healthy to eat vegetables and fruits, but we often forget that they don't need to come from a farm: wild plants are nutritional powerhouses. Purslane, for instance, a weed that thrives in many parts of the world, has six times more vitamin E than spinach and more omega-3 fatty acids than any other vegetable. As humans have selectively bred produce to be larger and sweeter and to withstand storage better, we've lost many of the vitamins, minerals, protein, fiber, and healthy fats that make wild plants so good for us.

In the recipe section, I've featured several wild plants, including the following:

Black Birch

(Birch Bark Sun Tea, page 200)

If you have kids, seek out a black birch tree and snap off a branch, then peel back the bark and have them smell it. It will blow their minds—it smells just like root beer! You can make a sun tea by stripping the bark of many branches—also a fun project for kids. An added benefit is that black birch is said to be a natural painkiller.

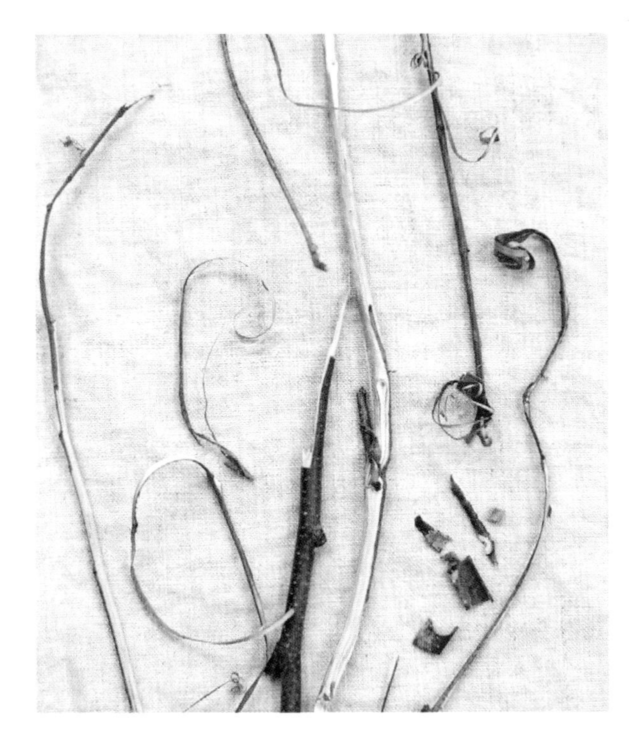

Dandelions

(Wilted Dandelion Greens with Balsamic Onions, page 170)

When harvested early in the spring, dandelion greens and their flower buds are very delicious. Avoid the ones growing in sidewalk cracks and instead look for young plants growing in a pesticide-free lawn, whose flowers haven't yet bloomed. They're very high in iron, manganese, potassium, riboflavin, thiamin, and vitamins B6 and C.

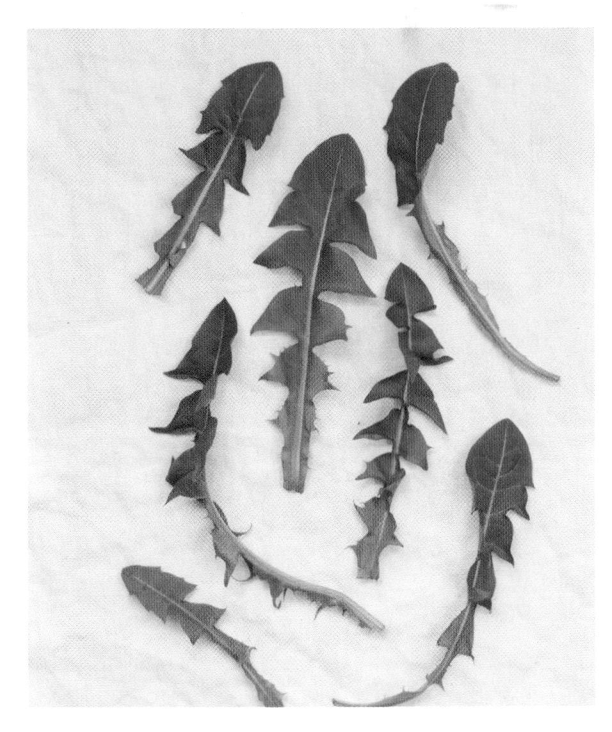

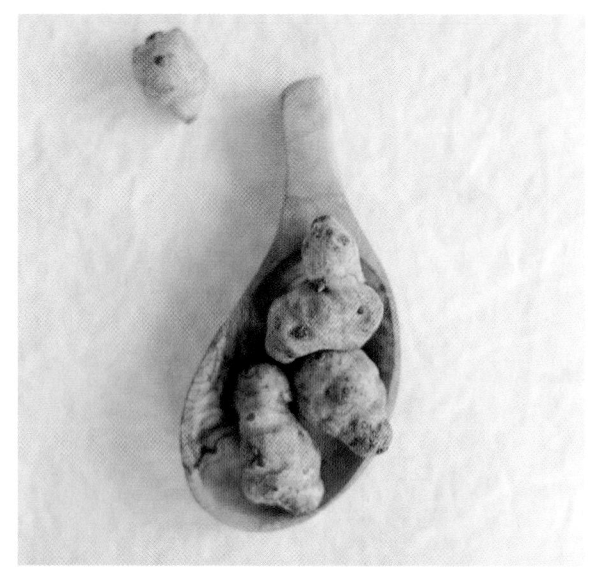

Jerusalem Artichokes

(Warm Asparagus with Jerusalem Artichokes, Smoked Ham, and Pastured Egg, page 178)

This tuber is a close relative of the sunflower. It can be cultivated or grow wild, but the wild version is a little more difficult to identify because they don't always show their classic, mini-sunflower blossoms. Jerusalem artichokes contain inulin, a carbohydrate that won't spike your insulin levels, which makes them a good alternative to potatoes in many dishes. They are also high in iron, phosphorus, potassium, and thiamin.

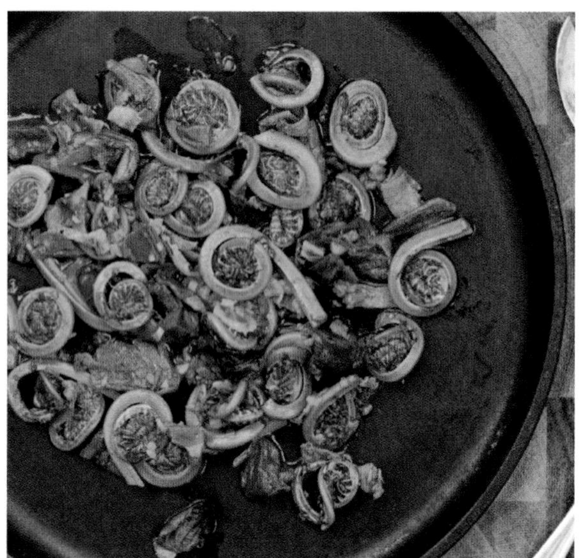

Fiddlehead Ferns

(Fiddlehead Ferns with Porcini and Prosciutto, page 176)

Spiral-coiled gifts of spring, fiddleheads are among the most beautiful things to put on a plate. Be sure to cook them well; they are not to be eaten raw. It's also important to get the sprouts from the ostrich fern and not other varieties. Look for a papery brown covering on the fiddlehead and a U-shaped groove on the inside of the stem. Fiddleheads can be found growing in clusters of three to twelve in damp soil, such as by rivers and streams. When harvesting, be considerate and only take half of the fiddleheads in a cluster, so the plant can still survive. They're very high in manganese, magnesium, phosphorus, iron, potassium, and vitamin C, and they have twice the amount of antioxidants in blueberries.

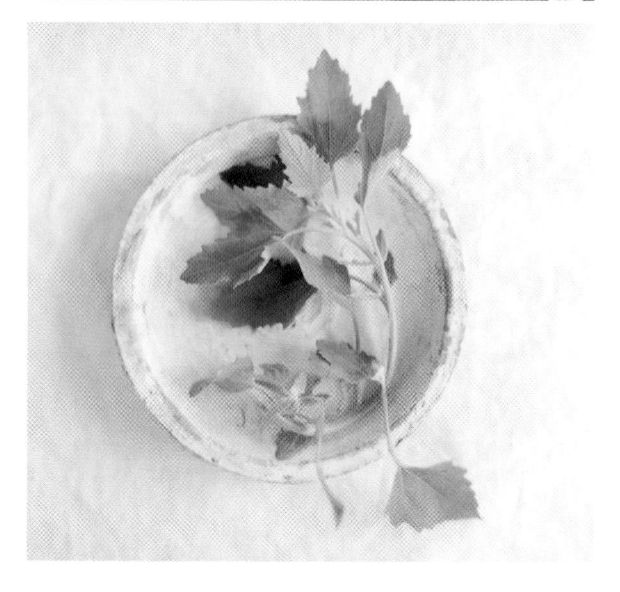

Lamb's Quarters

(Sea Scallops with Ramps and Wilted Lamb's Quarters, page 162)

Once you learn to identify this leafy plant with its powdery coating, you'll see it everywhere. Lamb's quarters are best eaten in early summer and can be used in place of spinach for cooking. They're a very good source of vitamins B6, C, and K, thiamin, riboflavin, calcium, potassium, copper, and manganese. Although they can be eaten raw, I much prefer them cooked—they're more flavorful then, with a taste similar to spinach but slightly earthier, and they have a lovely silky texture.

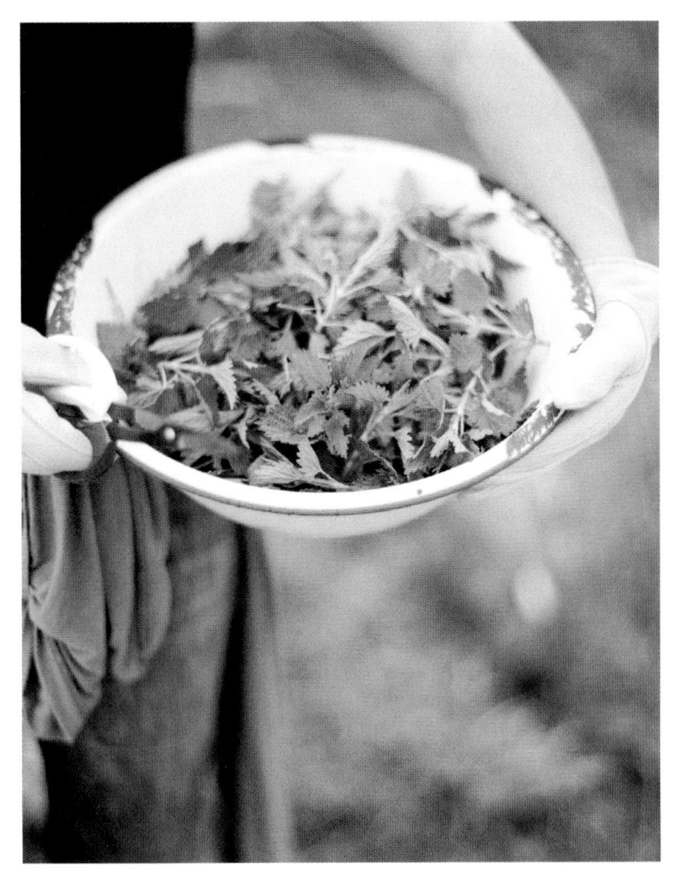

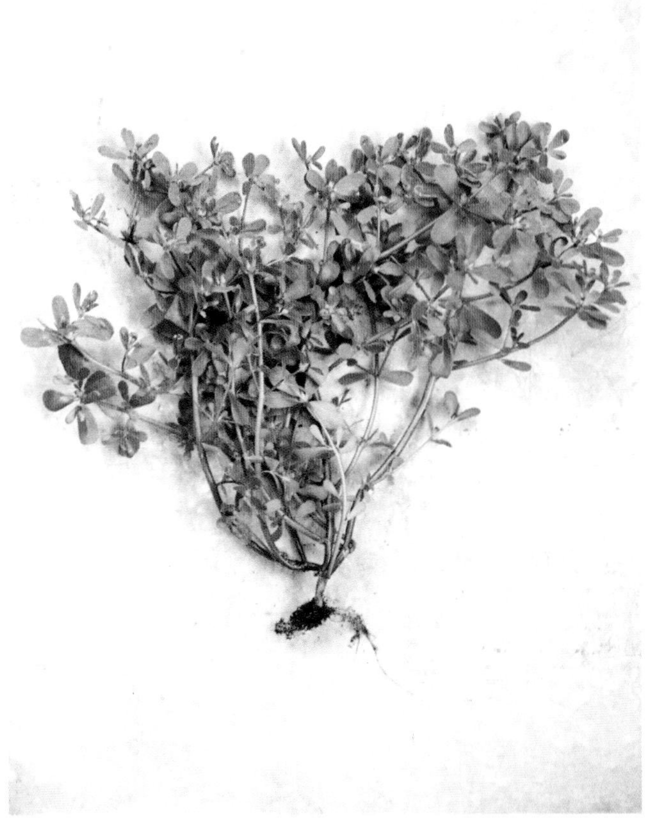

Nettles

(Stinging Nettle Soup with Lemon-Chive Crème Fraîche, page 154)

These spiny little buggers are found in early spring in New England. Seek out the smaller plants, and use gloves when harvesting. You'll commonly find them growing in large clumps in rich, moist soil. They're high in calcium, vitamins A and C, iron, magnesium, thiamin, and potassium. Naturopaths consider nettles useful for adrenal fatigue, arthritis, and general inflammation. Interestingly, the fiber from this plant is great for making ropes and clothes, and it was used in World War I when there was a cotton shortage.

Purslane

(Purslane Potato Salad with Bacon and Shallots, page 243)

Purslane plays the starring role in many cultures' traditional dishes, from saag to spanakopita. It has more omega-3 fatty acids than any other plant. Its mild, lemony taste is fantastic in a salad, and you can find it growing just about anywhere you look!

Ramps

(Sea Scallops with Ramps and Wilted Lamb's Quarters, page 162)

Sometimes called wild leeks, ramps can be cooked or eaten raw, just like onions. Their flavor is intense, so I suggest you try them sautéed or grilled first. They're high in vitamin C and iron.

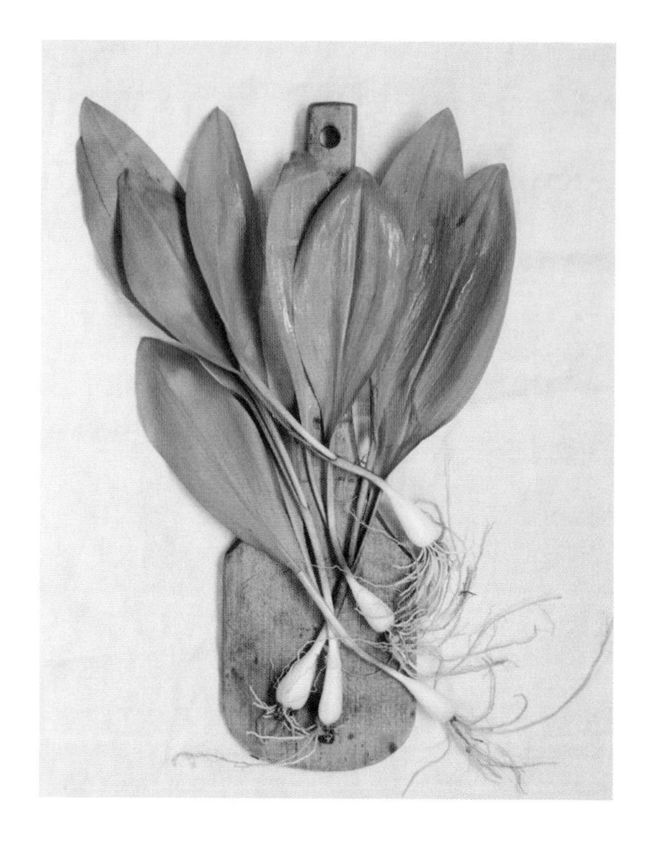

If you're interested in foraging, here are some tips to keep in mind:

Talk to an expert. Consider finding a local expert on foraging who knows what grows in your area. It's often much easier to learn about plants when someone points them out to you, rather than simply seeing photos in a book—and since it's particularly important to identify wild plants correctly if you're planning to eat them, it's worth making sure you learn from someone who knows their stuff. If you live in New England, Russ Cohen is a wonderful guide to wild edibles, and he leads walks all over, including at our farm.

Forage near an organic farm. The soil on and around organic farms is healthy, so you get a wide variety of wild edibles, and since they don't use chemical pesticides, you don't need to worry about ingesting them on your wild plants. You might even ask at the farm if you can harvest some purslane or lamb's quarters from their beds. I'll bet they will be thrilled to have you take them, for free!

Avoid certain areas. It's best to avoid plants growing along a roadside or questionable waterways, to avoid potential toxins.

Get permission. Don't just let yourself onto someone's property if you see a patch of special mushrooms or Concord grape leaves. Ask first.

Be sustainable. Don't yank out every ramp root or every single fiddlehead in the clump. Take just a few, no more than half. Also, check your state's list of endangered plants before you head out, and if you find an endangered plant, do not pick it.

Be aware of fakers. Be sure you can identify the poisonous look-alike plants for your favorite forage items. This is especially true of mushrooms; many of the most lethal varieties have an agreeable flavor. For safety, when you're new to foraging, start with easy-to-identify plants such as dandelions.

Start small. Some people are allergic to certain wild plants. Take a small taste first to see if it agrees with you. If you tend to have digestive issues with certain cultivated plants, it's likely that certain wild plants will disagree with you, too.

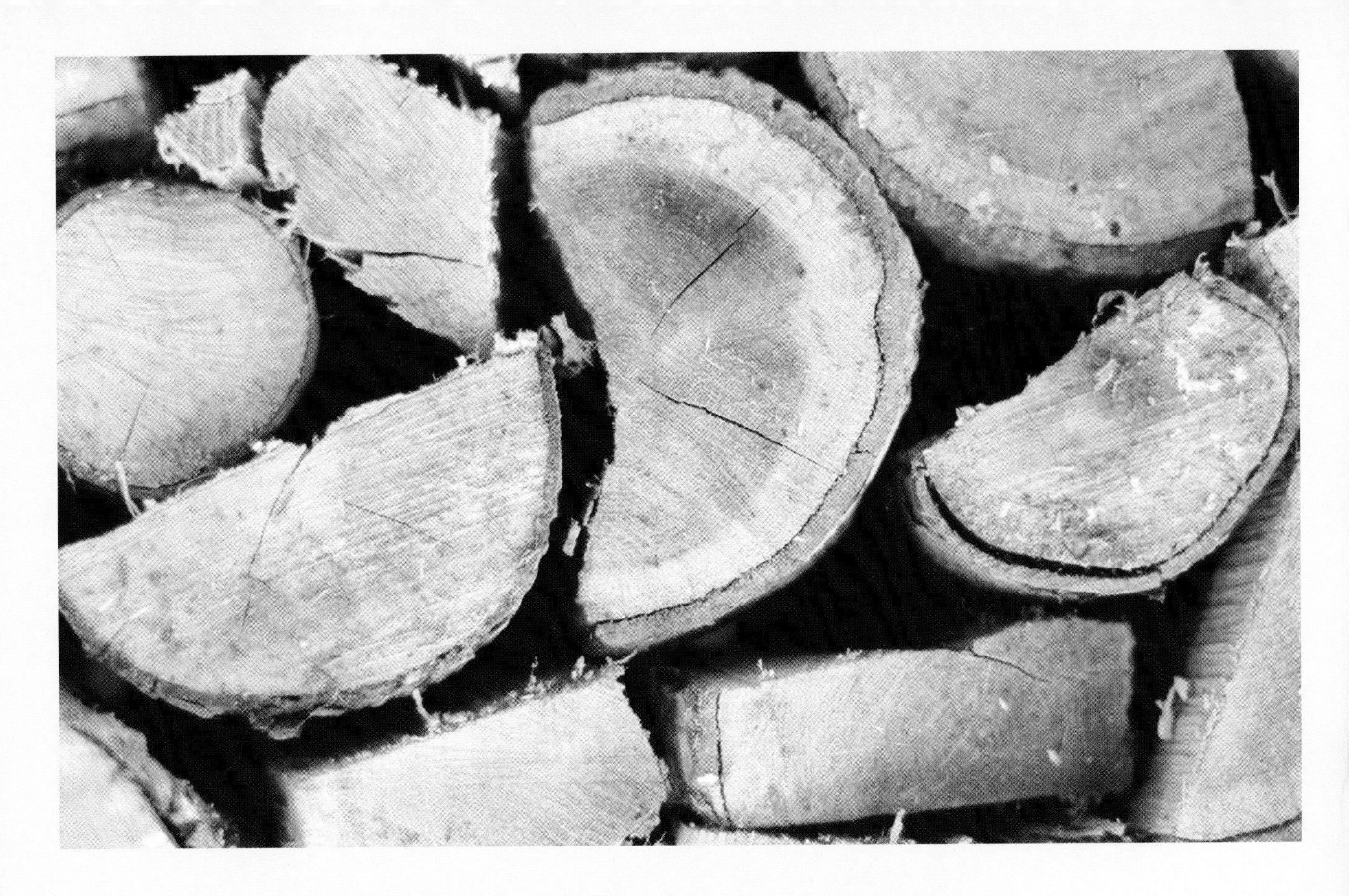

MANAGING A WOODLOT

If you're lucky enough to have forest on your property, you have easy access to a free, renewable fuel source: wood. In fact, wood is one of the most sustainable fuels we have.

Burning fossil fuels or coal frees ancient carbon dioxide that was circulating thousands of years ago, increasing the total amount of carbon in the atmosphere. Burning wood, on the other hand, is carbon-neutral—it releases just the amount of carbon dioxide that the growing tree absorbed. Harvesting diseased or older trees on your property and using them as a fuel source is the most eco-friendly way to heat your home.

Managing your woodlot to use that fuel wisely should be as much a priority for your homestead as producing food. The following steps are a good guide to managing your woodlot.

Step 1: Cleanup. Remove fallen and diseased trees, invasive (non-native) species,and other potentially dangerous trees and brush, such as ones that are leaning and may fall.

Step 2: Selective cutting. Now that you have removed what you don't want, it's time to thin the forest to give the trees you do want to keep room to grow. Think about what kind of trees you'll need for your homestead—both now and in twenty years, when today's saplings will have matured—and cut down the rest. Will you be building fencing? If so, keep more cedar. Do you need fuel and building material? Keep more oak. Want to have maple syrup? Keep more maple.

Step 3: Maintenance. If you have pigs, sheep,or goats, run them through the woodlot on a rotational pattern. They'll eat brush such as buckthorn, poison ivy, and brambles, so you'll have less work keeping the lot cleared, and their manure will keep the soil fertile. They also eat small saplings, allowing the bigger trees to thrive. After a storm, remove any fallen trees and use them for fuel. And finally, whenever you need wood for a project, thin the trees as needed.

THE IDEAL HOMESTEAD SETUP

THESE ARE A FEW IDEAS FOR SETTING UP YOUR HOMESTEAD, BASED ON LOT SIZE. YOU'LL PROBABLY NEED TO CUSTOMIZE THEM TO FIT YOUR PARTICULAR LOT, SO HERE ARE SOME GENERAL TIPS TO KEEP IN MIND:

- Place your vegetable beds in the sunniest spot on your land. In the U.S., that's usually wherever there's southern exposure.
- It may be wise to fence in your garden to shield it from deer, rabbits, and the numerous other animals that love free salad bars.
- If you have a hill, make sure that the animals aren't uphill from your vegetables, so that raw manure runoff doesn't get into your vegetable beds.
- If there's a lot of wind on your property, you may want to plant some bushes or trees as a windbreak, so that your tender transplants won't be blown away.
- If you live in an area that gets cold in the winter and you have more than just a handful of animals to keep watered, frost-free hydrants are a great investment.
- It's important to have a rotational grazing system (see page 61), so don't fill every field with animals. Allow some land to recover between grazings—it's healthier for the animals and for the land.
- Placing the barn in the middle of the 1-acre property gives you water, power, utilities, and feed close to all of the animals, and provides shelter for the animals in most of the fields if needed.
- On the 1-acre plot, the chickens can (and should) be moved into the other fields to eat parasites from the sheep poop and insects; not only does this provide great protein for the chickens, it helps keep your mini-farm clean. An electric fence keeps them contained and safe from predators—they'd likely be able to jump over a split-rail fence.

⅛ ACRE PLOT

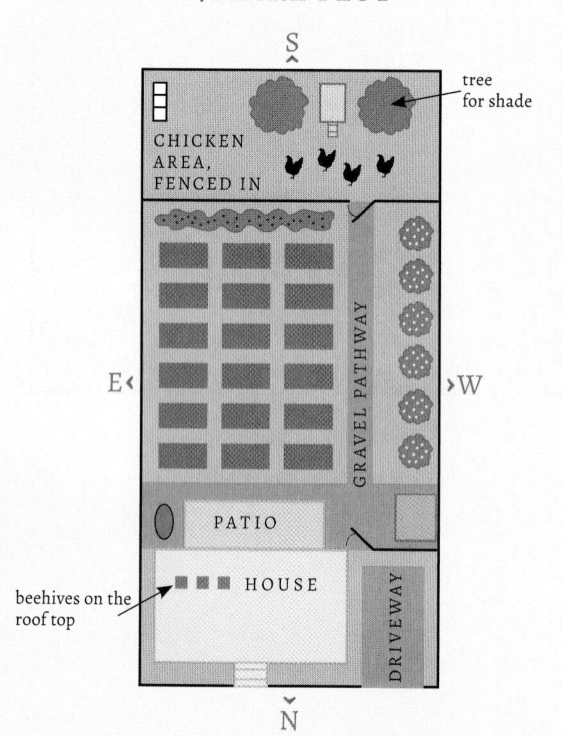

¼ ACRE PLOT

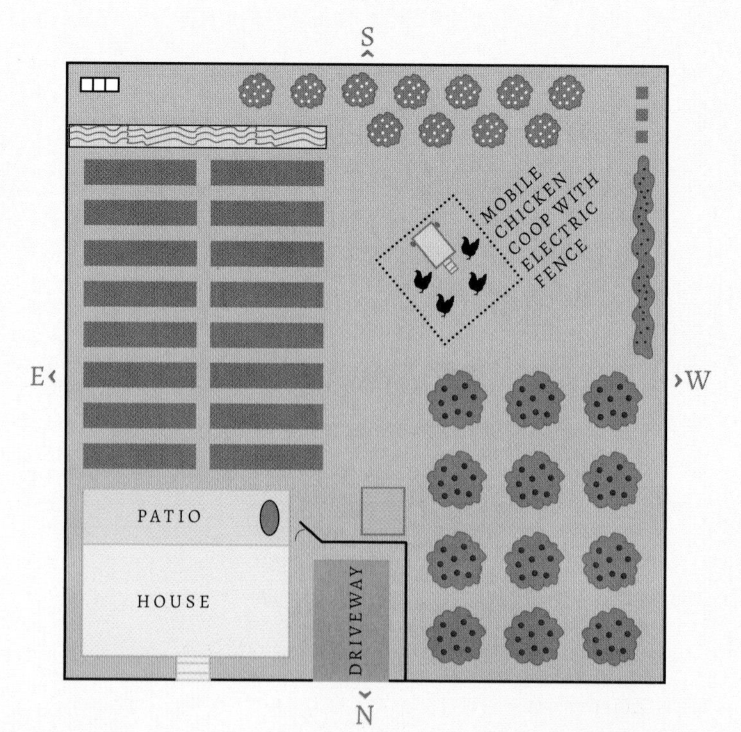

1 ACRE PLOT

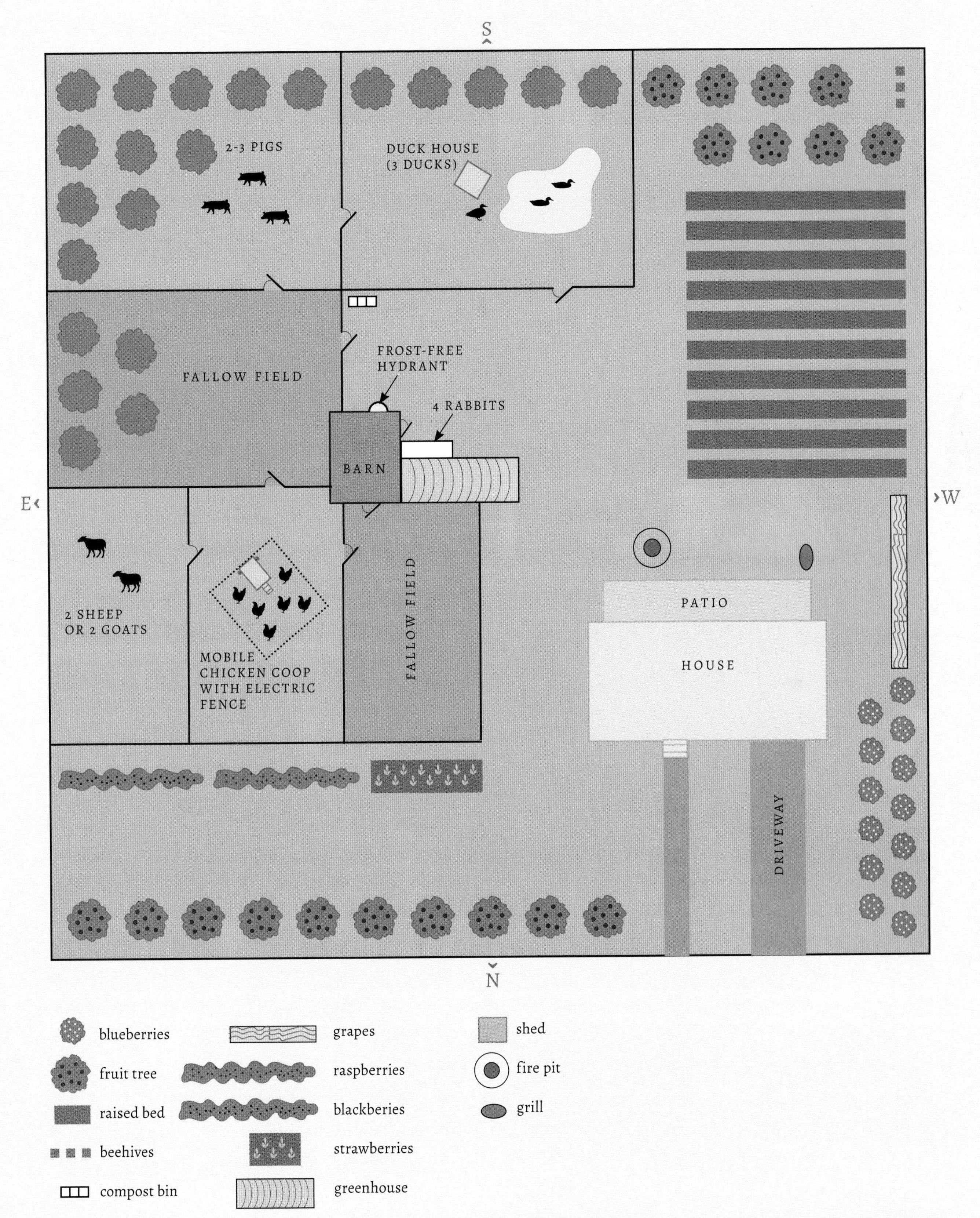
S
2-3 PIGS
DUCK HOUSE
(3 DUCKS)
FALLOW FIELD
FROST-FREE
HYDRANT
4 RABBITS
BARN
E
W
2 SHEEP
OR 2 GOATS
MOBILE
CHICKEN COOP
WITH ELECTRIC
FENCE
FALLOW FIELD
PATIO
HOUSE
DRIVEWAY
N
blueberries
fruit tree
raised bed
beehives
compost bin
grapes
raspberries
blackberies
strawberries
greenhouse
shed
fire pit
grill

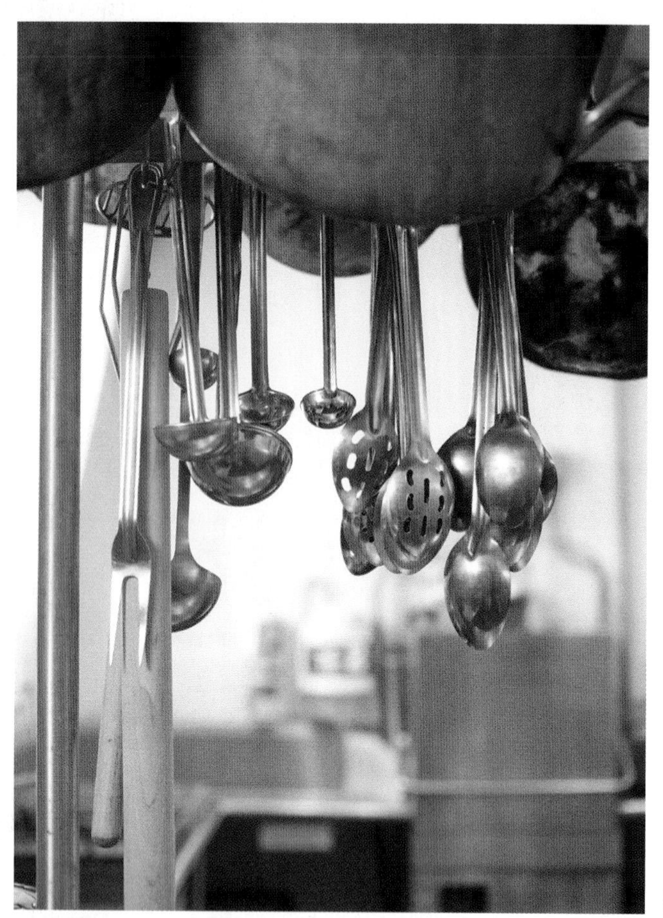
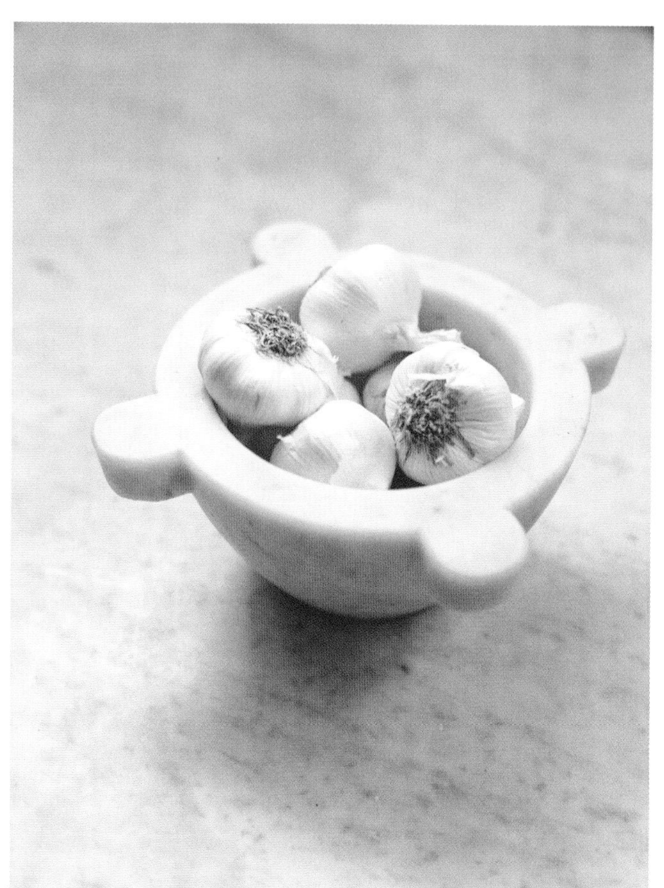
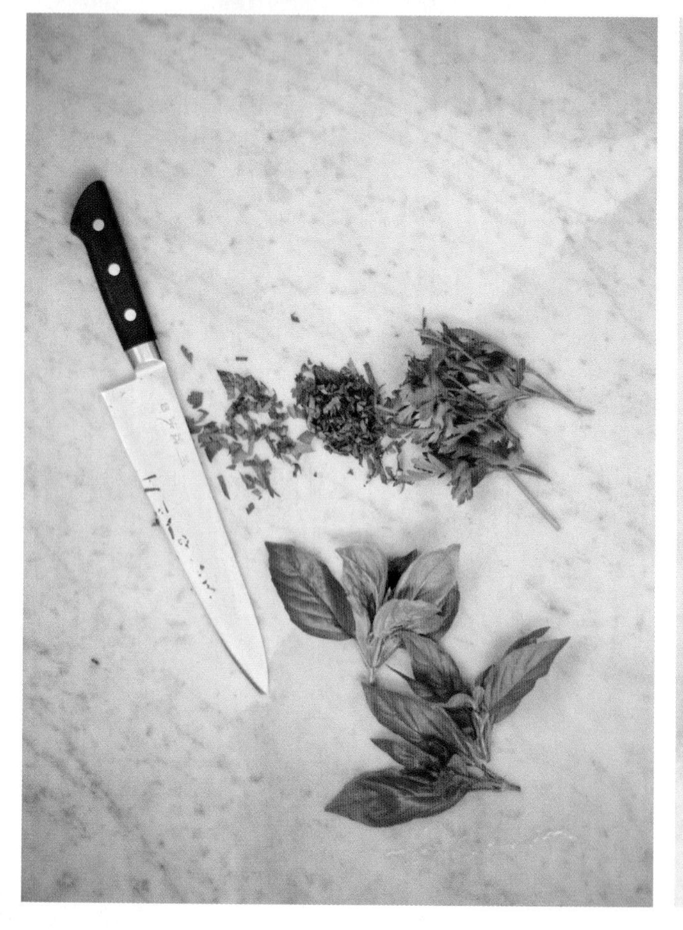
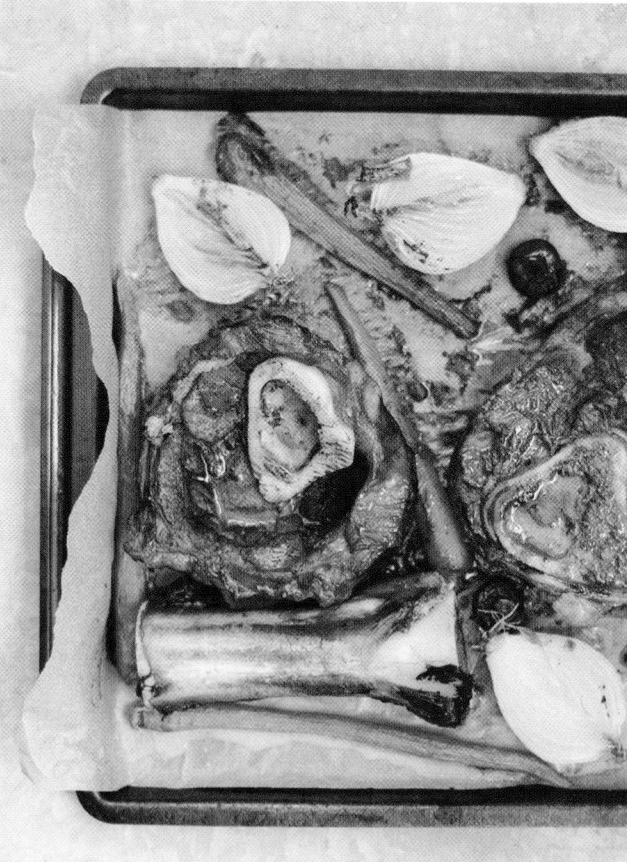

Cooking

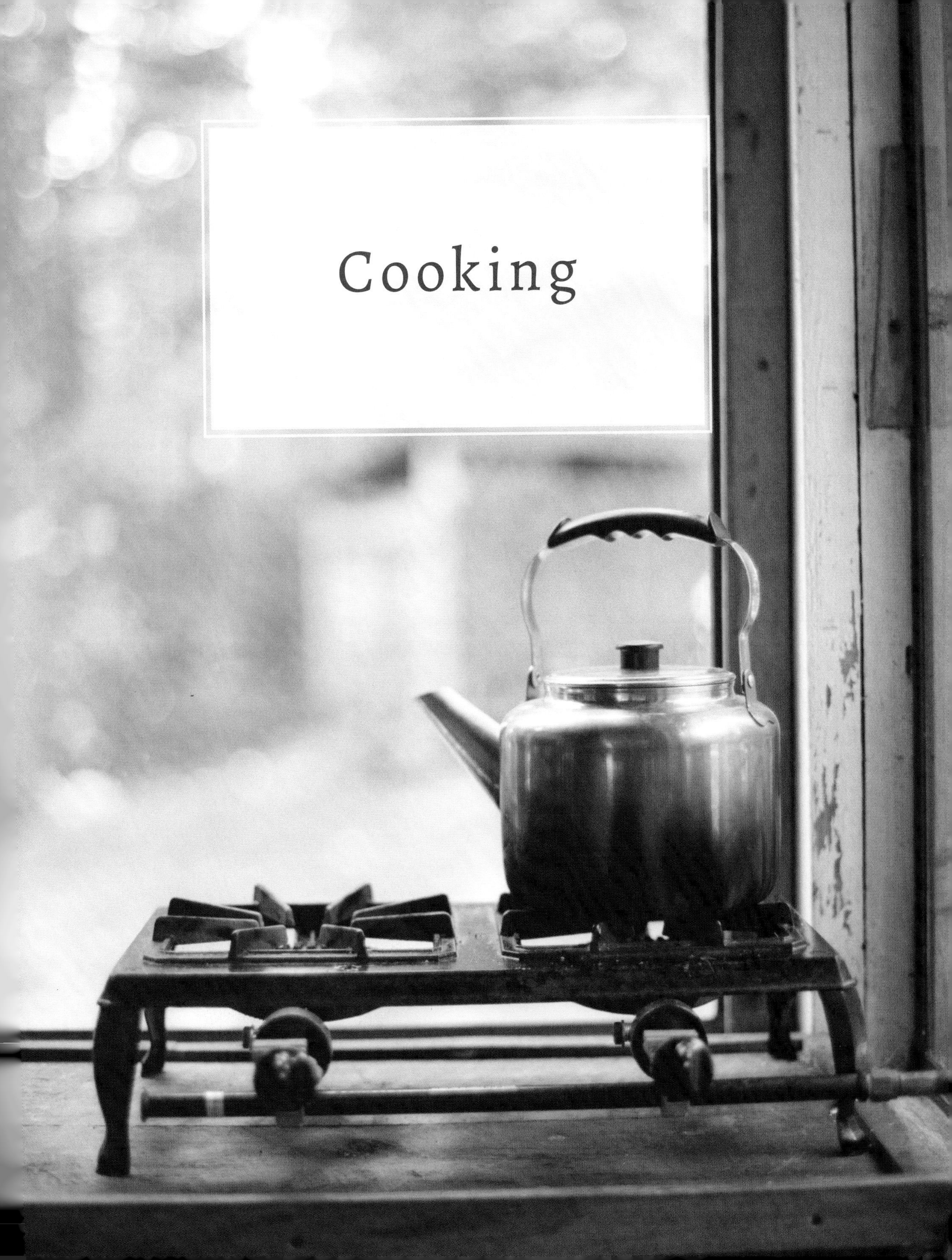

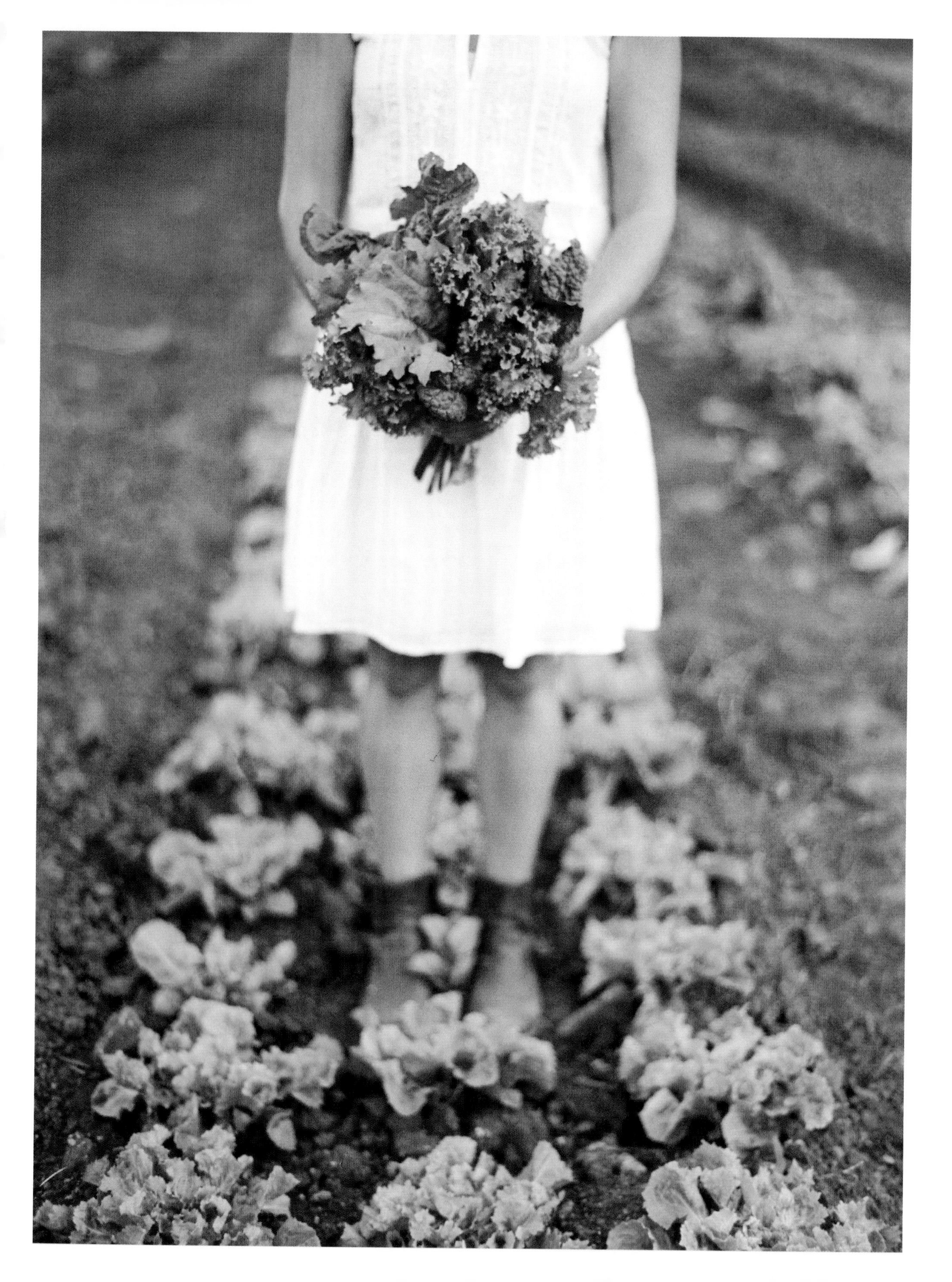

Using the Recipes

Because the way I eat is not just Paleo but also as local as possible, the chapters in this part of this book are organized according to the growing season of the produce coming in from the fields. But rather than group the recipes by the calendar-based seasons of spring, summer, and fall, I've broken them up into "Early Season," "Midseason," and "Late Season." This reflects the relative growing and/or harvest season of each produce item—regardless of region or growing zone.

For example, both rhubarb and asparagus are considered early-season crops, regardless of when on the calendar they pop out of the ground where you live. I've also tried to use only ingredients that are current with the season. For example, you won't find tomatoes and asparagus mingling together in the same recipe because they aren't in season at the same time. An exception to this seasonal focus is a collection of basic recipes for year-round staples, such as stocks and condiments, starting on page 327. (If you wish to find recipes by type or course, such as soups, salads, or desserts, please utilize the index.)

A few notes about the ingredients used in the recipes:

- **Eggs.** Use large eggs, preferably from pasture-raised chickens.
- **Salt.** I use fine-grain sea salt in all of my cooking.
- **Stock.** If you want to substitute store-bought broth for the homemade stock called for in my recipes, please use low-sodium broth and reduce the amount of salt (or salty ingredients, like fish stock and coconut aminos) that you use. In most of my recipes, salt is added "to taste," but you may not need to add any salt when using store-bought broth because it already contains salt (whereas my recipes for homemade stock do not).

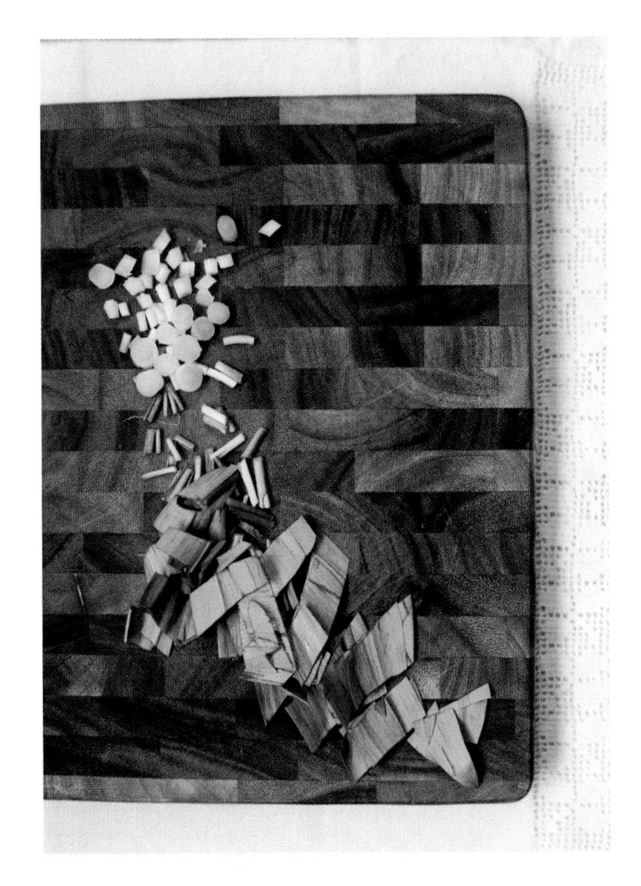

Modifying the Recipes for Your Dietary Needs

Paleo. On pages 13 to 18, you will find a detailed description of the Paleo diet and the specific key ingredients associated with it, such as preferred cooking fats, sources of protein, and vegetables.

Whole 30.* This thirty-day challenge is a bit stricter than the standard Paleo diet. On the Whole30, for example, there are no added sweeteners or dairy products (that means no butter, although ghee is okay). Almost all of my recipes are Whole30-compliant, often with no modifications needed. Only a handful of recipes cannot be used during the Whole30 regimen, and these are noted as such. After your Whole30 program, the rest of my recipes are fair game.

Nuts and eggs. Because many people are allergic to these ingredients, I indicate in each recipe whether it is free of nuts and/or eggs. I also indicate if the recipe can be modified to make it nut- or egg-free, and if substitute ingredients can be used.

AIP. This stands for the Autoimmune Protocol for the Paleo diet. Those with active autoimmune diseases should consider the additional removal of nuts, eggs, all dairy (including ghee), nightshades (peppers, eggplant, tomatoes, and white potatoes), and spices derived from seeds (black pepper, cardamom, cumin, coriander, fennel, mustard, and nutmeg). When possible, I've modified recipes to make them AIP-compliant; however, some recipes contain too many ingredients unsuitable for the AIP protocol.

Those with autoimmune conditions may find that after a month or so on this protocol, certain foods can be reintroduced. Start by reintroducing one ingredient at a time, and give your body three days to see if you notice any symptoms. Many people find that they can safely consume a standard Paleo diet after some time on the Autoimmune Protocol. However, I find that the 80/20 rule needs to be closer to 95/5 or even 100 percent for people with active autoimmune conditions.

Cooking and Eating Sustainably

As a nutritionist, I believe that a dish should be, above all other factors, good for your health. As a sustainability advocate, I also believe that food purchases should support local economies, living wages and fair working conditions for those who produce food, ethical treatment of the animals who produce food for you or give their lives for you, and good environmental practices, such as building healthy soil and promoting biodiversity. For consumers, supporting good environmental practices includes not buying food that travels long distances to reach you, has excessive packaging, or is treated with chemical pesticides or fertilizers. All of these things come into play when I prepare a meal for my family. Obviously, this is difficult to do 100 percent of the time, but the more you consider these factors when you eat, the easier it will be to make sustainable eating a habit.

The 80/20 Rule Applied to Sustainability

Sometimes, for the purpose of enhancing flavor in my cooking, I use ingredients that are not grown locally to me. I use organic citrus (to brighten soups and stews), organic black pepper and other spices, fair-trade dark chocolate, and occasionally organic coconut oil. Just as many folks living a Paleo lifestyle use the 80/20 rule (80 percent Paleo, 20 percent

---

The Whole30®, developed by my friends Dallas and Melissa Hartwig, is a great thirty-day introduction program to the Paleo diet. It is detailed on their website, whole30.com, and in their books, It Starts with Food *and* The Whole30.

non-Paleo), I like to think of my food choices as a ratio. The great majority of my food fits the criteria listed in the paragraph above, but I allow myself a few exceptions 20 percent of the time.

The bottom line is that you are in charge of your food choices. Use your money wisely, consider growing your own food, and support food producers who are conscious about sustainability. You will find that eating fresh, locally produced, nutrient-dense food is much easier to do when you grow your own, belong to a CSA, or shop at farmers markets.

Making It Work in Real Life

If you ask any of my friends what they've had to eat at my house, they will likely point to dishes found in this book. This is honestly how I eat on a daily basis. Of course there are times when we eat a simple roasted chicken with a side of veggies and a quick salad. I often cook in large batches, making sure that our fridge is packed with leftovers, which are easy to grab when we're running out the door to a kid's baseball game. I always tell my nutrition clients that it's just as easy to roast two or three chickens as it is to roast one, so try to make double or triple whenever possible. Having a kitchen full of healthy options greatly reduces your desire to spend lots of money on greasy takeout. It's all about making good food affordable and convenient, too. Here are some tips I've discovered for making a sustainable Paleo lifestyle work in real life.

- **Buy in bulk.** Get an extra freezer and fill it with frozen meat. Buying meat in bulk from local farmers can be very cost-effective.
- **Make leftovers.** It's nuts to cook three full meals for a family every single day. Cook in bulk so you don't have to cook every night and you'll have tons of great leftovers to guilt you out of getting takeout. When I grill steak, I grill at least three pounds. The same goes for roasting sweet potatoes—at least five or six go in the oven at once. This way, all I have to do on a busy night is make a fresh salad or a quick sauté of fresh veggies and heat up the meat and starch. Keep it simple for yourself and be prepared!
- **Keep fresh herbs close by.** Plant fresh herbs close to your house. It's great to be able to run outside and grab a bunch of fresh mint or basil to finish off a dish. Keeping herbs right outside your kitchen means that you have easy access. They grow well in containers (see page 136), and you'll have less waste if you simply use what you need from your plants instead of buying a whole bunch of basil just for the teaspoon required in one recipe.
- **Don't stress over using exact ingredients.** When making the recipes in this book, please substitute where you need to with what's available to you. Don't have any local Swiss chard? Use some kale or spinach. No access to goat meat? No problem; lamb is an easy-to-find substitute. I've listed substitution ideas with most of the recipes, but feel free to improvise if you don't tolerate, don't like, or can't find certain ingredients.

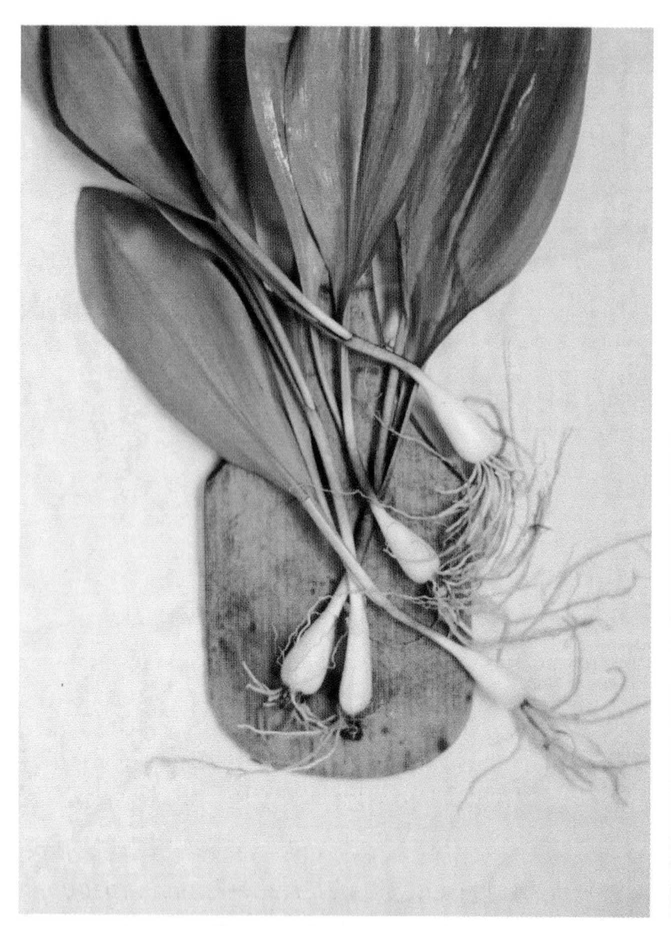
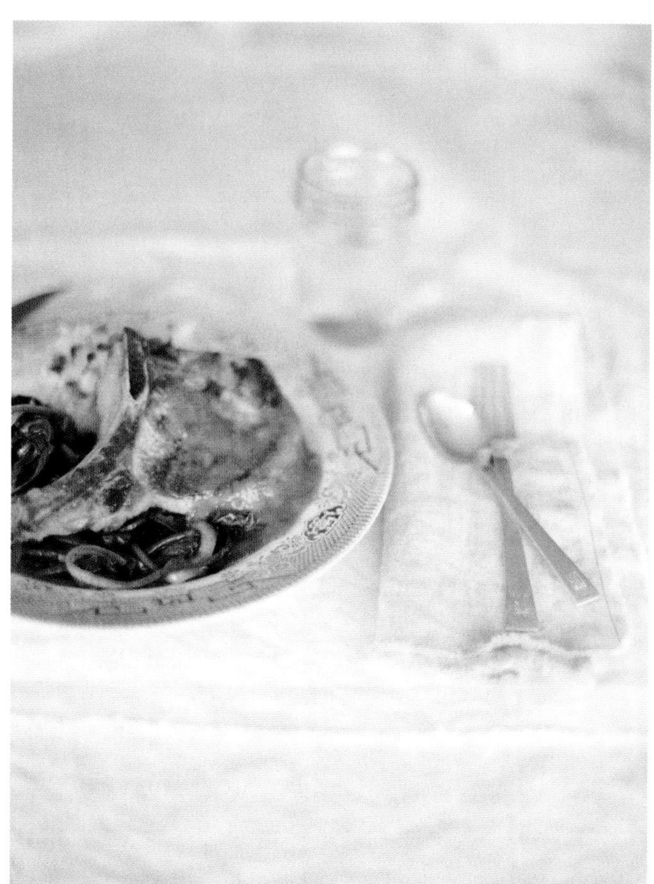
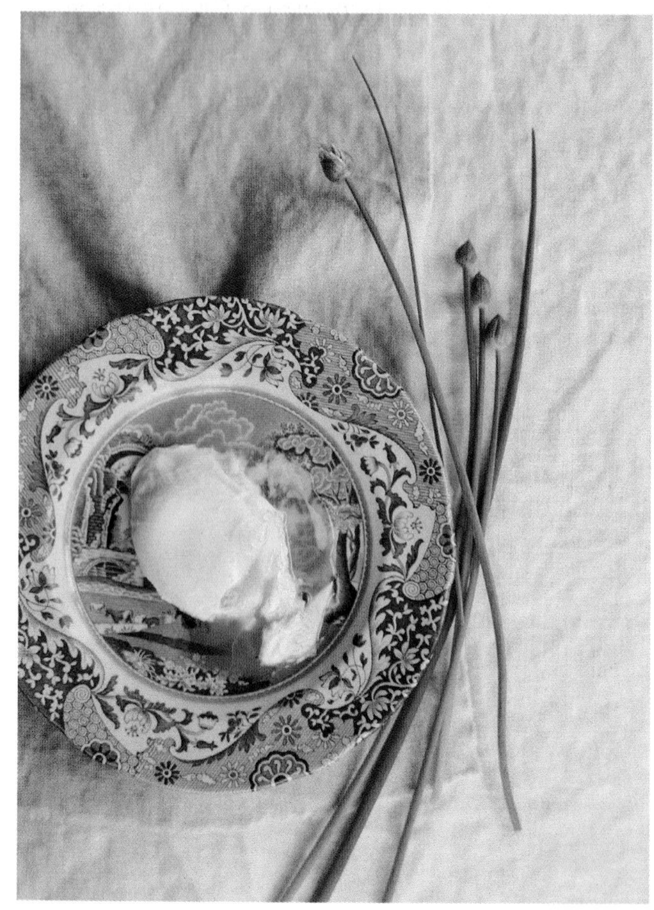
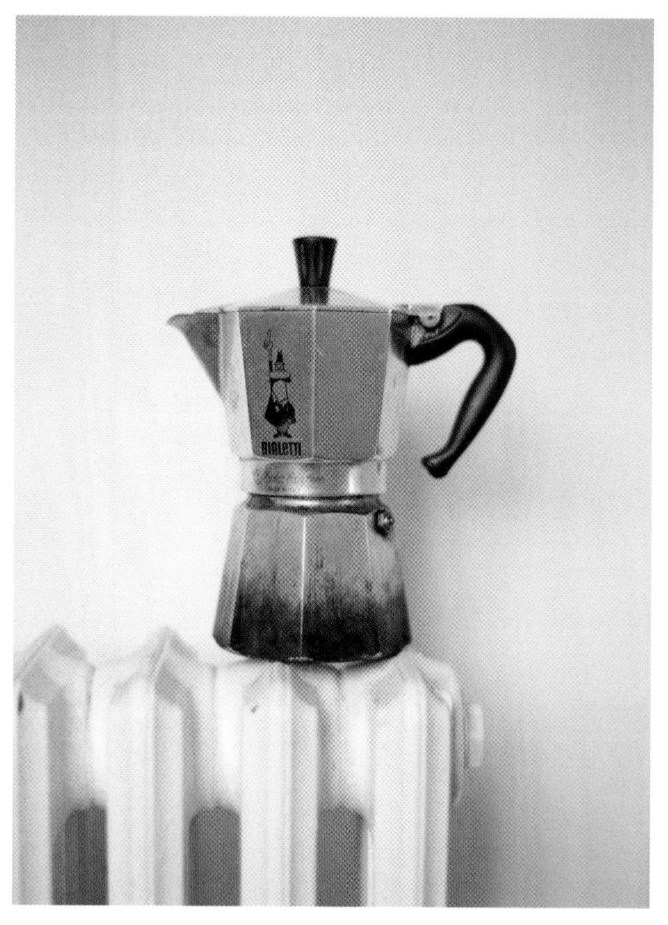
BIALETTI

Early Season Recipes

Spring brings with it chartreuse green colors and bright, light flavors. Nettles pop up from fertile soil, stalks of asparagus emerge, and baby greens make for fresh salads. While it can still be cold in New England, there is a new happiness to everyone's mood. It's a muddy and busy time. On the farm, we time our lambing to occur in mid-March so that the little ones don't face too much cold when they're ready to venture out of the barn. Seedlings are started in the greenhouse, and the pace of life really begins to pick up. By May, it's our busiest time of the year. Some of my favorite recipes from this season are Stinging Nettle Soup with Lemon-Chive Crème Fraîche (page 154), Chicken Saag with Turnip Greens (page 190), and Umami-Laden Spring Vegetables with Shiitake Mushrooms (page 188).

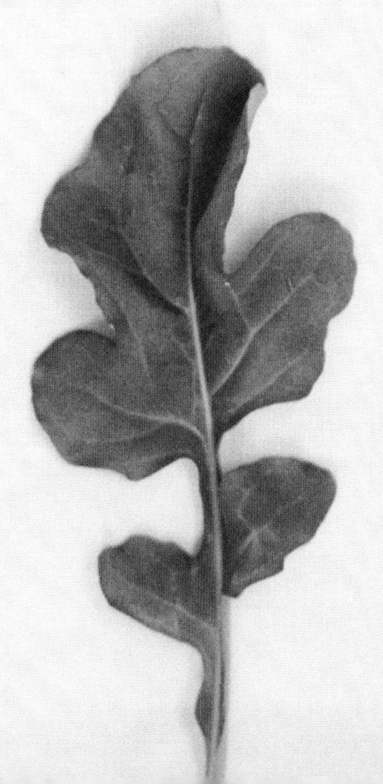

Stinging Nettle Soup with Lemon-Chive Crème Fraîche

This bright green, creamy soup is incredibly delicious. It's the reward for harvesting your own nettles, which is a bit of an adventure, but well worth it. Sting nettles are one of the first edibles to emerge in early spring. They like rich soil, and many old farmers know to plant their crops where nettles grow. Look for them near rivers or streams. Try harvesting nettles when they're four to twelve inches tall, and cut them down at the base. If you find them at a taller stage, just trim off the tops. You'll know you've found them if you step on them with bare feet; it feels like you've been stung by a ton of bees. Nettles have tiny needles that inject a stinging chemical and can stay in your skin for hours, reminding you of your mishap. Be sure to wear thick gloves when harvesting. The chemical responsible for the stinging sensation is rendered harmless by cooking. Historically, nettles have been used as a diuretic and to treat joint pain, and they are also said to be nourishing to the adrenal glands. For more on nettles and other wild edibles, see page 141.

Serves 6

- *1 tablespoon ghee (page 347)*
- *1 medium yellow onion, diced*
- *3 yellow potatoes or 2 pounds Jerusalem artichokes, peeled and diced*
- *1½ quarts homemade chicken stock (page 338)*
- *Big bowlful of nettle leaves (¼ to ½ pound), removed from the stalk and washed (handle with gloves until cooked)*
- *Sea salt and ground black pepper*
- *3 tablespoons crème fraîche (page 347) or canned, full-fat coconut milk*
- *2 tablespoons minced fresh chives*
- *Grated zest of 1 lemon*
- *2 tablespoons lemon juice*

1. In a large soup pot, heat the ghee over medium heat.
2. Add the diced onion and cook for 5 minutes, or until soft.
3. Add the diced potatoes and chicken stock and bring to a boil. Once at a boil, reduce the heat and simmer gently for 30 minutes.
4. Add the nettle leaves and cook until wilted.
5. Remove the soup from heat and purée with an immersion blender.
6. Season to taste with salt and pepper.
7. In a small bowl, combine the crème fraîche with the chives, lemon zest, and lemon juice. Mix well.
8. Serve the soup in shallow bowls with a swirl of the crème fraîche mixture on top.

Whole30	Substitute coconut milk or coconut cream for the crème fraîche.
Nut-free	Yes
Egg-free	Yes
AIP	Substitute coconut oil for the ghee. Use Jerusalem artichokes or sweet potatoes instead of yellow potatoes. Omit the black pepper. Substitute coconut milk or coconut cream for the crème fraîche.

NOTES: *You can substitute nettles in any recipe that calls for spinach. They are fantastic in a frittata or pureed into a pesto with olive oil and nuts of your choice. Nettles also make a great tea. If you can't find nettles, use spinach or Swiss chard.*

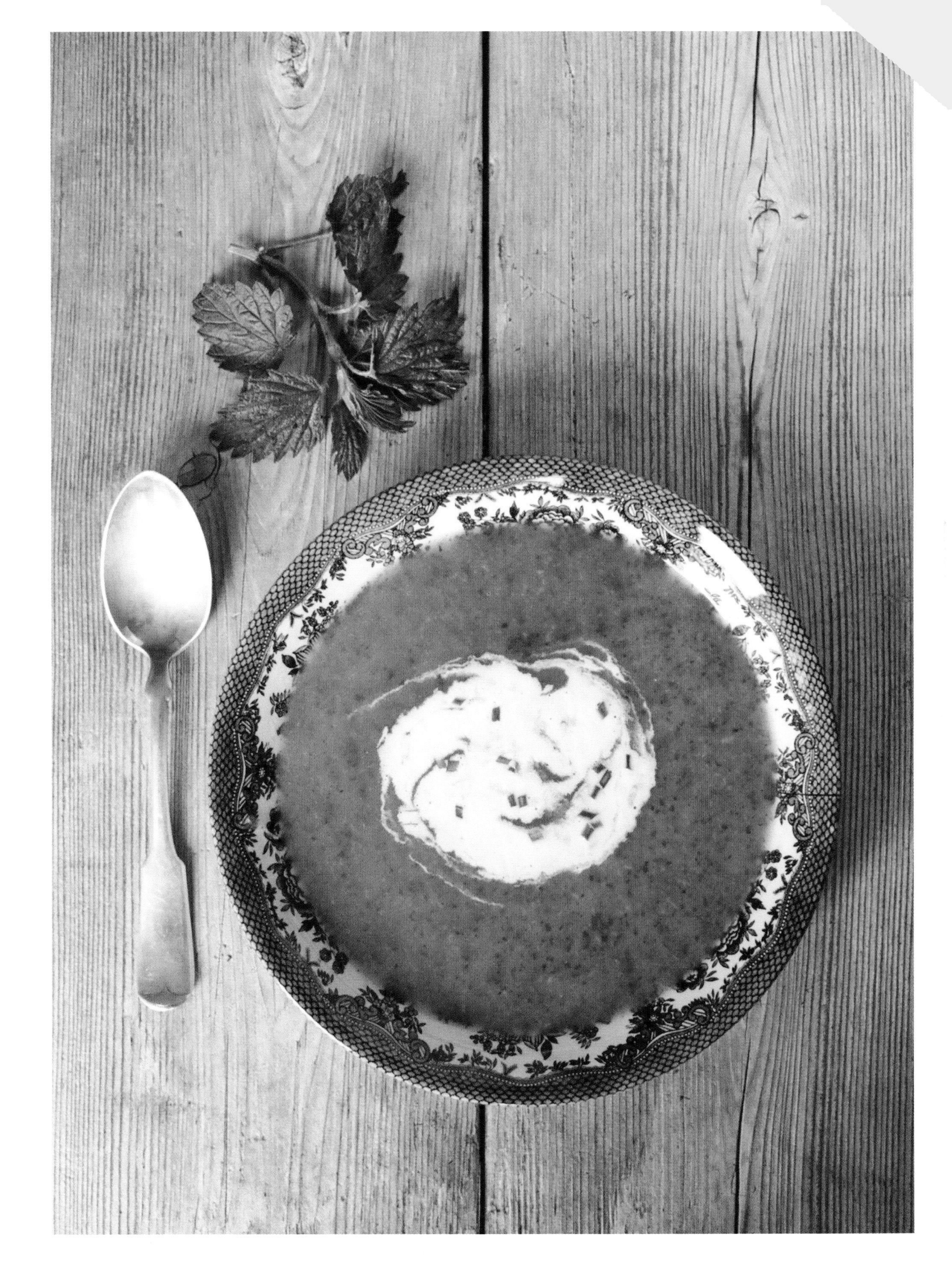

Escarole Frittata

This frittata is absolutely lovely! You can substitute virtually any green for the escarole, but I really love how light the escarole is in this nourishing and delicious dish. Frittatas are economical, simple to make, and packed with nutrients. On the farm, we alternate who cooks for lunch and eat together, and this is my go-to dish when I need something for a crowd. The combination of sweet onions, salty pancetta, and bright fresh herbs is particularly wonderful. Serve it with a side of fruit or potatoes or a fresh green salad.

Serves 4

- *8 ounces pancetta, bacon, or bacon ends, trimmed of excess fat and diced small*
- *2 cups thinly sliced white onion (about 1 medium onion)*
- *5 cremini mushrooms, diced small*
- *2½ cups coarsely chopped escarole (1 medium head)*
- *8 eggs*
- *3 tablespoons canned, full-fat coconut milk or heavy cream*
- *2 tablespoons chopped fresh parsley leaves*
- *2 tablespoons chopped fresh basil leaves*
- *Ground black pepper*

1. Preheat the oven to 350°F.
2. In a large ovenproof skillet, sauté the pancetta for 10 minutes, or until browned and crispy. Remove from the heat.
3. Pour off most of the fat so that only a thin coating remains in the pan. Reserve the rest of the fat for later use. Add the onion and cook on medium-low heat for about 15 minutes, until caramelized.
4. Add the mushrooms, about 1 teaspoon of the reserved fat (if needed), and the escarole. Bring the heat up to medium and sauté for about 5 minutes, until the escarole is wilted.
5. In a medium bowl, beat the eggs with the coconut milk, parsley, basil, and a pinch of black pepper.
6. Pour the eggs into the pan with the escarole mixture and cook over medium heat for about 3 minutes to allow the bottom to set.
7. Transfer the pan to the oven and bake for 10 minutes.
8. Turn the oven to the broil setting and finish off the frittata by broiling the top for 2 to 3 minutes, until light brown.
9. Allow to cool slightly, then serve. Frittatas are also excellent cold or at room temperature.

NOTES: *Escarole is a bitter green. You can substitute any hearty green, like collards, kale, Swiss chard, or mustard greens.*

Whole30	Yes
Nut-free	Yes
Egg-free	No
AIP	No

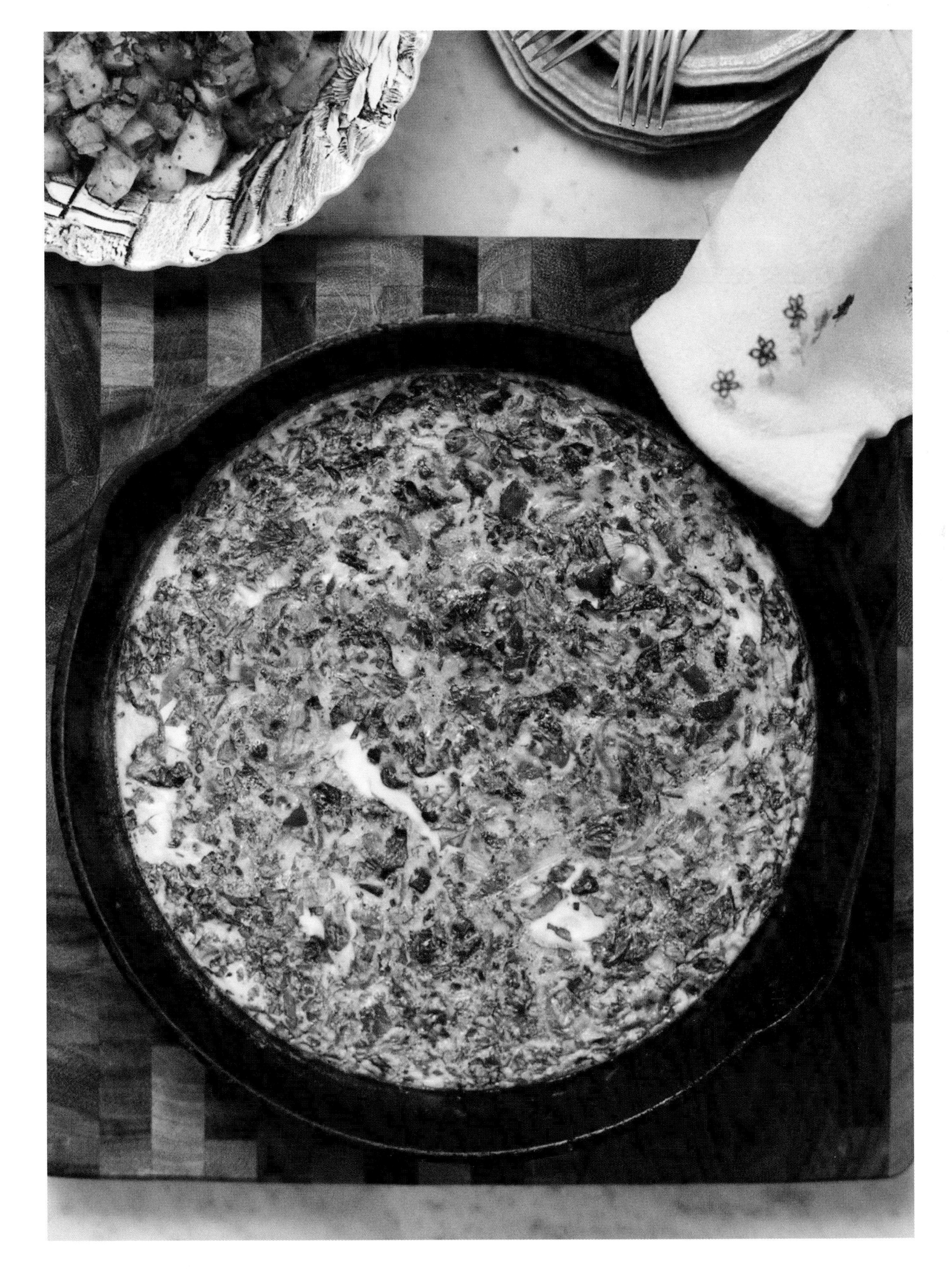

Garlic Scape Pesto over Steamed Eggs

Garlic scapes are heaven for garlic lovers. These curly tops of hardneck garlic are the plant's flowers, and they can be found about the same time strawberries are in season. This intense pesto is amazing on hard-boiled pasture-raised eggs. Fresh eggs are notoriously hard to peel—and I have tried numerous techniques. Follow the instructions here for steaming eggs, which will make peeling them much easier. You can also try the pesto over steak, mix it with zucchini noodles, spread it on Salted Herb Crackers (page 298), or mix a teaspoon into scrambled eggs.

Serves 6 as an appetizer (with extra pesto for another use)

For the Garlic Scape Pesto

(Makes about 1½ cups)

- *½ pound garlic scapes (about 8 to 10), cut into 2-inch pieces*
- *½ cup raw almonds*
- *¾ cup grated Parmesan cheese*
- *¼ teaspoon sea salt*
- *1 tablespoon lemon juice*
- *1 cup fresh parsley leaves*
- *1 cup cold-pressed, extra-virgin olive oil*
- *6 eggs*

1. Combine all of the ingredients for the pesto in a food processor and blend until smooth. Set aside.
2. Place a metal colander or steaming basket in a large pot so that the lid will fit tightly.
3. Add the eggs to the colander and then add enough water so that it just touches the bottom of the eggs, but they are not fully submerged. Cover with a tight-fitting lid.
4. Bring the water to a boil, then reduce the heat to medium. Steam the eggs for 20 minutes.
5. Using oven mitts or tongs, carefully remove the colander or steaming basket from the pot.
6. Immediately transfer the eggs to the empty bowl and shake it so that the shells crack a bit.
7. Pour ice-cold water over the eggs and allow them to cool for about 10 minutes.
8. Peel the eggs in the sink, under running water. Compost the shells.
9. Slice each egg in half and place ½ teaspoon of the pesto on each half.

NOTES: *Garlic scapes really mellow out when you cook them. Try them tossed in a stir-fry or boiled lightly, like string beans. Or try blanching them and tossing them with balsamic or red wine vinegar and sautéed mushrooms. If you can't find garlic scapes, try making the pesto with a bunch of arugula and a few cloves of garlic.*

Whole30	Omit the cheese.
Nut-free	Omit the nuts.
Egg-free	Omit the eggs and serve the pesto over roasted vegetables.
AIP	Omit the nuts and cheese. Omit the eggs and serve the pesto over roasted vegetables

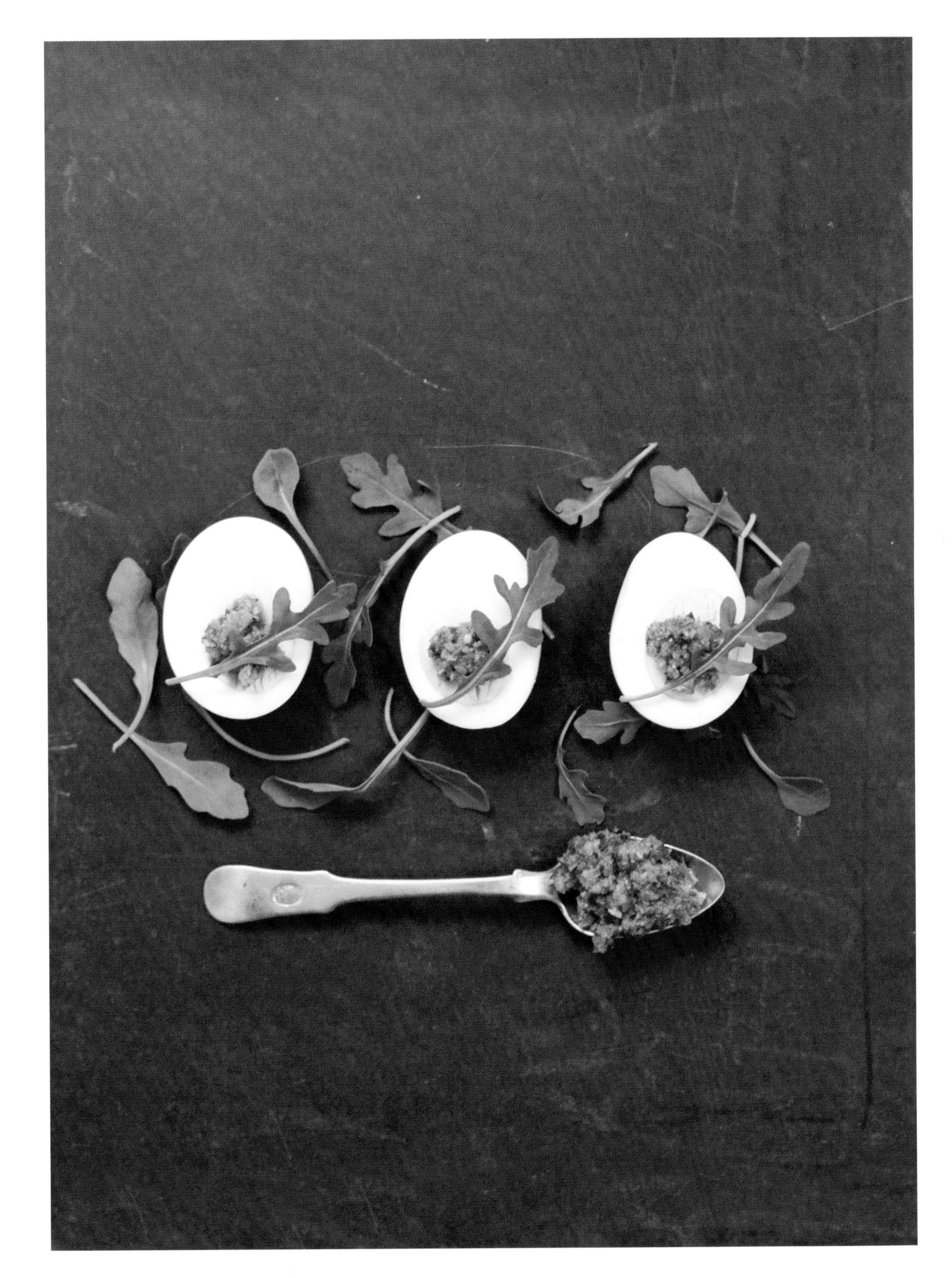

Grilled Leg of Lamb with Garlic Scape Pesto and Mint

Lamb is my favorite meat. Although many people associate it with springtime, I like to eat it throughout the year. I know you'll love it in this recipe, grilled with a mixture of Garlic Scape Pesto (page 158) and fresh mint. Garlicky, moist, and fresh-tasting, this simple dish is a total crowd-pleaser. Serve it with Umami-Laden Spring Vegetables with Shiitake Mushrooms (page 188).

Serves 6

- *½ cup Garlic Scape Pesto (page 158)*
- *½ cup cold-pressed, extra-virgin olive oil*
- *½ cup finely chopped fresh mint leaves*
- *Juice of ½ lemon*
- *1 (2½- to 3-pound) boneless leg of lamb*

1. Mix together the pesto, olive oil, mint, and lemon juice in a small bowl. Thoroughly cover the lamb with the mixture and allow to marinate in the refrigerator for a few hours or overnight.
2. Heat a grill to medium heat (see page 362 for grilling tips).
3. Place the lamb on the hot grill and cook for about 10 minutes. Flip and cook until the internal temperature reaches 125°F (for rare), about 8 to 14 minutes. Remove from the heat, cover with foil, and allow to rest for at least 20 minutes before slicing.

Whole30	Yes
Nut-free	Yes
Egg-free	Yes
AIP	Yes

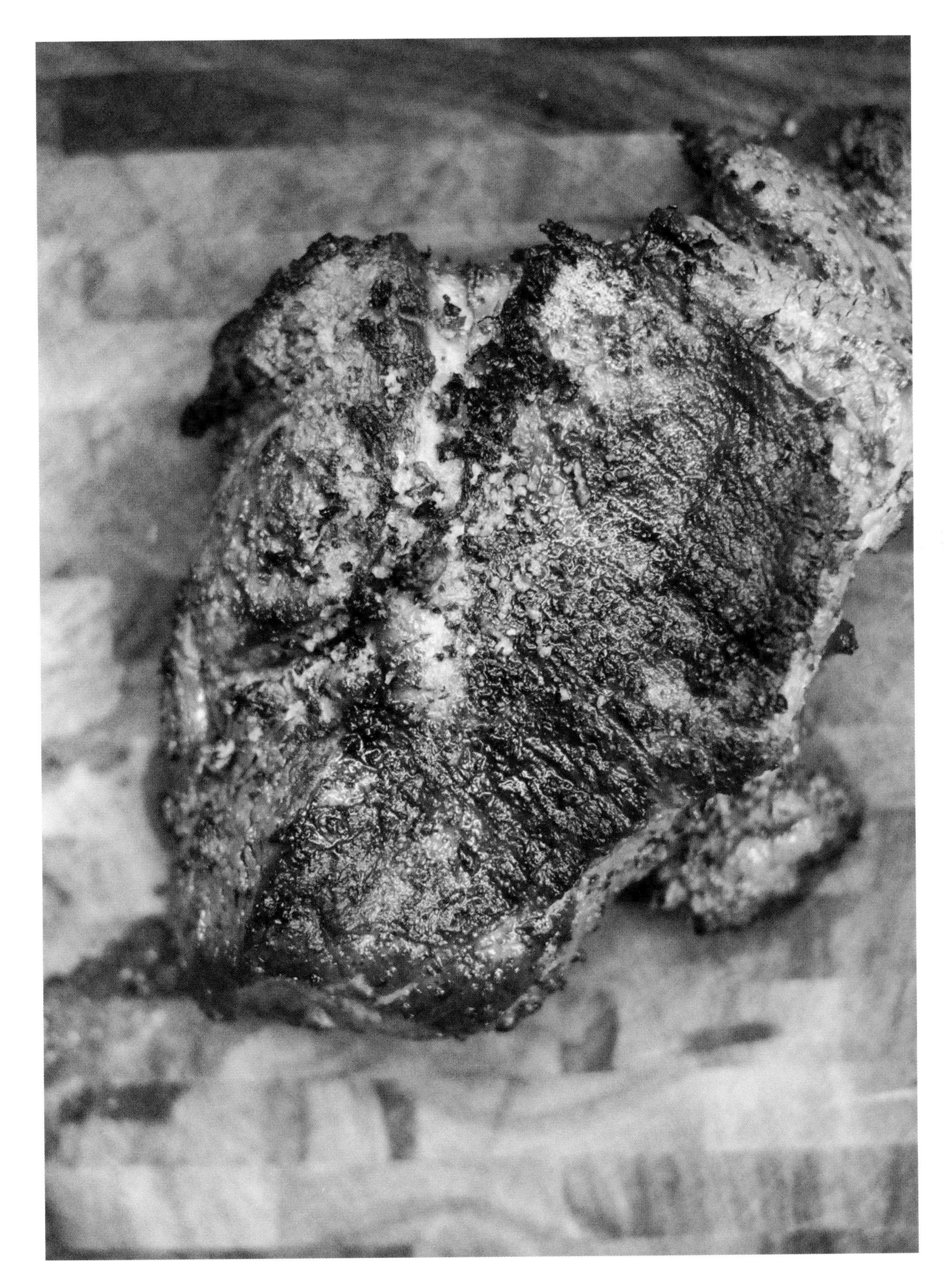

Sea Scallops with Ramps and Wilted Lamb's Quarters

Lamb's quarters are simply amazing. They're weeds that you've probably seen growing on the edge of your property, but they taste a bit like spinach—only much better and less bitter—and they're free! I was not impressed with the taste of them when raw, but when cooked lightly, I couldn't believe how amazing they are. Lamb's quarters have a poisonous lookalike called nettleleaf goosefoot, but you'll know that plant by the strongly unpleasant odor it gives off when crushed between your fingers. Lamb's quarters do not have this scent. Wash the greens well to remove all of the pollen from the leaves. Ramps are a common wild edible and have a garlicky onion taste. For more on lamb's quarters, ramps, and other wild edibles, see pages 140 to 142. Sea scallops are among the most sustainable seafood choices—see page 85 for more information on sustainable seafood.

Serves 2

- *5 strips bacon*
- *6 sea scallops*
- *Sea salt and ground black pepper*
- *4 ramps, chopped, green and white parts separated*
- *Big bowlful of lamb's quarters, washed well*
- *Juice of 1 lemon*
- *Grated zest of 1 lemon*

1. In a skillet over medium heat, cook the bacon. Once done, remove it from the pan and set aside to drain on paper towels. Pour off most of the fat from the pan into a cup, keeping about a tablespoon in the pan for the scallops.

2. Remove the feet from the scallops. (The foot is the inch-long tough piece on the side of the scallop, and it's no fun to eat.) Pat the scallops dry and sprinkle with salt and pepper.

3. Heat the skillet over medium-high heat. When the pan is nice and hot, add the scallops to the pan and let them sizzle for about 2 minutes per side. Remove from the pan and set aside.

4. Lower the heat slightly and add about a tablespoon of the reserved bacon fat. Add the white parts of the ramps and let them cook for a few minutes.

5. Add the ramp greens and lamb's quarters. Cook until bright green and wilted, about 2 minutes.

6. Now that the bacon is cool, crumble it into small pieces.

7. On each plate, place half the greens. Sprinkle with 1 teaspoon of the lemon juice. Add three scallops, top with about 2 tablespoons of crumbled bacon, and finish with a sprinkle of lemon zest, salt, and pepper.

NOTES: *If scallops aren't your thing or are hard to find, substitute 4 to 6 ounces of shrimp or monkfish. If you can't find ramps, substitute scallions or green garlic. If you are lucky enough to find a patch of ramps, please be sustainable in the way you harvest them. You don't need to pluck out the entire bed. Pull a few from the center of the patch, and save the rest so you can have some again next year. Substitute spinach or Swiss chard for the lamb's quarters if you can't find them.*

Whole30	Yes
Nut-free	Yes
Egg-free	Yes
AIP	Omit the black pepper.

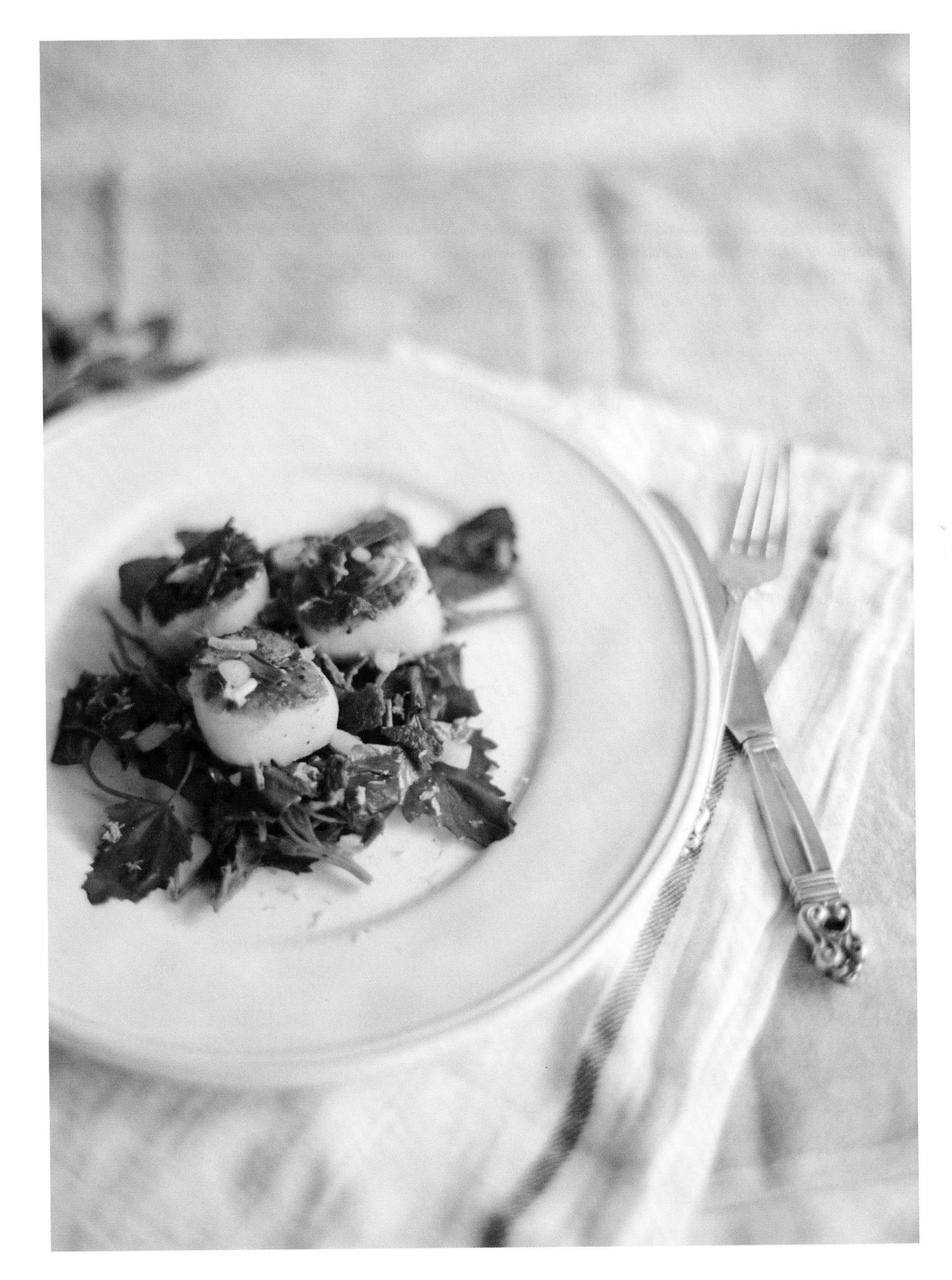

Spring Egg Drop Soup with Lemon-Ginger Meatballs

This is sort of a hybrid of an Asian egg drop soup and stracciatella, a delicious Italian egg "ribbon" soup made with chicken stock. The result is light and refreshing, yet really satisfying and comforting. I love to eat it for breakfast! It's also special enough to serve to guests. If you want to make it ahead of time, just complete the recipe through Step 4, let cool, and refrigerate. Ten minutes before you'd like to serve it, warm it up and continue with the rest of the steps. This will keep the spinach a brighter green.

Serves 6

- *1 tablespoon unsalted butter (page 348) or ghee (page 347)*
- *1 medium yellow onion, diced*
- *1 tablespoon minced fresh ginger*
- *2 quarts homemade chicken stock (page 338)*
- *1 batch Lemon-Ginger Meatballs (page 166), cooked*
- *3 cups minced spinach, Swiss chard, lamb's quarters, or other greens*
- *2 eggs, beaten*
- *2 tablespoons fish sauce*
- *2 tablespoons coconut aminos (see Notes)*
- *1 teaspoon lemon juice (or to taste)*

1. Melt the butter in a soup pot over medium heat.
2. Add the onion and sauté for 5 minutes.
3. Add the ginger and sauté for another few minutes.
4. Add the chicken stock and meatballs and simmer for 10 minutes.
5. Add the spinach and cook for about 5 minutes.
6. After about 5 minutes, slowly add the eggs to the soup in a light stream. Stir the soup as you do so to produce strands of eggs instead of one large poached egg.
7. Add the fish sauce, coconut aminos, and finally the lemon juice to brighten the soup.
8. Check the seasoning and season with salt or more coconut aminos, if needed.

NOTES: *If you're using store-bought stock, use less coconut aminos; otherwise, it may be too salty.*

Whole30	Use ghee, not butter.
Nut-free	Yes
Egg-free	Omit the eggs.
AIP	Omit the eggs. Substitute coconut oil for the butter.

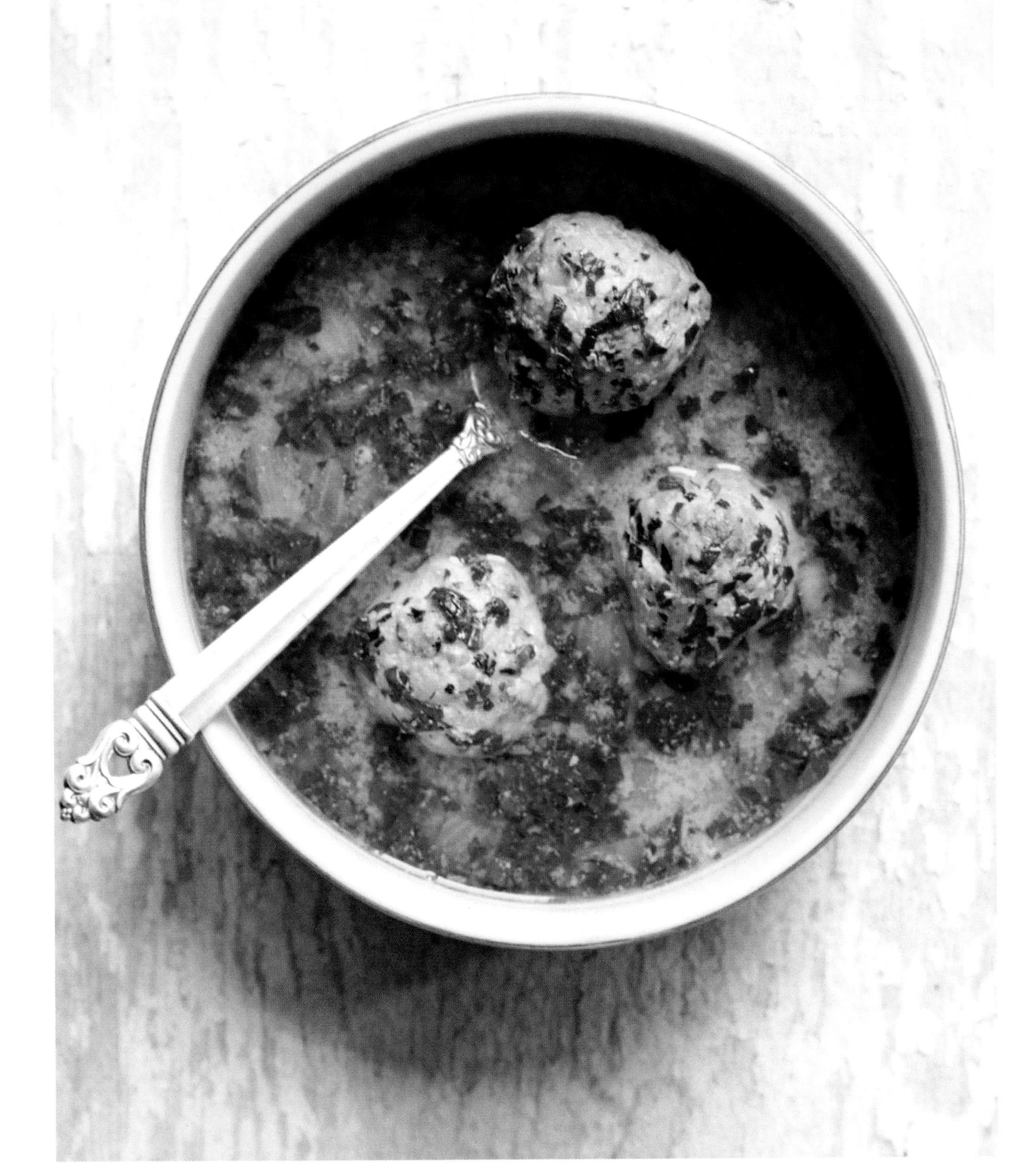

Lemon-Ginger Meatballs

The lemon and bright herbs give these meatballs an unexpected fresh and light taste. I originally made them for the Spring Egg Drop Soup with Lemon-Ginger Meatballs (page 164), but they are so good on their own that I feel they deserve their own recipe. Serve them as an appetizer, or double the recipe and have them with some mashed sweet potatoes and a little salad for a meal.

Makes 25 to 30 little meatballs or 18 golf ball–sized meatballs

- *1 pound ground pork or ground turkey*
- *4 shiitake mushrooms, stemmed and minced*
- *1 tablespoon minced fresh mint leaves*
- *1 tablespoon minced fresh basil leaves*
- *1 tablespoon minced fresh parsley leaves*
- *1 egg white*
- *1½ teaspoons grated fresh ginger*
- *2 teaspoons grated lemon zest*
- *¼ teaspoon sea salt*
- *¼ teaspoon ground black pepper*

1. Preheat the oven to 425°F.
2. In a large bowl, combine all of the ingredients and mix well.
3. Line a rimmed baking sheet with parchment paper.
4. Using your hands, form the mixture into 25 to 30 little meatballs or about 18 golf ball–sized meatballs.
5. Place the meatballs on the lined baking sheet and bake for 12 to 15 minutes, until light brown.

Whole30	Yes
Nut-free	Yes
Egg-free	Omit the egg.
AIP	Omit the egg and black pepper.

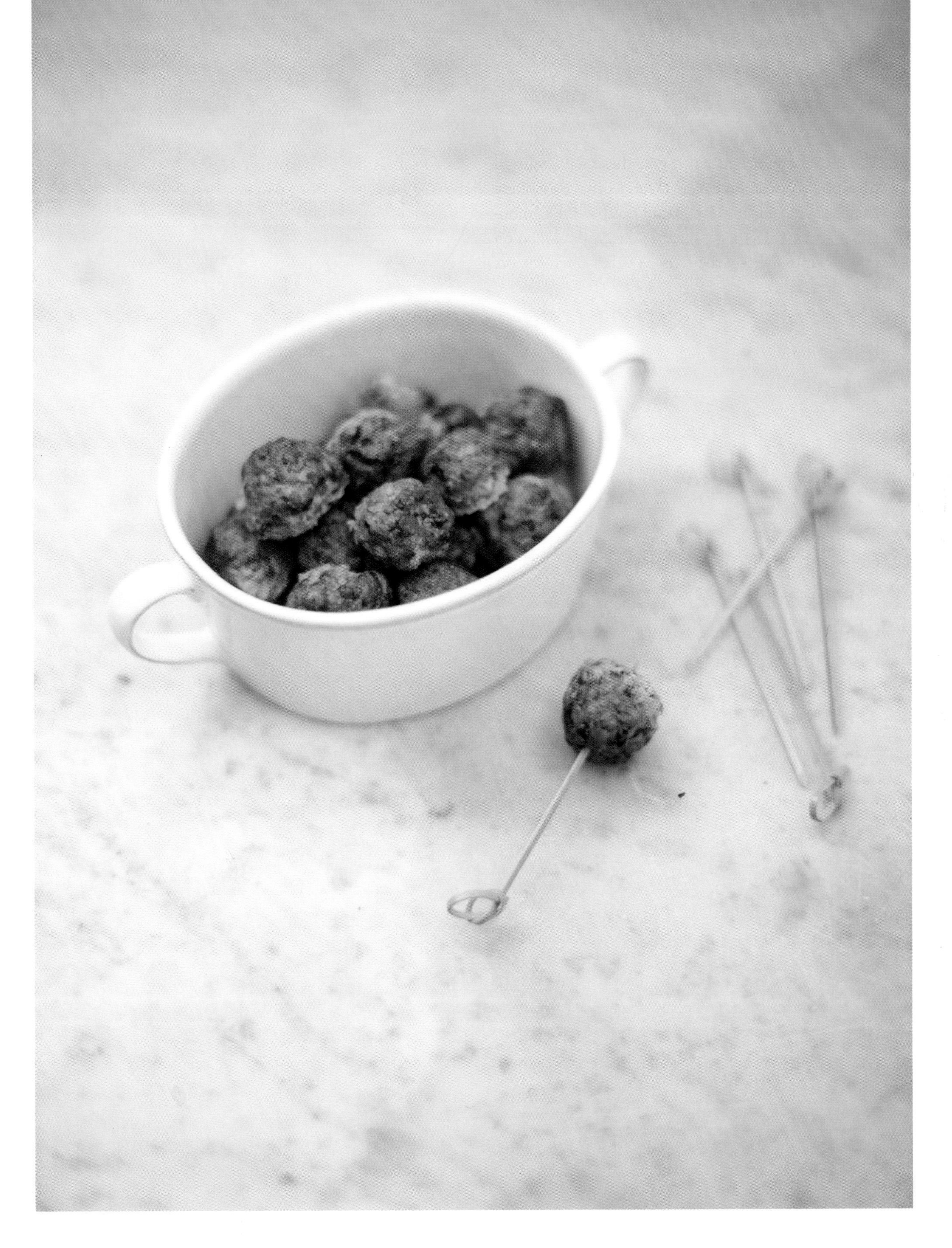

Pan-Seared Pork Chop with Rhubarb-Ginger Sauce

Of all the meat we raise on the farm, I have to say that our pork is the most different from its grocery store counterpart. The flavor is richer and, well, just more heavenly. With pork chops, I often don't do much more than season them with salt and pepper and sear them in a pan. If I want to take it a step further, I'll pair them with a sweet-tart accompaniment like the Rhubarb-Ginger Sauce on page 172. It's an absolutely amazing combination.

Serves 4

- *4 pork chops, 1½ inches thick*
- *2 tablespoons bacon fat, ghee (page 347), or coconut oil*
- *Sea salt and ground black pepper*
- *1 cup Rhubarb-Ginger Sauce (page 172), warmed*

1. Bring the chops to room temperature.
2. In a large heavy skillet, melt the bacon fat over medium heat.
3. Dry off the pork chops and generously season them on both sides with salt and pepper.
4. Working in batches so as to not overcrowd the pan, sear the pork chops for about 4 minutes on the first side (don't touch, just leave them in the pan for the entire 4 minutes to get a nice sear). After 4 minutes, flip the chops. Cook them until the internal temperature reaches 145°F.
5. Remove from the heat and allow to rest for 5 minutes or so before cutting into the meat.
6. Serve each chop with ¼ cup of the warmed Rhubarb-Ginger Sauce.

NOTES: *If you don't have rhubarb, try using apples or pears to make the sauce. This sauce is great on a variety of grilled meats; try it with chicken or fish.*

Whole30	Yes
Nut-free	Yes
Egg-free	Yes
AIP	Use bacon fat or coconut oil, not ghee. Omit the black pepper.

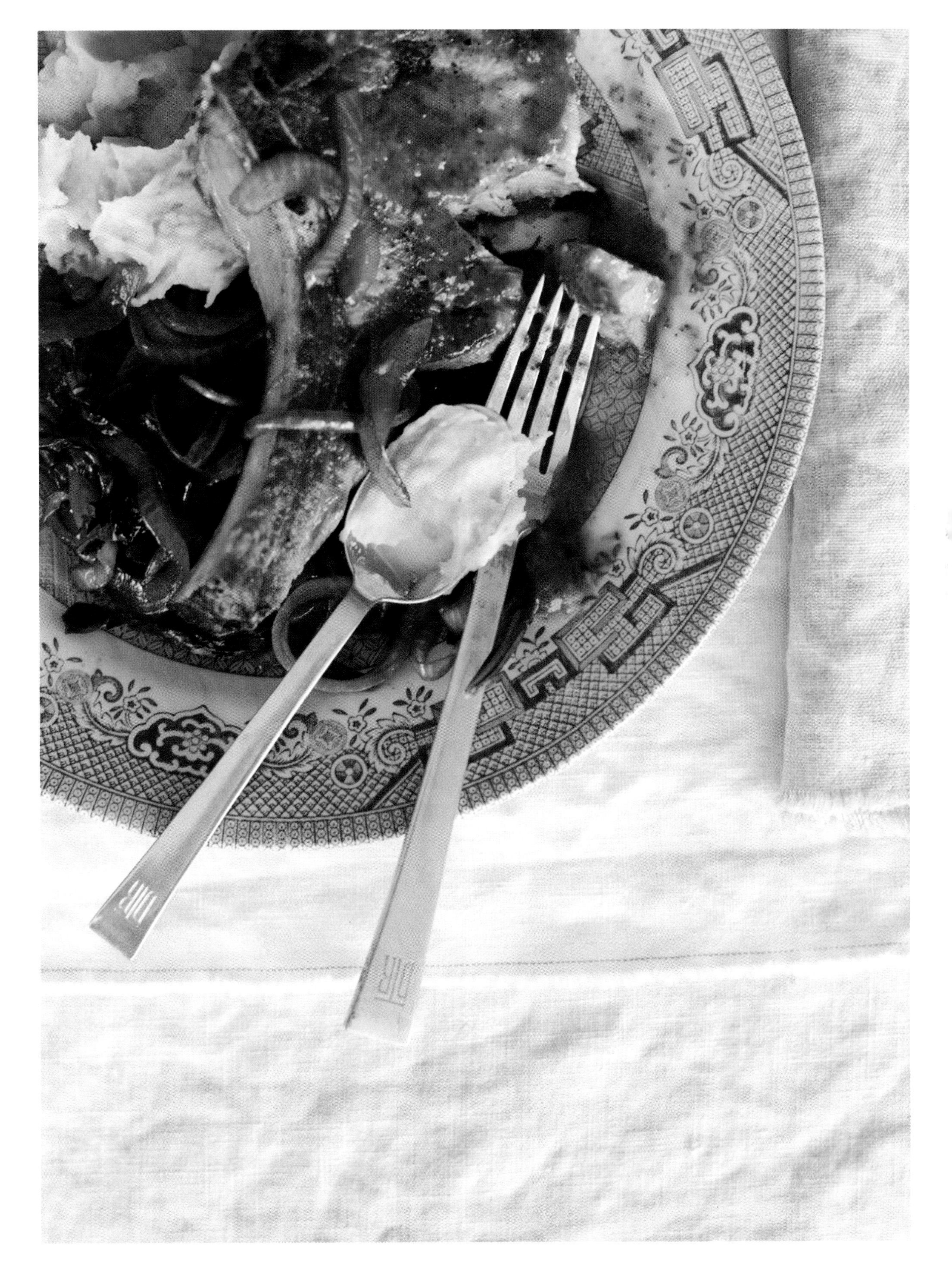

Wilted Dandelion Greens with Balsamic Onions

For the best-tasting dandelion greens, harvest them in the early spring. Very young, shade-grown dandelion greens are the best for eating. Leaves from plants growing in direct sun tend to be more bitter. Also, try to seek out plants growing on the edge of a lawn or farm instead of those growing in sidewalk cracks. The healthier the soil, the healthier the plant is for you to eat. For more on dandelions and other wild edibles, see page 139.

Serves 4

- *1 teaspoon bacon fat, ghee (page 347), or coconut oil*
- *1 medium yellow onion, sliced thin*
- *2 tablespoons balsamic vinegar*
- *1 big bunch dandelion greens (2 large handfuls), washed*
- *1 tablespoon lemon juice*
- *Sea salt and ground black pepper*

NOTES: *Dandelion flowers are edible, too. Some people say that they taste like a combination of corn, spinach, and Brussels sprouts. Try blanching them for 60 seconds and then add them to an omelet or soup. Dandelion roots can be harvested, dried, and ground to brew a beverage that is even more delicious than coffee. If you want to use a substitute for the greens, try any bitter green, like kale or Swiss chard.*

Whole30	Yes
Nut-free	Yes
Egg-free	Yes
AIP	Omit the black pepper and use bacon fat or coconut oil, not ghee.

1. In a large skillet, melt the bacon fat over medium-low heat.
2. Add the onion and cook until translucent, about 10 minutes. Do not brown or the dish will be bitter.
3. Add the balsamic vinegar and cook for another couple of minutes, until the onion absorbs most of the vinegar and turns dark.
4. Add the dandelion greens, still wet from washing. The water on the leaves will allow them to steam slightly as they wilt. Cook for about 2 minutes, until they are lightly wilted but not completely cooked down.
5. Sprinkle on the lemon juice and season to taste with salt and pepper.

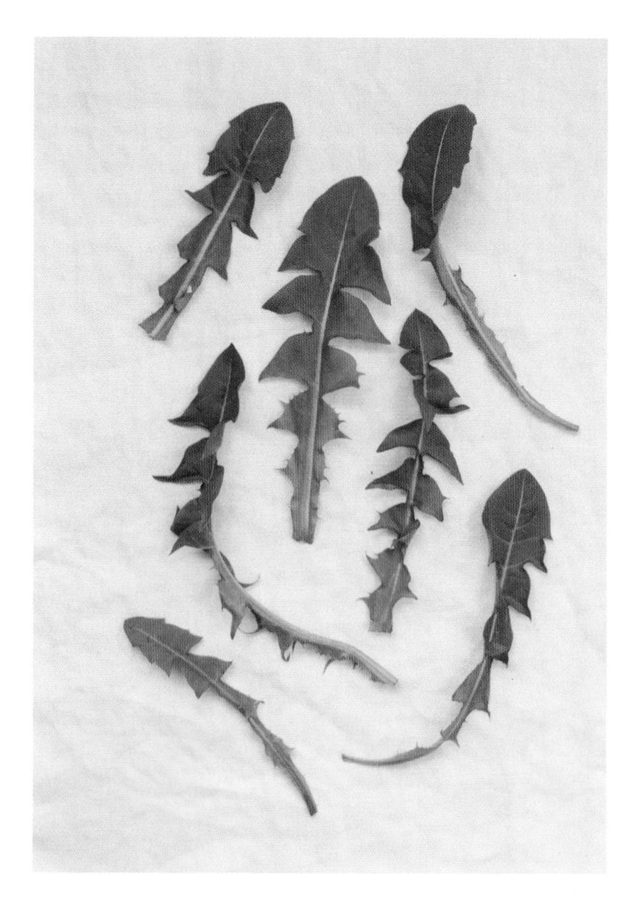

Simple Mashed Sweet Potatoes with Chives

Although they're harvested in the fall, sweet potatoes store so well that they can be eaten year-round. Sweet, silky, and incredibly comforting, these mashed sweet potatoes are lovely. They don't need much added to them because their flavor is perfect as is. They are fantastic alongside a seared pork chop or the meat of your choice. I like to serve them to my guests and see their reaction when they first try them. They're always a big hit!

Serves 4

- *3 pounds sweet potatoes, peeled and chopped into 2-inch chunks (white or orange flesh)*
- *½ cup canned, full-fat coconut milk*
- *Sea salt and ground black pepper*
- *2 tablespoons minced fresh chives, for garnish*

Whole30	Yes
Nut-free	Yes
Egg-free	Yes
AIP	Omit the black pepper.

1. In a large soup pot filled with water, bring the sweet potatoes to a boil.
2. Simmer for approximately 25 minutes, or until they are fork-tender.
3. Add the coconut milk and mash by hand or whip with a handheld electric mixer.
4. Add salt and pepper to taste and garnish with fresh chives.

NOTES: *If you eat dairy, try using heavy cream or whole, raw milk instead of coconut milk for ultra-decadent mashed sweet potatoes.*

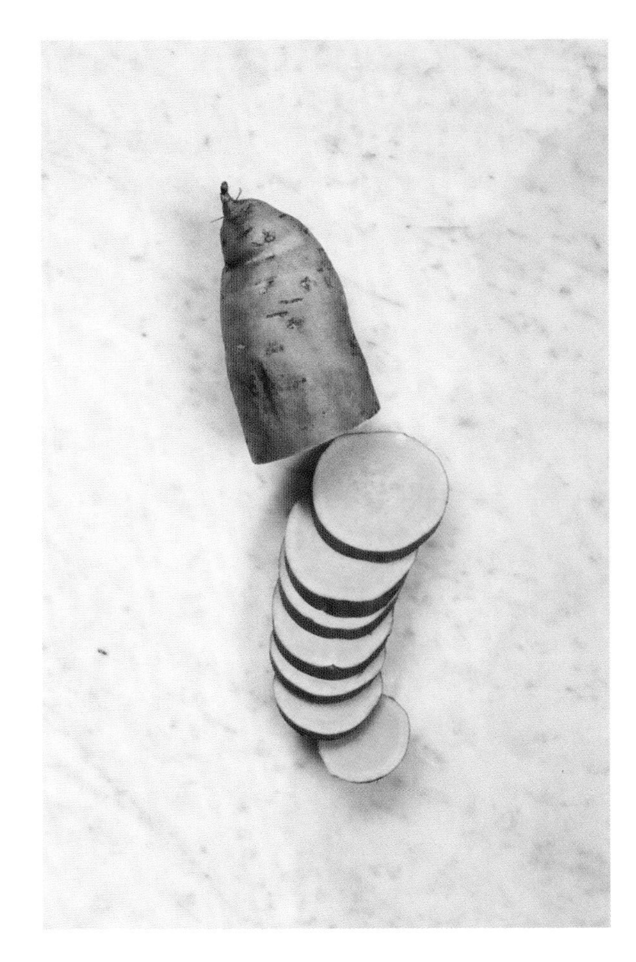

Rhubarb-Ginger Sauce

This simple sauce is to die for. It's tangy and a little spicy from the large amount of ginger, but the raisins calm it down and sweeten it up—no need to add sugar. It can transform an average cut of meat into something very special. It's also fantastic with scallops and adds a zippy kick to vanilla ice cream.

Makes about 2 cups

- *3 stalks rhubarb, chopped into ½-inch pieces*
- *2 cups apple juice*
- *1 tablespoon grated fresh ginger*
- *½ cup raisins*

1. In a medium saucepan, combine all of the ingredients.
2. Bring to a simmer over medium-low heat, then reduce the heat to low and continue to cook for 25 minutes, or until the rhubarb is very soft and the sauce has reduced a bit.
3. Purée the mixture in a blender or with an immersion blender. Serve warm with meat or atop vanilla ice cream.

NOTES: *If you don't have rhubarb, try using apples or pears. This sauce is great on a variety of grilled meats; try it with chicken or fish.*

Whole30	Yes
Nut-free	Yes
Egg-free	Yes
AIP	Yes

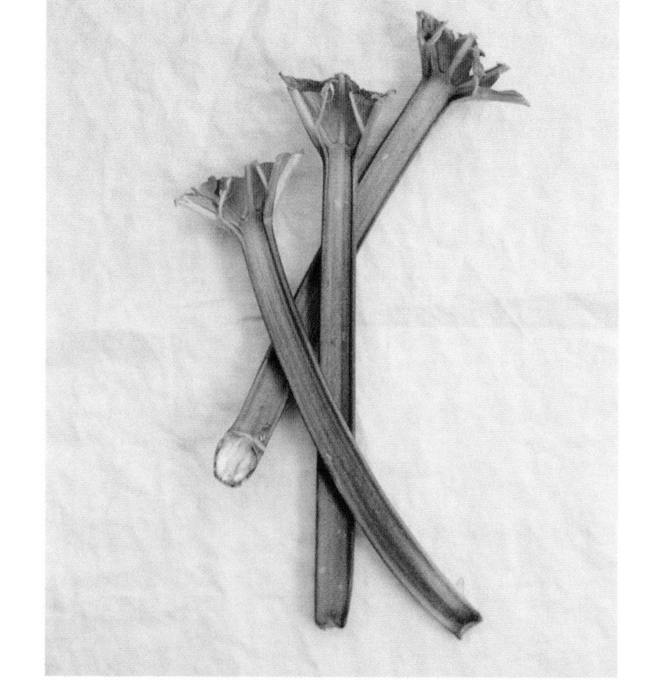

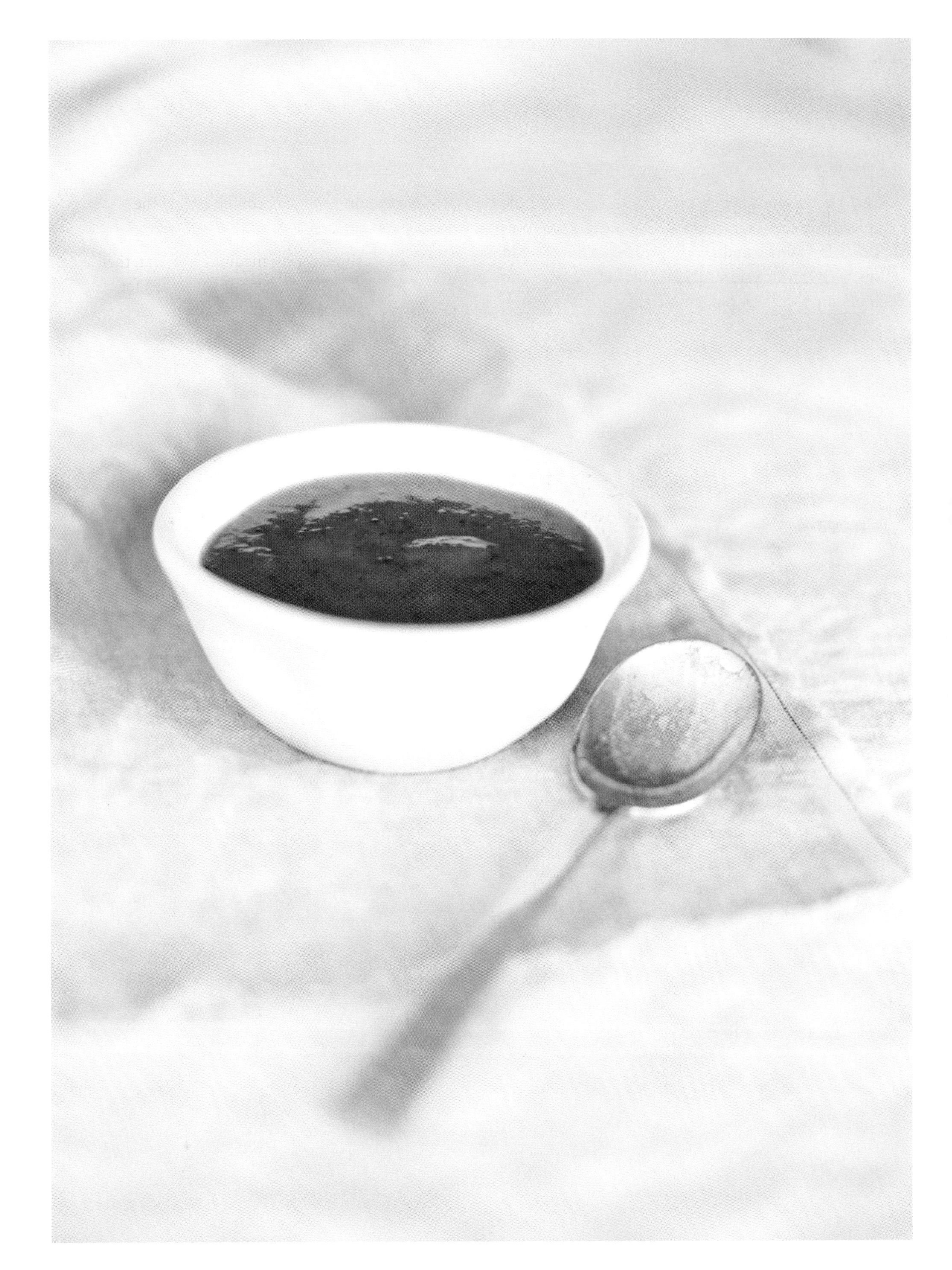

Spring Salad with Dill, Flowers, and Champagne Vinaigrette

What a gift it is when fresh lettuce from the garden is ready to eat! I wait for it all winter. Adding fresh dill to a green salad really brings it to life. The little spice from the radishes and red onion gives this salad a nice bite, and the flowers make it beautiful. The dressing is a bit like honey mustard dressing, but not as sweet or overpowering. This is the perfect salad for grilled lamb, fresh fish, or roasted chicken.

Serves 8

- *12 cups torn fresh spring lettuce (about 3 heads)*
- *6 radishes, sliced very thin*
- *½ medium red onion, sliced very thin*
- *1 cup chopped fresh dill*
- *Handful of edible flowers, such as pansies, Johnny-jump-ups, or nasturtiums*

For the dressing

(Makes about 1 cup)

- *½ cup cold-pressed, extra-virgin olive oil*
- *¼ cup champagne vinegar*
- *2 tablespoons lemon juice*
- *1 tablespoon Dijon mustard*
- *2 teaspoons honey*
- *½ teaspoon sea salt*
- *½ teaspoon ground black pepper*

1. Place the lettuce in a large bowl.
2. Top with the radishes, onion, dill, and flowers.
3. In a small pint jar with a lid, such as a mason jar, combine all of the dressing ingredients, then cover and shake.
4. Dress the salad right before serving.

NOTES: *For the lettuce mix, I like to use a combination of Boston, red leaf, arugula, and a little romaine for crunch.*

Whole30	Omit the honey from the dressing.
Nut-free	Yes
Egg-free	Yes
AIP	Omit the black pepper from the dressing.

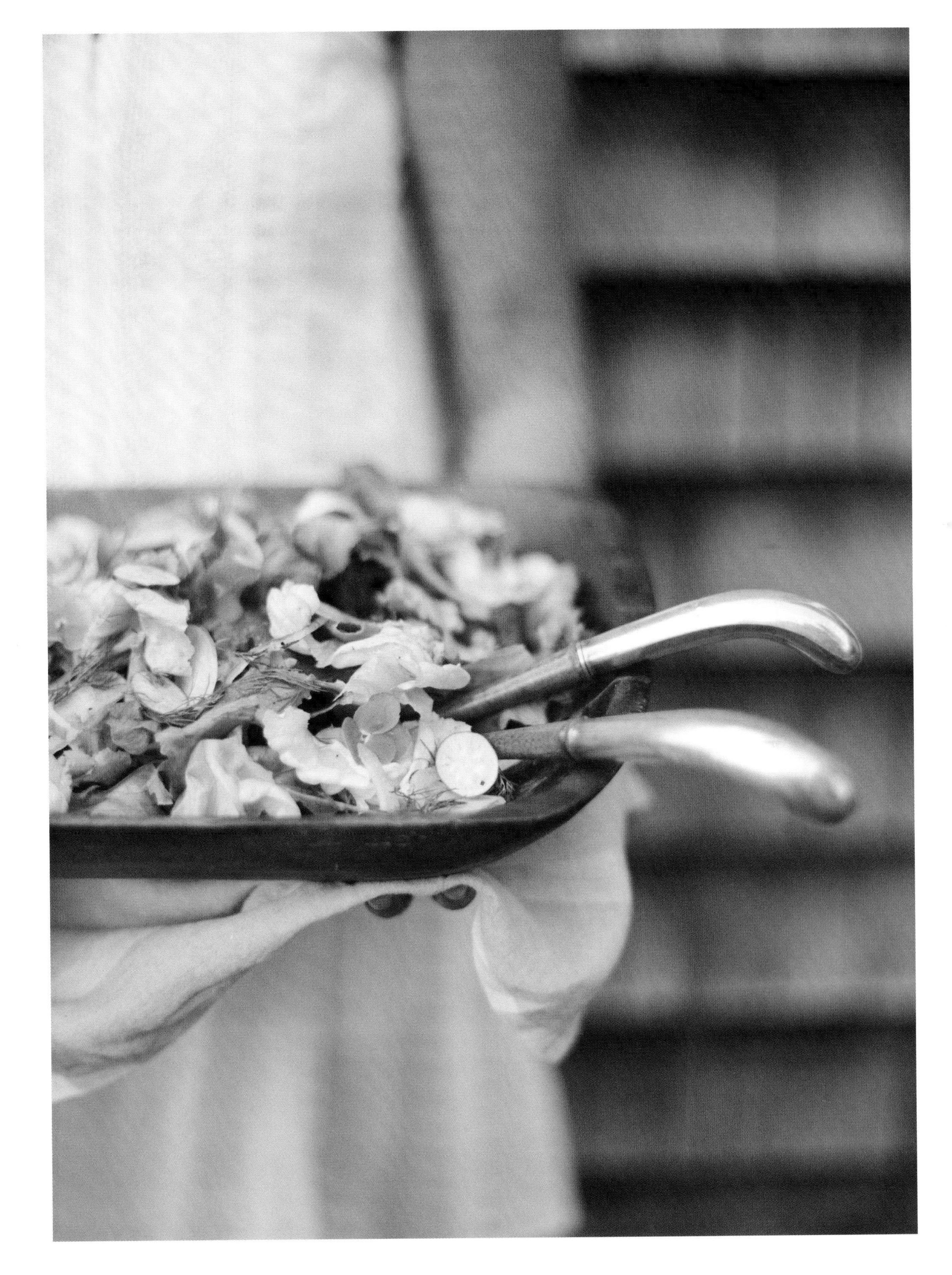

Fiddlehead Ferns with Porcini and Prosciutto

Is there any vegetable more beautiful than a fiddlehead fern? These little spirals are what early spring in New England is all about. They're here and then *poof,* they vanish so quickly that it's easy to miss them. If you're lucky enough to get your hands on some, you'll love them. They taste a lot like asparagus, and they're delicious here with prosciutto and porcini mushrooms. You can also try them with hollandaise sauce or in other dishes in place of asparagus. Nutritionally, fiddleheads have twice the antioxidants of blueberries. Foodborne illness has been associated with raw and undercooked fiddleheads, so be sure to cook them well—boil or steam for 15 minutes. It's also important to get the sprouts from the ostrich fern and not from other varieties. Look for a brown, papery covering on the fiddlehead and a U-shaped groove on the inside of the stem. They can be found growing in clusters of three to twelve in damp soil, such as by rivers and streams. When harvesting, be considerate and take only half of the fiddleheads in a cluster so that the plant can survive. For more on fiddleheads and other wild edibles, see page 140.

Serves 4

- *¾ cup dried porcini mushrooms*
- *¾ pound fiddlehead ferns, trimmed and washed*
- *3 teaspoons unsalted butter (page 348) or ghee (page 347), divided*
- *5 slices prosciutto, cut into small strips*
- *6 cloves garlic, minced*
- *2 tablespoons lemon juice*
- *Sea salt and ground black pepper*

Whole30	Use ghee instead of butter.
Nut-free	Yes
Egg-free	Yes
AIP	Omit the black pepper. Use coconut oil in place of the butter or ghee.

1. Place the mushrooms in a bowl and cover with 2 cups of warm water; set aside to soak.
2. Place the fiddleheads in a medium saucepan and cover with 2 inches of water. Bring to a boil, then reduce the heat to maintain a simmer. Continue to cook for 15 minutes.
3. When the fiddleheads are done, drain the water and fill the pot with very cold water to stop them from cooking further. Set aside.
4. In a skillet over medium heat, melt 1 teaspoon of the butter.
5. Add the prosciutto strips and sauté for a few minutes until crisp. Remove the prosciutto from the pan and set aside.
6. Melt the remaining 2 teaspoons of butter in the skillet over medium-low heat. Add the garlic and cook for 5 minutes. Do not let it burn.
7. Drain the mushrooms, reserving 2 tablespoons of the juice. Add the mushrooms and reserved juice to the pan, along with the fiddleheads. Cook for about 3 minutes.
8. Remove the pan from the heat and add the lemon juice.
9. Sprinkle the top with the prosciutto strips, and add salt and pepper to taste.

NOTES: *If fiddleheads are difficult to find, try using asparagus (trimmed and cut into 2-inch lengths) instead, reducing the cooking time to 5 minutes. You can substitute bacon or pancetta for the prosciutto.*

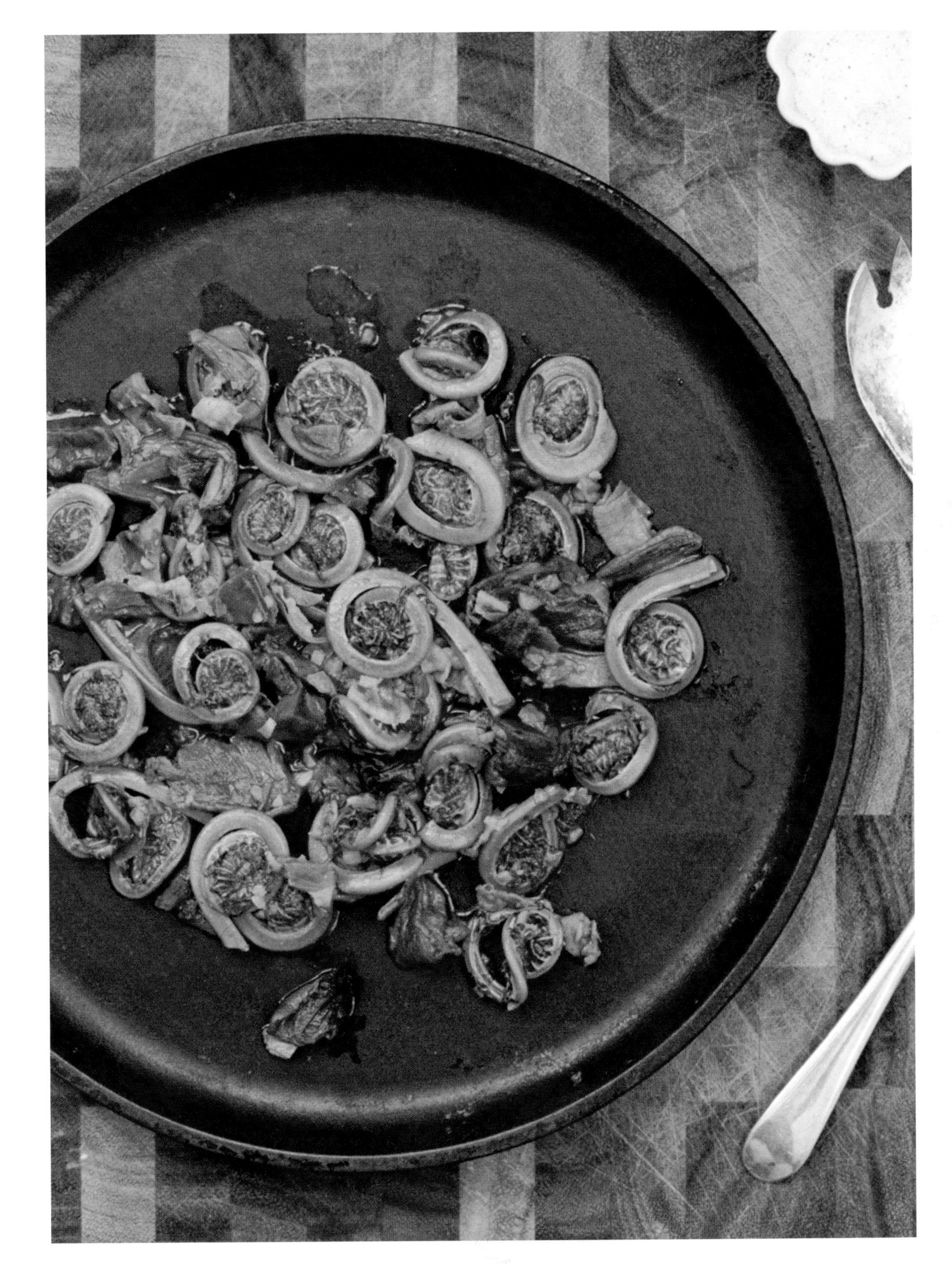

Warm Asparagus Salad with Jerusalem Artichokes, Smoked Ham, and Pastured Eggs

This is one of my favorite ways to eat asparagus: simply roasted with some good ham and a farm-fresh egg. We get a lot of "double yolkers" here on the farm, which my kids think means they'll have a lucky day. We tend to see them more often in the spring, when our young hens have just started producing eggs and double-ovulate more frequently. Jerusalem artichokes, also called "sunchokes," are the tubers of a beautiful, sunflower-like plant that gets quite tall. They are available in the fall through the spring and are best when dug up after a frost. Peeling Jerusalem artichokes can be difficult, so look for ones that are less knobby to make the task easier. In this dish, they are a nice way to soak up the bright orange egg yolk from omega-3-rich pastured eggs. For more on Jerusalem artichokes, see page 140.

Serves 2

- *½ to ⅔ pound asparagus, cleaned and bottom third snapped off*
- *6 Jerusalem artichokes, peeled and sliced into ¼-inch coins*
- *1 tablespoon melted bacon fat or coconut oil*
- *Sea salt and ground black pepper*
- *½ teaspoon Dijon mustard*
- *1 teaspoon lemon juice*
- *2 teaspoons cold-pressed, extra-virgin olive oil*
- *1 teaspoon red wine vinegar*
- *2 eggs*
- *4 ounces good-quality ham, sliced ¼ inch thick*
- *1 teaspoon unsalted butter (page 348)*

NOTES: *Steamed or roasted white or sweet potatoes can be used instead of Jerusalem artichokes.*

Whole30	Substitute ghee for the butter.
Nut-free	Yes
Egg-free	Omit the eggs.
AIP	No

1. Preheat the oven to 425°F.
2. Place the asparagus in a bowl with the Jerusalem artichokes and toss with the bacon fat and a sprinkle of salt and pepper.
3. Line a baking sheet with parchment paper. Spread the asparagus and Jerusalem artichokes out on the baking sheet and roast for 30 minutes.
4. While the asparagus and Jerusalem artichokes are roasting, mix up the dressing by combining the mustard, lemon juice, and olive oil in a small bowl. Set aside.
5. Fill a medium saucepan halfway with water. Add the vinegar and bring to a boil. Reduce the heat to maintain a simmer.
6. Crack each egg into a small bowl or ramekin. With a spoon, make a swirl in the center of the simmering water (this will help the egg stay together once you slide it in).
7. Gently slide an egg into the swirl in the water. Turn off the heat and cover the pan. For a super-runny egg, cook for only about 3 minutes. The longer you leave it in the water, the more the yolk will cook.
8. Remove the egg from the water with a slotted spoon and set it on a plate. Repeat with the second egg and set both aside until you are ready to serve.
9. Stack the ham slices and slice them into matchsticks.
10. In a skillet, heat the butter and sauté the ham for just a few minutes, until lightly browned.
11. Toss the asparagus and Jerusalem artichokes with the dressing.
12. To serve, divide the asparagus and Jerusalem artichokes between two plates, add the ham, and top each plate with a poached egg. Sprinkle a little salt and pepper over each egg and serve.

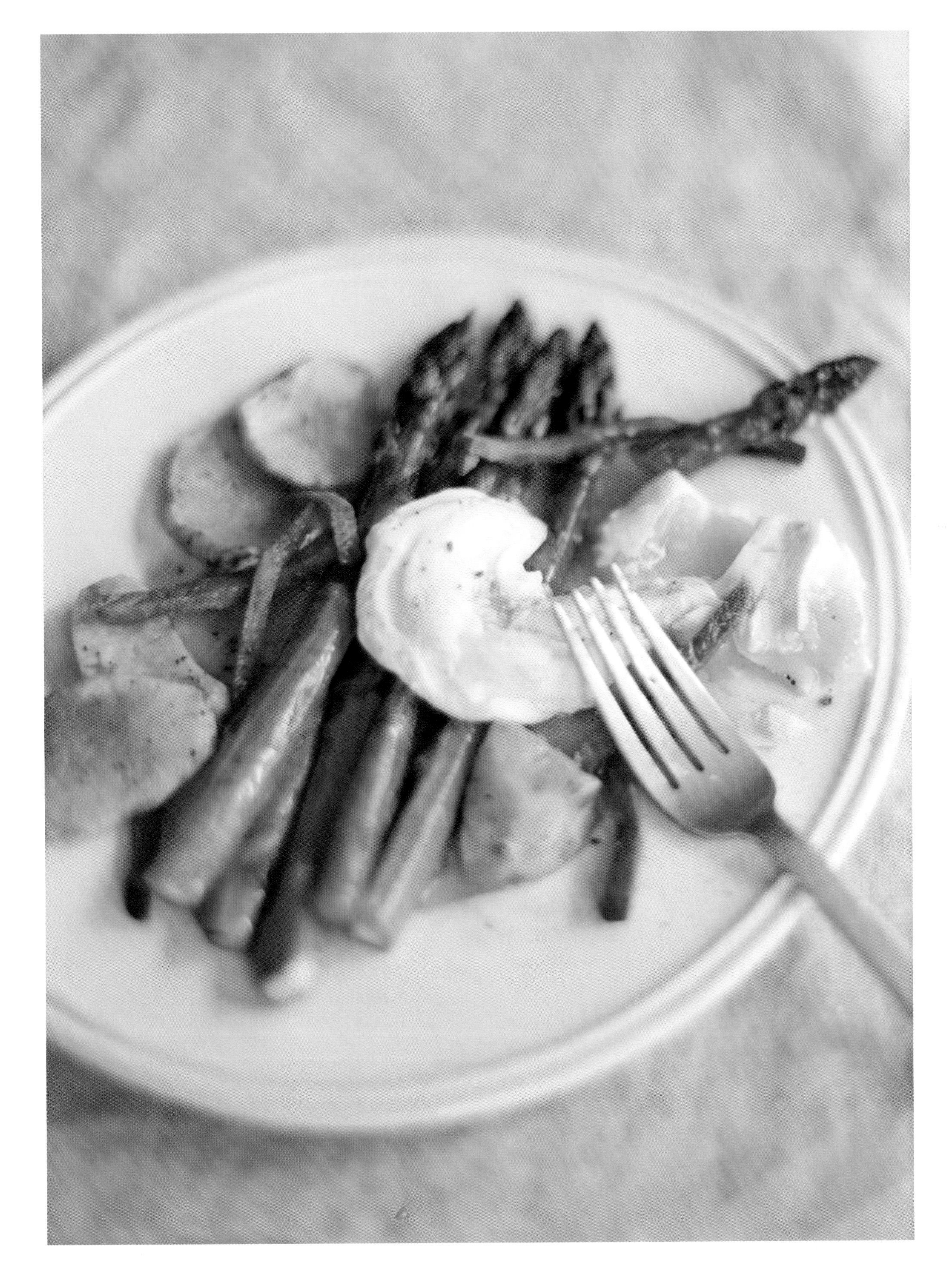

Roasted Asparagus Soup with Trumpet Mushrooms and Sorrel

This thick, rich soup is perfect for a cool, rainy spring day. Roasting the asparagus intensifies its flavor, and the sweet potato both gives the soup sweetness and thickens it. The addition of sorrel, an often-overlooked herb that has a bright, lemony flavor, gives the soup a nice zing. Finally, I love the sautéed trumpet mushrooms for their meaty texture and umami flavor.

Serves 4 to 6

- *1½ pounds asparagus*
- *3 tablespoons ghee (page 347), divided*
- *Sea salt and ground black pepper*
- *1 large yellow onion, chopped*
- *1 medium white-fleshed sweet potato, peeled and cut into large chunks*
- *1 to 2 pinches of cayenne pepper*
- *1½ quarts homemade chicken stock (page 338)*
- *¼ pound trumpet mushrooms (see Notes)*
- *Juice of ½ lime*
- *2 to 3 fresh sorrel leaves, cut into thin ribbons (see Notes)*
- *White truffle oil, for serving (optional)*

NOTES: *If trumpet mushrooms are hard to find, substitute another type of mushroom, such as oyster or button. You can substitute an orange-fleshed sweet potato for the white-fleshed one, but it will change the color of the soup. If you are unable to find sorrel, use a squirt of fresh lemon juice.*

Whole30	Yes
Nut-free	Yes
Egg-free	Yes
AIP	Omit the black pepper and cayenne pepper.

1. Preheat the oven to 425°F. Line a rimmed baking sheet or other baking dish with parchment paper.
2. Wash the asparagus well to make sure that all of the grit is removed (you don't want a crunchy soup) and snap off the bottom third of the stalks. Reserve the bottom portion of the stalks for use in Step 7.
3. Melt 1 tablespoon of the ghee. In a large bowl, toss the asparagus with the melted ghee and a sprinkling of salt and pepper.
4. Spread the asparagus on the prepared baking sheet. Place in the oven and roast for 30 minutes, or until the asparagus is tender.
5. While the asparagus is roasting, melt 1 tablespoon of the ghee in a large soup pot over medium heat.
6. Add the onion and sauté for about 10 minutes, until soft.
7. Add the sweet potato, cayenne pepper, reserved pieces of asparagus stalk, and stock. Simmer for 30 minutes, or until the sweet potato is soft.
8. While the soup is simmering, cut the trumpet mushrooms into small coins, about ⅛ inch thick. Sauté them in the remaining tablespoon of ghee over medium-high heat for about 5 minutes per side, until lightly browned. Drain on a paper towel and set aside.
9. Remove the asparagus stalks from the soup and discard. Cut the roasted asparagus into 2-inch pieces and add to the soup. Simmer for about 5 minutes.
10. Remove the soup from heat and blend with an immersion blender. You can also blend with a food processor or blender, working in batches.
11. Add the lime juice and season with salt and pepper to taste.
12. When ready to serve, ladle the soup into bowls and garnish with the mushrooms, sorrel, and a drizzle of truffle oil, if desired.

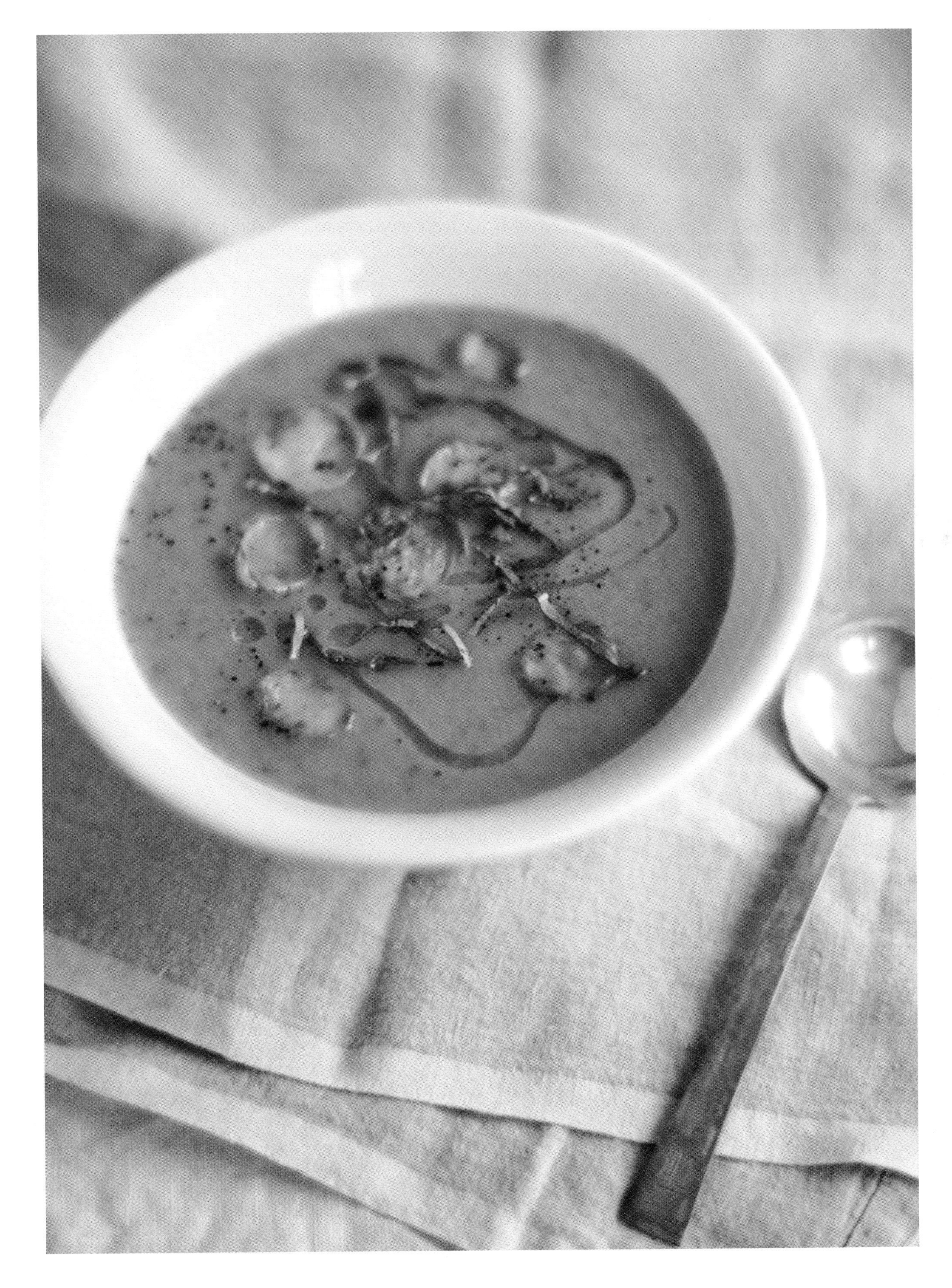

Primal Spring Turnip, Beet, and Carrot Gratin

This is a lovely, earthy twist on potatoes gratin. It is a rich side that goes equally well with lamb or fish and a lightly dressed salad. I like to eat leftovers for breakfast with an over-easy egg. Any combination of golden and red beets would work well, and including at least a few red beets makes for an intense color combination. You can also skip the beets altogether and just use more turnips.

Serves 4 to 6

- *2 teaspoons ghee (page 347), melted*
- *3 medium to large hakurei turnips, sliced very thin, divided*
- *⅓ cup minced fresh parsley leaves, divided*
- *1 medium yellow onion, sliced very thin, divided*
- *1 teaspoon sea salt, divided*
- *2 medium beets, peeled and sliced very thin*
- *1 medium carrot, peeled and sliced very thin*
- *Pinch of cayenne pepper*
- *½ cup half-and-half or canned, full-fat coconut milk*
- *⅔ cup grated Parmesan cheese (optional)*

1. Preheat the oven to 450°F. Grease the bottom of a gratin dish or other 10-inch baking dish with the ghee.
2. Spread half of the turnip slices across the bottom of the baking dish in an overlapping layer.
3. Top the turnip layer with a sprinkle of parsley, half of the onion slices, and a pinch of salt.
4. Add a layer of beets, followed by more parsley, the remaining onion slices, and a pinch of salt.
5. Add the carrot slices. Sprinkle this layer with a pinch of cayenne, more parsley, and a pinch of salt.
6. Finish with the remaining turnips.
7. Cover the baking dish and bake for 20 minutes.
8. Pour in the half-and-half and continue baking, covered, for 20 minutes.
9. Remove the cover, sprinkle with the Parmesan cheese, if using, and bake, uncovered, for 15 more minutes, until browned.

NOTES: *If you can't find hakurei turnips, you can substitute another turnip, but the flavor will be more bitter (hakurei turnips are very sweet). You can also try other root crops, like rutabagas, in this dish.*

Whole30	Omit the half-and-half and cheese.
Nut-free	Yes
Egg-free	Yes
AIP	Omit the half-and-half, cheese, and cayenne. Use coconut oil instead of ghee.

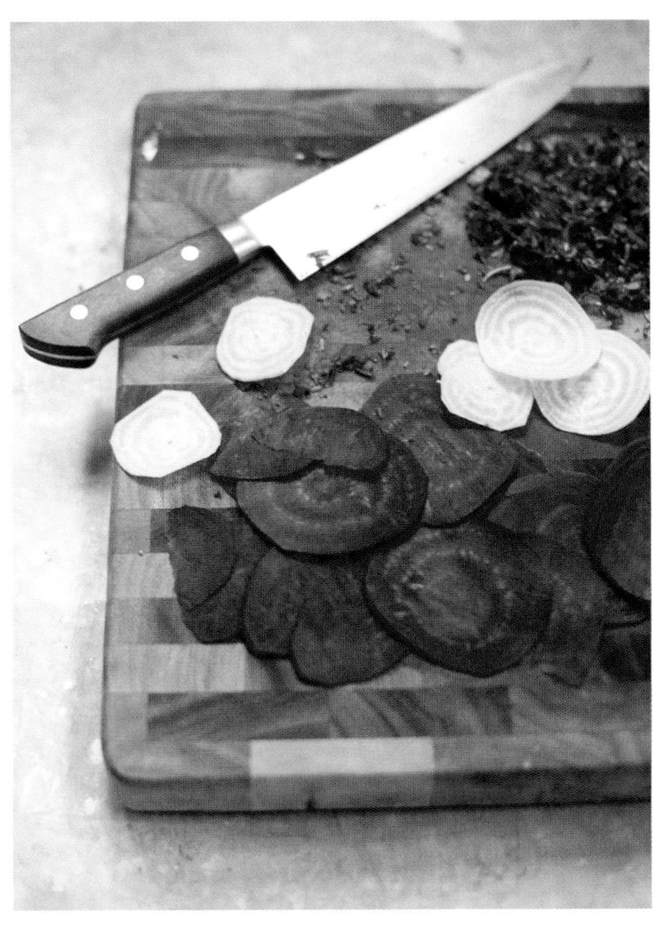
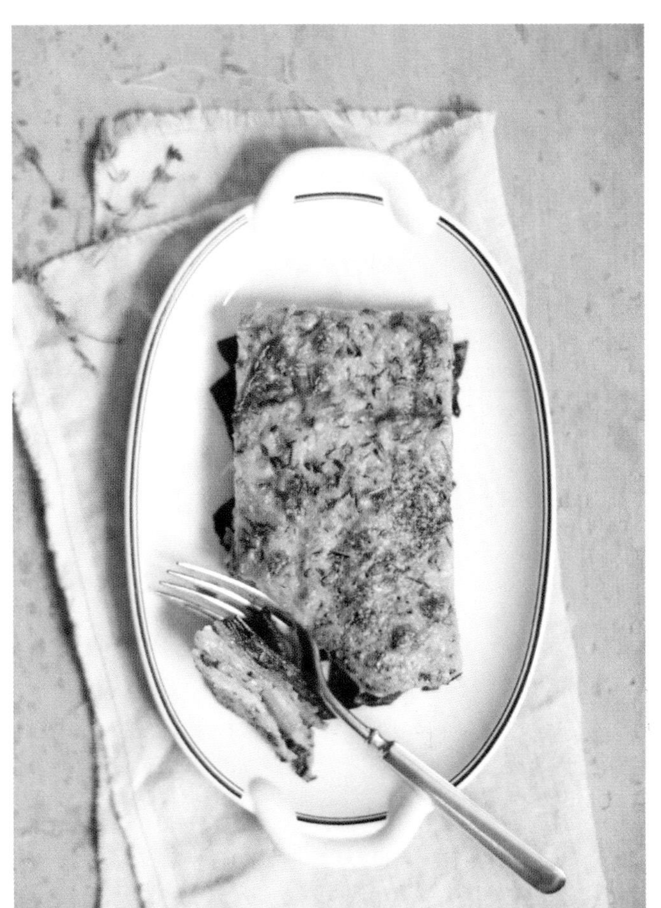
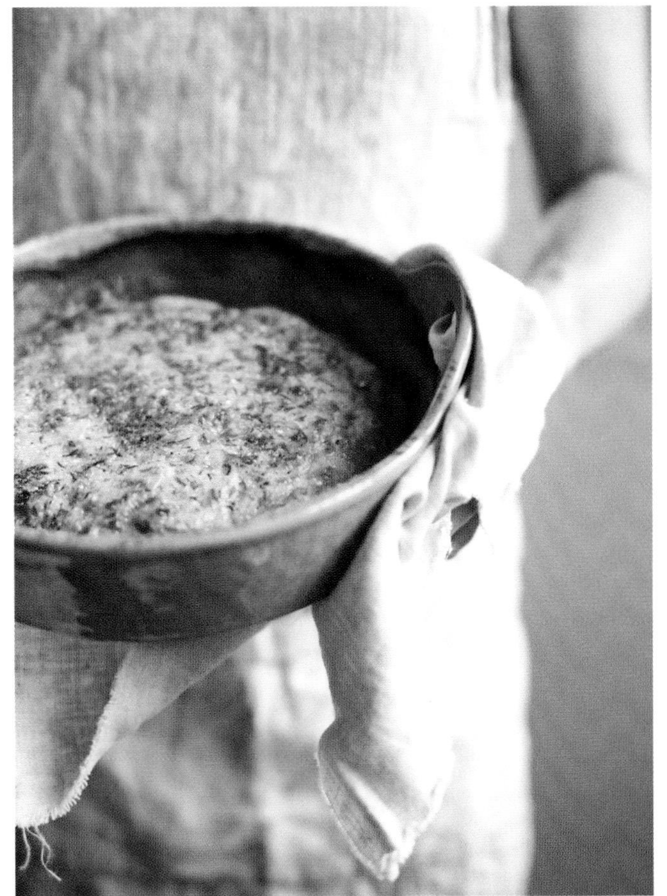
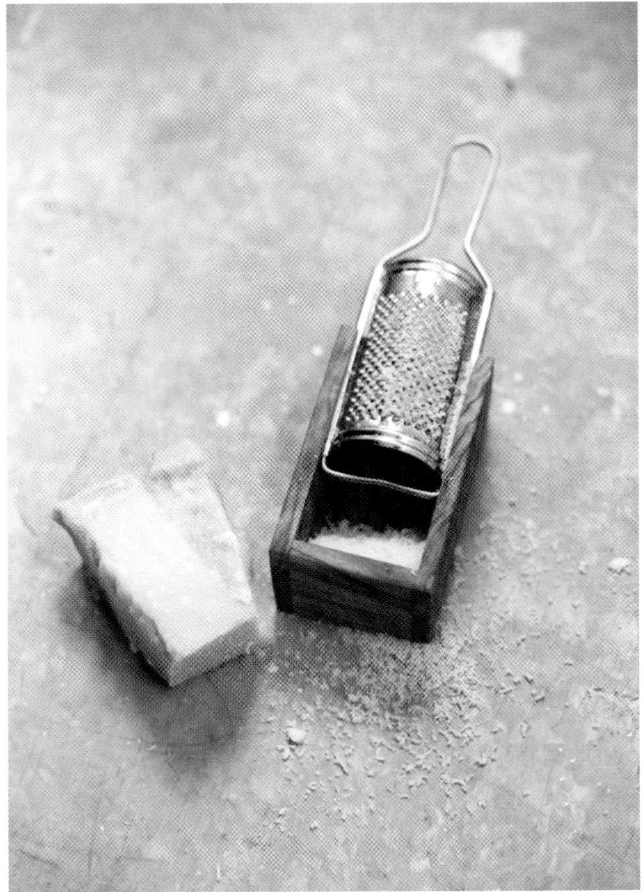

Spring Salad of Arugula, Radishes, and Grilled Steak

This peppery salad is a spring wake-up call for your mouth. It's simple enough for a weeknight meal, yet special enough to serve to guests. I absolutely love radishes in a salad: they provide crunch and a spicy, fresh, crisp taste that is almost a little fizzy on your tongue. If you don't want to grill your steak outdoors, try using a cast-iron grill pan for the stovetop. I really love mine. Just remember to turn on your exhaust fan or you'll set off all your smoke detectors and have fire trucks racing to your house (yes, this actually happened to me).

Serves 4 as a main dish, 8 as an appetizer

- *2 pounds flank steak*
- *Sea salt and ground black pepper*
- *6 cups arugula, washed*
- *1 large bunch radishes (about 15), sliced very thin*
- *¼ medium red onion, sliced very thin*
- *1 batch Creamy Horseradish Herb Dressing (page 186)*

Whole30	Yes
Nut-free	Yes
Egg-free	Omit the horseradish dressing, and in its place use a simple dressing of lemon juice and olive oil.
AIP	Omit the horseradish dressing, and in its place use a simple dressing of lemon juice and olive oil. Omit the black pepper.

1. Heat a grill to a medium-high heat (see page 362 for grilling tips).
2. Bring the steak to room temperature. Dry off any extra moisture with a towel and sprinkle the steak with salt and pepper.
3. Place the steak on the hot grill and cook for about 3 minutes per side (for rare, longer if you don't like it red).
4. Remove the steak from the heat and set aside to rest while you make the rest of the salad.
5. In a large salad bowl, combine the arugula, radishes, and red onion.
6. Slice the steak against the grain, very thin. Top the salad with the steak slices.
7. Dress the salad, sprinkle with a bit more salt and pepper, and serve.

NOTES: *You can use strip steak instead of flank steak if you wish. If radishes are too peppery for you, try a hakurei turnip—you'll be surprised at how mild the flavor is. You can also substitute your favorite lettuce for the arugula.*

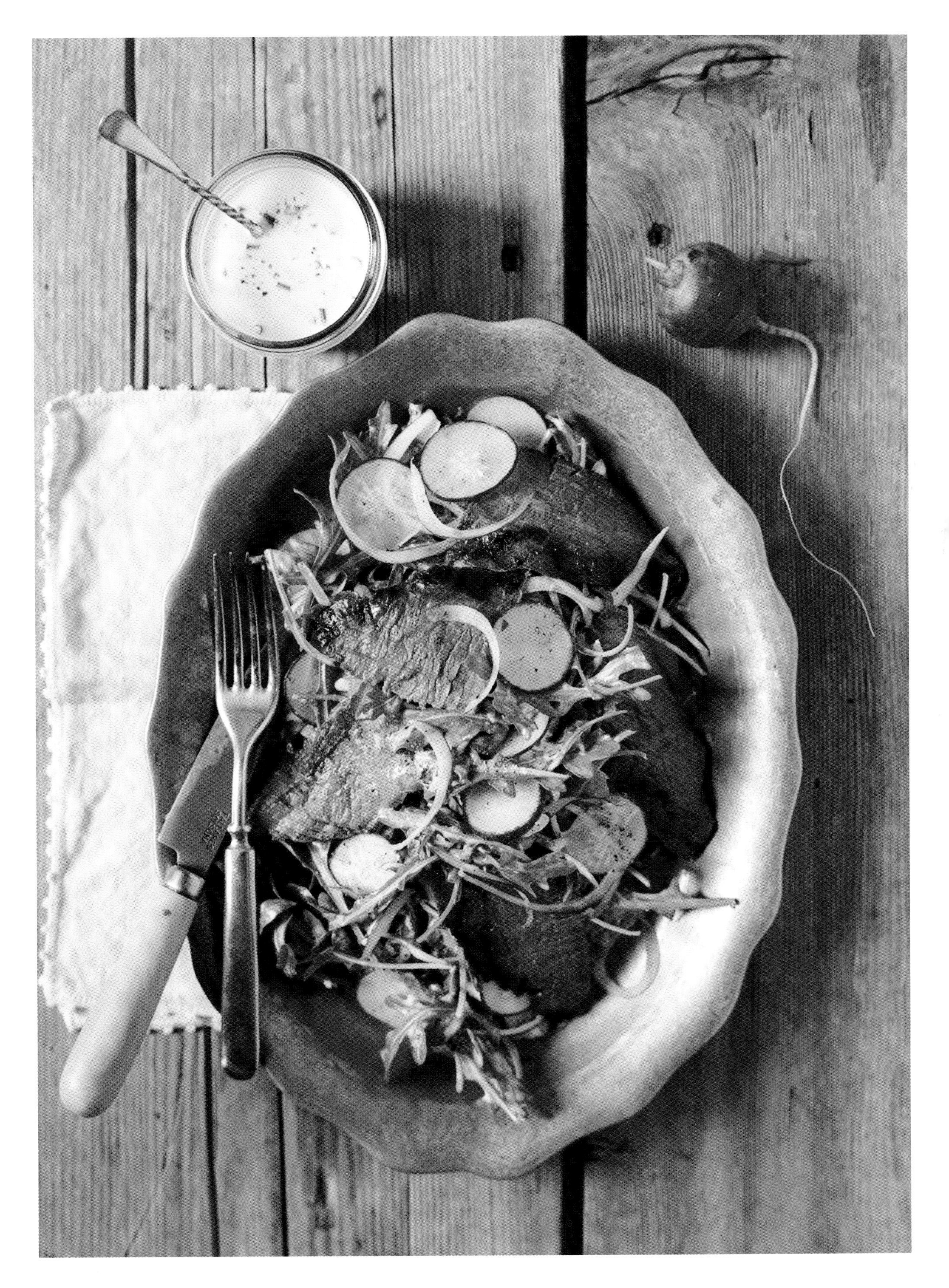

Creamy Horseradish Herb Dressing

This dressing was originally made for the Spring Salad of Arugula, Radishes, and Grilled Steak (page 184), but it was so incredibly good that I ended up eating it on just about everything I could. (In fact, I could just drink this stuff.) It's lovely as a dip for artichokes or on a lettuce wrap with your favorite meat for a quick lunch. If you want to make the dressing a bit thinner, add a little coconut milk and thin to the desired consistency.

Makes ⅔ cup

- *½ cup homemade mayonnaise (page 344)*
- *2 teaspoons lemon juice*
- *1 tablespoon minced fresh chives*
- *1 tablespoon minced fresh mint leaves*
- *1 tablespoon minced fresh parsley leaves*
- *1 tablespoon Dijon mustard*
- *2 tablespoons all-natural, prepared horseradish*
- *1 clove garlic, minced*
- *Sea salt and ground black pepper to taste*

1. Combine all of the ingredients in a small bowl and mix well. This dressing will keep for 1 week in a sealed container in the fridge.

Whole30	Yes
Nut-free	Yes
Egg-free	No
AIP	No

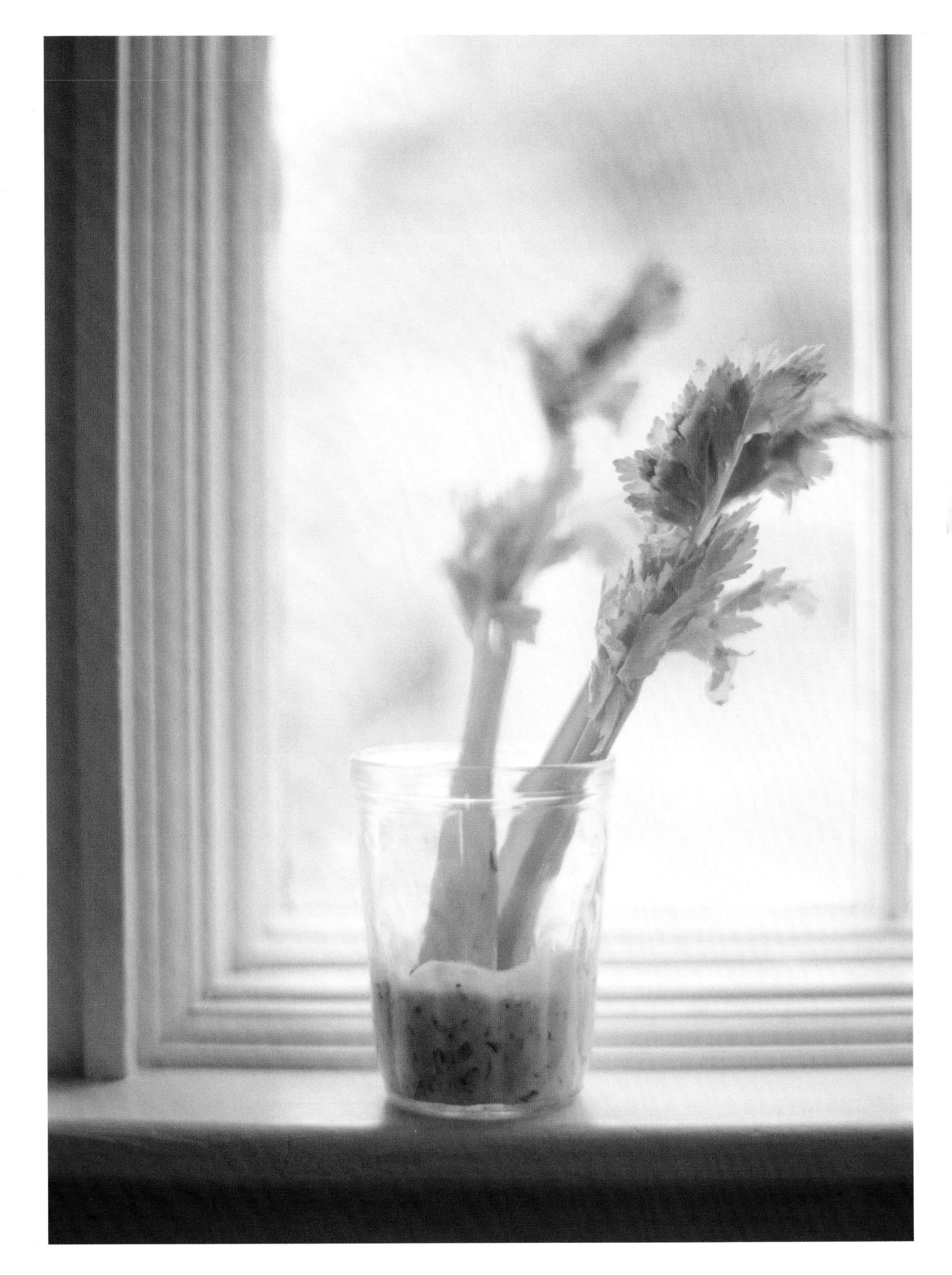

Umami-Laden Spring Vegetables with Shiitake Mushrooms

In late June, our farm fields finally come alive and are bursting with greens and crunchy snow peas. This is the best way to highlight their textures and flavors—with lots of umami, the fifth taste that the tongue can perceive (in addition to the familiar tastes of sweet, salty, bitter, and sour). In this four-star veggie dish, the umami comes from mushrooms and fish sauce, which are added at the end. This is a fantastic side to any protein. I particularly love it with Grilled Leg of Lamb with Garlic Scape Pesto and Mint (page 160), but fish is also a wonderful companion.

Serves 4

- *4 tablespoons coconut oil, divided*
- *10 garlic scapes, scallions, or green garlic, cut into 1- to 2-inch pieces*
- *1 pinch to ⅛ teaspoon red pepper flakes*
- *½ pound Swiss chard or other tender braising greens, stems cut into ½-inch pieces and leaves into 2-inch chunks (see Notes)*
- *¾ pound snow peas, tops and strings snapped off*
- *8 ounces shiitake mushrooms, stemmed and cut into slices ½ inch thick*
- *2 tablespoons fish sauce*

1. Heat 2 tablespoons of the coconut oil in a large, heavy skillet. Add the scapes and red pepper flakes and cook for 5 minutes.
2. Add the Swiss chard stems and cook for 3 minutes.
3. Add the snow peas and chard leaves and cook for another 3 to 5 minutes, until the snow peas are cooked but not mushy. Remove to a platter.
4. Heat the remaining 2 tablespoons of coconut oil in the skillet and fry the shiitakes for 3 minutes, or until softened and browned.
5. Return the rest of the veggies to the pan and add the fish sauce, cooking just until heated through.

NOTES: *If using spinach, leave the leaves whole and the stems on. Other mushrooms, such as oysters, can be substituted for the shiitakes.*

Whole30	Yes
Nut-free	Yes
Egg-free	Yes
AIP	Omit the red pepper flakes.

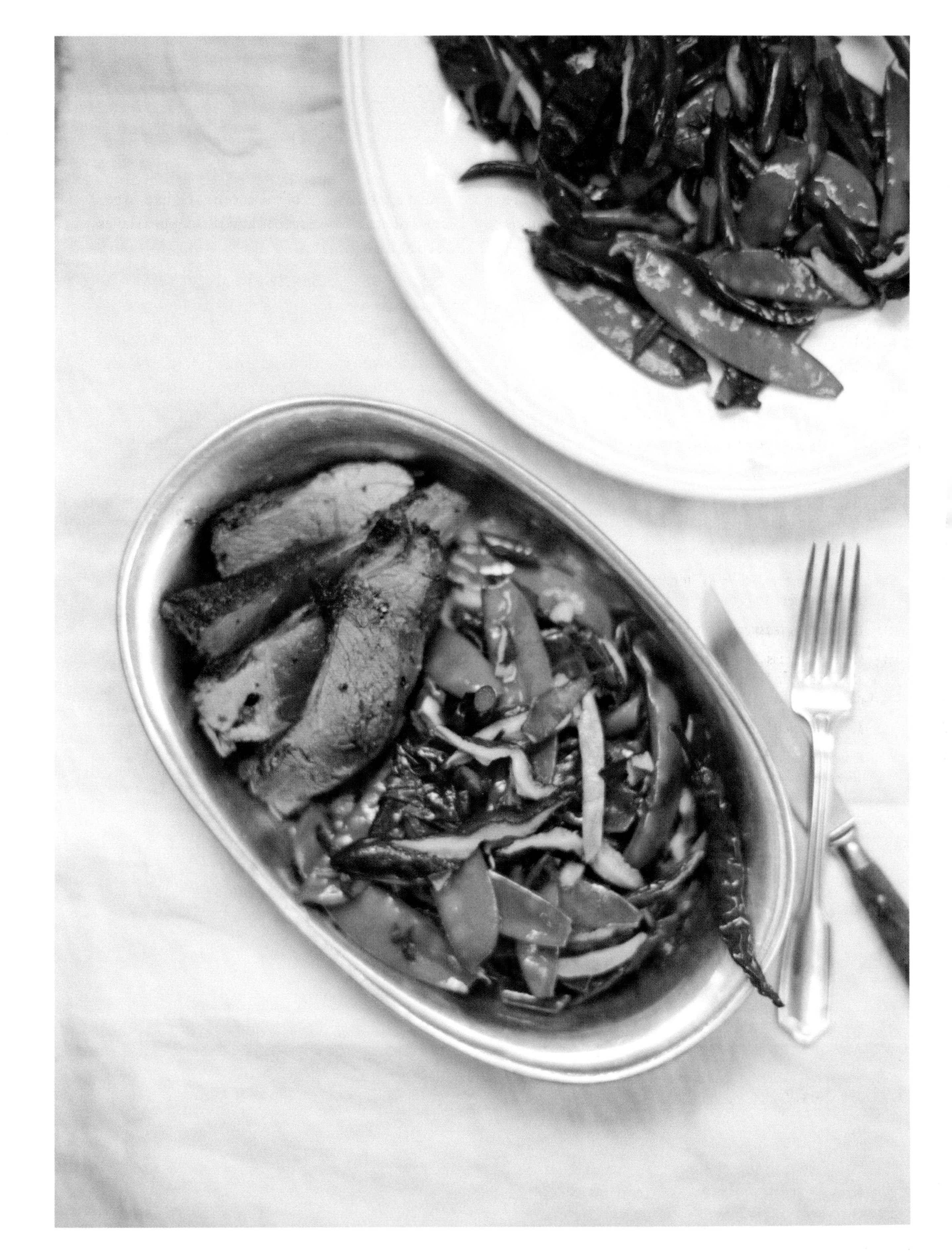

Chicken Saag with Turnip Greens

This rich and comforting dish will make your house smell amazing! This is a great recipe to use after you've made a roasted chicken or chicken stock. Traditionally, saag is made with all kinds of greens and cooked for hours. Here in the United States, most of the saag dishes we encounter are made with spinach, but I think something amazing happens when you make it with turnip greens. The slightly mustard flavor of the greens transforms into a sweet complement to the Indian spices. I also much prefer the firmer texture of turnip greens to spinach, which can get mushy since this dish simmers for a while. Don't be intimidated by the long list of spices here—this dish is very easy to make.

Serves 4

- *½ cup ghee (page 347)*
- *1 tablespoon turmeric*
- *2 teaspoons cumin seeds*
- *1 teaspoon ground cumin*
- *1 teaspoon ground coriander*
- *½ teaspoon garam masala*
- *1 serrano chile, seeded and chopped*
- *4 cloves garlic, minced*
- *1 tablespoon grated fresh ginger*
- *1 teaspoon sea salt*
- *1½ pounds turnip greens (from about 9 or 10 turnips) or 2 bunches other braising greens (see Notes), chopped fine*
- *1 cup homemade chicken stock (page 338)*
- *4 cups shredded roasted chicken (page 336)*
- *½ cup whole-milk yogurt, heavy cream, or coconut cream (optional)*
- *¼ cup chopped fresh cilantro leaves, for garnish*
- *1 batch Coconut Crêpes (page 192), for serving*

1. Melt the ghee in a large pot over medium heat. Add the spices, serrano chile, garlic, ginger, and salt and cook for 10 minutes.
2. Add the chopped turnip greens in batches, stirring into the mixture a little at a time until well incorporated.
3. Add the chicken stock and simmer, covered, for 1 hour.
4. Remove the cover and simmer for another 10 minutes to allow the sauce to reduce slightly.
5. Add the chicken and adjust salt to taste.
6. At this point, if you are avoiding dairy, you can simply garnish with the cilantro and serve. It's delicious this way, but adding the yogurt adds a creaminess that brings it to a whole new level. So, if you like a little dairy, turn off the heat, add the yogurt, and stir well.
7. Serve in bowls, garnished with cilantro, with coconut crêpes.

NOTES: *If you can't find turnip greens, you can substitute a variety of greens, like spinach, kale, chard, or mustard greens, or even wild edibles like lamb's quarters or purslane.*

Whole30	Use coconut cream instead of yogurt or heavy cream. Serve with steamed potatoes, white or sweet, in place of the crêpes.
Nut-free	Yes
Egg-free	Yes, but serve with steamed potatoes, white or sweet, in place of the crêpes.
AIP	No

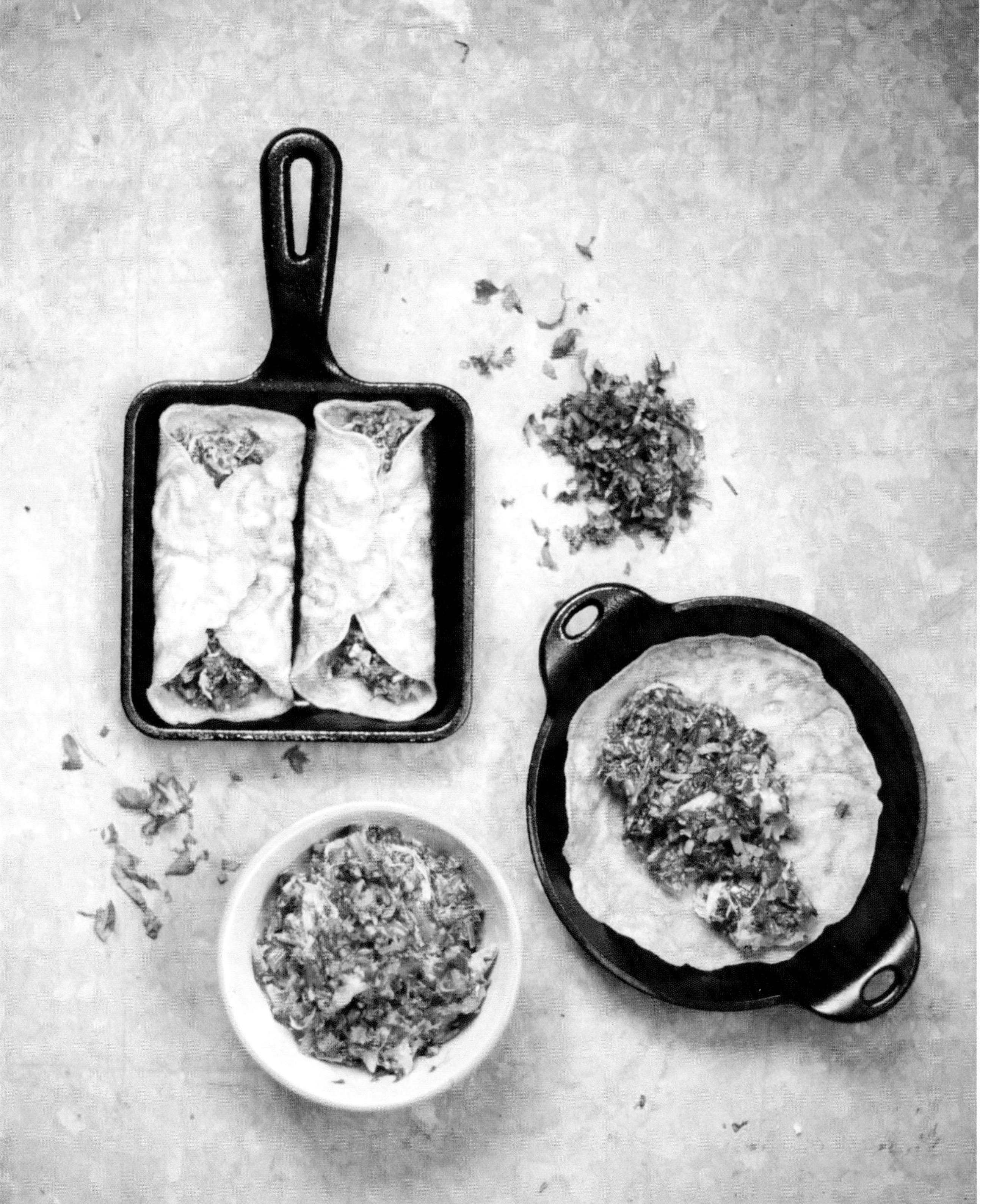

Coconut Crêpes

These crêpes are light and sort of remind me of injera, the traditional Ethiopian bread. They are fantastic with Chicken Saag with Turnip Greens (page 190) or any savory stew, and they don't have a strong coconut taste. They're also very simple to make.

Makes about 15 crêpes

- *⅔ cup tapioca starch*
- *⅓ cup coconut flour*
- *¼ teaspoon baking soda*
- *½ teaspoon sea salt*
- *2 eggs*
- *1½ cups canned, full-fat coconut milk*
- *2 tablespoons coconut oil, divided, plus extra as needed for the pan*
- *Up to ½ cup water (optional)*

Whole30	No
Nut-free	Yes
Egg-free	No
AIP	No

1. In a large bowl, whisk the dry ingredients until blended.

2. Combine the eggs, coconut milk, and 1 tablespoon of the coconut oil in a separate bowl. (Melt the coconut oil first if it's not already liquid.)

3. Add the wet ingredients to the dry ingredients and mix until well combined.

4. Check the consistency of the batter—it should be like a very thin pancake mix, but different coconut milks can yield different consistencies, so add up to ½ cup water if needed.

5. Warm a skillet over medium heat.

6. Melt the remaining tablespoon of coconut oil in the skillet. Then, using a large spoon, pour about ¼ cup of the batter onto the skillet.

7. Flip the crêpe after about 3 minutes, when the bottom is very lightly browned, and cook on the other side for another 1 to 2 minutes.

8. Transfer the finished crêpe to a warm plate and cover with a towel until ready to serve. Repeat with the rest of the batter, adding more coconut oil to the pan if needed.

See photo on page 191.

Sunny Parsley Potatoes

My family and I much prefer the taste of white potatoes to sweet potatoes. I'm so glad that the greater Paleo community is starting to accept peeled white potatoes, even though cavemen didn't eat them. They're incredibly nutrient-dense, a good source of starch, and a great prebiotic to feed your intestinal flora. In the morning, I often use leftover potatoes to make this dish, which fuels my busy family's day. It is also great to make in a double batch and have on hand as a starchy side to any meat dish you're serving for lunch or dinner. These potatoes are mild enough not to overpower the main dish.

Serves 4

- *2 pounds yellow potatoes, peeled and diced*
- *1 tablespoon bacon fat or ghee (page 347)*
- *1 medium yellow onion, diced small*
- *1 teaspoon smoked paprika (sweet or hot, depending on your taste)*
- *2 teaspoons lemon juice*
- *Sea salt and ground black pepper*
- *2 tablespoons minced fresh parsley leaves, for garnish*

Whole30	Yes
Nut-free	Yes
Egg-free	Yes
AIP	Omit the paprika and black pepper. Use sweet potatoes instead of yellow potatoes, and use coconut oil instead of bacon fat or ghee.

1. Boil the potatoes in a large pot of water until tender, about 20 minutes. Drain and set aside.
2. Heat the bacon fat in a skillet over medium heat.
3. Add the onion and cook until translucent, about 5 to 7 minutes.
4. Add the potatoes to the pan and sauté until browned.
5. Sprinkle with the paprika, lemon juice, and salt and pepper to taste.
6. Remove from the heat and sprinkle with the parsley. Serve with any egg dish, or even with chicken or fish for dinner.

NOTES: *You can also make this dish with sweet potatoes.*

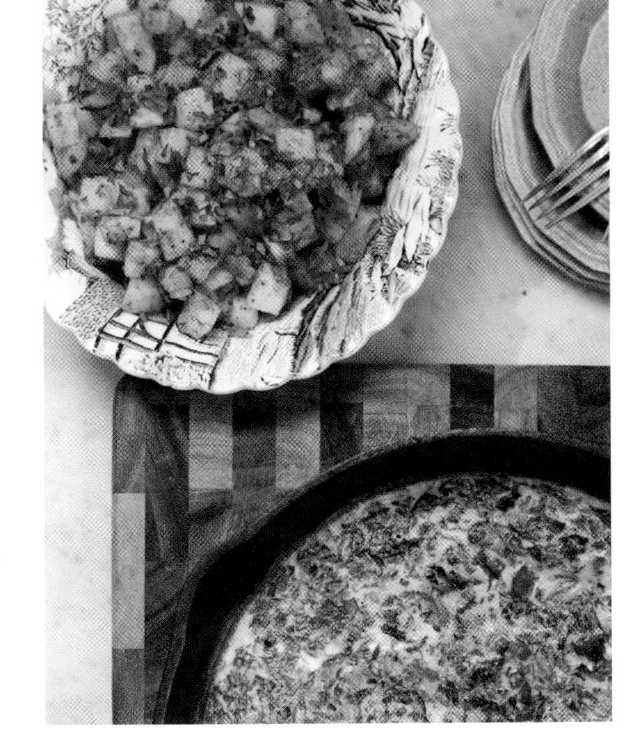

Snap Pea and Radish Salad with Roasted Chicken and Gingery Herb Dressing

We often have impromptu communal suppers with our farm crew. The first night I made this salad, we were headed over to my neighbor Talie's house after a hard day of farm work with temperatures in the nineties. Heat that high early in the season is unusual and can be very stressful for the newly planted seedlings, drying them out and potentially stunting their growth. That meant the radishes were ready to be harvested extra early, and the spinach was at the perfect stage for salad. This refreshing salad has lots of protein and a nice crunch from the snap peas. The gingery dressing cools the crunchy, spicy radishes. It's a great combination of spring's bright flavors. We had a lovely evening swimming and learning all about Peru from our farm interns. Make this salad the next time you are invited to a potluck!

Serves 4 as a main dish, 8 as a side

- *1 pound snap peas, tops snapped off and cut in half crosswise*
- *½ head of butter lettuce, leaves torn*
- *4 cups loosely packed fresh baby spinach leaves*
- *1 (3- to 4-pound) roasted chicken (page 336), sliced or shredded*
- *¼ medium red onion, sliced very thin*
- *1 large bunch of radishes (about 15), washed and sliced very thin*

For the dressing

- *Juice of 1 lime*
- *Juice of 1 lemon*
- *1 tablespoon minced fresh cilantro leaves*
- *1 tablespoon minced fresh mint leaves*
- *1 teaspoon grated fresh ginger*
- *⅓ cup cold-pressed, extra-virgin olive oil*
- *Sea salt and ground black pepper to taste*

1. Steam the snap peas over boiling water for about 3 minutes. Remove from the heat and refrigerate for 20 minutes.
2. In a very large bowl, combine the butter lettuce and spinach.
3. Add the chicken meat, then the red onion, the radishes, and finally the chilled snap peas.
4. Make the dressing: Combine the dressing ingredients in a food processor and blend until smooth. Alternatively, place the ingredients in a tall container and blend with an immersion blender.
5. Dress the salad right before serving.

NOTES: *Arugula would also be fantastic in this salad.*

Whole30	Yes
Nut-free	Yes
Egg-free	Yes
AIP	Omit the black pepper.

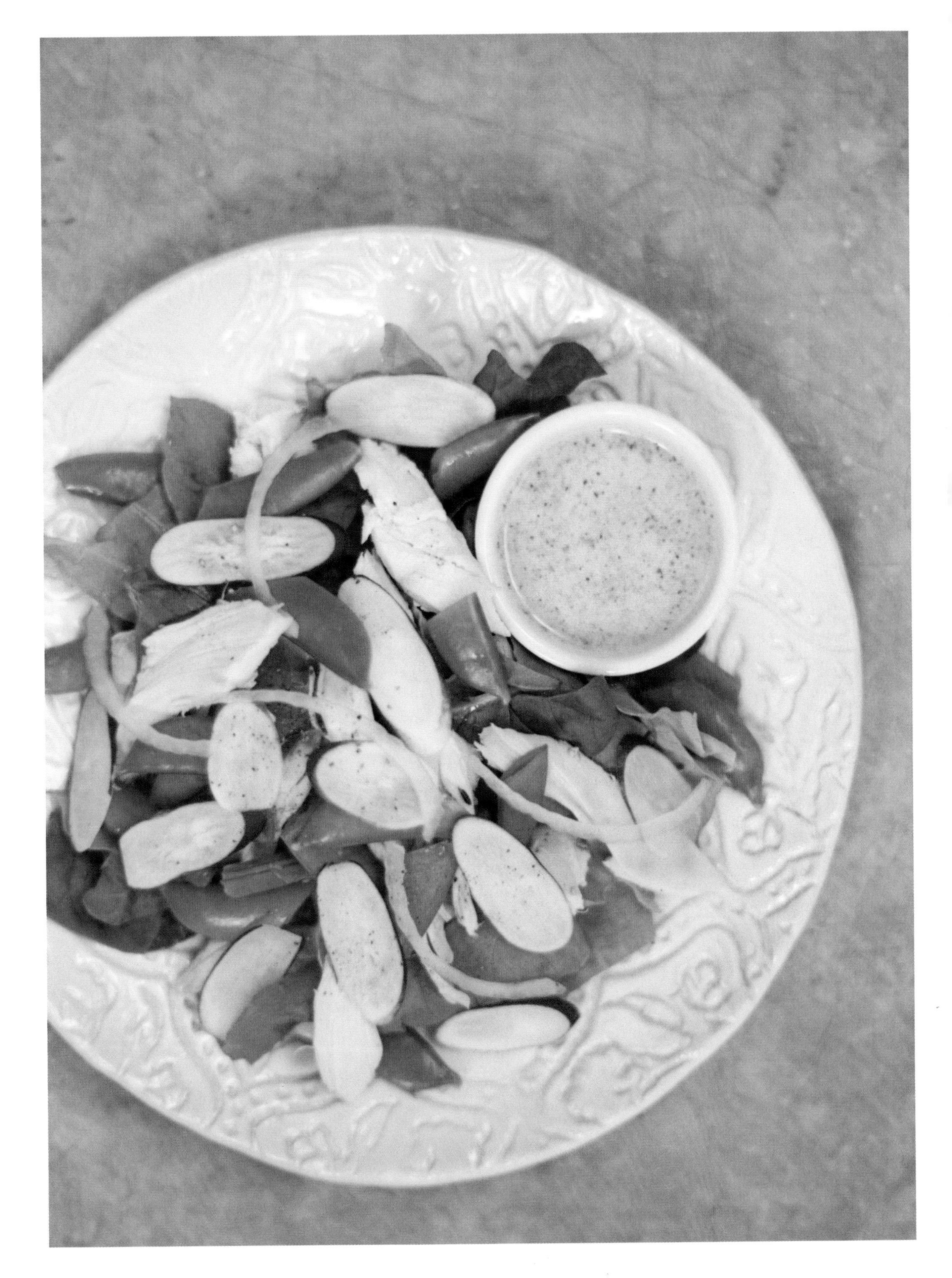

Baby Bok Choy Curry

This simple yet delicious recipe takes just a few minutes to make and is my absolute favorite way to prepare bok choy. We grow a ton of Asian greens on our farm. They are easy to grow and incredibly nutrient-dense. All you need is some protein on the side to turn this into a fantastic, simple weeknight dinner.

Serves 4

- *1 tablespoon coconut oil*
- *1 medium yellow onion, sliced thin*
- *1 teaspoon curry powder*
- *1 pound baby bok choy, chopped*
- *1 teaspoon fish sauce*
- *1 tablespoon coconut aminos*
- *⅓ cup canned, full-fat coconut milk*
- *2 tablespoons minced fresh cilantro leaves, for garnish*

Whole30	Yes
Nut-free	Yes
Egg-free	Yes
AIP	No

1. In a large skillet over medium-high heat, warm the coconut oil. Add the onion and cook for 3 minutes, or until the onion begins to soften.
2. Stir in the curry powder and cook for another few minutes, until well incorporated.
3. Add the bok choy and cook until wilted, about 5 minutes.
4. Add the fish sauce, coconut aminos, and coconut milk. Cook for just a few more minutes, then garnish with the cilantro and serve.

NOTES: *If bok choy is hard to find, try using shredded savoy, green, or napa cabbage.*

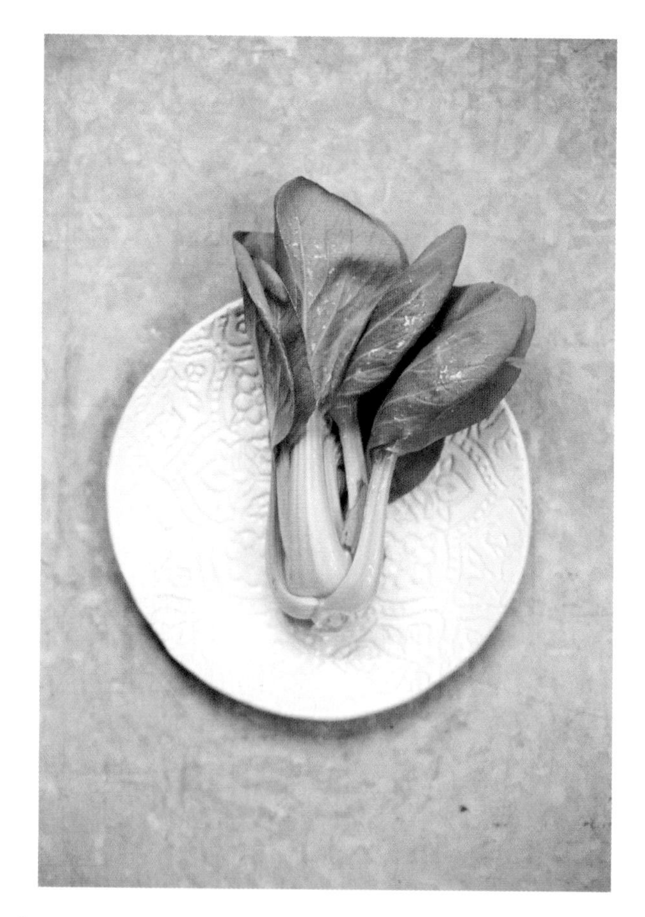

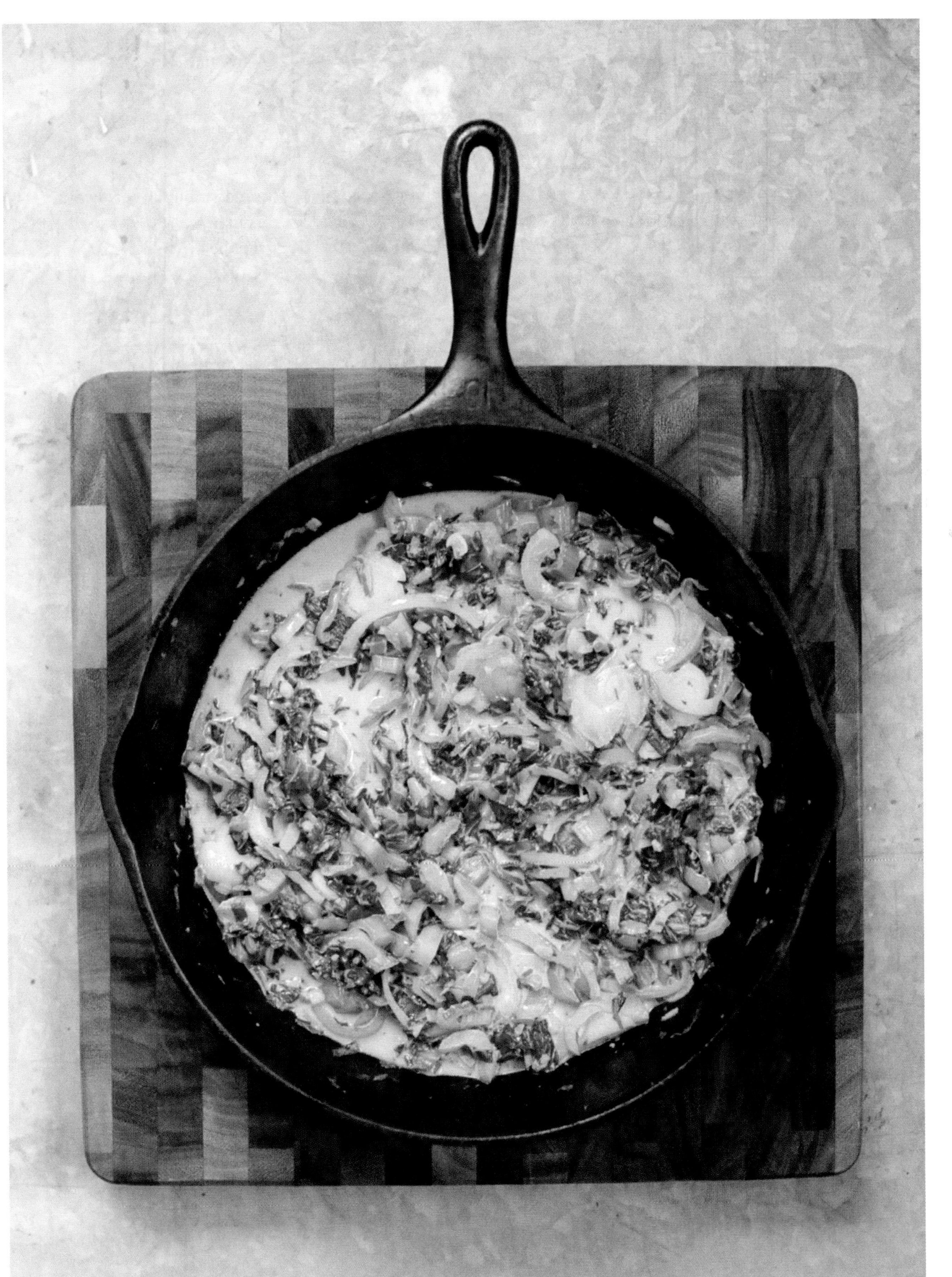

Almond Panna Cotta with Roasted Strawberries

Panna cotta, an Italian dessert, literally means "cooked cream." It's fantastic made with cream, but after much experimenting, I found the perfect ratio of coconut and almond milk to really highlight the flavor of the strawberries. This easy-to-make, light dessert can be served with a simple topping of sliced fresh fruit, but roasting the strawberries with balsamic vinegar really livens them up and brings this dish to a whole new level.

Serves 6

- *¼ cup water*
- *1 tablespoon gelatin (see Notes)*
- *1½ cups almond milk*
- *½ cup canned, full-fat coconut milk or heavy cream*
- *¼ cup honey*
- *Seeds scraped from ½ vanilla bean or 1 teaspoon vanilla extract*

For the roasted strawberries

- *2 cups fresh strawberries, hulled and halved or quartered*
- *2 tablespoons aged balsamic vinegar*
- *1 teaspoon vanilla extract*
- *2 tablespoons honey*

Whole30	No
Nut-free	Omit the almond milk and increase the amount of coconut milk to 2 cups.
Egg-free	Yes
AIP	Omit the almond milk and increase the amount of coconut milk to 2 cups.

1. Make the panna cotta: Place the water in a small cup and sprinkle the gelatin over it. Set aside.
2. In a small saucepan, heat the almond milk, coconut milk, and honey until the mixture begins to steam (it is not necessary to bring it to a boil).
3. Remove the pan from the heat and stir in the vanilla bean seeds and gelatin mixture.
4. Pour into ramekins, teacups, or small mason jars.
5. Cover and refrigerate overnight.
6. Make the roasted strawberries: Preheat the oven to 350°F.
7. In a glass baking dish, combine the strawberries, balsamic vinegar, vanilla, and honey. Roast for 30 minutes.
8. Resist the urge to eat it now.
9. Strain the sauce and set the strawberries aside. In a small saucepan over medium heat, simmer the sauce for about 5 minutes, or until it thickens into a syrup. Pour the sauce back over the strawberries.
10. Serve warm or cold with the panna cotta.

NOTES: *I like to use grass-fed gelatin in my cooking. Two good sources are Bernard Jenson and Great Lakes. If you'd like to be super fancy and invert the panna cotta cups, simply place them in very hot water for a few minutes. Place a dish on top of the cup and then flip it over, and the panna cotta will slide right out.*

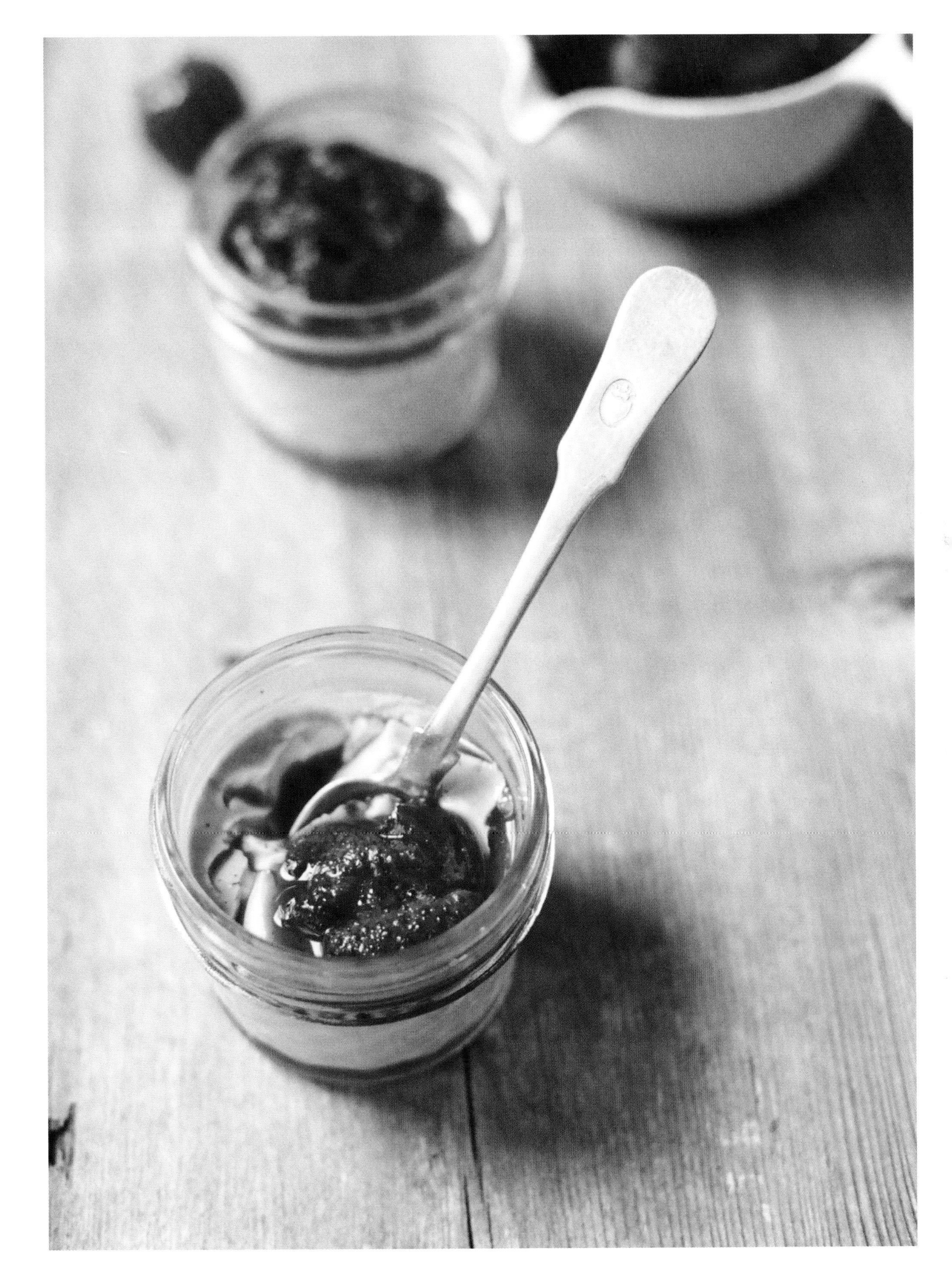

Birch Bark Sun Tea

This tea is one of my kids' favorites. If you've got a black birch tree nearby, you must try it. I learned about this tea from Russ Cohen, a wild edibles specialist. He came to my farm one day in early spring and helped me identify the edible wild plants growing around the farm. Russ noticed a black birch tree, snapped off a twig, peeled back the bark, and handed it to me to smell. I couldn't believe it—the scent is root beer! When brewed, it creates a refreshing and lightly root beer–scented tea that we all love. We also put this tea in our SodaStream to carbonate it. Fantastic! My kids even love the process of peeling the bark. Look for live growth, which should reveal light-colored twigs and bark with a green inner skin.

Makes 1 quart

- *20 black birch twigs, a little shorter than the height of a 1-quart mason jar*

1. Strip the bark off the twigs. Place the twigs and their peeled-off bark in a 1-quart mason jar.
2. Fill the jar with water, cover, and allow to sit in the warm sun for two days. Serve cold and carbonate, if you wish!

NOTES: *Stripping the bark off the branches is a great project for kids. It doesn't require a knife, but it's time-consuming. Set them to work! Kids also love the taste of this tea.*

Whole30	Yes
Nut-free	Yes
Egg-free	Yes
AIP	Yes

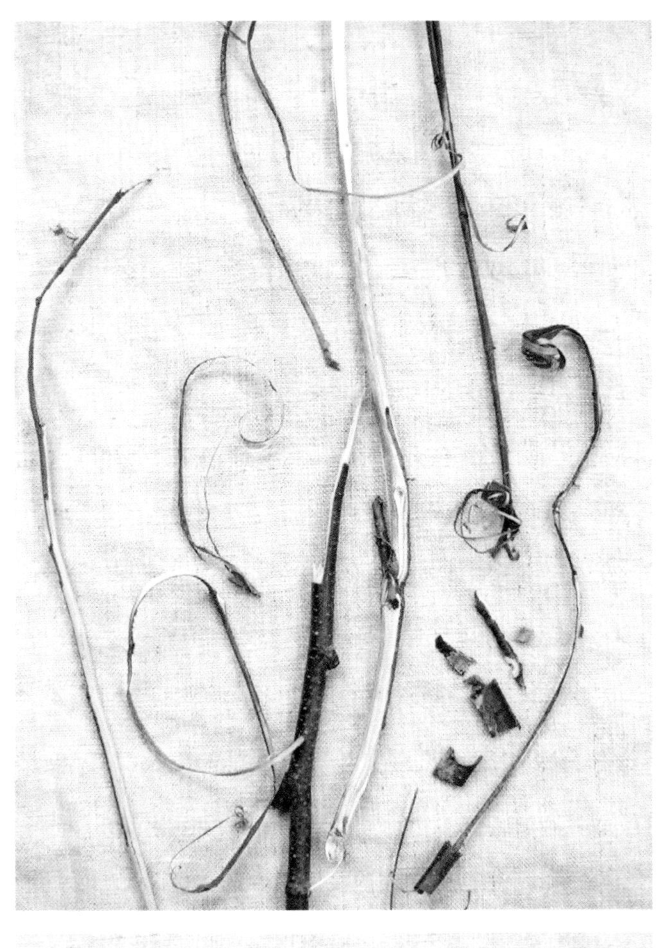

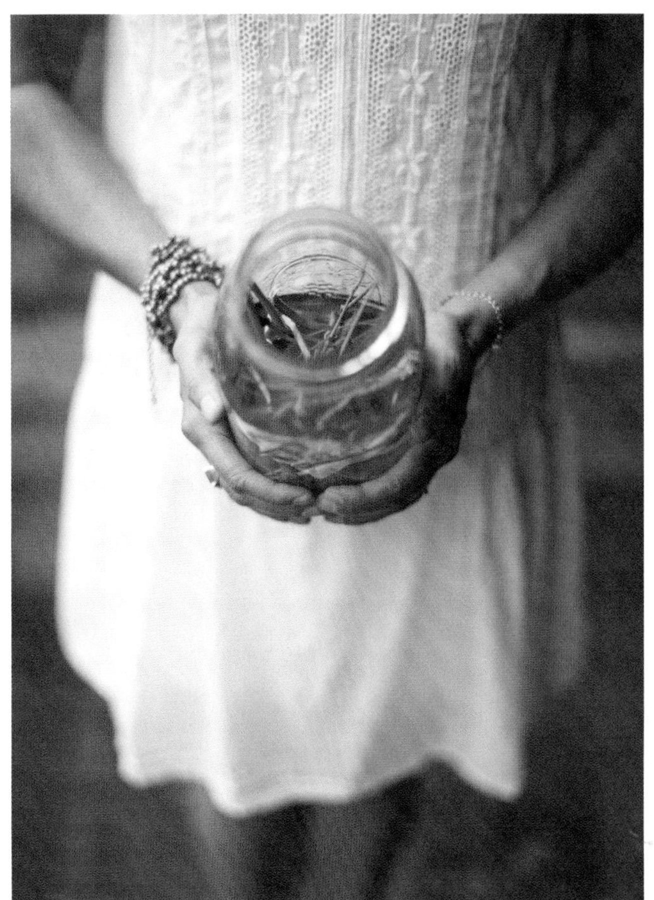

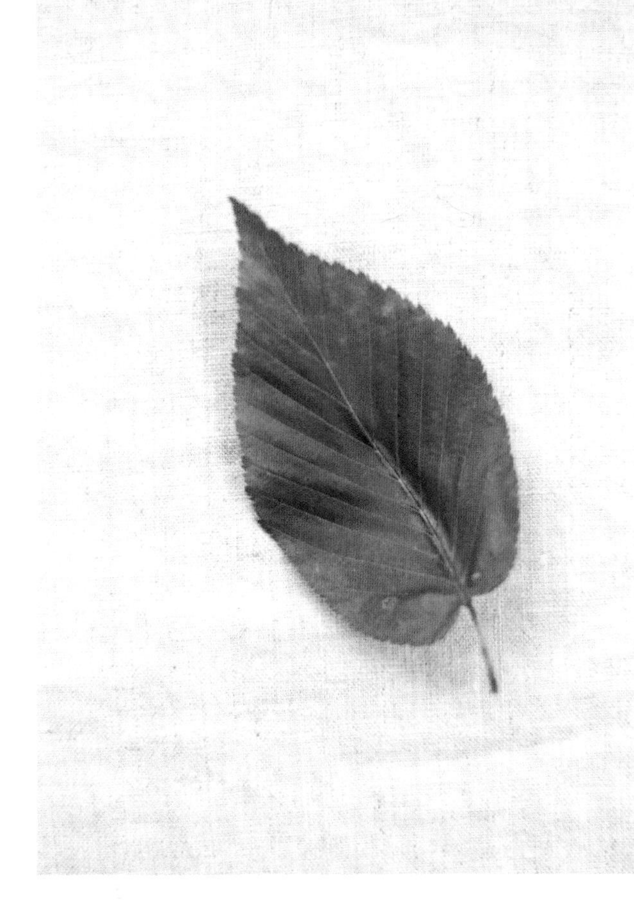

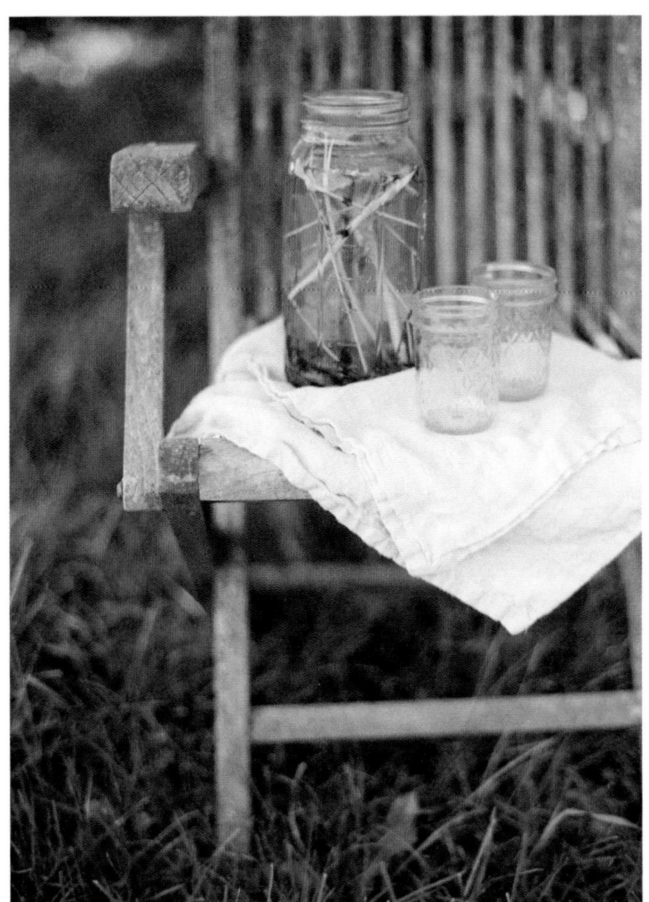

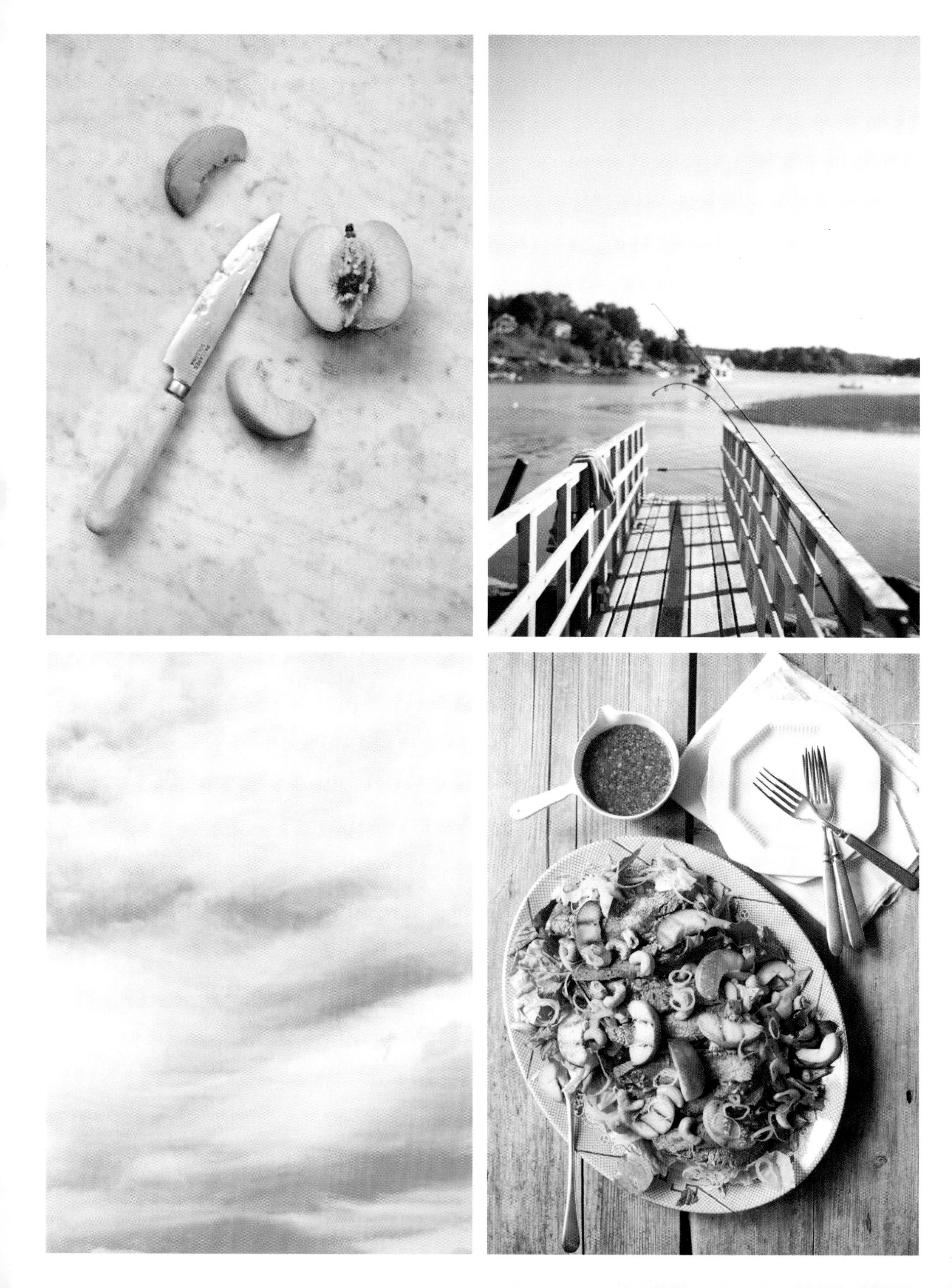

Midseason Recipes

From July through September on our farm, our vegetables are really producing. Strawberries have just passed, and we're on to the full bounty of leafy greens like kale and chard, plus zucchini and everybody's favorite: summer tomatoes! Aside from short camping trips or day trips to the beach, we're usually very busy running our farm during this season, and it can be hard to keep up with the abundance of vegetables coming out of the fields. I do try to spend a few days canning tomatoes and freezing some of the greens (see pages 352 and 354). I also often make a double or triple batch of starchy carbs and grill large amounts of meat at once to save time. Then, on hot and busy days, all I have to do to for a complete meal is prepare a simple fresh salad or stir-fry for dinner, and reheat the protein and starch for a quick and stress-free supper.

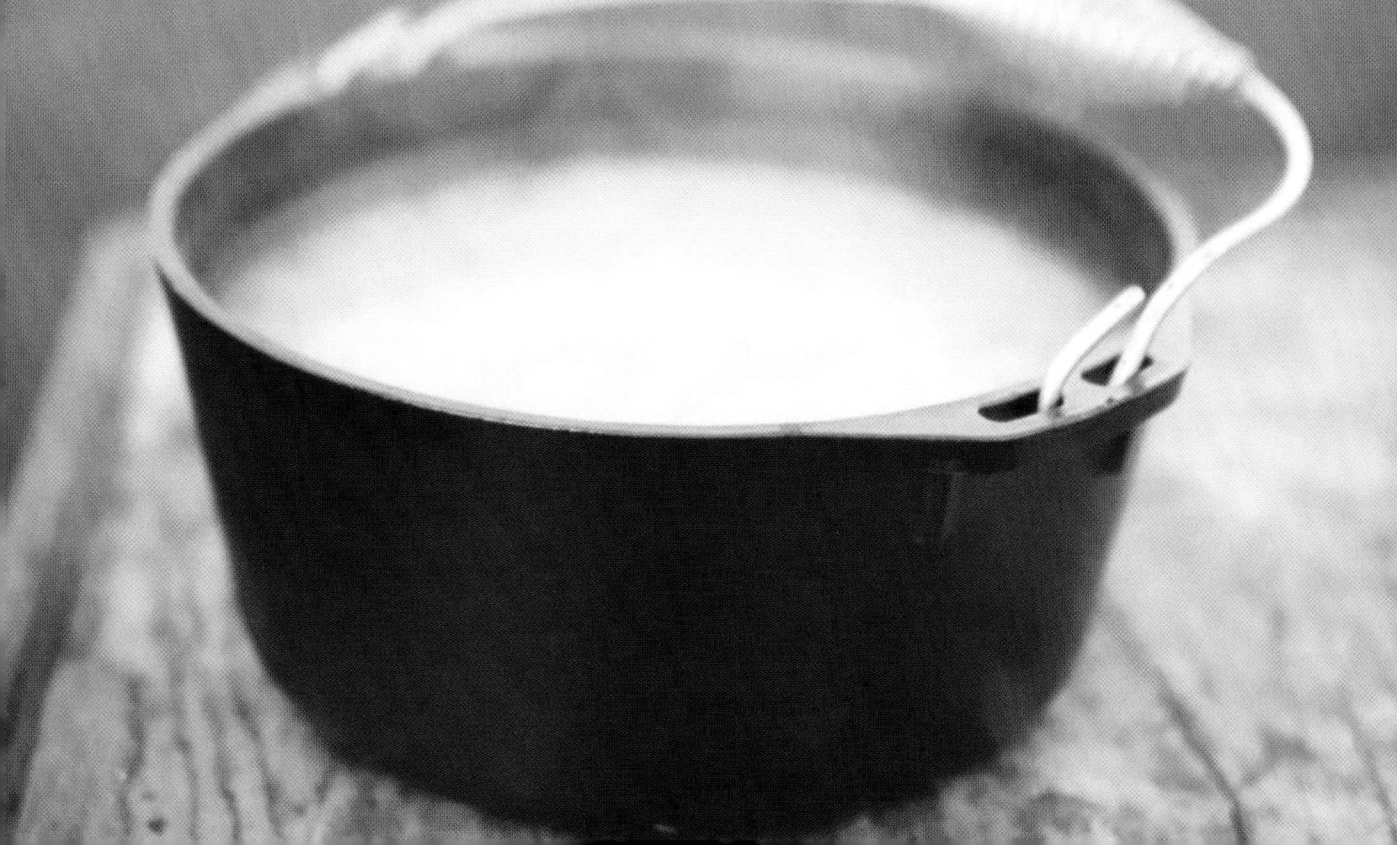

Cinnamon-Basil Breakfast Sausages

My family loves eating homemade sausages, and I tend to invent a new combination almost once a week. This batch was too good not to share. These bright and happy sausages are wonderful on a summer morning. Serve with scrambled eggs or Perfect Pastured Paleo Omelet (page 222), Speedy Summer-Fresh Tomato Sauce (page 222), and a strong cup of coffee.

Serves 4

- *1 pound ground pork*
- *2 tablespoons minced fresh basil leaves*
- *1 tablespoon Cinnamon Dry Rub (page 224)*
- *2 teaspoons minced fresh ginger*
- *½ teaspoon sea salt*
- *½ teaspoon ground black pepper*

1. Combine all of the ingredients in a bowl and mix well with your hands.
2. Form the mixture into small patties, using about 1 to 2 tablespoons per patty.
3. Heat a skillet over medium heat.
4. Working in batches, fry the sausages for about 5 minutes on the first side, until browned, then flip and continue cooking until the second side is browned and the meat is no longer pink inside. Serve warm.

NOTES: *Fresh mint or chives make a great substitute for basil in this recipe.*

Whole30	Yes
Nut-free	Yes
Egg-free	Yes
AIP	No

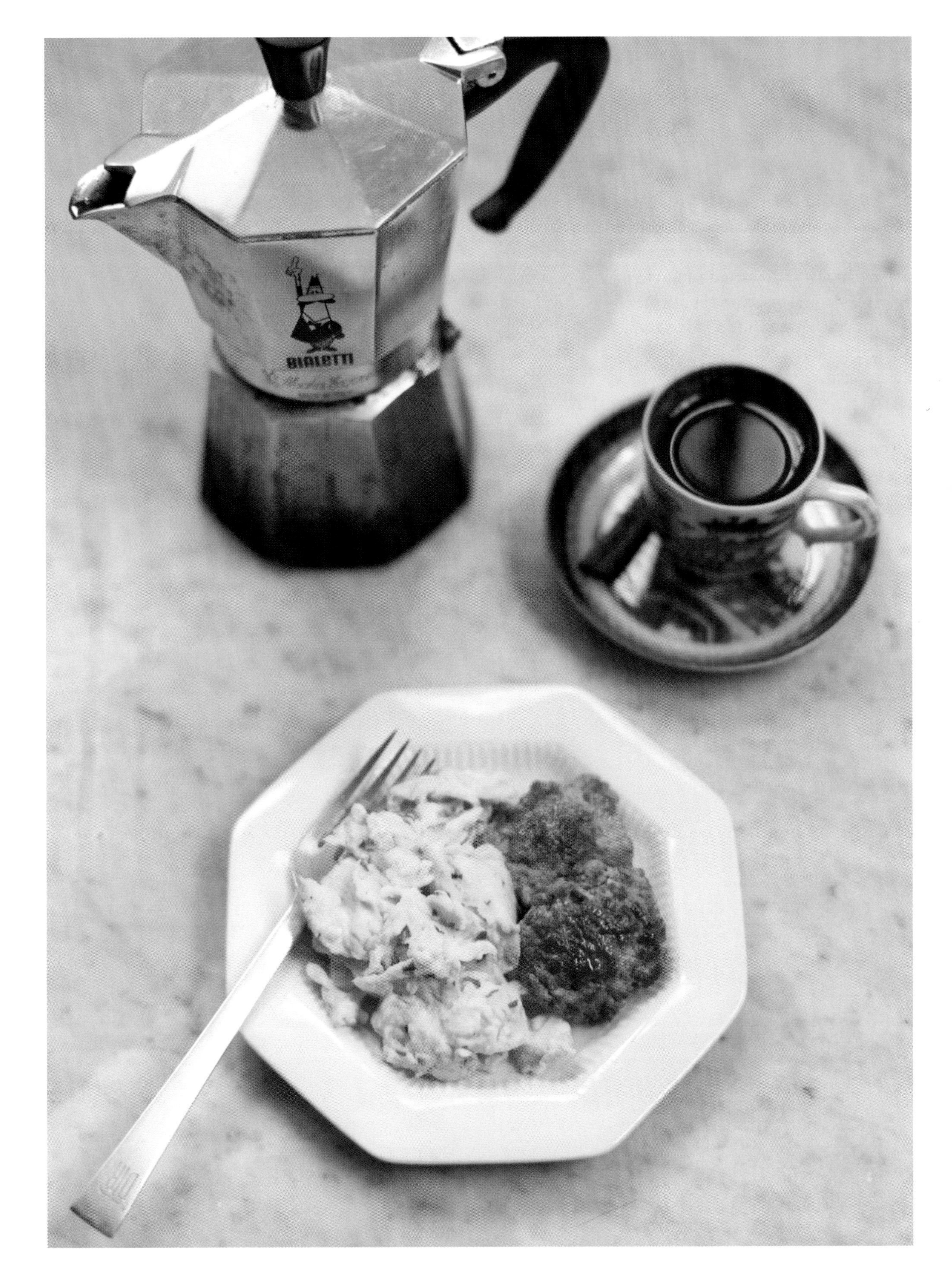
BIALETTI

Kohlrabi Cakes with Bacon and Dill

These cakes are incredible! Really, please try them. They're creamy and very dense, similar to the Bubble and Squeak recipe in my first cookbook, *Paleo Lunches and Breakfasts on the Go*, except that here I use kohlrabi and dill, making them much more herby and fresh-tasting. Kohlrabi is a pretty standard vegetable in Europe, but this alien-looking veggie hasn't really caught on in the United States. It tastes like a mix between a broccoli stem and a turnip. If you're not a fan of smoked fish, try these cakes with a fried or poached egg, or as a side dish to any protein.

Makes about 12 cakes, serving 6

- *1 pound yellow potatoes (about 4 small), peeled and quartered*
- *1 pound kohlrabi (about 2 heads), peeled and cut the same size as the potatoes*
- *½ pound bacon ends, bacon pieces, or pancetta, diced small*
- *1 small yellow onion, diced*
- *3 cloves garlic, minced*
- *½ cup whole milk or canned, full-fat coconut milk*
- *½ teaspoon ground white pepper*
- *1¼ cups potato starch*
- *3 tablespoons minced fresh dill (plus sprigs for garnish, if desired)*
- *10 ounces smoked trout or white fish or 6 fried or poached eggs, for serving (optional)*
- *2 tablespoons crème fraîche (page 347), for garnish (optional)*

Whole30	Omit the milk and crème fraîche.
Nut-free	Yes
Egg-free	Yes
AIP	Substitute sweet potatoes for the yellow potatoes. Omit the milk, crème fraîche, and white pepper.

1. Boil the potatoes and kohlrabi in a pot of water for about 20 to 30 minutes, until tender. Drain and transfer to a large bowl. Set aside.

2. In a skillet, cook the bacon over medium heat until brown and crispy.

3. Add the onion and garlic to the pan and continue cooking until the onion is translucent.

4. Using a slotted spoon, transfer the bacon mixture to a paper towel to drain. Pour off all but 1 tablespoon of the bacon fat from the skillet. Set the skillet with the bacon fat aside (you will use it again in Step 6). Save the rest of the bacon fat for another use.

5. In the large bowl, mash the drained potatoes and kohlrabi with the milk, pepper, and potato starch, then add the bacon mixture and mix well. Add the dill and mix to combine.

6. Heat the skillet with the reserved bacon fat over medium heat.

7. Working in batches, place three or four burger-sized clumps of the kohlrabi mixture in the pan. (Do not overcrowd the pan; the number of cakes you cook at a time depends on the size of your pan.) Cook for about 5 minutes, until the bottoms are lightly browned. Flip, lightly press down with the back of a spatula, and continue cooking until the second side is browned. Transfer the finished cakes to a plate, and repeat with the rest of the kohlrabi mixture.

8. Serve two cakes per person with a piece of smoked fish or a fried or poached egg, and garnish with crème fraîche and a sprig of fresh dill, if you like.

NOTES: *Kohlrabi is also excellent shredded raw into salads, cut into "fries" and roasted, or steamed. If you can't find kohlrabi for this recipe, substitute hakurei turnips or broccoli stems.*

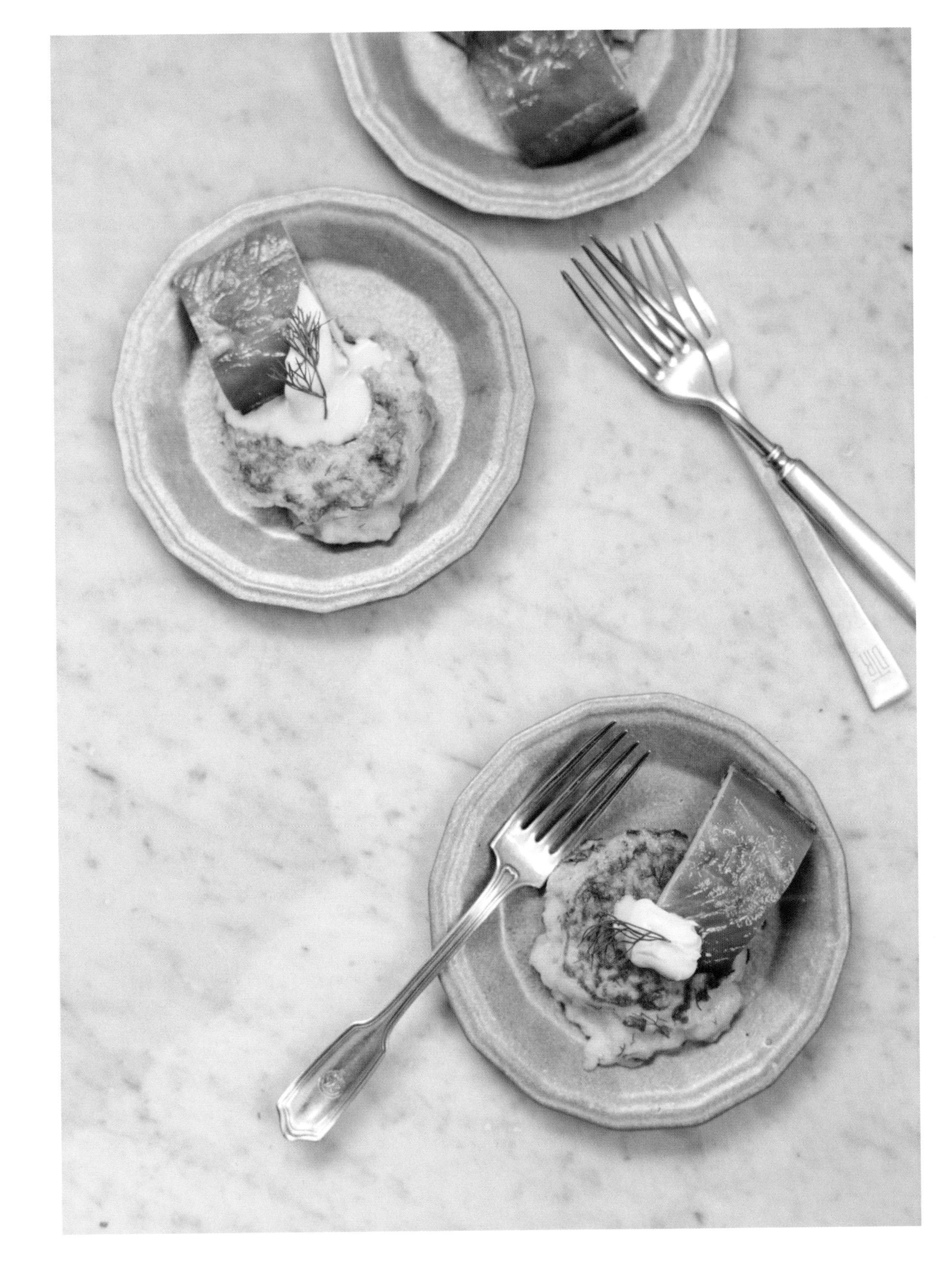

Maple-Spiced Venison Jerky

This jerky is a perfect power snack or quick breakfast on the run when paired with dried pears and soaked and sprouted hazelnuts with dried pears and soaked and sprouted hazelnuts. I tried quite a few jerky recipes before I landed on this one, which my kids and I love. I read once to slice nearly frozen beef on a mandoline, which I tried the first time I made jerky. I sliced the beef way too thin and ended with crunchy "beef chips" instead of soft jerky. Learn from my mistake and make the slices about ⅛ inch thick. If you can't get your hands on venison, use flank steak instead.

Makes about ½ pound jerky

- *1 pound venison steak or beef flank steak*
- *¼ cup coconut aminos*
- *2 tablespoons Worcestershire sauce*
- *2 tablespoons maple syrup*
- *1 tablespoon all-natural liquid smoke*
- *1 tablespoon onion powder*
- *½ teaspoon ground white pepper*
- *½ teaspoon minced fresh ginger*
- *¼ teaspoon cayenne pepper*

1. Slice the steak against the grain into strips about ⅛ inch thick (not paper thin). Slightly frozen meat is a bit easier to slice.

2. Place the meat in a container or bag with the remaining ingredients and marinate overnight in the refrigerator.

3. Remove the meat from the marinade and place on paper towels to dry. Placing either in a dehydrator set to high or on racks in the oven set on the lowest possible heat setting (150°F to 170°F).

4. Start checking the jerky after 3 hours. If it still seems too moist, leave it in the dehydrator or oven to continue dehydrating. The ideal texture is like a soft leather. In my experience, it can take as little as 3 hours and as long as 8 hours to get to the right dryness.

5. After removing it from the dehydrator or oven, allow the jerky to cool at room temperature before storing it in refrigerator. If you refrigerate it while it's still warm, condensation will develop and create unwanted moisture on the jerky, causing it to spoil. It will keep for several weeks when stored in an airtight container.

Shown with Simple Dried Pears (page 210) and Crispy Almonds (page 211).

Whole30	Omit the maple syrup and Worcestershire sauce.
Nut-free	Yes
Egg-free	Yes
AIP	No

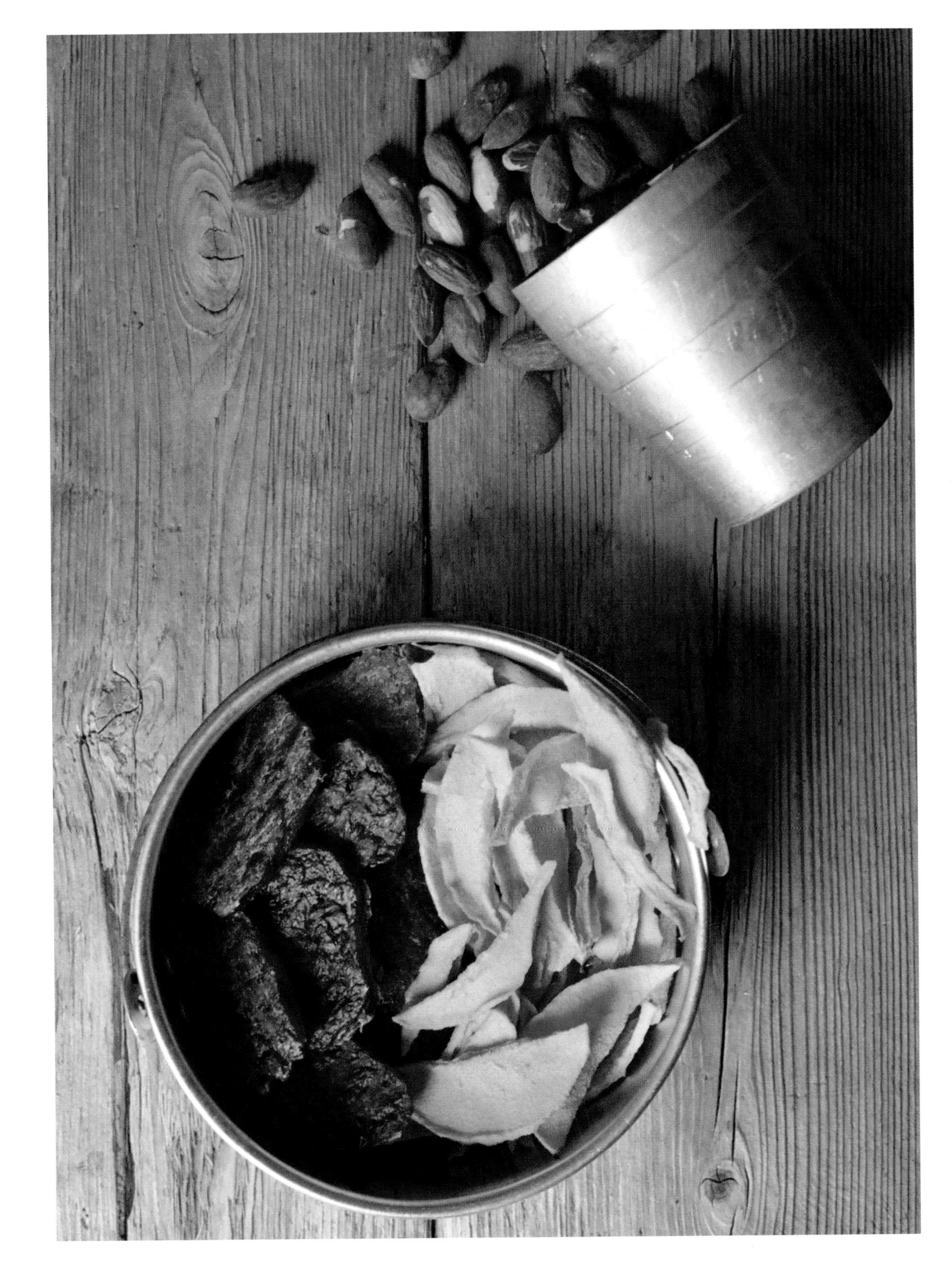

Simple Dried Pears

I don't know why it's so hard to find dried pears in the store. They are so much more interesting to me than other dried fruit. They have an amazing sugary taste that is much more flavorful than the leathery dried apples you find in supermarkets. If you don't already have a food dehydrator, you should get one. It's lots of fun to experiment with your garden bounty by drying fruits and making jerky. Once you've had a dried pear, you'll see what I mean. I like to combine these with jerky and soaked and sprouted nuts to make mini snacks for my family.

Makes about 2 cups

- *1 tablespoon lemon juice*
- *6 Bartlett pears*

1. Fill a large bowl about two-thirds full with cold water. Add the lemon juice.
2. Peel the pears. You don't always have to peel fruit, but pears benefit from being peeled before you dehydrate them.
3. Core the pears and cut into slices about ½ inch thick, placing the pieces in the bowl of lemon water as you work to keep them from browning.
4. Dry the pears and place in a dehydrator on low or on racks in the oven set on the lowest possible heat setting (150°F to 170°F).
5. Allow the pears to dehydrate until they are completely dry, about 8 hours. After removing them from the dehydrator or oven, allow them to come to room temperature before storing—otherwise they could sweat and spoil.
6. Try not to eat them all at once. They're that good! They will keep for months in a sealed container.

See photo on page 209.

NOTES: *You can also make dried apples this way.*

Whole30	Yes
Nut-free	Yes
Egg-free	Yes
AIP	Yes

Crispy Almonds

Soaking nuts in salted water before dehydrating them not only makes them extra tasty but also enhances their nutritional benefits. This recipe is very easy to make, but it does take some time: at least 7 hours for soaking and 12 to 24 hours for dehydrating the nuts.

Makes 4 cups

- *1 tablespoon sea salt*
- *2 quarts filtered water, plus more if needed*
- *4 cups raw almonds (organic if possible)*

1. Dissolve the salt in the water, then pour it over the nuts. If you need to, add more water to cover the nuts. Cover and leave in a warm place for at least 7 hours, or overnight.

2. Drain the soaked nuts in a colander and spread on a stainless-steel rimmed baking sheet. Place in a warm oven (no warmer than 150°F) or a dehydrator set to low and dehydrate, turning occasionally, until thoroughly dry and crisp, about 12 to 24 hours. Make sure that they are completely dry; otherwise, they could develop mold and won't have that wonderful crispy texture. Dehydrating may take less time in an oven than in a dehydrator, so check frequently to ensure that they don't burn. Oven temperatures can vary, especially in gas ovens.

3. After removing the almonds from the oven or dehydrator, allow to cool to room temperature before placing in a jar or other container. They will keep for months.

See photo on page 209.

NOTES: *Be sure to buy raw (not roasted) almonds for this recipe. This method works with a variety of seeds and most nuts. (I love crispy pecans!) Generally, the denser the nut, the longer the soaking time, and the longer it takes to dehydrate them. Just keep checking the nuts or seeds in the oven or dehydrator, as drying times vary depending on the thickness of the food being dehydrated.*

Whole30	Yes
Nut-free	No
Egg-free	Yes
AIP	No

Grilled Calamari with Tomatoes and Aged Balsamic

Squid is quite sustainable and delicious, and it's usually one of the least expensive options at the seafood counter. It doesn't have to be coated in breadcrumbs, either. When grilled and tossed with balsamic vinegar, it takes on a sweet taste, which is highlighted here by the summery flavors of tomato and basil. This dish is super simple and fast to prepare. Try serving it as an appetizer the next time you have friends over. My son Anson loves the tentacles, so I always make sure to have the fishmonger toss in a few just for him. He absolutely adores this dish!

Serves 2 to 3

- *1 pound squid, cleaned and gutted*
- *1 tablespoon bacon fat or coconut oil, melted*
- *Sea salt and ground black pepper*
- *1 shallot, sliced thin*
- *2 tablespoons aged balsamic vinegar*
- *1 cup cherry tomatoes, cut in half*
- *½ cup ribbon-sliced fresh basil leaves*
- *2 tablespoons cold-pressed, extra-virgin olive oil*
- *Juice of ½ lemon*

1. Heat a grill to medium-high heat (see page 362 for grilling tips).
2. Rinse and dry the squid. Cut the bodies down the middle to make one flat piece. You can use tentacles, but try to stick with larger ones so they don't fall through the grates of the grill. I like to use a grill basket for them.
3. Coat the squid with the bacon fat and a large pinch each of salt and pepper.
4. Grill for just a few minutes, until no longer translucent. Set aside.
5. In a medium-sized bowl, toss the shallot with the balsamic vinegar.
6. Add the tomatoes, basil, olive oil, lemon juice, and squid and toss to combine.
7. Season to taste with salt and pepper. Serve warm.

NOTES: *You can also pan-fry the squid indoors. Cook over high heat for just a few minutes to prevent it from becoming rubbery and chewy.*

Whole30	Yes
Nut-free	Yes
Egg-free	Yes
AIP	Omit the tomatoes and black pepper. Substitute grilled zucchini for the tomatoes.

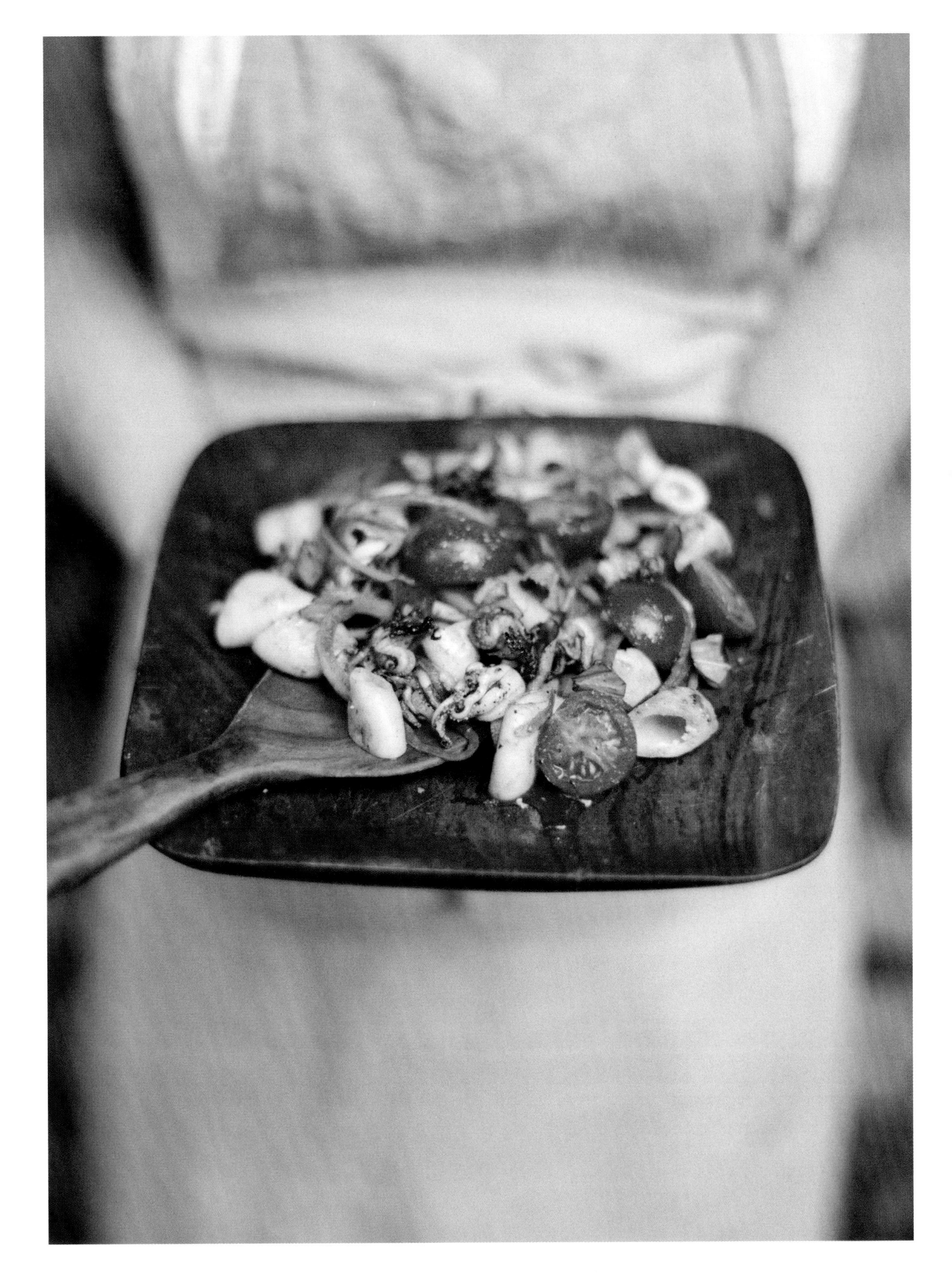

Lamb Chops with Fresh Ginger Herb Sauce

I love lamb in any form. You don't really need to do much to bring out its flavor, but this lovely lemony herb sauce takes the meat to a new level of deliciousness. The sauce is also a fantastic dressing for grilled vegetables like zucchini or eggplant. The chops are shown here with Shirazi Noodle Salad (page 216).

Serves 4

- *12 lamb loin chops or 8 shoulder chops, about ¾ inch thick*
- *Sea salt and ground black pepper*

For the sauce

- *1 cup roughly chopped fresh mint leaves*
- *1 cup roughly chopped fresh parsley leaves*
- *½ cup chopped fresh cilantro leaves*
- *½ teaspoon minced fresh ginger*
- *1 teaspoon minced jalapeño pepper*
- *1 teaspoon minced garlic*
- *⅓ cup cold-pressed, extra-virgin olive oil*
- *Juice of 2 lemons*

1. Heat a grill to medium heat (see page 362 for grilling tips). Allow the lamb to come to room temperature while the grill heats up. Season the lamb with salt and pepper.
2. Grill the lamb for about 4 minutes on the first side, then flip and continue cooking until medium-rare (145°F on a digital thermometer), about 4 more minutes. Set the chops on a platter.
3. Make the sauce: Combine the mint, parsley, cilantro, ginger, jalapeño pepper, garlic, olive oil, and lemon juice in a food processor and pulse until blended.
4. Top each chop with a spoonful of the sauce right before serving.

Shown with Shirazi Noodle Salad (page 216).

NOTES: *This sauce also goes great with grilled beef and chicken!*

Whole30	Yes
Nut-free	Yes
Egg-free	Yes
AIP	Omit the jalapeño pepper and black pepper.

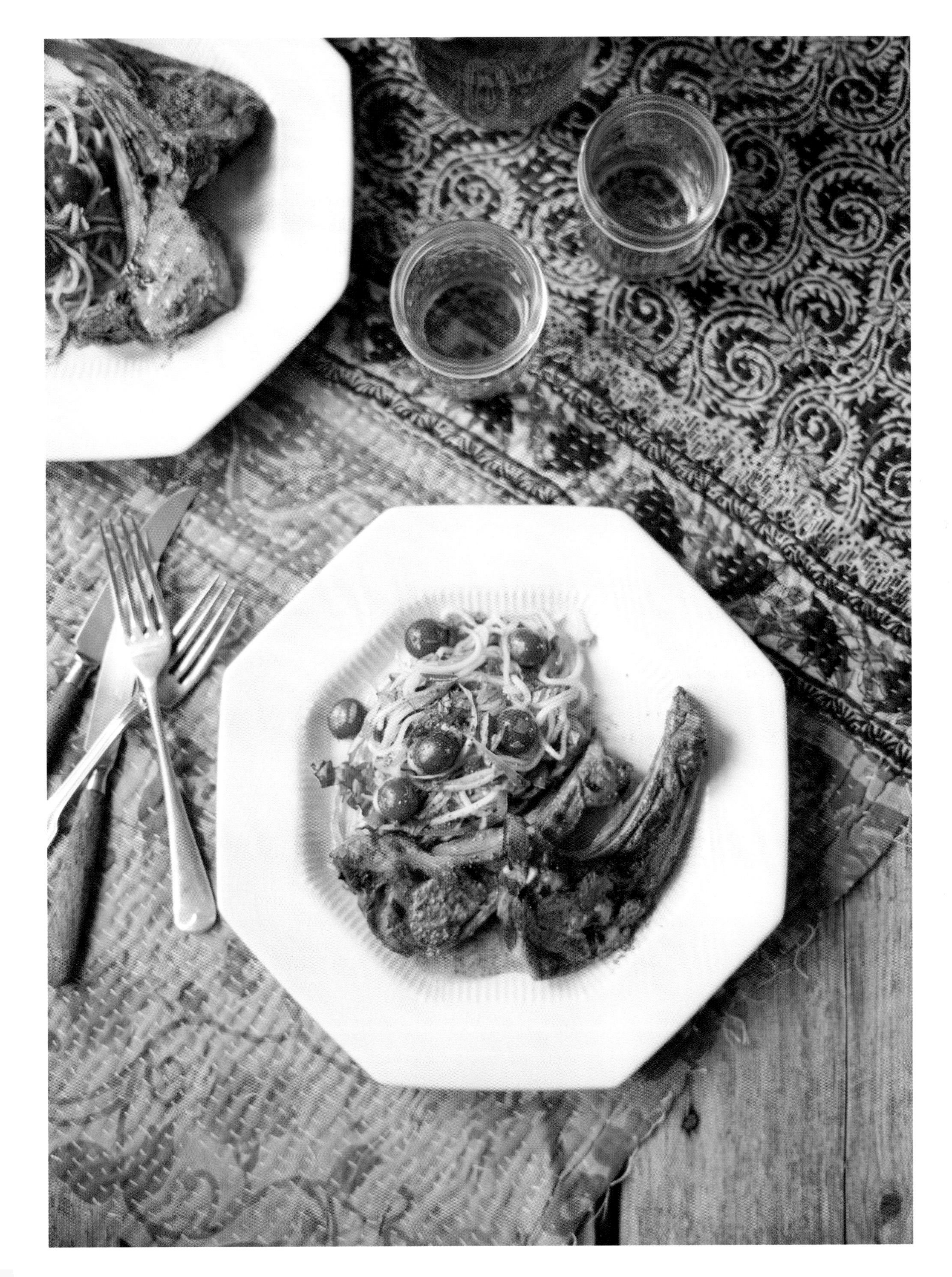

Shirazi Noodle Salad

Some friends of mine host a "gourmet night" once a month. Each month, they pick a theme and ask guests to bring one dish to serve to the crowd. When my husband and I were invited and I needed a last-minute Persian dish, I emailed my friend Arsy Vartanian, an Iranian cookbook author. She suggested this side dish, which traditionally looks like a salsa but is eaten like a salad. Luckily, I had all of the ingredients either in the kitchen or growing in the fields, so I didn't even need to run to the store to make it. I decided to turn the traditionally chopped cucumbers into noodles, added some zucchini to help the texture a bit, and added some mint to liven it up. It was a great dish to bring to the dinner party, and everyone loved it. Its light and refreshing flavors complement so many other stronger dishes.

Serves 4 to 6

- *2 medium cucumbers*
- *1 medium zucchini*
- *Juice of 1 lemon*
- *¼ cup cold-pressed, extra-virgin olive oil*
- *2 cups cherry tomatoes*
- *½ cup minced fresh parsley leaves*
- *¼ cup minced fresh mint leaves*
- *¼ cup very thinly sliced red onion (best done on a mandoline)*
- *Sea salt and ground black pepper*

1. With a spiral slicer, slice the cucumbers and zucchini into noodles and place in a bowl.
2. Toss with the lemon juice, olive oil, cherry tomatoes, parsley, mint, and red onion. Season with salt and pepper to taste.

See photo on page 215.

NOTES: *If you don't have a spiral slicer, you can use a vegetable peeler or mandoline to make long strips of cucumber and zucchini. We grow a yellow zucchini called Goldy from High Mowing Seeds—different from a summer squash—which is an incredibly bright color and is very fun for this dish.*

Whole30	Yes
Nut-free	Yes
Egg-free	Yes
AIP	Omit the tomatoes and black pepper.

Creamy Coleslaw with Fresh Dill

This slaw is based on the classic slaw you probably ate (or refused to eat) as a kid, but when you use homemade mayonnaise, you'll taste firsthand how much better coleslaw can be. The addition of lots of fresh dill also gives it a fresh, summery taste. Serve this side dish along with a spicy grilled steak, smoked brisket, or fried fish. It's also perfect to double or triple for a party! If you're making it a day ahead, consider using all green cabbage, as red cabbage likes to bleed all over the rest of the salad as it sits in the fridge. However, it makes for a beautiful presentation the day it's made.

Serves 6 to 8

- *½ small head green cabbage, shredded*
- *½ small head red cabbage, shredded*
- *1 cup peeled and shredded carrots*
- *½ cup chopped fresh dill*
- *⅓ cup minced fresh chives*
- *¼ cup thinly sliced red onion*
- *1⅓ cups homemade mayonnaise (page 344)*
- *⅓ cup apple cider vinegar*
- *2 tablespoons honey (optional)*
- *Sea salt and ground black pepper*

1. Combine the cabbage, carrots, dill, chives, and red onion in a large bowl.
2. Mix together the mayo, vinegar, and honey, if using, in a small bowl.
3. Toss the cabbage mixture with the dressing.
4. Add salt and pepper to taste. Serve.

See photo on page 218.

NOTES: *This slaw can sit overnight and still tastes great! Try adding some fresh or rehydrated seaweed.*

Whole30	Omit the honey.
Nut-free	Yes
Egg-free	Substitute ⅔ cup olive oil for the mayonnaise.
AIP	Substitute ⅔ cup olive oil for the mayonnaise, and omit the black pepper.

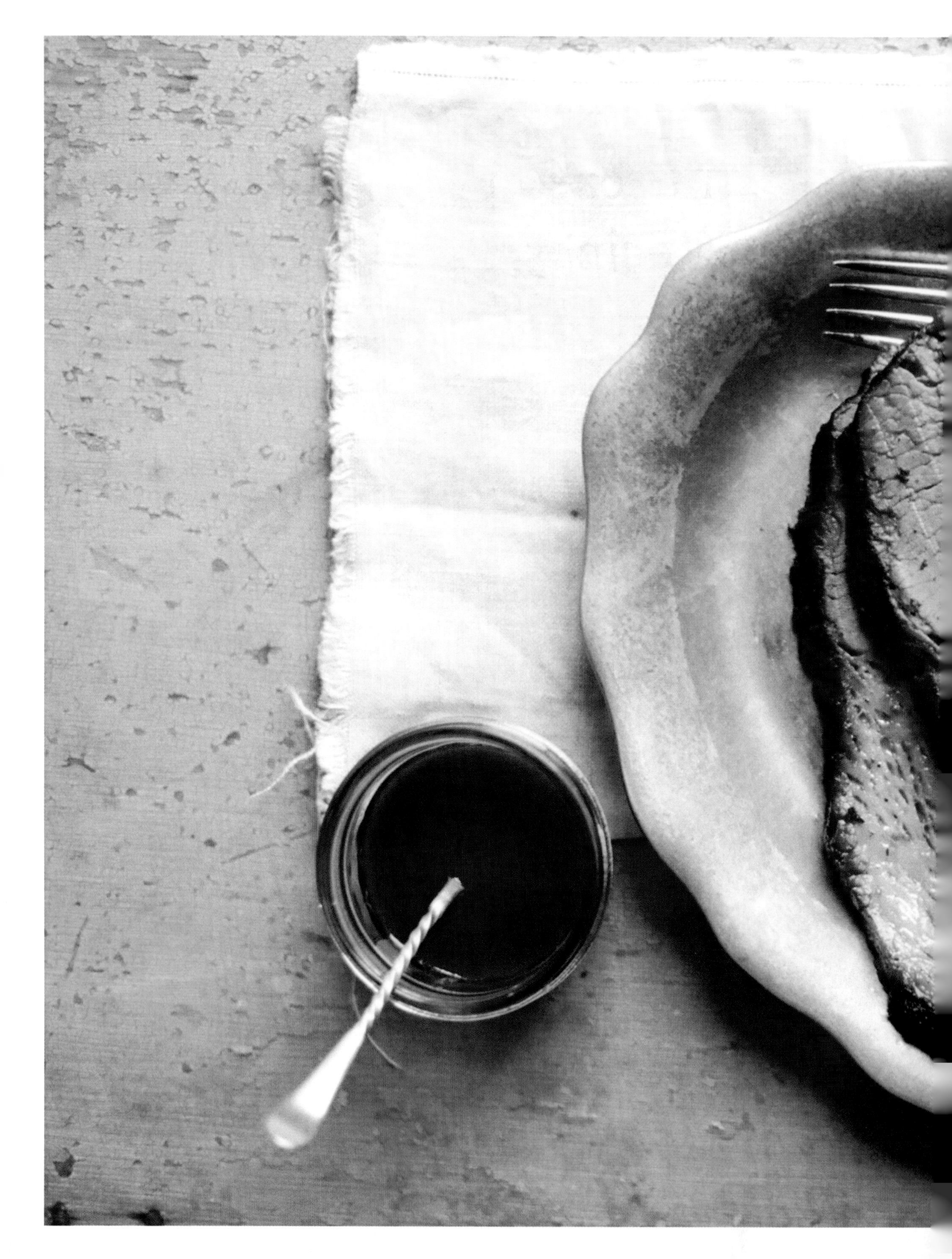

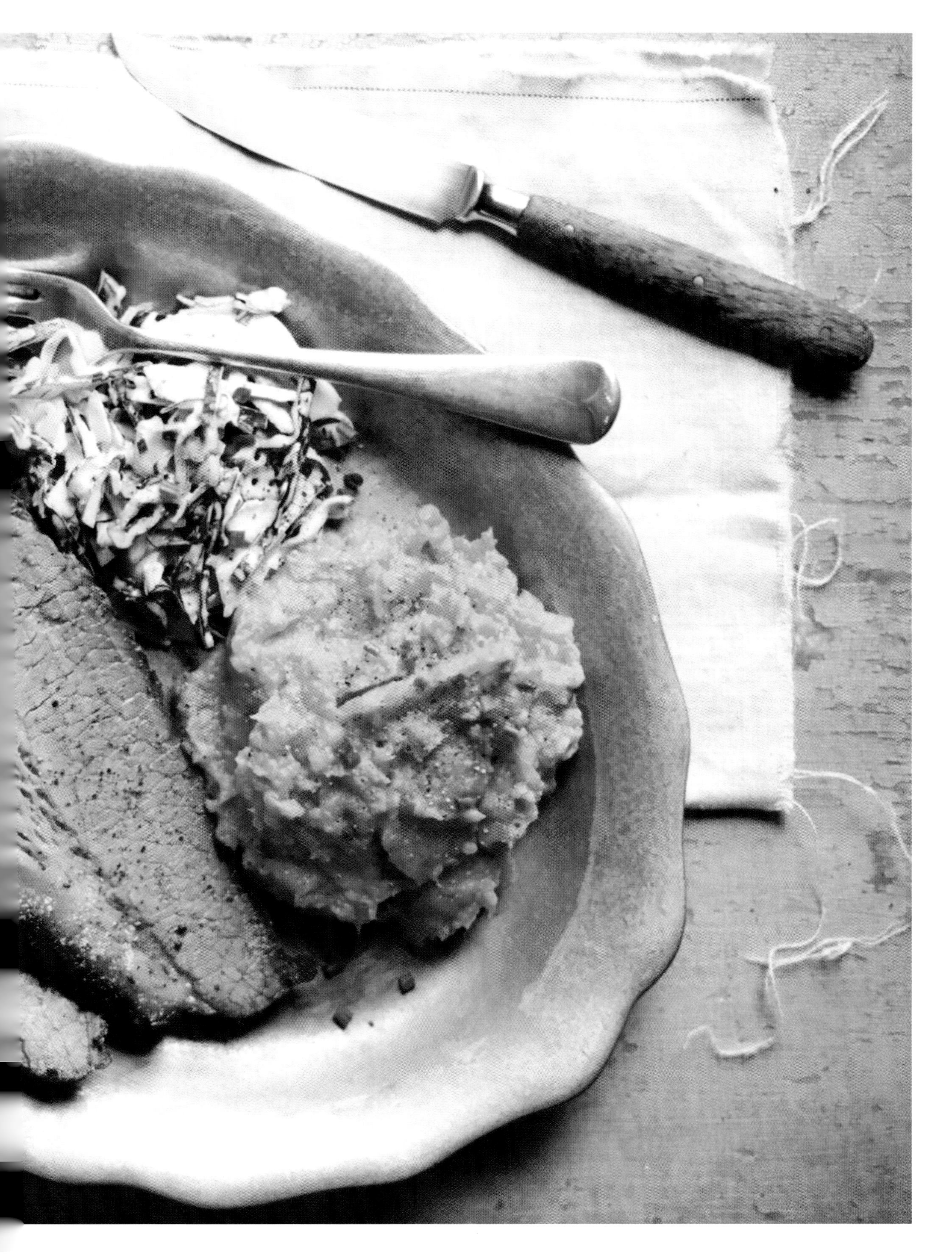

Frank's Hickory-Smoked Brisket

Frank is the resident foodie on our farm, especially when it comes to grilling, smoking, curing, or really doing anything with meat. He almost went to cooking school but then took a path as a builder, and he has a shop on our farm where he rebuilds doors, builds new spaces, and helps me taste-test my recipes. When I told him I wanted to smoke a brisket, he told me exactly how to do it. I then had him to dinner to ensure that the rub, barbecue sauce, and side dishes were what he expected, and I received gold stars from him and everyone else in the room. This dish was also a huge hit at the Open Door Food Pantry dinner (see page 395). If you'd like to seriously impress someone, make this recipe. Although it takes a while, it requires little hands-on time: it marinates overnight; the 7 to 8 hours of slow cooking are largely unattended; and it rests for 30 to 60 minutes. Trust me, the flavor is unbelievable and worth the time spent.

Shown on page 218 with Creamy Coleslaw with Fresh Dill (page 217) and Simple Mashed Sweet Potatoes with Chives (page 171).

Serves about 15 to 20

- *1 (10-pound) side of brisket (full brisket if possible)*
- *1 cup Spiced Dry Rub (page 221)*
- *6 cups hickory wood chips, divided*
- *1 batch Smoky BBQ Sauce (page 346) or your favorite barbecue sauce*

NOTES: *This recipe makes a lot, but you can purchase a smaller brisket and follow the same steps—just adjust the slow-roasting time at the end by checking the temperature with a meat thermometer about 2 hours after you place the meat in the oven (in Step 10). Try experimenting with other wood chips for a different flavor.*

Whole30	Yes
Nut-free	Yes
Egg-free	Yes
AIP	No

1. Coat the brisket all over with the dry rub and wrap tightly with wax paper, parchment paper, or tin foil. Leave in the refrigerator overnight.

2. When you're ready to start slow cooking, remove the brisket from the fridge and bring it to room temperature. I suggest starting this at about 8 or 9 a.m.

3. Soak 2 cups of the hickory chips in water for at least 20 minutes. Set aside.

4. Preheat a grill set up for indirect grilling (see page 362) to 200°F. (You can also set up a smoker if you have one, but it is not necessary. Frank used his infrared grill and warmed it to 200°F.) You can make the brisket on a regular gas grill, too, if the grill has multiple burners that enable you to create a two-zone cooking area.

5. When the grill is warm, place the soaked hickory chips in a metal tray. Top the wet chips with 1 cup of dry chips and place the tray under the grilling rack.

6. Unwrap the meat and place it over the cool portion of the grill, fat side up. Close the lid and let it cook for about 4 hours, or until it reaches an internal temperature of 150°F. Make sure that the

temperature of the grill stays at 200°F to 220°F (you may need to crack the lid an inch to moderate the temperature).

7. After 2 hours, add 2 more cups of soaked wood chips topped with 1 cup of dry chips.

8. Preheat the oven to 220°F. When the meat reaches an internal temperature of 150°F, after about 4 hours, it's time to move it to the oven.

9. Place the brisket in a large dish with a lid (such as an enameled cast-iron braising dish) or wrap it in foil (a less-sustainable but functional option) and place it on a rimmed baking sheet in the oven.

10. Roast for about 3 to 4 hours, or until the internal temperature reaches 185°F.

11. Remove the brisket from the oven and allow it to sit on the counter, covered, for 30 to 60 minutes before thinly slicing it against the grain.

12. Serve with barbecue sauce.

Spiced Dry Rub

This all-purpose dry rub can be used on beef, pork, lamb, and goat before grilling to give the meat a warm, spicy flavor. I like to make a double batch and store it in my cabinet so I have it on hand.

Makes ¾ cup

- *3 tablespoons sea salt*
- *2 tablespoons garlic powder*
- *2 tablespoons onion powder*
- *1 tablespoon cayenne pepper*
- *1 tablespoon coriander*
- *1 tablespoon freshly ground black pepper*
- *1 tablespoon smoked hot paprika*
- *1 tablespoon mustard powder*
- *1 tablespoon ginger powder*

1. Combine all of the ingredients in a bowl and mix well.

NOTES: *Try to allow the rub to sit on the meat for at least 4 hours. Overnight is ideal.*

Whole30	Yes
Nut-free	Yes
Egg-free	Yes
AIP	No

Speedy Summer-Fresh Tomato Sauce

When your garden is bursting with tomatoes, try this super-quick sauce over eggs to start your day off right. It also goes great with zucchini noodles or spaghetti squash.

Makes just under 1 quart

- *4 pounds tomatoes*
- *¼ cup ghee (page 347)*
- *½ medium yellow onion, diced small*
- *2 cloves garlic, minced*
- *3 tablespoons chopped fresh basil leaves*
- *Sea salt and ground black pepper*

Whole30	Yes
Nut-free	Yes
Egg-free	Yes
AIP	No

1. Chop the tomatoes into 1-inch dice and place them in a colander to drain.
2. In a large skillet, melt the ghee over medium heat. Add the onion and cook for 5 minutes, or until soft.
3. Add the garlic and cook for another 2 minutes.
4. Squeeze out any remaining juice from the tomatoes and then add them to the pan. Cook for about 10 minutes, until cooked down and very soft.
5. Remove from the heat and add the basil and salt and pepper to taste.

NOTES: *If you would like to make this sauce when tomatoes are out of season, use a 28-ounce can of diced or crushed tomatoes (or better yet, use 2 pints of your own canned tomatoes, drained; see page 354).*

Perfect Pastured Paleo Omelet

I tried a dish similar to this in Morocco and couldn't believe how delicious it was. This is a basic omelet recipe is intended to be topped with Speedy Summer-Fresh Tomato Sauce (above). Serve it with Cinnamon-Basil Breakfast Sausages (page 204).

Serves 1

- *3 eggs*
- *½ teaspoon coconut flour*
- *1 teaspoon fish sauce*
- *1 teaspoon bacon fat*
- *Speedy Summer-Fresh Tomato Sauce (above), for serving*

1. Combine the eggs, coconut flour, and fish sauce in a bowl and mix well.
2. Melt the bacon fat in a skillet over medium-high heat.
3. Pour the egg mixture into the pan and cook for a few minutes, until it looks mostly done.
4. Flip the two sides into the middle and cook for another minute, top with tomato sauce, and serve.

Whole30	Yes
Nut-free	Yes
Egg-free	No
AIP	No

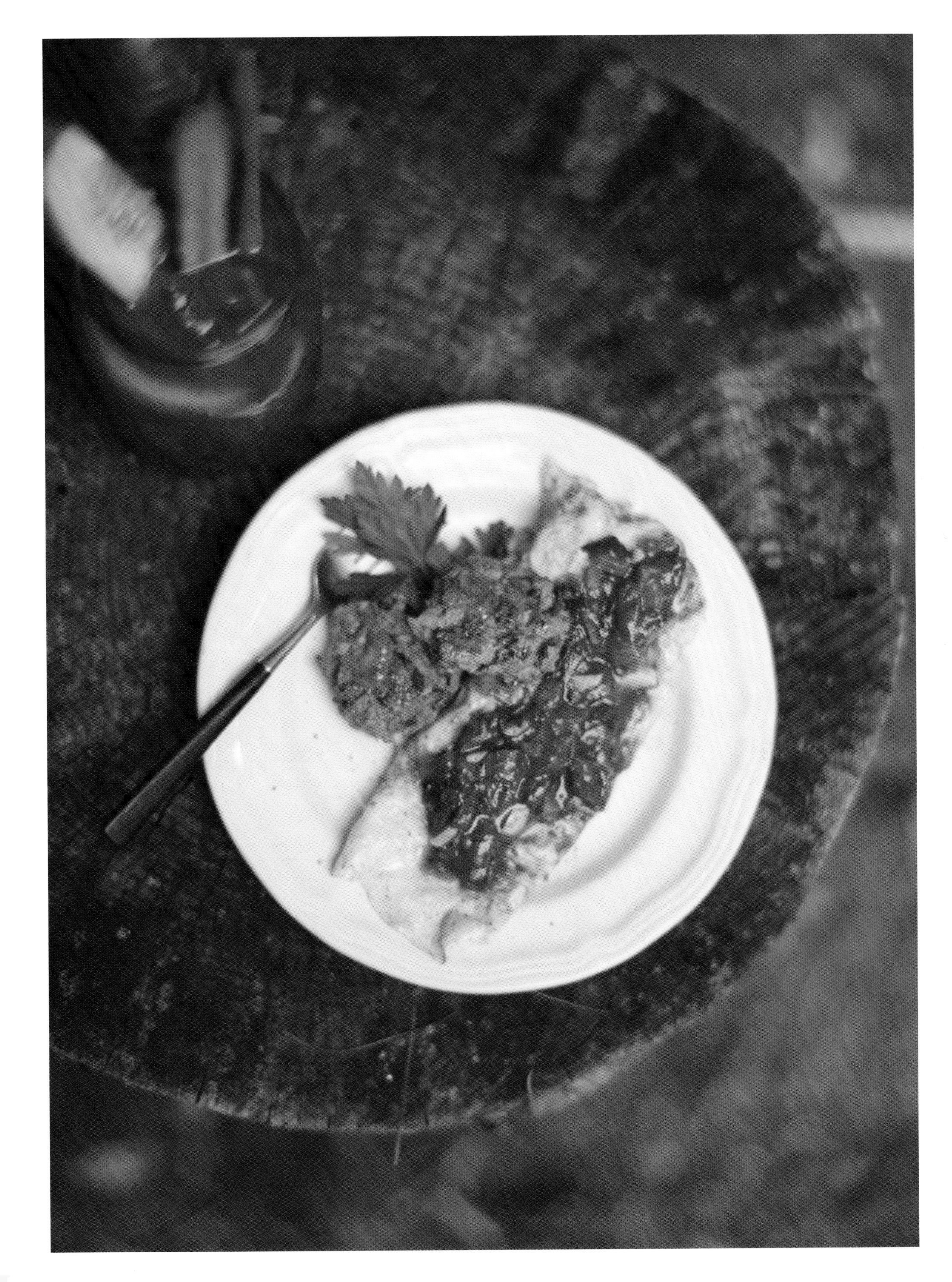

Grilled Cinnamon Steak

I often just season steak with salt and pepper, but sometimes I coat the meat in a dry rub, and I'm always happy when I do. The meat is tender, and the flavor is warm and slightly exotic. I made this steak for the Fourth of July and served it with Simple and Sweet Sugar Snap Peas (page 227) and Carrot Daikon Ribbon Salad (page 226), as shown. All of the dishes played off each other really nicely. Do yourself a favor and get a digital meat thermometer. You'll never regret it. While you can judge a perfectly done steak by look and feel, having a digital thermometer ensures that you'll remove the steak from the heat at just the right time. For rare steak, remove the meat at 125°F, medium-rare at 130°F, medium at 140°F, and medium-well at 155°F. The temperature will increase about 5°F as it rests off the grill.

Serves 4 to 6

For the cinnamon dry rub

- *1 tablespoon ground cinnamon*
- *1 tablespoon onion powder*
- *1 tablespoon garlic powder*
- *1 tablespoon dry mustard*
- *1 teaspoon Chinese five-spice powder*
- *1 teaspoon sea salt*
- *½ teaspoon ground black pepper*

- *2 pounds grass-fed steak, such as filet mignon, skirt steak, or rib eye, about 2 inches thick*

Whole30	Yes
Nut-free	Yes
Egg-free	Yes
AIP	No

1. Mix the dry rub spices together in a small bowl. Rub over both sides of the steak and allow to marinate in the refrigerator for at least 4 hours or overnight.

2. Heat a grill to medium heat (see page 362 for grilling tips). Remove the steak from the refrigerator to let it come to room temperature while the grill heats up.

3. Place the steak on the hot grill and cook for about 7 minutes. Then flip and cook for another 5 minutes for medium-rare to medium doneness, or until the temperature reaches between 130°F and 140°F (my preferred level of doneness). Cook for more or less time according to how you like your steaks.

4. Let the steak rest for 10 minutes before slicing and serving.

Shown with Carrot Daikon Ribbon Salad (page 226) and Simple and Sweet Sugar Snap Peas (page 227).

NOTES: *I recently discovered a cut called beef fillet tail that I really like—it's the tail end of the fillet. Lamb and pork—especially pulled pork or ribs—work really well with this rub, too.*

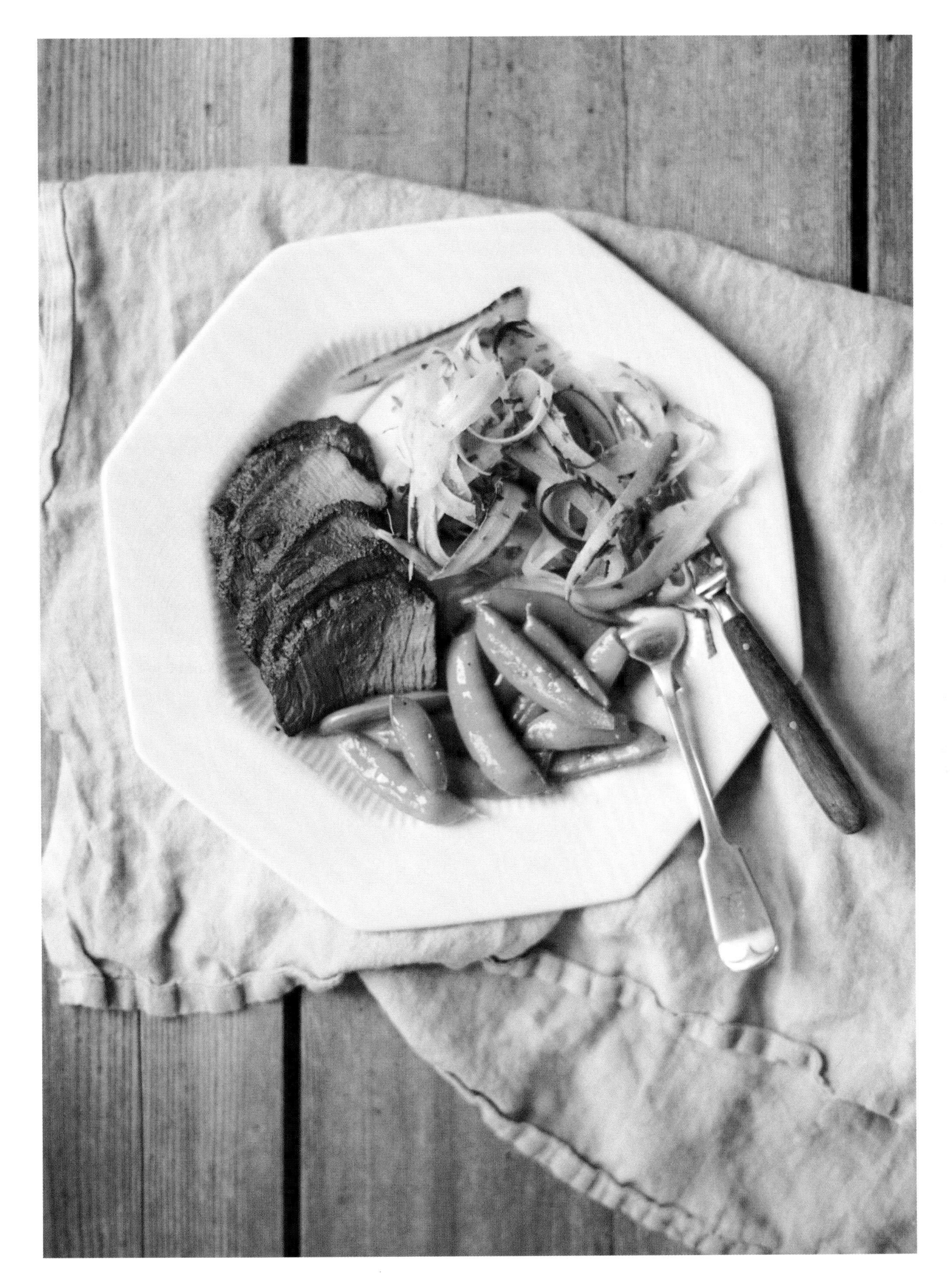

Carrot Daikon Ribbon Salad

This lovely and light salad is almost like a slaw. It's crisp and gingery, and it's fantastic alongside many different meats. Try it with Grilled Cinnamon Steak (page 224) or with any grilled meat on a hot summer evening. It's great the next day, too!

Serves 4

- *½ pound carrots*
- *1 daikon radish*
- *⅓ cup chopped fresh parsley leaves*
- *⅓ cup chopped fresh basil leaves*
- *1 teaspoon chopped fresh mint leaves*
- *1 teaspoon minced fresh ginger*
- *Juice of ½ lime*
- *¼ cup cold-pressed, extra-virgin olive oil*

NOTES: *Get the freshest and best-looking carrots you can for this dish. If you can't find daikon, grate some turnips or parsnips.*

Whole30	Yes
Nut-free	Yes
Egg-free	Yes
AIP	Yes

1. With a vegetable peeler, peel the carrots and daikon into ribbons. Toss together in a large bowl.
2. In a smaller bowl, combine the other ingredients and mix well.
3. Toss the carrots and daikon in the dressing, and serve.

See photo on page 225.

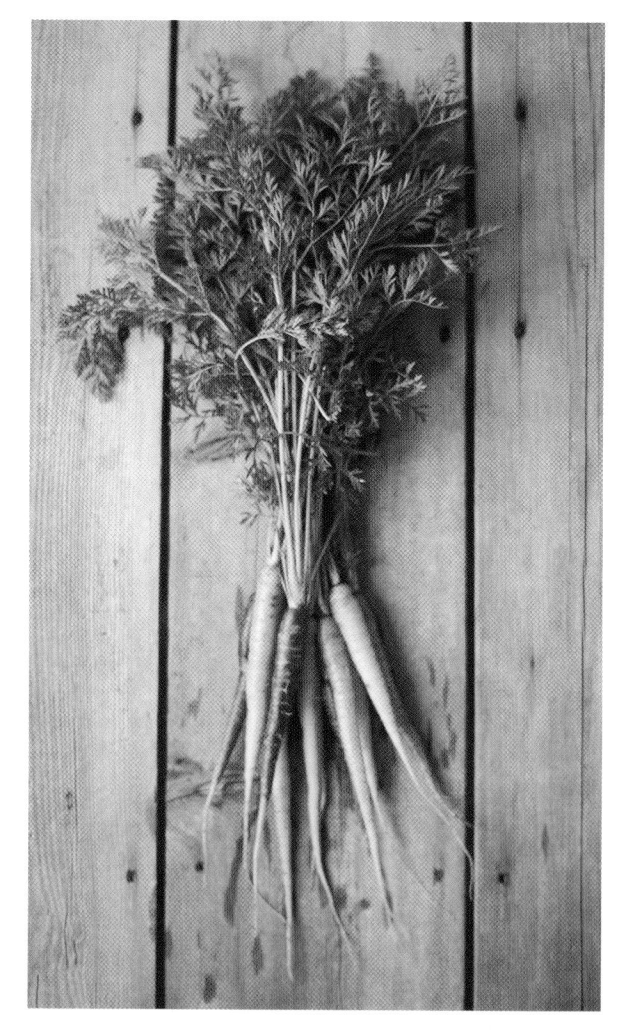

Simple and Sweet Sugar Snap Peas

This side dish is as easy as it gets. I like to serve it with grilled meat or seafood. Snap peas can be eaten raw, but if you cook them lightly, they're more easily digested, and I think the flavor really improves. They don't require much fuss to transform into one of my favorite vegetables. Pick bright green snap peas that are fresh, as opposed to eating them out of season. They're at their peak in New England in late June through early July.

Serves 6

- *1 pound sugar snap peas*
- *1 teaspoon cold-pressed, extra-virgin olive oil*
- *Sea salt and ground black pepper*

1. Snap the tops off the peas, removing the little string that runs down the pea.
2. Fill a medium saucepan with about 2 cups of water and bring to a boil.
3. Toss in the snap peas and boil for 2 to 3 minutes.
4. Drain the peas in a colander. Rinse with cold water for a minute until they are no longer hot.
5. Toss the peas with the olive oil and add salt and pepper to taste.

See photo on page 225.

NOTES: *Although snap peas are technically legumes and therefore not part of the Paleo diet, the protein portion of this vegetable is immature, so I don't really have an issue with snap or snow peas.*

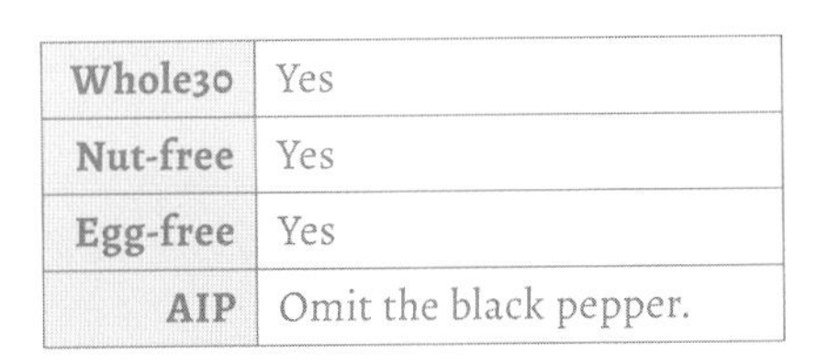

Whole30	Yes
Nut-free	Yes
Egg-free	Yes
AIP	Omit the black pepper.

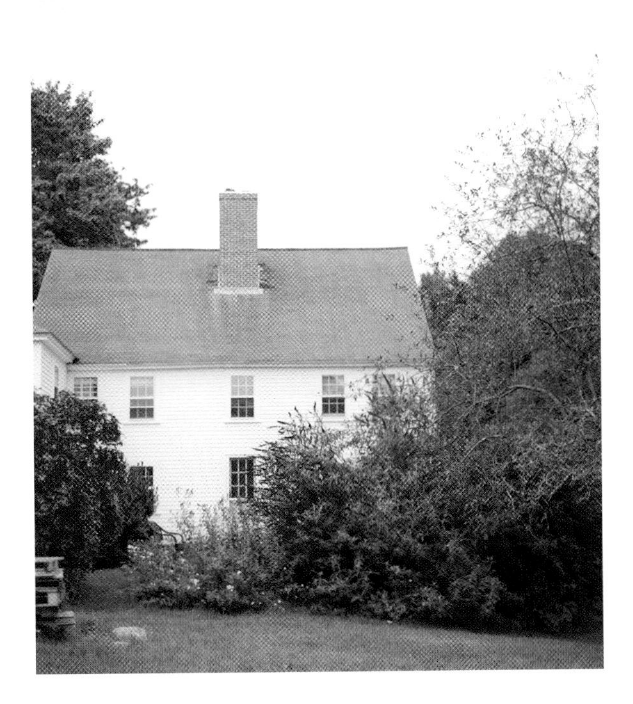

Light and Crispy Pan-Fried Fish with Lemony Basil Sauce

I used to love fried fish as a kid, and I really missed it when I realized that I couldn't eat gluten anymore—the gluten-free alternatives I found always left me feeling awful. This fish is very light, and my whole family devours it every time I make it! The lemon-basil mayonnaise is a great summery accompaniment. Not only does it go great with fried fish, but it's also a tasty dipping sauce for raw veggies or condiment for a lettuce wrap with your favorite meat. Yeah, it's that good! Try serving this fish with a side of Creamy Coleslaw with Fresh Dill (page 217).

Serves 4

For the sauce

- *1 cup homemade mayonnaise (page 344)*
- *1 cup loosely packed fresh basil leaves*
- *Juice of ½ lemon*
- *1 tablespoon Dijon mustard*
- *1 teaspoon sea salt*

For the fish

- *2 pounds firm white fish fillets, about 1 inch thick*
- *2 cups potato starch*
- *2 tablespoons onion powder*
- *2 teaspoons ground white pepper*
- *2 teaspoons sea salt*
- *2 eggs*
- *1½ cups canned, full-fat coconut milk*
- *½ cup bacon fat, lard, or coconut oil, for frying*

Whole30	No
Nut-free	Yes
Egg-free	No
AIP	No

1. Make the sauce: Combine all of the ingredients and blend with an immersion blender or in a food processor. You can also finely chop the basil and simply stir it into the sauce. Place the sauce in the fridge while you prepare the fish.

2. Cut the fish into strips about 2 inches long and ¾ to 1 inch wide. Set aside.

3. Combine the potato starch, onion powder, white pepper, and salt in a bowl, and mix well. Transfer to a plate so you can easily dip the fish in the mixture. Set aside.

4. In a shallow bowl, beat the eggs. Set aside.

5. Pour the coconut milk in another shallow bowl. Set aside.

6. Now you're ready to fry. In a deep sauté pan, heat the fat for frying over medium-high heat until it shimmers. Preheat the oven to 350°F, and line a rimmed baking sheet with parchment paper.

7. Working in batches, dip the fish strips in the coconut milk, then in the potato starch mixture, then in the eggs, and finally back in the potato starch mixture. Place the coated strips in the skillet, making sure not to overcrowd the pan, and fry for 2 minutes on each side, until golden brown.

8. When the fish is done, place it on the prepared baking sheet and place in the oven to finish cooking. Bake for about 8 minutes (depending on thickness).

9. Serve with the chilled sauce.

NOTES: *Try this recipe with swordfish, cod, halibut, or monkfish.*

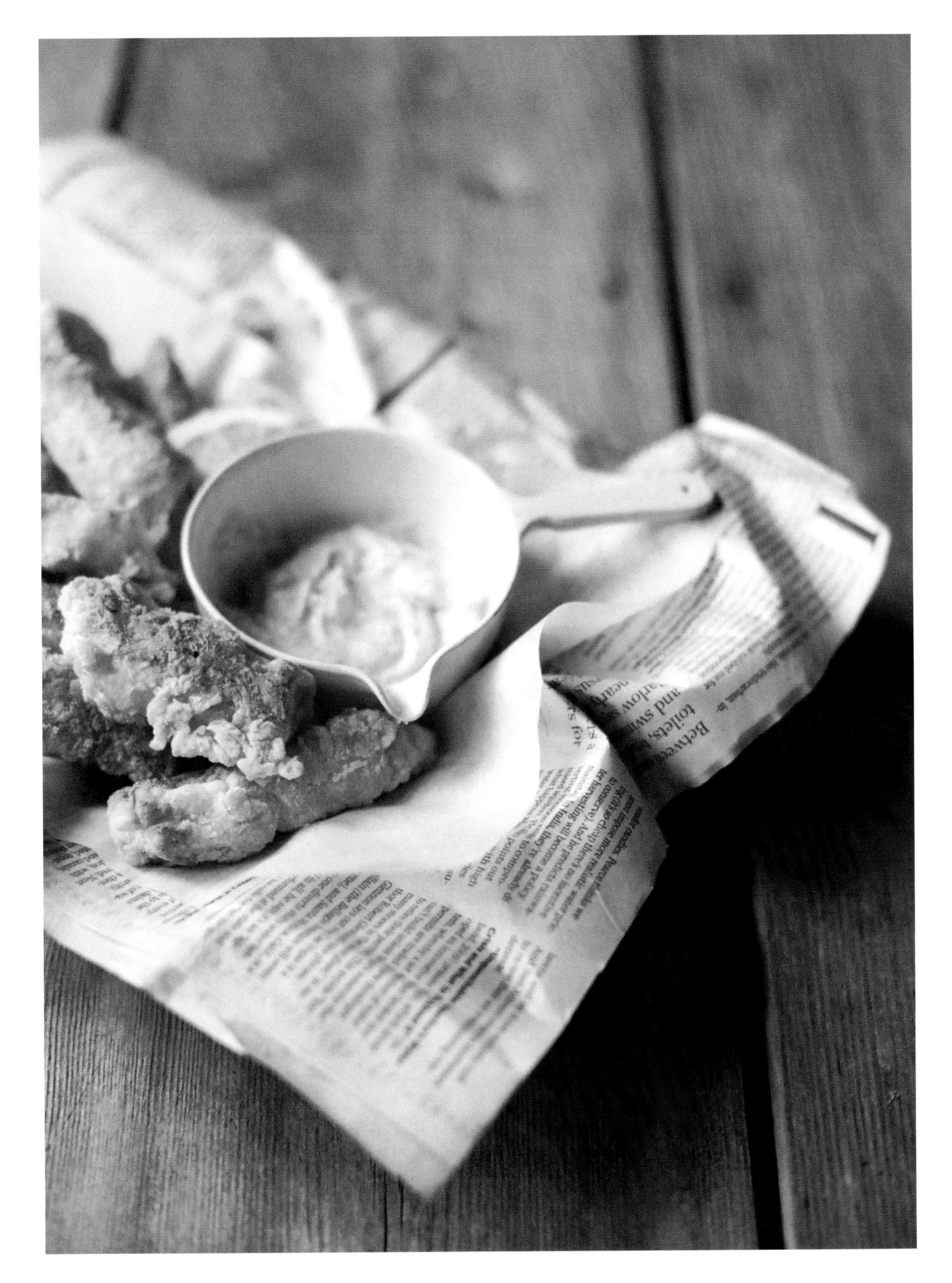

Deconstructed BLT Soup

I served this dish at BaconPalooza down in Virginia with my friend Kristin Canty, who directed the film *Farmageddon*. We needed a dish that was fast to make, delicious, and could showcase the incredible bacon from farmer Mark Baker's Mangalitsa pigs. It got rave reviews! Normally, I'm not a fan of gazpacho, which tends to be bitter and acidic. After lots of attempts to befriend gazpacho, I struck gold with this recipe. I use a lot more cucumber and black pepper than most recipes, which gives the soup a light, fresh, and spicy taste. Top it with some bacon and microgreens, and you've got a total winner!

Serves 4

- *8 large plum tomatoes*
- *1 cup roughly chopped red onion*
- *1 large clove garlic, chopped*
- *1 small jalapeño pepper, seeded and chopped*
- *⅓ cup loosely packed basil leaves*
- *2 cups peeled and roughly chopped cucumber (1 English cucumber)*
- *Juice of 1 lime*
- *2 teaspoons balsamic vinegar*
- *2 teaspoons Worcestershire sauce*
- *½ teaspoon sea salt*
- *¾ teaspoon ground black pepper*
- *4 strips bacon, diced and cooked until crispy*
- *Large handful of microgreens, washed*

1. Bring a large pot of water to a boil, and set up an ice water bath.
2. Score an X on the bottom of each tomato. Drop the tomatoes into the boiling water for 15 to 30 seconds, then move them to the ice bath.
3. In a blender, combine all of the ingredients except the bacon and microgreens and puree.
4. Pour into four bowls and top each bowl with bacon and microgreens. Serve cold.

NOTES: *If you would like to make this recipe when tomatoes are out of season, use a 28-ounce can of peeled whole tomatoes (or better yet, use 2 pints of your own canned tomatoes; see page 354).*

Whole30	Omit the Worcestershire sauce.
Nut-free	Yes
Egg-free	Yes
AIP	No

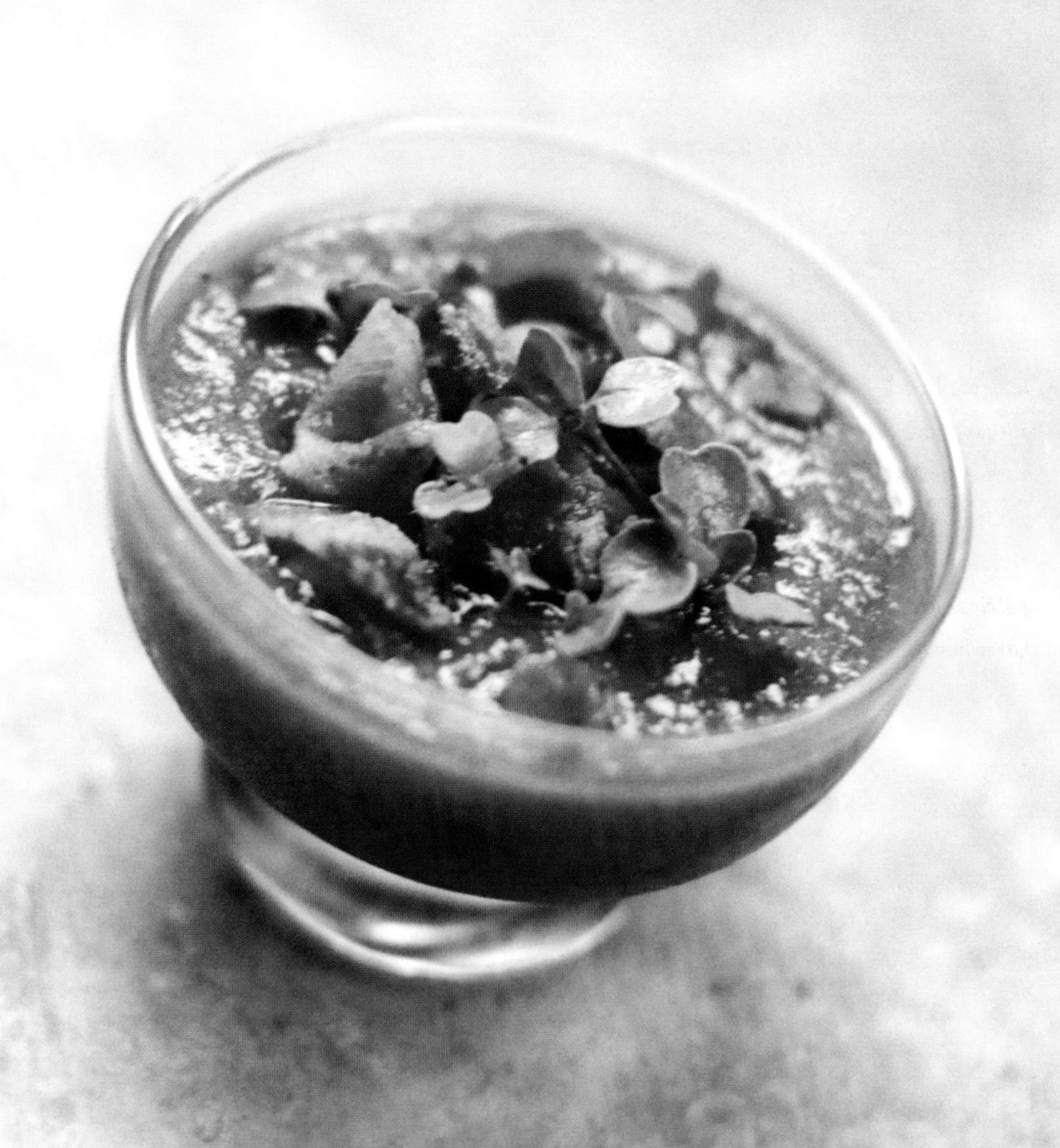

Spiced Okra

I first tried a version of this recipe down in Atlanta, Georgia, when I had dinner with my friends Julie and Charles Mayfield. It blew me away. If you don't think you like okra or are afraid of this odd-looking vegetable, please make these spicy little treats and you'll fall in love. The basic idea is to cover the okra with spices and roast them quickly in a hot oven. They aren't gummy at all, as can happen with okra in stew recipes. This dish makes a great side, or you can serve it as an appetizer before a summer meal.

Serves 6 as an appetizer, 3 as a side

- *1 pound okra*
- *⅓ cup ghee (page 347) or bacon fat, melted*
- *1 tablespoon ground cumin*
- *1 teaspoon onion powder*
- *½ teaspoon ground white pepper*
- *¼ teaspoon smoked hot paprika*
- *¼ teaspoon sea salt*

1. Preheat the oven to 400°F. Line a rimmed baking sheet with parchment paper.
2. Place the okra in a large bowl. Drizzle with the ghee.
3. Combine the spices and salt in a small bowl and mix well with your hands. Sprinkle the spice mixture over the okra.
4. Lay the okra on the prepared baking sheet and place in the oven. Bake for 5 minutes, flip them, and continue baking another 5 minutes. Serve warm or at room temperature.

NOTES: *Small okra, about the size of your pinky finger, is best for this recipe.*

Whole30	Yes
Nut-free	Yes
Egg-free	Yes
AIP	Omit the cumin, white pepper, and paprika. Use bacon fat instead of ghee.

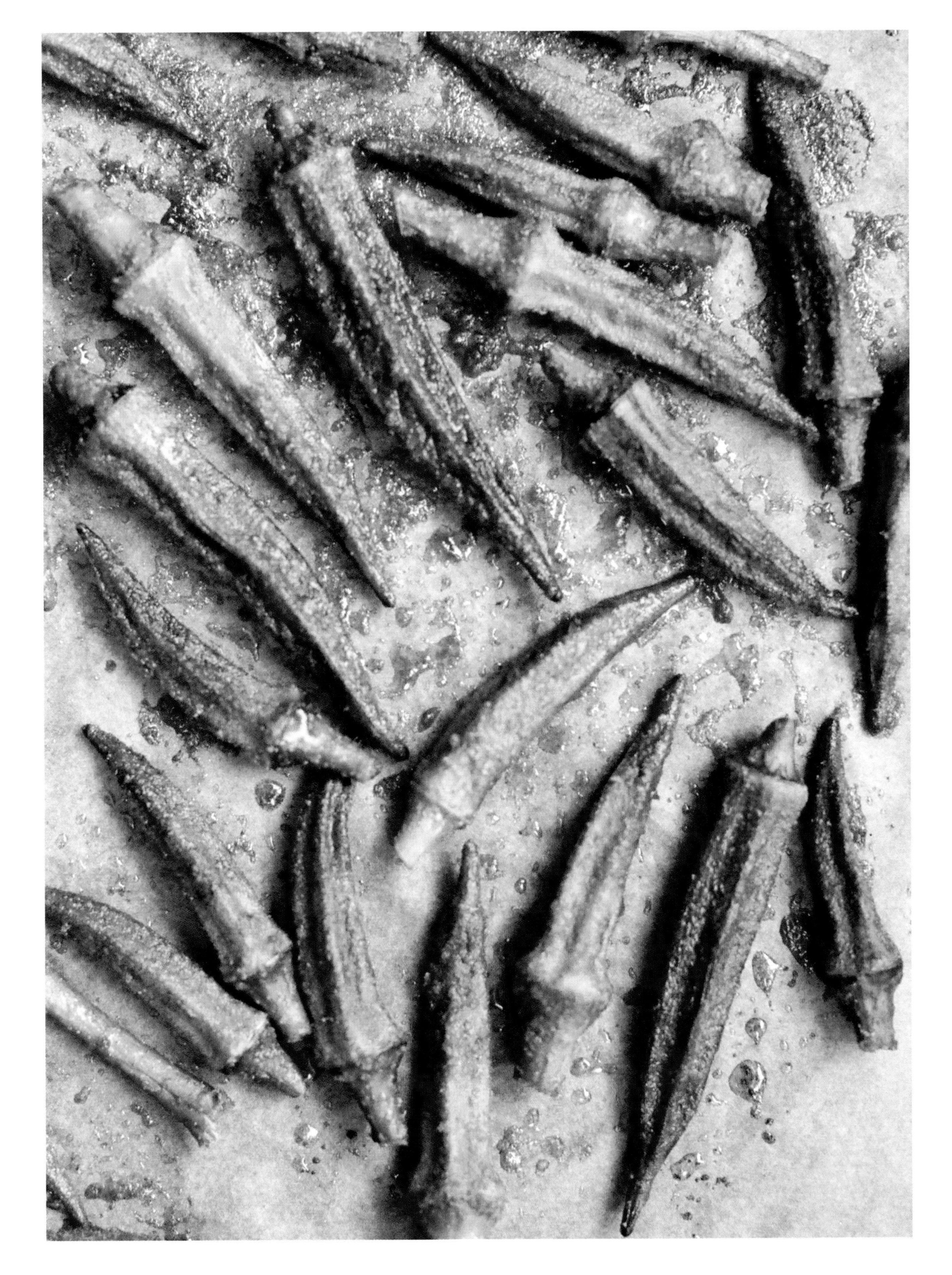

Vietnamese Beef Salad with Peaches and Herbs

After having this salad at my friend's house, I asked her for the recipe and then proceeded to make it three times for dinner that same week. I was obsessed with the dressing on the grilled beef, which is so good I could drink it from a glass. It's easy enough to make on a weeknight, yet show-stopping enough to serve to guests, and I guarantee that they will be asking you for the recipe, too. It's a perfect summer meal on one plate.

Serves 6

- *2 pounds flank steak*
- *Sea salt and ground black pepper*
- *2 peaches, sliced into wedges (not peeled)*
- *Juice of 2 limes*
- *¼ cup fish sauce*
- *1 jalapeño pepper, minced*
- *1 tablespoon honey*
- *3 cloves garlic, minced*
- *½ cup minced fresh cilantro leaves*
- *10 cups chopped mixed lettuce, such as romaine and red leaf*
- *1 cup chopped fresh mint leaves*
- *1 cup chopped fresh basil leaves*
- *1 cucumber, peeled, seeded, and sliced*
- *⅔ cup roasted, unsalted cashews*
- *2 shallots, sliced thin*

1. Bring the steak to room temperature and season on both sides with salt and pepper.
2. Heat a grill to medium-high heat (see page 362 for grilling tips). Grill the steak for 10 to 15 minutes or until medium-rare, flipping it two-thirds of the way through the cooking process.
3. When the steak is almost done, grill the peach wedges for about 2 minutes on each side. Watch them carefully, as they can burn easily if the grill is too hot.
4. Set the finished steak and peaches on separate plates while you make the dressing.
5. Make the dressing: Combine the lime juice, fish sauce, jalapeño, honey, garlic, and cilantro in a large bowl.
6. After the steak has rested for at least 5 minutes, cut it in half down the middle (with the grain), then slice the meat crosswise and at an angle into ¼-inch-thick strips. Place the strips in the bowl with the dressing.
7. To arrange the salad, place the lettuce, mint, basil, and cucumber on a large serving tray.
8. Remove the steak from the dressing and pour about half of the dressing over the salad fixings.
9. Top the salad fixings with the sliced steak and peaches and sprinkle with the cashews and shallots.

NOTES: *Feel free to substitute steak tips for the flank steak and the nuts of your choice for the cashews.*

Whole30	Omit the honey.
Nut-free	Omit the cashews.
Egg-free	Yes
AIP	Omit the black pepper, jalapeño, and cashews.

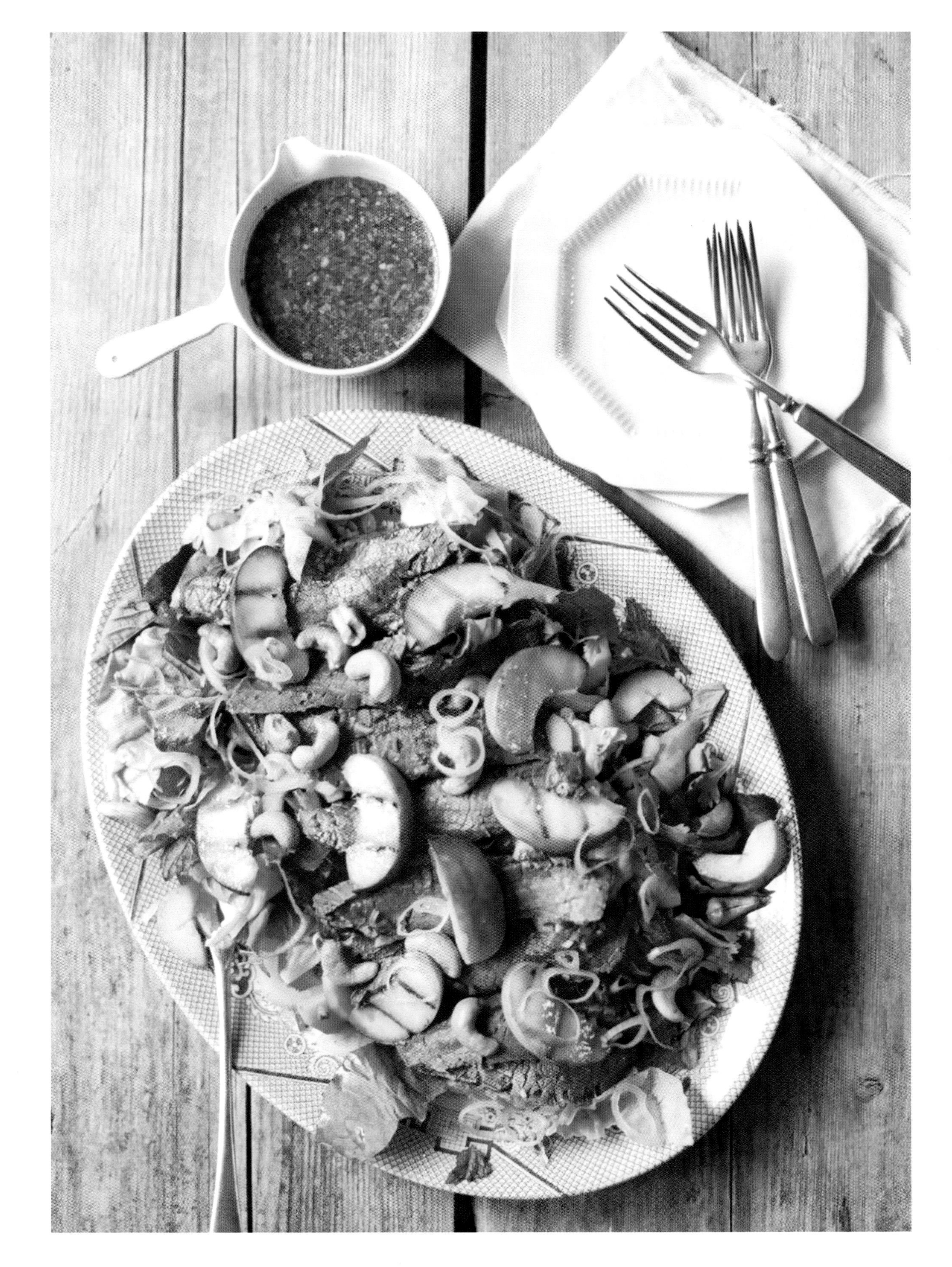

Steamed Lobsters

Lobster was once considered "poor man's food," but I also remember when it was so expensive that it was a special-occasion food. These days, at least in New England, you can get lobster at a pretty reasonable price. In my family, we always have at least one summer lobster dinner, and we also celebrate New Year's Day with lobster. Steaming lobster is my favorite way to prepare it at home. Take a deep breath; it's not as hard as you think!

Serves 4

- *4 lobsters, 1 to 2 pounds each (leave the rubber bands on for cooking)*
- *2 lemons, quartered*
- *¼ cup unsalted butter (page 348), melted, for dipping*

1. Fill a large stockpot about one-quarter full with water. Bring the water to a boil over high heat.

2. Once the water is boiling, add the lobsters and quickly cover the pot. It will take about 12 minutes to cook a 1- to 1¼-pound lobster, about 13 minutes for a 1½- to 2-pound lobster.

3. The shells will turn bright red when the lobsters are done. Place them on a serving tray and remove the rubber bands. It's nice to crack the claws for your guests.

4. Place the lemon quarters and melted butter on the table for folks to dip the meat in.

5. To eat, twist off the claws and crack them open using a nutcracker. The knuckle meat can be accessed with kitchen shears. You will probably have to get in there with your hands and do a little digging as well, which is part of the fun. The tiny little legs are fun to suck on, and there's a little meat in there, too. Pull off the tail and rinse the exposed meat under water to get rid of the "green stuff" from the cavity of the lobster. With a knife, cut down the middle of the underside of the shell and remove the meat. It's also helpful to remove the central little flipper at the end of the tail and push out the meat from that end.

6. Save the shells for compost or stock (see page 342). Chickens really enjoy picking at the leftovers, and there's some great nutrients for them in the shells.

Whole30	Use melted ghee instead of butter for dipping.
Nut-free	Yes
Egg-free	Yes
AIP	Omit the butter.

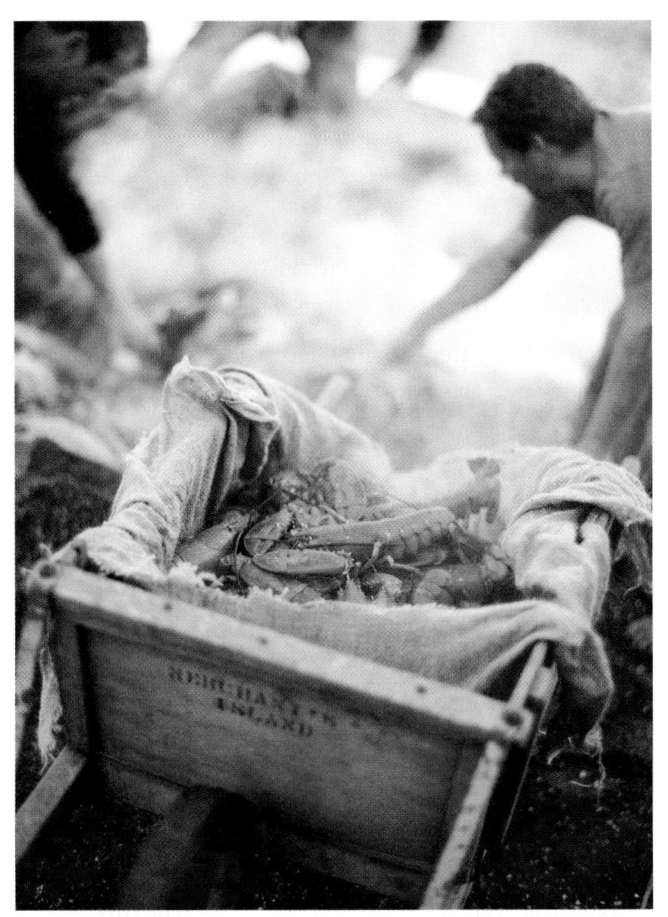

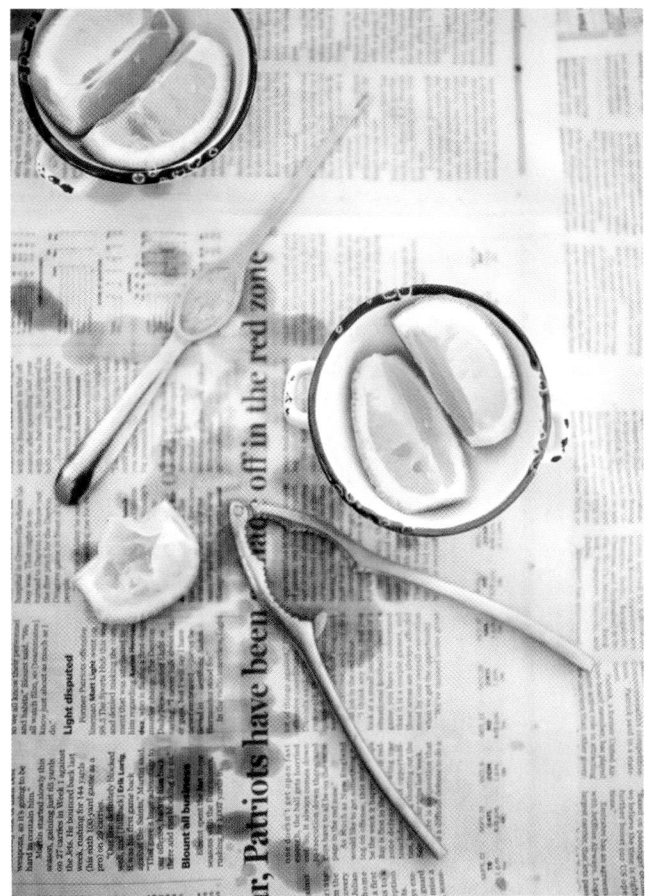
Patriots have been
off in the red zone
Light disputed
Blount all business

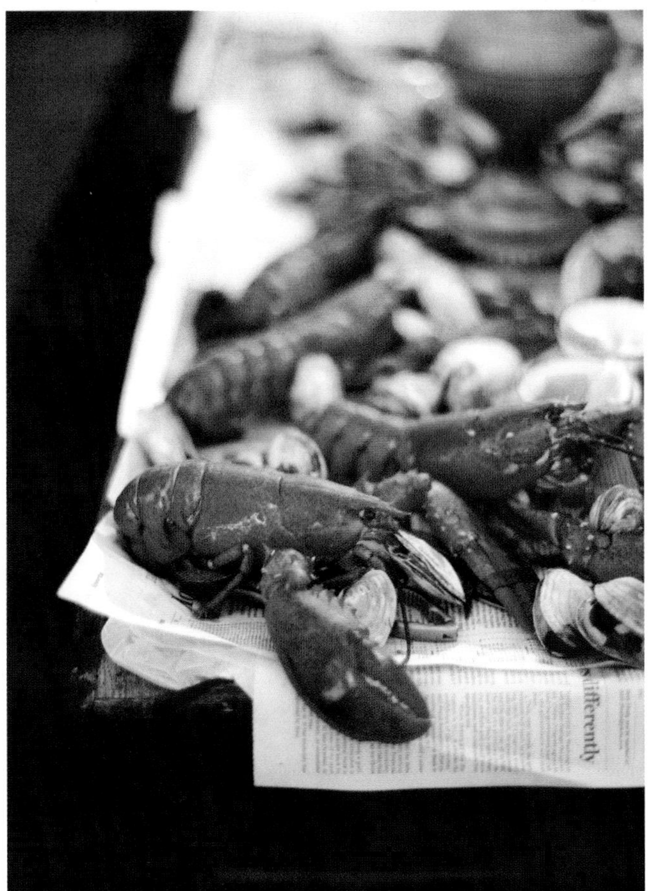
differently

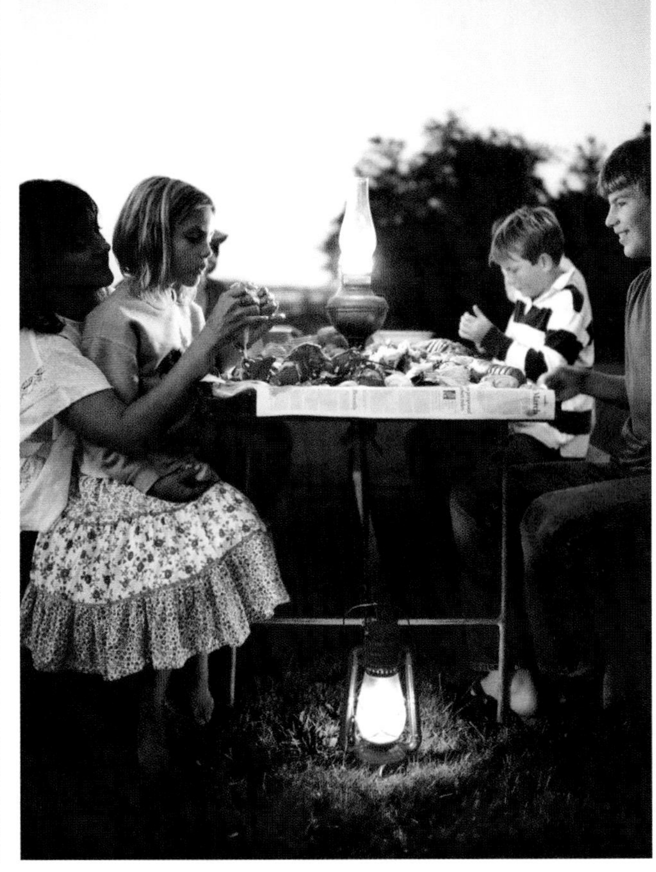

Steamed Clams

I realize that not everyone has access to the beach for a clambake (page 380), so here is the kitchen version.

Serves 4

- *2 pounds steamer clams*
- *¼ cup unsalted butter (page 348), melted, for dipping*

1. Place a steamer basket in a tall pot with 1 inch of water in the bottom. Bring the water to a boil.

2. Examine the clams to determine which are still alive. If any are open and nonresponsive (for example, if they don't snap shut when you touch their shells), toss them out, as they are dead and could make you sick if you eat them.

3. Place the clams in the boiling steam bath, cover, and steam for about 5 to 7 minutes. They're ready when the clams are mostly open. Remove from the heat and discard any clams that did not open. Do not discard the broth.

4. To serve, distribute the steamed clams among four bowls. Serve with the melted butter and clam broth, and provide a bowl for the empty shells.

5. To eat, pull a clam out of its shell by its "foot" (the siphon). Using your fingers, remove the skin covering the foot of the clam. Using the foot as a handle, first dip the clam in the broth—this "initial dip" will help to rinse off any sand that still might be on the clams. Then dip it in the melted butter, then pop it into your mouth. This is a messy process but oh so worth it.

6. The leftover shells are fantastic for getting a little extra calcium into your backyard hens or as a soil amendment in your compost. Don't throw them out!

NOTES: *Instead of steamer clams, you can use another type of small clam or even mussels (with beards removed).*

Whole30	Use melted ghee instead of butter for dipping.
Nut-free	Yes
Egg-free	Yes
AIP	Omit the butter.

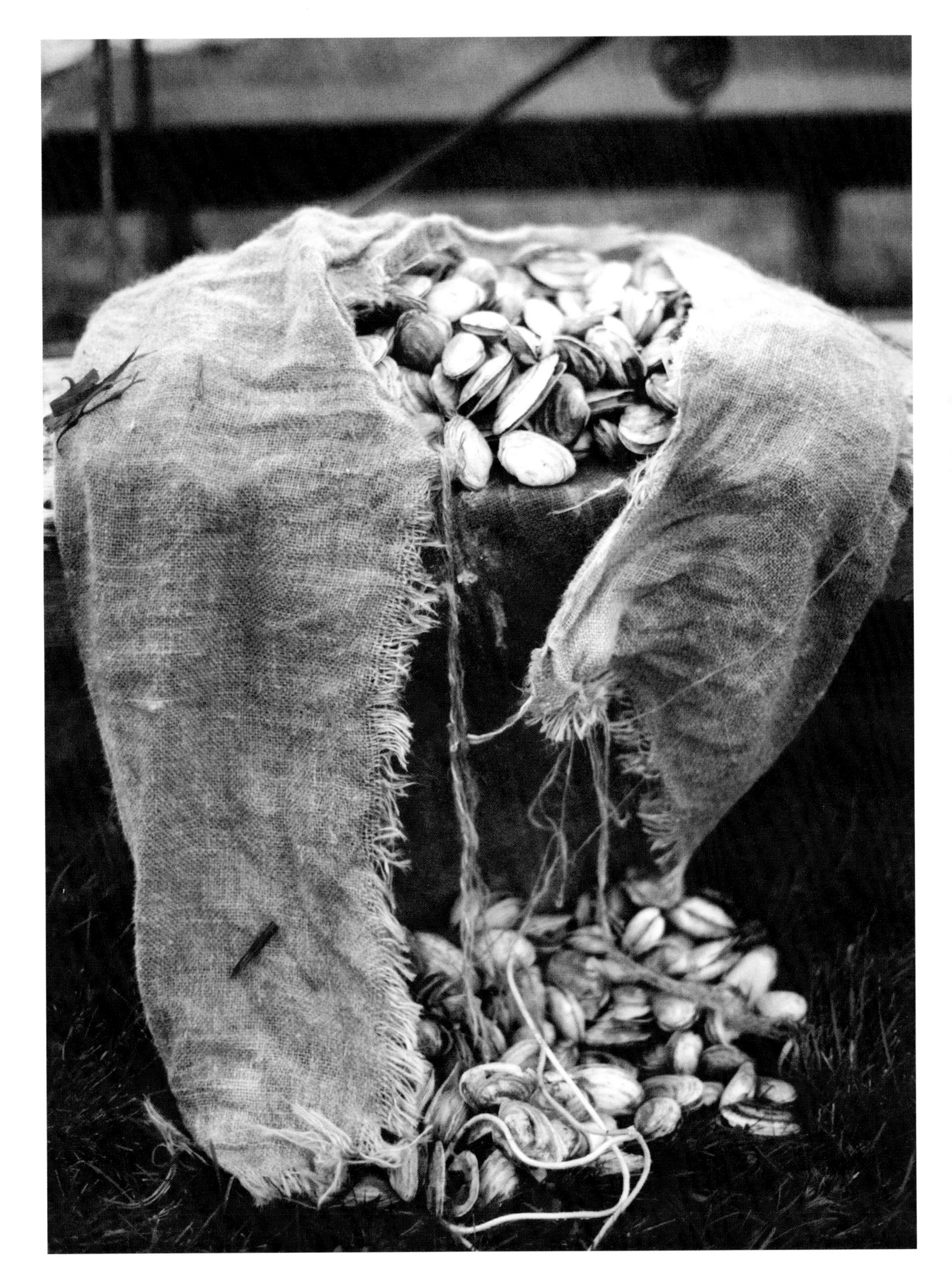

Provençal Seafood Chowder with Fennel and Tarragon

For one of our clambakes, I wanted to make a chowder that was a little more upscale than a typical clam chowder. This lighter blend of fresh fish and scallops with aromatic fennel and generous amounts of tarragon was a huge hit with all of our guests, and it's certainly a new favorite of mine. I guarantee you'll love it! I've tried it both with and without the cream added at the end, and it's fantastic either way. Serve with Bacon Chive Biscuits (page 242).

Serves 6

- *1 pound sea scallops*
- *½ pound bacon, diced*
- *1 large yellow onion, diced*
- *2 stalks celery, diced*
- *2 bulbs fennel, diced*
- *Pinch of cayenne pepper*
- *2 cups diced tomatoes, with juices*
- *2 quarts homemade fish stock (page 342)*
- *1½ pounds firm white fish fillets, such as striped bass or cod, cut into bite-sized pieces*
- *⅓ cup heavy cream or coconut cream (optional)*
- *Sea salt and ground black pepper*
- *3 tablespoons chopped fresh tarragon leaves, for garnish*
- *3 tablespoons chopped fresh chives, for garnish*

1. Remove and discard the small side muscle, called the "foot," from each scallop. Cut the scallops into quarters. Set aside.
2. In a large soup pot, brown the bacon over medium heat.
3. Add the onion, celery, fennel, and cayenne pepper and sauté for 10 minutes.
4. Add the tomatoes and fish stock and bring to a simmer over medium-low heat. Continue to simmer for 30 minutes.
5. Add the fish and scallops and continue cooking for 5 to 10 minutes, just until the fish is cooked through.
6. Turn off the heat and add the cream, if you wish.
7. Season to taste with salt and pepper.
8. Serve in bowls and garnish with the fresh tarragon and chives.

Shown with Bacon Chive Biscuits (page 242).

NOTES: *Not a seafood fan? Use roasted chicken instead of the scallops and fish and chicken stock (page 338) instead of the fish stock.*

Whole30	Use coconut cream or coconut milk instead of heavy cream.
Nut-free	Yes
Egg-free	Yes
AIP	Omit the cayenne pepper, tomatoes, and black pepper, and use coconut cream or coconut milk instead of heavy cream.

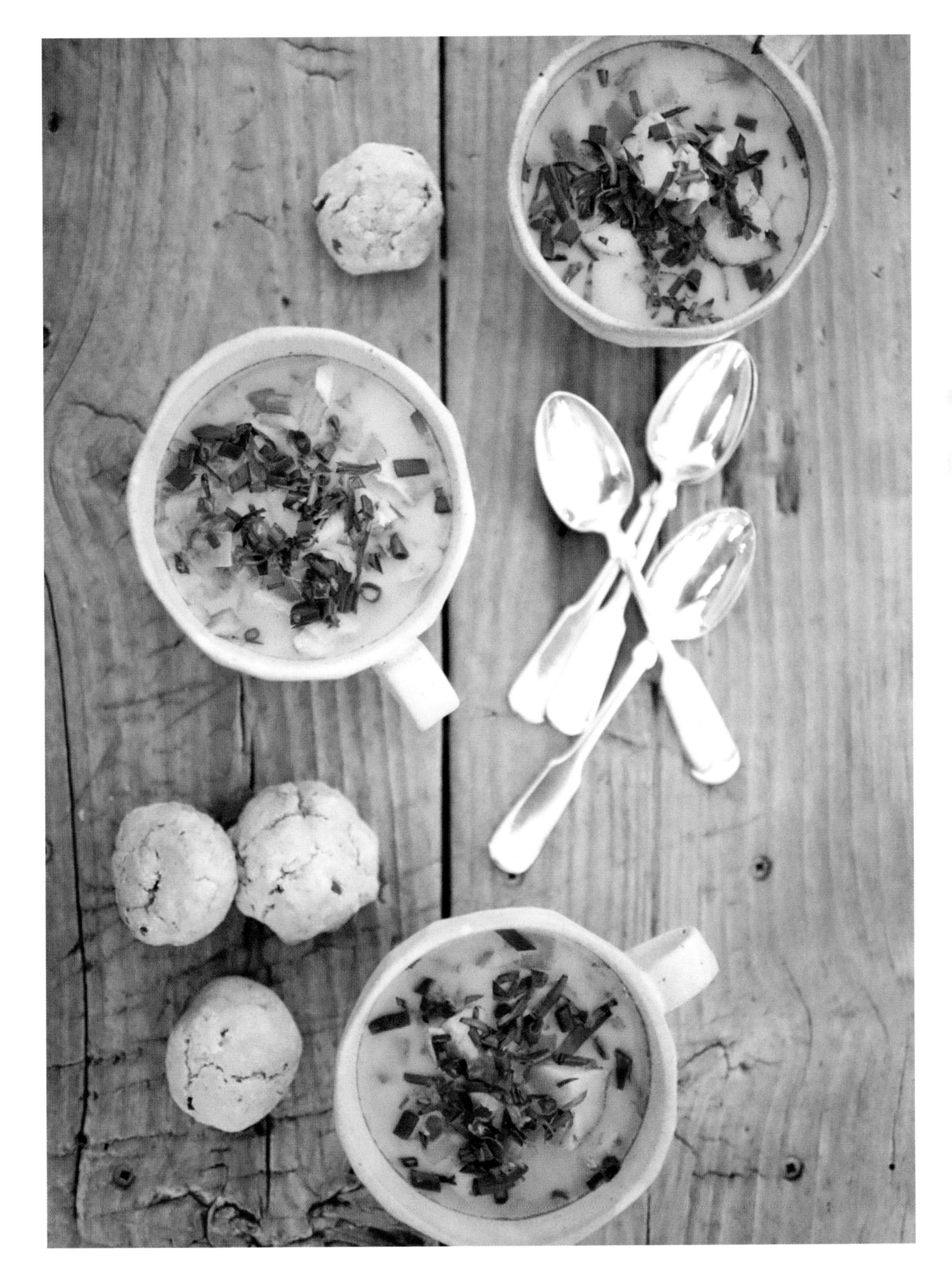

Bacon Chive Biscuits

These biscuits are the perfect accompaniment to any soup or stew. When I started eating gluten-free, I became a huge fan of Chebe Bread, a tapioca-based baking mix to which you add tons of cheese. You can get these little cheese rolls at Brazilian restaurants, too. I tried making these with just tapioca and they didn't quite work, but with the other flours mixed in, they're perfect!

Makes about 18 golf ball–sized biscuits

- *½ cup ghee (page 347), melted*
- *2 eggs*
- *¼ cup water*
- *1 tablespoon lemon juice*
- *2 cups tapioca starch*
- *⅓ cup potato flour*
- *¼ cup coconut flour*
- *½ teaspoon baking powder*
- *½ teaspoon sea salt*
- *1 teaspoon cream of tartar*
- *½ cup crumbled, cooked bacon (about 5 strips bacon)*
- *2 tablespoons minced fresh chives*

1. Preheat the oven to 350°F. Line a baking sheet with parchment paper.
2. Combine the ghee, eggs, water, and lemon juice in a small bowl.
3. In a large bowl, whisk the tapioca starch, flours, baking powder, salt, cream of tartar, bacon crumbles, and chives until blended.
4. Add the wet ingredients to the dry ingredients and mix until incorporated.
5. Using your hands, form the dough into golf ball–sized balls and place them on the lined baking sheet, 2 inches apart.
6. Bake for about 18 minutes, until light brown. They'll be a bit gooey inside because of the tapioca starch, but that's normal.

See photo on page 241.

NOTES: *For a twist on this recipe, replace the chives with other herbs, like fresh rosemary.*

Whole30	No
Nut-free	Yes
Egg-free	No
AIP	No

Purslane Potato Salad with Bacon and Shallots

Purslane is a weed that is found all over the globe. In fact, it's the eighth most distributed plant in the world. It looks like a succulent, with its small, thick leaves. It doesn't have a strong taste and can be substituted for parsley or spinach in most recipes. It has more omega-3s than any other vegetable, and it's free! You can find it growing in your garden or at a local organic farm. Just ask the farmer if you can harvest some purslane, and they'll be thrilled to let you have as much as you like—I guarantee it! For more on purslane and other wild edibles, see page 141.

Serves 6

- *¾ pound bacon*
- *2 pounds red potatoes, peeled and diced*
- *⅔ cup minced fresh parsley leaves*
- *⅓ cup cold-pressed, extra-virgin olive oil*
- *⅓ cup lemon juice*
- *1 large or 2 small shallots, sliced thin*
- *½ cup purslane leaves (from a very large bunch)*
- *Sea salt and ground black pepper to taste*

1. Preheat the oven to 350°F. Line a rimmed baking sheet with parchment paper.

2. Lay out the bacon on the prepared baking sheet. Bake the bacon for about 20 minutes, or until done. Drain the bacon on a towel-lined plate. Set aside.

3. While the bacon is baking, cook the potatoes: Fill a large pot halfway with water and bring it to a boil. Add the potatoes to the boiling water. Cook for 15 minutes, or until a fork can be easily inserted into the potatoes, then drain them.

4. Crumble the cooked bacon and place it in a large bowl. Add the potatoes and the rest of the ingredients to the bowl and mix well. Serve lukewarm or cold.

See photo on page 245.

NOTES: *If you can't find purslane, use more parsley. You can also substitute sweet potatoes for the red potatoes.*

Whole30	Yes
Nut-free	Yes
Egg-free	Yes
AIP	Substitute sweet potatoes for the red potatoes. Omit the black pepper.

Grilled Chicken with Raspberry-Chipotle Glaze

Raspberry season marks the height of summer to me. Instead of baking sweet desserts, I like to incorporate fruit into meat dishes. This fantastic glaze is smoky and sweet at the same time, and if you didn't know what's on the chicken, it would be difficult to put your finger on exactly which ingredients are working here to make it taste so great. Serve with a green salad, sliced watermelon, and a potato salad, like my Purslane Potato Salad with Bacon and Shallot (page 243). The chicken can be served hot or cold for a refreshing mid-summer dinner. The glaze also works well on roasted pork.

Serves 6

For the chicken

- *2 tablespoons ground cumin*
- *1 teaspoon ground white pepper*
- *2 teaspoons onion powder*
- *1 teaspoon sea salt*
- *3 to 4 pounds bone-in chicken parts*

For the sauce

- *3 cups fresh raspberries*
- *3 tablespoons chipotle peppers in adobo sauce, minced*
- *½ cup unsalted butter (page 348)*
- *Juice of 1 lime*

Whole30	Use ghee instead of butter for the sauce.
Nut-free	Yes
Egg-free	Yes
AIP	No

1. Heat a grill to a medium-low heat (see page 362 for grilling tips).

2. In a small bowl, combine the spices and salt. Coat the chicken pieces with the spice blend.

3. Grill the chicken skin side down for 10 to 15 minutes (making sure that the skin does not burn), then flip and continue cooking until the chicken reaches 165°F, about 10 to 15 minutes. When done, remove the chicken to a platter and allow to rest.

4. While the chicken is grilling, make the sauce: Combine the raspberries, chipotle peppers, butter, and lime juice in a saucepan and bring to a simmer over medium heat. Allow the mixture to gently bubble for about 10 minutes, stirring to break up the raspberries.

5. Strain the sauce with a fine-mesh sieve over a medium-sized bowl, using a spoon to press the sauce through the sieve.

6. Serve the sauce warm or cold with the chicken.

Shown with Purslane Potato Salad with Bacon and Shallots (page 243).

NOTES: *You can also use another berry, like blackberries or pitted cherries, in place of the raspberries.*

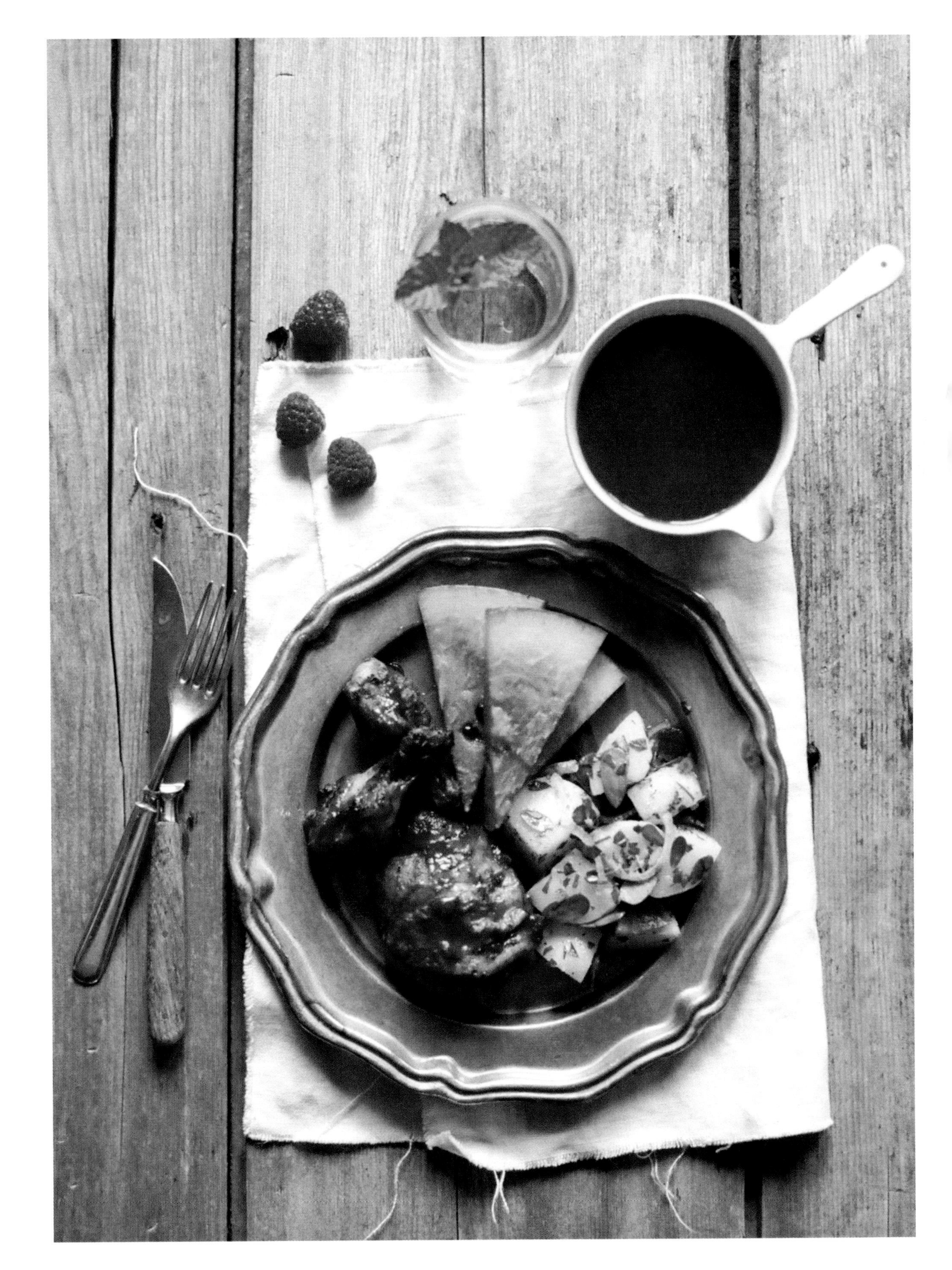

Summer Garden Salad with Seaweed and Lemon-Ginger Dressing

It's a good idea to incorporate some seaweed into your diet on a regular basis when you're eating Paleo. Industrial table salt is fortified with iodine, but if you've switched to natural sea salt (which I hope you have!), you may not be getting as much iodine as you need, which can affect thyroid health. Seaweed is a great, natural way to get more iodine. But did you know that the bright green seaweed salad found at most Asian restaurants is full of chemical dyes and corn syrup? Make this salad at home instead. The simple lemon dressing lets the fresh vegetables and lettuce shine through without weighing them down. Look for dried seaweed in the Japanese section of a better grocery store.

Serves 8

- *1 large head green lettuce, torn into small pieces*
- *1 head radicchio, torn into small pieces*
- *2 carrots, peeled and grated or shaved with a peeler*
- *1 small beet, peeled and grated*
- *1 small kohlrabi, peeled and grated*
- *3 radishes, sliced very thin*
- *¼ cup thinly sliced red onion*

For the Dressing

- *Juice of 1 lemon*
- *⅓ cup cold-pressed, extra-virgin olive oil*
- *⅛ teaspoon grated fresh ginger*
- *½ teaspoon sea salt*
- *⅛ teaspoon ground black pepper*

- *1 tablespoon untoasted, cold-pressed sesame oil*
- *½ cup shredded nori seaweed*

1. In a large bowl, mix the green lettuce with the radicchio.
2. Top with the carrots, beet, kohlrabi, radishes, and onion.
3. In a small bowl, combine the lemon juice, olive oil, and ginger with the salt and pepper. Mix well.
4. Just before serving, toss the salad with the dressing.
5. Drizzle with the sesame oil and sprinkle the top with the seaweed.

NOTES: *I also love to top this salad with arame seaweed. Before using it, soak it in warm water for 15 minutes, then drain it well. You can also get frozen kelp strips from Ocean Approved to top your salad.*

Whole30	Yes
Nut-free	Yes
Egg-free	Yes
AIP	Omit the black pepper and sesame oil.

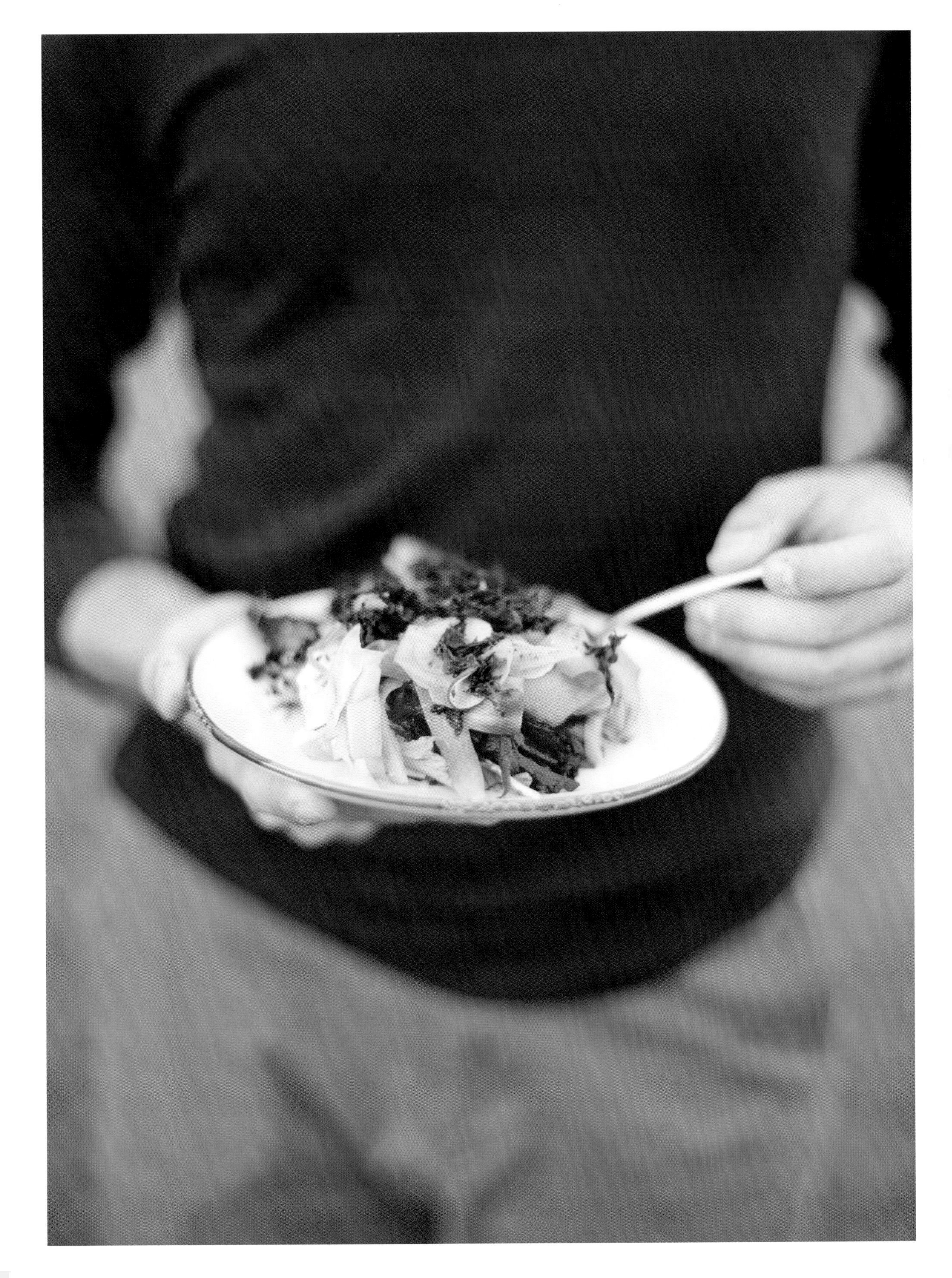

Red Curry Mussels with Ginger and Cilantro

I love collecting mussels. If you collect them yourself, go for the ones that spend the majority of their time in the water, as opposed to the ones farther up on the beach, which are exposed to air most of the time. Also, the more barnacles on the mussels, the less healthy they are. They can have some, but they should not be completely covered in barnacles. Mussels are very nutrient-dense and contain lots of minerals not commonly found in other foods. Plus, they taste great. My whole family loves them. If they're local to you, bivalves are among the most sustainable foods you can consume. I used to steam them open with just some stock and garlic until I tinkered around with this winning recipe. This broth is also fantastic as a soup base for any combination of vegetables and meat.

Serves 2 as a main dish, 4 to 6 as an appetizer

- *1 pound mussels*
- *1 cup homemade fish stock (page 342) or chicken stock (page 338)*
- *1 cup canned, full-fat coconut milk*
- *2 teaspoons Thai red curry paste*
- *1 teaspoon Sriracha (all-natural), or more, according to taste*
- *2 teaspoons minced fresh ginger*
- *1 tablespoon coconut aminos or wheat-free tamari*
- *1 tablespoon minced fresh cilantro leaves, for garnish*

1. Rinse the mussels under cool water and remove the beards, if any. Set aside.

2. In a large pot, combine the stock, coconut milk, curry paste, Sriracha, ginger, and coconut aminos and bring to a simmer over medium heat, stirring to mix well.

3. Once the mixture is simmering, add the mussels and cover the pot. Cook for 5 minutes, or until all of the shells open. You may have a few that don't open; this means they're dead and should be tossed out.

4. Transfer the mussels to a platter or individual shallow bowls and ladle some of the cooking liquid over the top. Garnish with the cilantro.

5. When you're done, compost the shells or feed them to your chickens—they love picking at the shells!

NOTES: *This light and delicious sauce is also incredible with cooked vegetables or meat.*

Whole30	Omit the Sriracha.
Nut-free	Yes
Egg-free	Yes
AIP	No

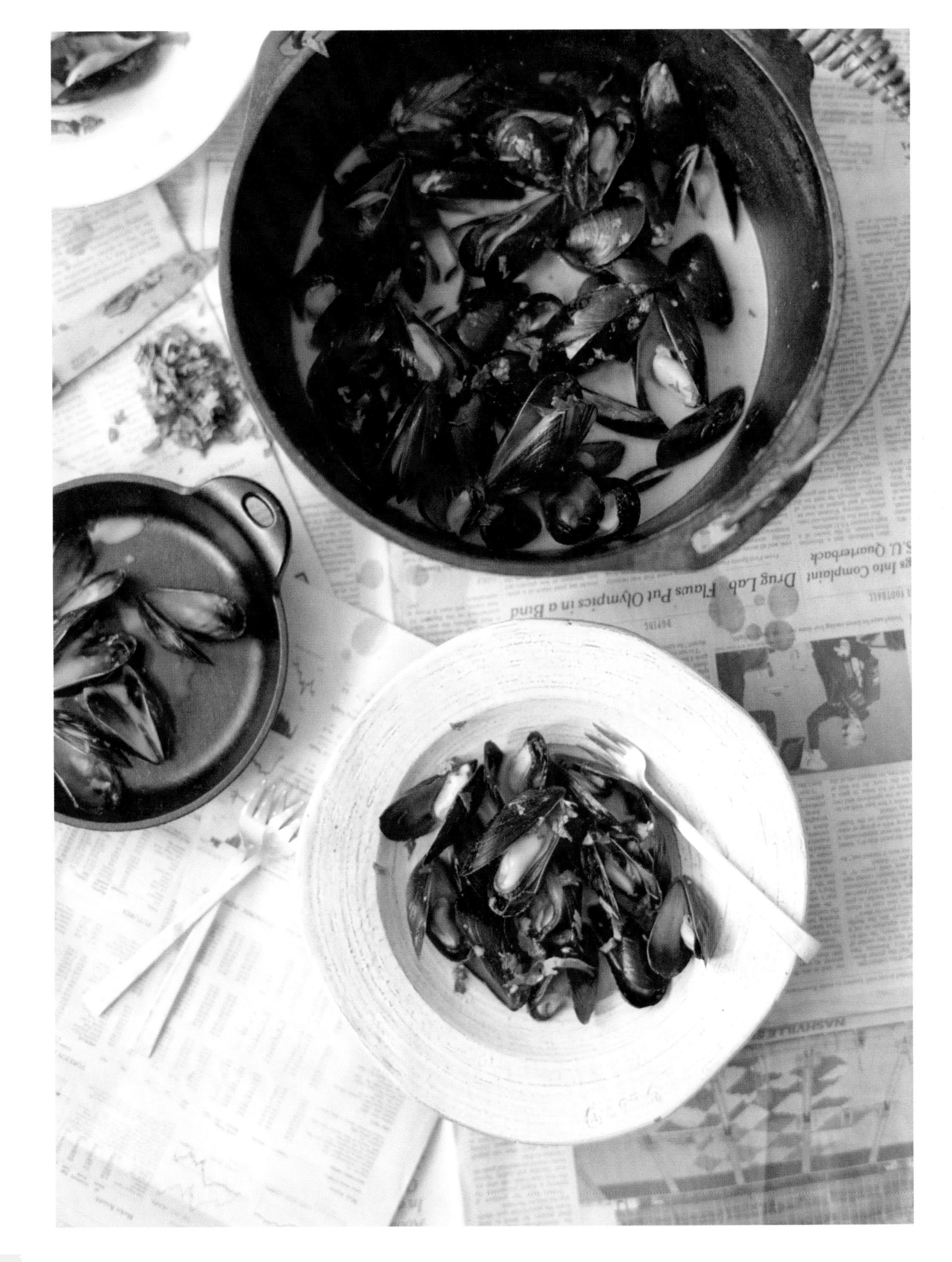

Garlic Green Beans with Tomatoes and Thyme

The inspiration for this simple dish came from my friend Katherine Morrison, whose recipe I've adapted here. The beans are infused with the garlic, tomatoes, and thyme and become meltingly delicious. It's wonderful served with an easy roasted chicken for a summery meal that's sure to please everyone at the table. I used a mixture of purple and green beans for the photo, which shows the blanched beans and the rest of the ingredients in the pan ready to be slow-cooked—the purple beans turn green once cooked. Any mixture of green, purple, or even yellow wax beans would work well.

Serves 4

- *1½ pounds green beans, stems removed*
- *½ cup cold-pressed, extra-virgin olive oil*
- *4 cloves garlic, minced*
- *¾ teaspoon fresh thyme leaves or 2 teaspoons dried thyme leaves*
- *1 cup diced tomato, red and/or yellow (I used a striped German tomato)*
- *1 shallot, sliced thin*
- *Pinch of cayenne pepper*
- *Sea salt and ground black pepper*

1. Bring a large pot of water to a boil. Add the beans and blanch for 2 minutes, then drain and rinse with cold water.

2. In a large cast-iron skillet, combine the olive oil, garlic, and green beans. Top with the thyme, tomato, shallot, cayenne, and a sprinkle of salt and pepper.

3. Warm the pan over very low heat, barely cooking it. Cover tightly and allow to cook on low for 45 minutes, stirring occasionally.

4. When done, the beans will be shriveled up and slightly caramelized. Stir and cook for another 5 minutes, uncovered, breaking up the tomato a bit. Turn off the heat and serve warm.

NOTES: *Try other beans, like yard-long Asian beans, red noodle beans, or my favorite, Italian flat green beans, in this recipe.*

Whole30	Yes
Nut-free	Yes
Egg-free	Yes
AIP	No

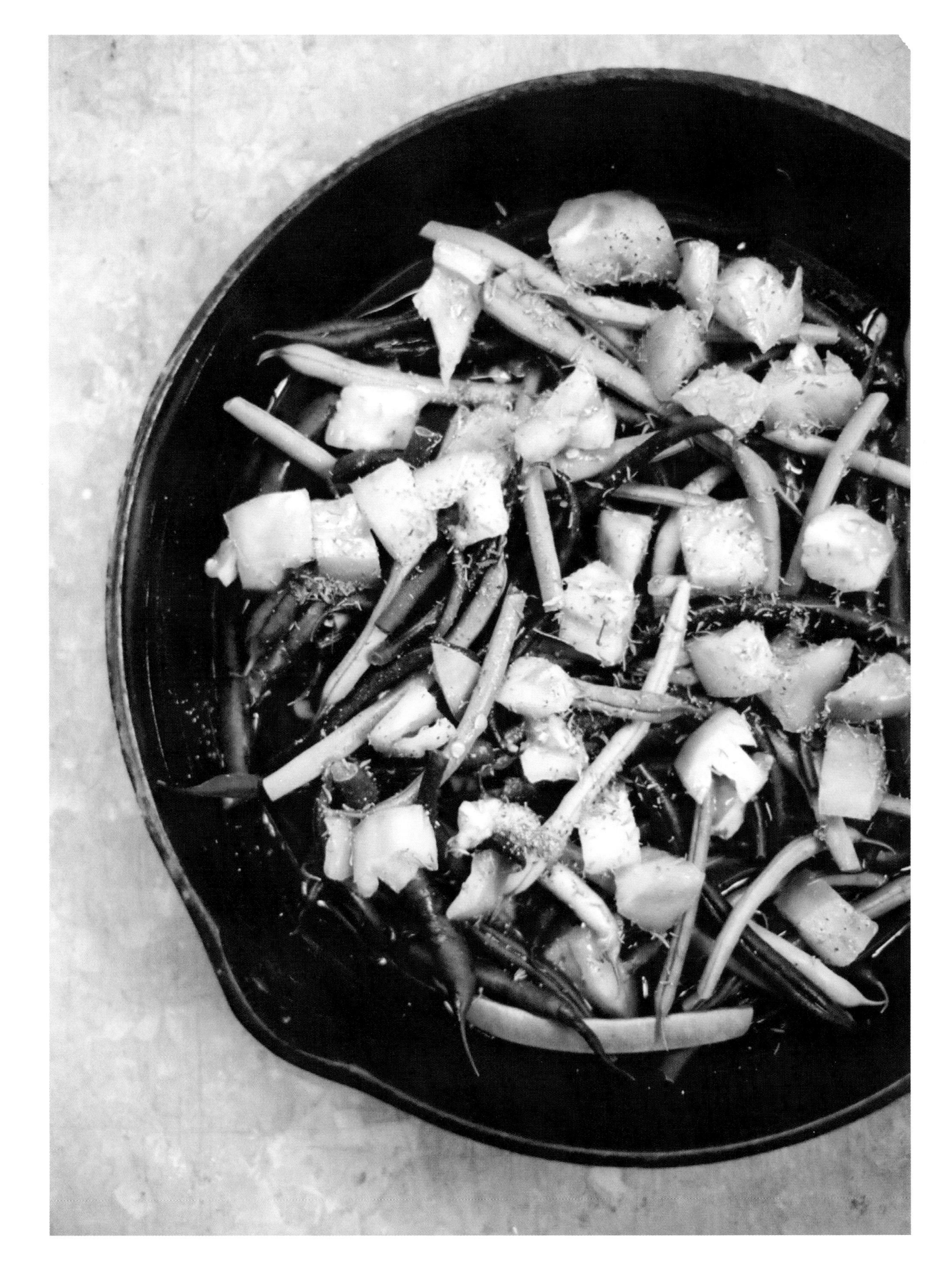

Zucchini Andouille Cakes with Lemon-Chive Sauce

I love a spicy breakfast, but these cakes are also great for lunch or an easy dinner. The egg whites give them a very light and fluffy texture. I'm always looking for new, creative ways to use the prolific zucchini that comes at me like an avalanche starting in early July and continuing throughout the summer. Sometimes they even get too big for me to tackle. When we have super-huge, baseball bat–sized squash, we feed them to the pigs, who joyfully devour them.

Makes about eight 3-inch cakes

For the sauce

- *¾ cup homemade mayonnaise (page 344)*
- *1½ teaspoons grated lemon zest*
- *1 teaspoon lemon juice*
- *2 tablespoons minced fresh chives*

For the cakes

- *2 tablespoons bacon fat or coconut oil, divided*
- *1 all-natural andouille sausage link, diced small (about ⅔ cup)*
- *½ cup minced yellow onion*
- *1 medium zucchini, grated (about 1½ cups)*
- *3 tablespoons chopped fresh cilantro leaves*
- *3 tablespoons chopped fresh basil leaves*
- *3 tablespoons coconut flour*
- *½ teaspoon ground black pepper*
- *6 eggs, separated*

1. Make the sauce: In a small bowl, combine the mayo, lemon zest, lemon juice, and chives and mix well. Place in the fridge while you prepare the cakes.

2. In a skillet, heat 1 tablespoon of the bacon fat over medium heat. Add the sausage and cook for a few minutes, until browned. Remove from the pan with a slotted spoon and place in a bowl. (Do not clean the skillet; you will use it later.)

3. To the bowl, add the minced onion, grated zucchini, and herbs. Mix well.

4. Add the coconut flour and pepper and mix well.

5. Add the egg yolks and mix until incorporated.

6. Beat the egg whites until firm (not stiff, just so that there is no loose liquid in the bowl). Gently fold them into the zucchini mixture. Don't overmix, or the eggs will fall (and defeat the purpose of whipping them, which is to give the cakes a nice loft).

7. Warm the remaining tablespoon of bacon fat in the same skillet you used to cook the sausage.

8. Working in batches, drop ¼-cup amounts of the zucchini batter into the pan. Don't overcrowd the pan. Fry for about 3 minutes, or until browned on the bottom, then flip, press down lightly with the back of a spatula, and continue cooking until the other side is browned. Serve warm with the sauce.

NOTES: *If you don't like the heat of andouille sausage, substitute a milder sausage such as kielbasa or sweet Italian-style sausage.*

Whole30	Yes
Nut-free	Yes
Egg-free	No
AIP	No

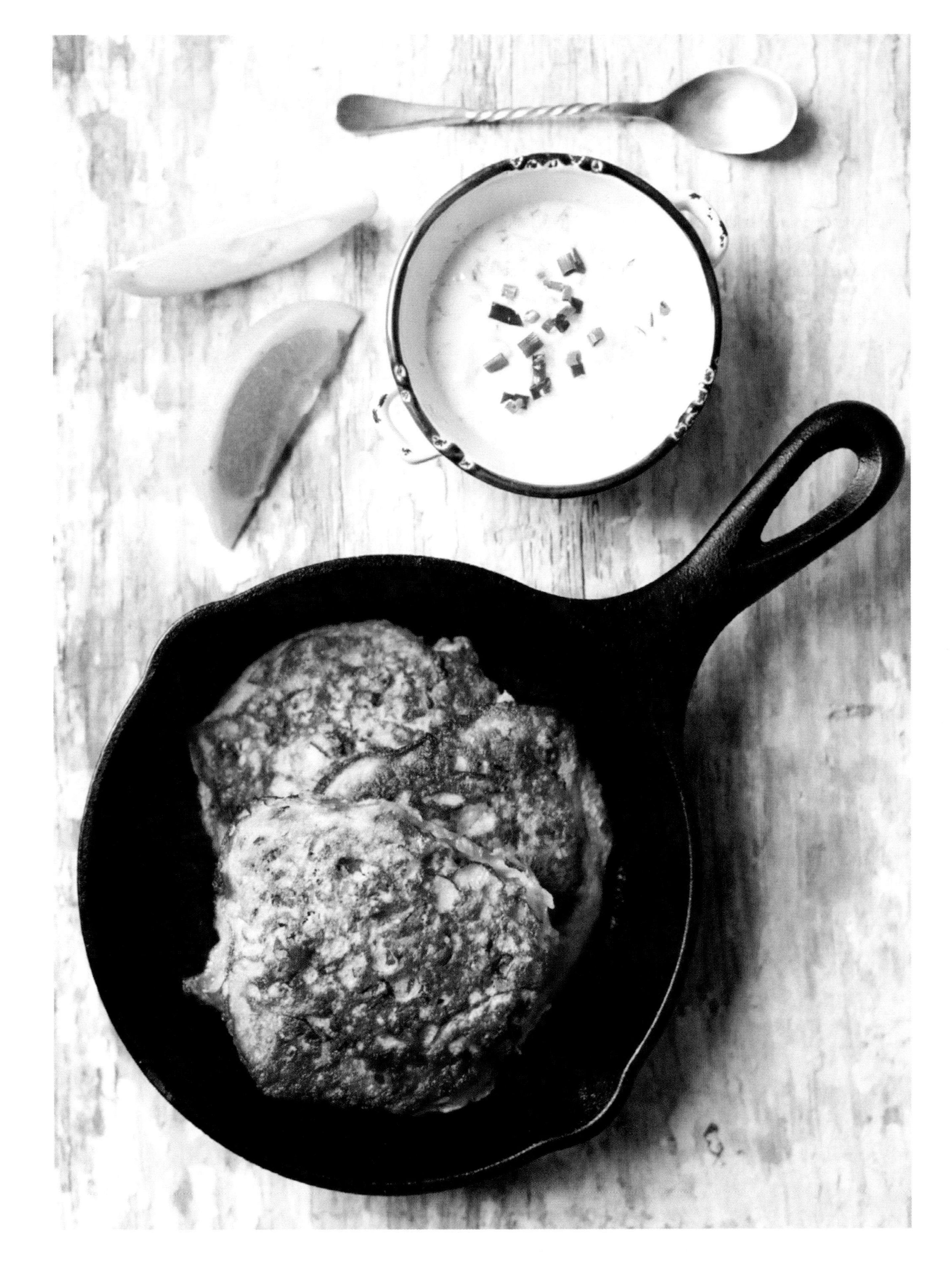

Grilled Eggplant Stacked with Indian-Spiced Beef

To me, grilling eggplant is the best way to eat this wonderful summer vegetable. Stacks of eggplant layered with spicy beef (also called "kheema") makes for a warm and comforting dish on a cool late-summer evening. I know you'll love this elegant and simple dish as much as I do. I like to use a combination of eggplant varieties. Feel free to use any eggplant you like, though the smaller ones taste less bitter.

Serves 4

For the beef

- *3 tablespoons ghee (page 347)*
- *2 cups diced white onion*
- *3 cloves garlic, minced*
- *1 tablespoon minced fresh ginger*
- *2 teaspoons ground coriander*
- *1 teaspoon smoked sweet paprika*
- *1 teaspoon ground cumin*
- *1 teaspoon garam masala*
- *1 pound ground beef*
- *2 cups diced tomatoes*
- *1 tablespoon seeded and chopped jalapeño pepper*
- *½ teaspoon sea salt*
- *½ teaspoon ground black pepper*
- *½ cup water*
- *2 teaspoons apple cider vinegar*
- *¼ cup chopped fresh cilantro leaves, plus more for garnish*

For the eggplant

- *2 large eggplants, sliced crosswise into ½-inch-thick rounds or lengthwise into ½-inch-thick planks*
- *¼ cup ghee (page 347), melted*
- *Sea salt and ground black pepper*

1. Make the spiced beef: In a large skillet, heat the ghee over medium heat. Add the onion and cook until translucent, about 5 to 7 minutes.
2. Add the garlic, ginger, coriander, paprika, cumin, and garam masala and cook for another 3 minutes.
3. Add the beef, breaking up the clumps with a spatula. Cook until the beef is no longer pink.
4. Stir in the tomatoes, jalapeño, salt, pepper, and water. Cover the pan and cook for 5 minutes.
5. Add the vinegar and turn off the heat. Set aside.
6. Stir in the cilantro and adjust the seasoning with more salt and pepper if needed.
7. Make the eggplant: Heat a grill to medium heat (see page 362 for grilling tips).
8. Rub the ghee over the eggplant slices and sprinkle them with salt and pepper.
9. Place the eggplant on the grill. Cook for about 3 minutes on one side, then flip and continue cooking for another 5 minutes or so, until the eggplant softens.
10. To assemble the dish, start by placing one eggplant slice at the bottom, cover with a layer of the beef mixture, then add another eggplant slice, one more layer of beef, and top with a final slice of eggplant. Garnish with cilantro.

NOTES: *I also love this dish with grilled zucchini instead of eggplant and ground lamb instead of beef.*

Whole30	Yes
Nut-free	Yes
Egg-free	Yes
AIP	No

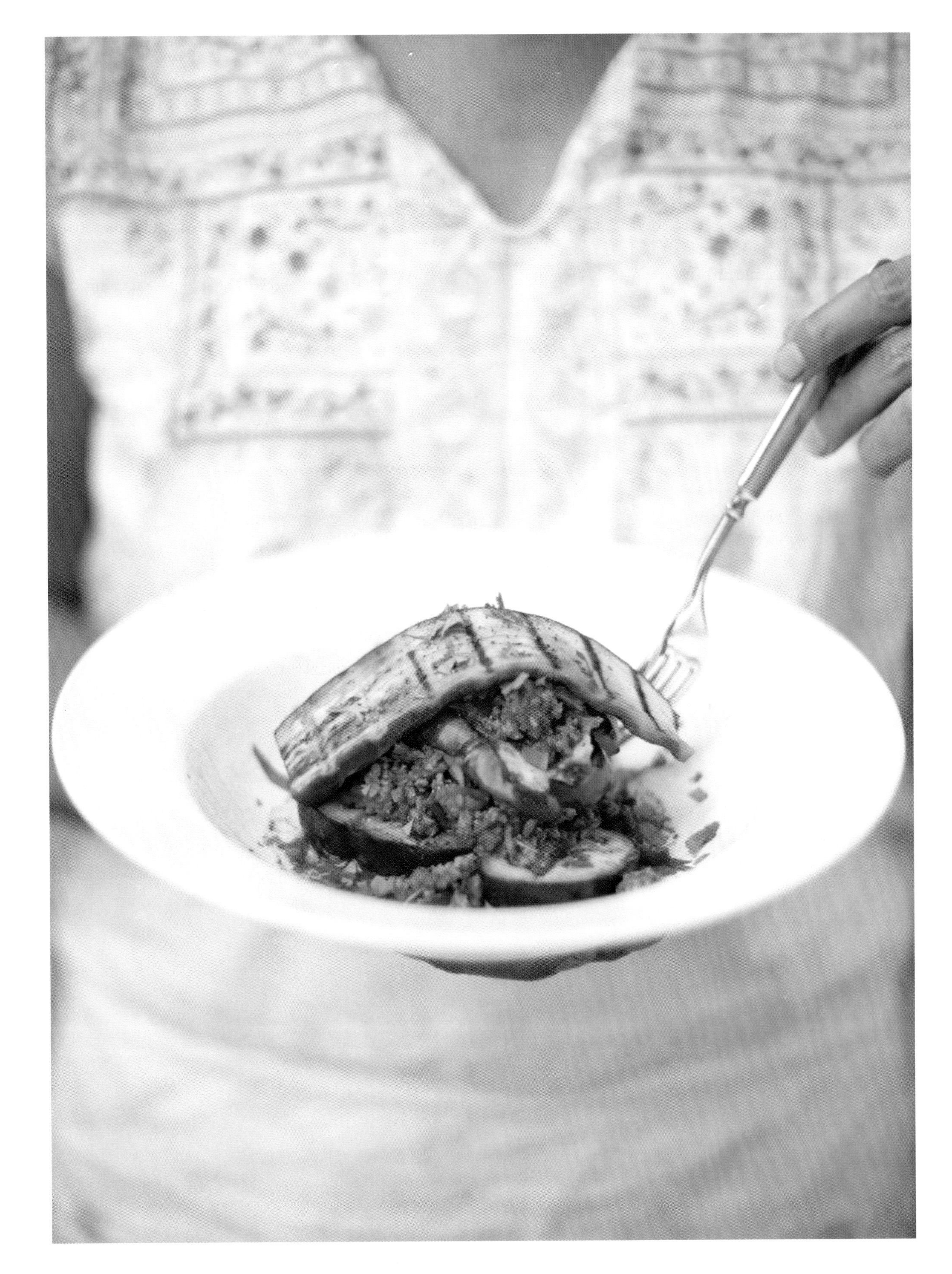

Creamy Cucumber Noodle Salad with Cherry Tomatoes

Long strings of cucumbers mixed with a creamy herb dressing and cherry tomatoes are so much fun served as a side with fish or grilled meat in the summer. My favorite cherry tomatoes are the Sun Gold variety, which we grow every year at the farm. They are less acidic than red tomatoes and have the most beautiful yellow-orange color, which has been my favorite hue since I was a little kid. If you've never used a spiral vegetable slicer before, you'll be amazed at how easy it is to make noodles out of all kinds of vegetables. Just please watch out for the very sharp blades.

Serves 4

- *½ cup homemade mayonnaise (page 344)*
- *Juice of 1 lemon*
- *½ cup minced fresh dill*
- *¼ cup minced fresh mint leaves*
- *2 medium cucumbers, peeled*
- *¼ cup very thinly sliced red onion*
- *1 pint cherry tomatoes, halved*
- *Sea salt and ground black pepper*

1. Mix the mayo, lemon juice, dill, and mint together in a small bowl. Set aside.
2. Using a spiral vegetable slicer, cut the cucumbers into noodles.
3. Place the cucumbers and red onion in a large bowl and toss with the dressing.
4. Top with the halved cherry tomatoes and season with salt and pepper to taste.
5. Serve at once—this dish does not like to wait.

NOTES: *This salad is also great with zucchini instead of cucumber.*

Whole30	Yes
Nut-free	Yes
Egg-free	Use ⅓ cup olive oil in place of the mayonnaise.
AIP	Use ⅓ cup olive oil in place of the mayonnaise. Omit the tomatoes and black pepper.

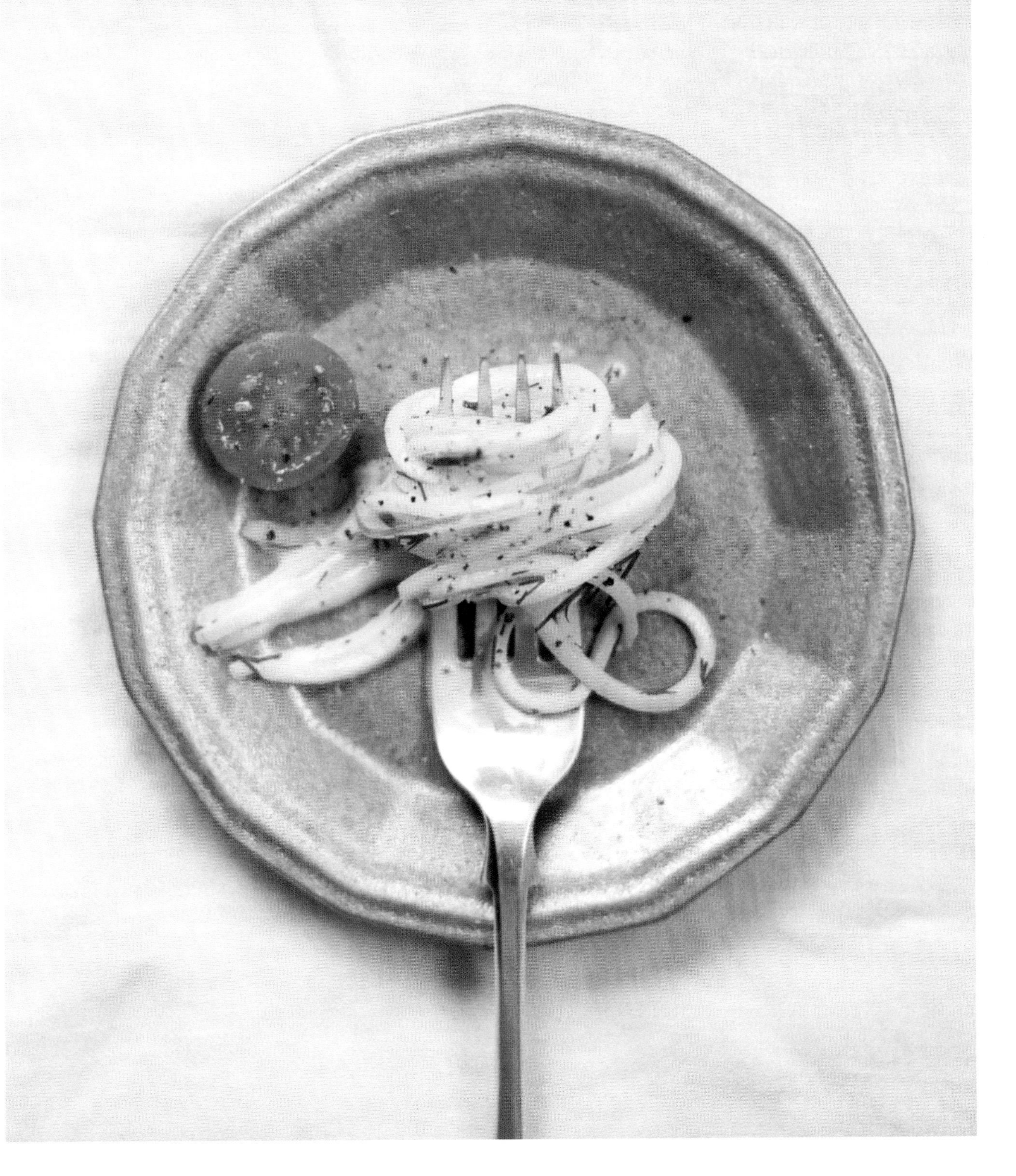

Lemon Crêpes with Blackberries and Peaches

I'm in love with these crêpes! They have no sweetener, but the addition of vanilla and fresh lemon makes them a refreshing treat. They're wonderful as a light summery dessert or as a brunch dish served with a side of sausages. If you don't have blackberries and white peaches on hand, try these with blueberries, strawberries, or your favorite seasonal fruit.

Makes about 12 crêpes

- *⅔ cup tapioca starch*
- *⅓ cup coconut flour*
- *¼ teaspoon baking soda*
- *½ teaspoon sea salt*
- *2 eggs*
- *1½ cups canned, full-fat coconut milk*
- *1 teaspoon vanilla extract*
- *Grated zest of 1 lemon*
- *1 tablespoon melted coconut oil, plus more for the pan*
- *Up to ½ cup water*
- *1 cup blackberries*
- *2 peaches, white or yellow, sliced*
- *1 tablespoon minced fresh mint leaves, for garnish (optional)*

1. In a large bowl, whisk together the tapioca starch, coconut flour, baking soda, and salt until blended.
2. In a separate bowl, whisk together the eggs, coconut milk, vanilla, lemon zest, and coconut oil.
3. Pour the wet ingredients into the dry ingredients and mix until thoroughly combined.
4. Check the consistency of the mixture—it should be like a very thin pancake batter. Add up to ½ cup water if needed.
5. Warm a skillet over medium heat.
6. Melt a tablespoon of coconut oil in the pan, then, using a large spoon, pour in about ¼ cup of the batter.
7. Flip the crêpe after about 3 minutes, when the bottom is very lightly browned, and continue to cook for another 1 to 2 minutes.
8. Transfer the finished crêpes to a warm plate and cover with a towel until ready to serve.
9. Repeat with the rest of the batter, adding more coconut oil to the skillet if it becomes dry.
10. To serve, place 2 or 3 crêpes on each plate and top with fresh blackberries and peach slices. Garnish with fresh mint, if desired.

Whole30	No
Nut-free	Yes
Egg-free	No
AIP	No

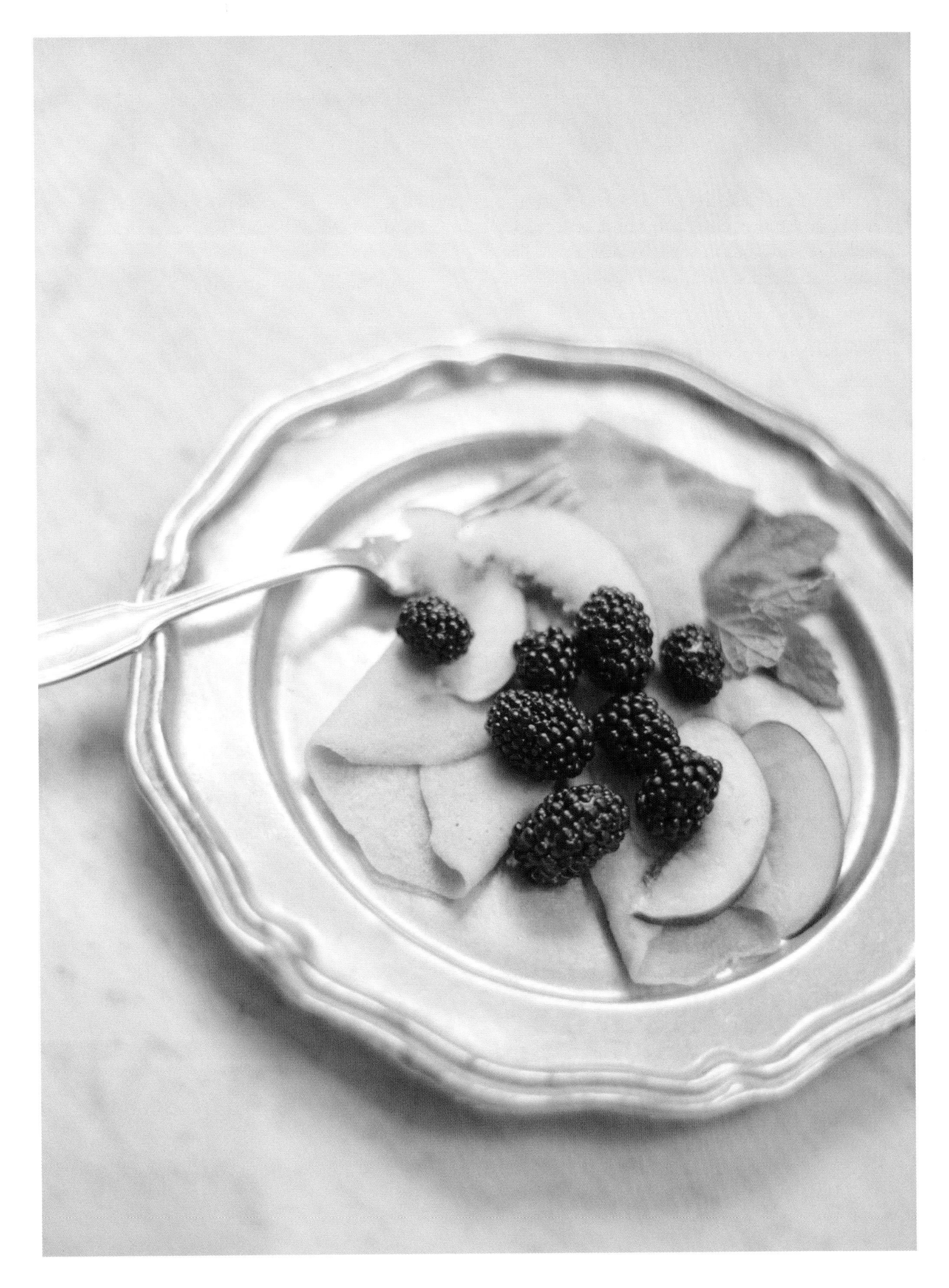

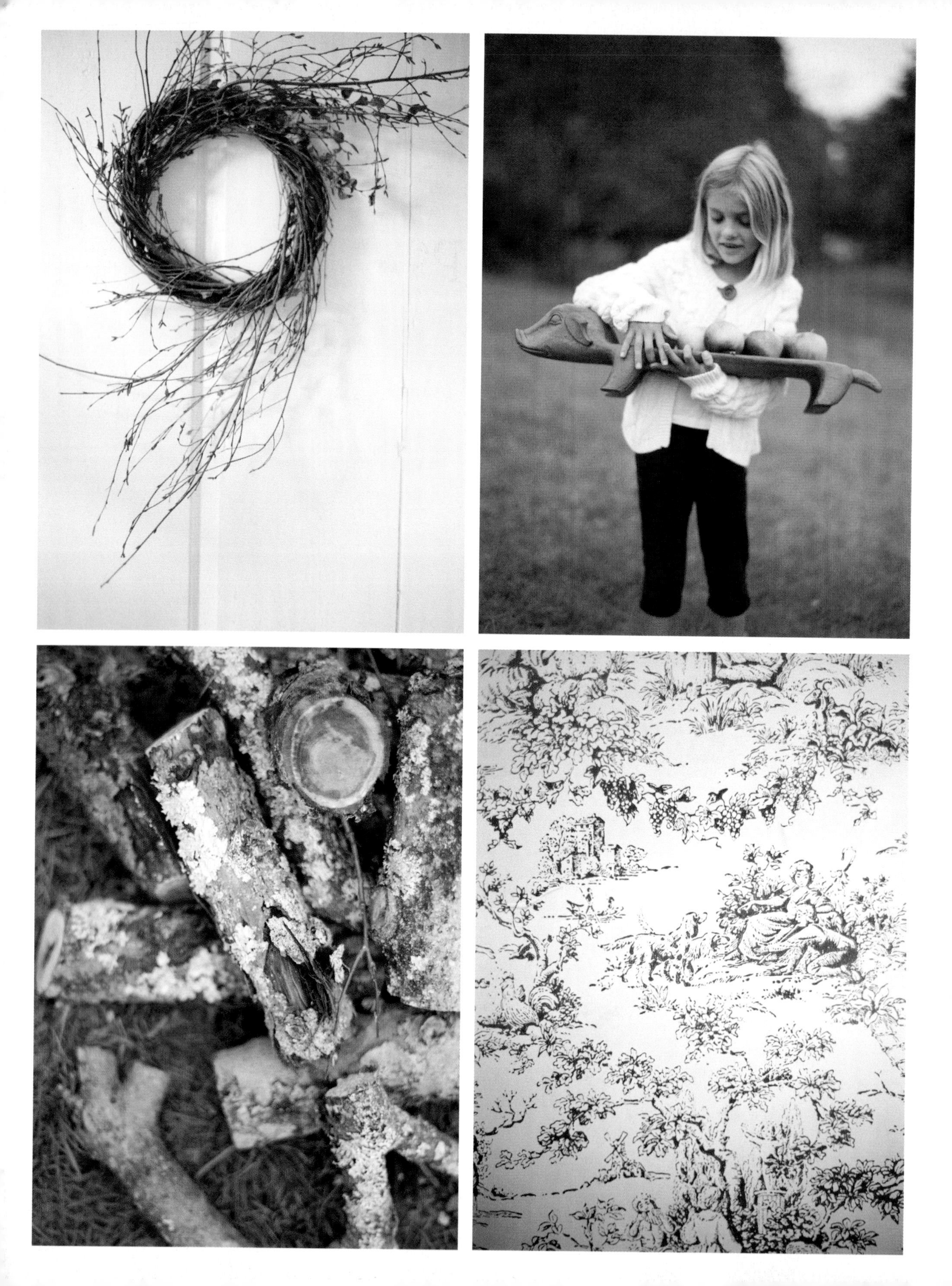

Late Season Recipes

One of my favorite times of the year is when summer finally breaks in late September and October. I suddenly have new motivation to spend more time in the kitchen making broths, soups, and stews. In the fields, we spend less time planting new crops and more time just harvesting. In New England, we can still harvest carrots, spinach, Brussels sprouts, and some other crops into mid-December if the conditions are good. Carrots in particular get much sweeter after the first frost. We celebrate the harvest with a big pig roast and make hard cider with apples from our friend's farm. The animals are processed, and our freezers are stocked for the winter. This is my favorite time of year to be cooking!

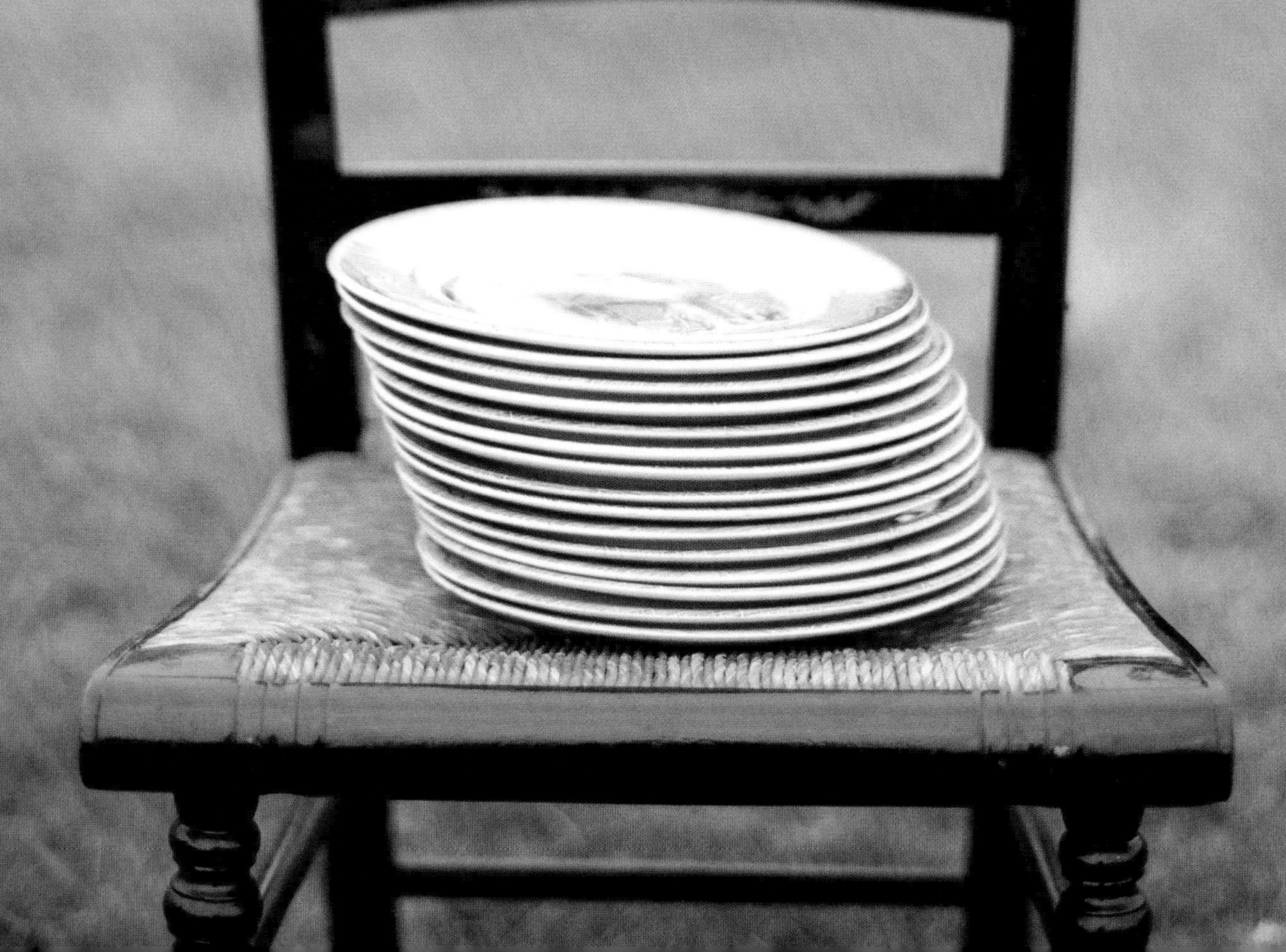

Big Bad Rooster Soup

This soup is legendary in my house. The story starts when my son Anson was four and figured out how to pick up hens and toss them back over the chicken wire into their pen. A rooster was watching him do this and decided he didn't like anyone messing with his girls. So the rooster took action. Imagine a bird almost as big as you coming straight for you, ready to fight. Anson was scared. After that, he needed a grown-up to walk with him every time he left the house, or else the Big Bad Rooster would come at him. The rooster, meanwhile, got cocky (pun intended!) and started to go after all the little kids on the farm. After a couple of weeks, Anson realized that if he walked with his Star Wars lightsaber, the bird left him alone, and he managed to save some of his friends from attack, too. But parents were complaining that their kids were scared to come to the farm because of this mean rooster. Eventually we were able to catch the Big Bad Rooster and Anson ordered me to cook him up, so I invented this soup. Anson found huge satisfaction in eating his archnemesis. I wrote about the soup in the farm newsletter and re-created the recipe to serve to customers in our farm stand. Everybody loved it, and it became a regular offering. Now, whenever we have a troublesome rooster, this soup is his fate. Feel free to substitute regular roasted chicken if you don't have a Big Bad Rooster hanging around.

Serves 6

- *1 tablespoon ghee (page 347)*
- *2 cups diced yellow onions*
- *2 cups peeled and diced carrots*
- *1 cup diced celery*
- *1½ teaspoons minced garlic*
- *1 teaspoon minced ginger*
- *2 quarts homemade chicken stock (page 338; see Notes)*
- *1 cup diced red bell pepper*
- *5 cups shredded napa cabbage*
- *3 cups chopped cooked chicken or rooster*
- *2 tablespoons coconut aminos or wheat-free tamari (see Notes)*
- *2 tablespoons fish sauce*
- *1 tablespoon lime juice*
- *1 tablespoon minced fresh mint leaves, for garnish*
- *1 tablespoon minced fresh cilantro leaves, for garnish*
- *1 tablespoon minced fresh basil leaves, for garnish*
- *Sriracha (all-natural), for garnish*

1. In a large soup pot, melt the ghee over medium heat. Add the onions and cook for 5 minutes, or until the onions soften.
2. Add the carrots, celery, garlic, and ginger and cook for 10 minutes, or until fragrant.
3. Add the chicken stock and bring to a simmer, then continue to simmer for 30 minutes.
4. Add the bell pepper, cabbage, and chicken and cook for about 2 minutes.
5. Turn off the heat and add the coconut aminos, fish sauce, and lime juice.
6. Ladle the soup into bowls and top with a generous helping of the fresh herbs and a squeeze of Sriracha to taste.

Whole30	Omit the Sriracha.
Nut-free	Yes
Egg-free	Yes
AIP	Substitute coconut oil for the ghee. Omit the bell pepper and Sriracha.

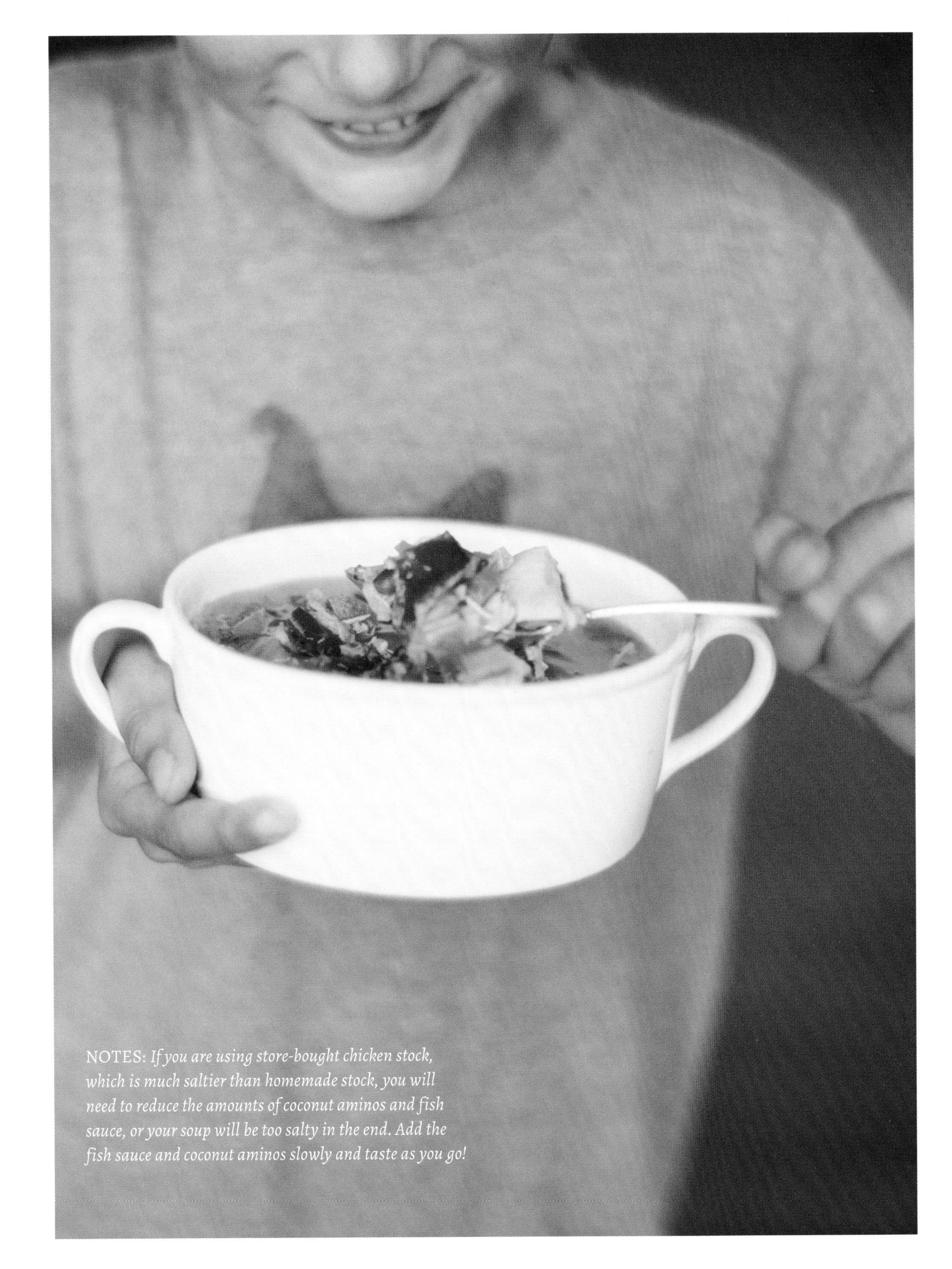

NOTES: *If you are using store-bought chicken stock, which is much saltier than homemade stock, you will need to reduce the amounts of coconut aminos and fish sauce, or your soup will be too salty in the end. Add the fish sauce and coconut aminos slowly and taste as you go!*

Wilted Mustard Greens with Warm Bacon Dressing and Ground Cherries

I had you at "bacon dressing," didn't I? Mustard greens and other dark leafy greens can be pretty bitter, but combining them with this warm and rich dressing and topping them with ground cherries transforms them into an amazing and beautiful side dish. I learned about this combination from my friends Emily and Diane, who are professional caterers and frequently host our family for dinner. Eating great meals with good friends in their home is even better than going out. Their cooking inspired several dishes in this cookbook.

Serves 4 to 6

- *1 cup ground cherries (see Notes)*
- *1 tablespoon bacon fat*
- *1 cup diced red onion*
- *5 strips bacon, cooked and crumbled*
- *¼ cup cold-pressed, extra-virgin olive oil*
- *2 tablespoons apple cider vinegar*
- *1 teaspoon Dijon mustard*
- *¼ teaspoon sea salt*
- *⅛ teaspoon ground black pepper*
- *1 pound tender young mustard greens*

1. Peel back the papery husks on the ground cherries. Rinse the fruits and set aside.
2. In a medium saucepan over medium heat, warm the bacon fat. Add the onion and sweat it for 15 minutes, lowering the heat if needed. Do not brown.
3. Add the cooked bacon crumbles to the pan and stir well.
4. Add the olive oil, vinegar, mustard, salt, and pepper and stir to combine. Remove from the heat and set aside.
5. On a platter, arrange the mustard greens. Drizzle the warm dressing over the greens.
6. Top with the ground cherries.

NOTES: *Ground cherries look like small tomatillos but taste sweeter, like a cross between a tomato and a pineapple. They fall to the ground, then ripen into a golden fruit covered with a papery skin. You'll find them at farmers markets in late summer and early fall. To store, keep them in their husks at room temperature for up to a week. If ground cherries are unavailable, feel free to substitute sweet cherry tomatoes.*

Whole30	Yes
Nut-free	Yes
Egg-free	Yes
AIP	No

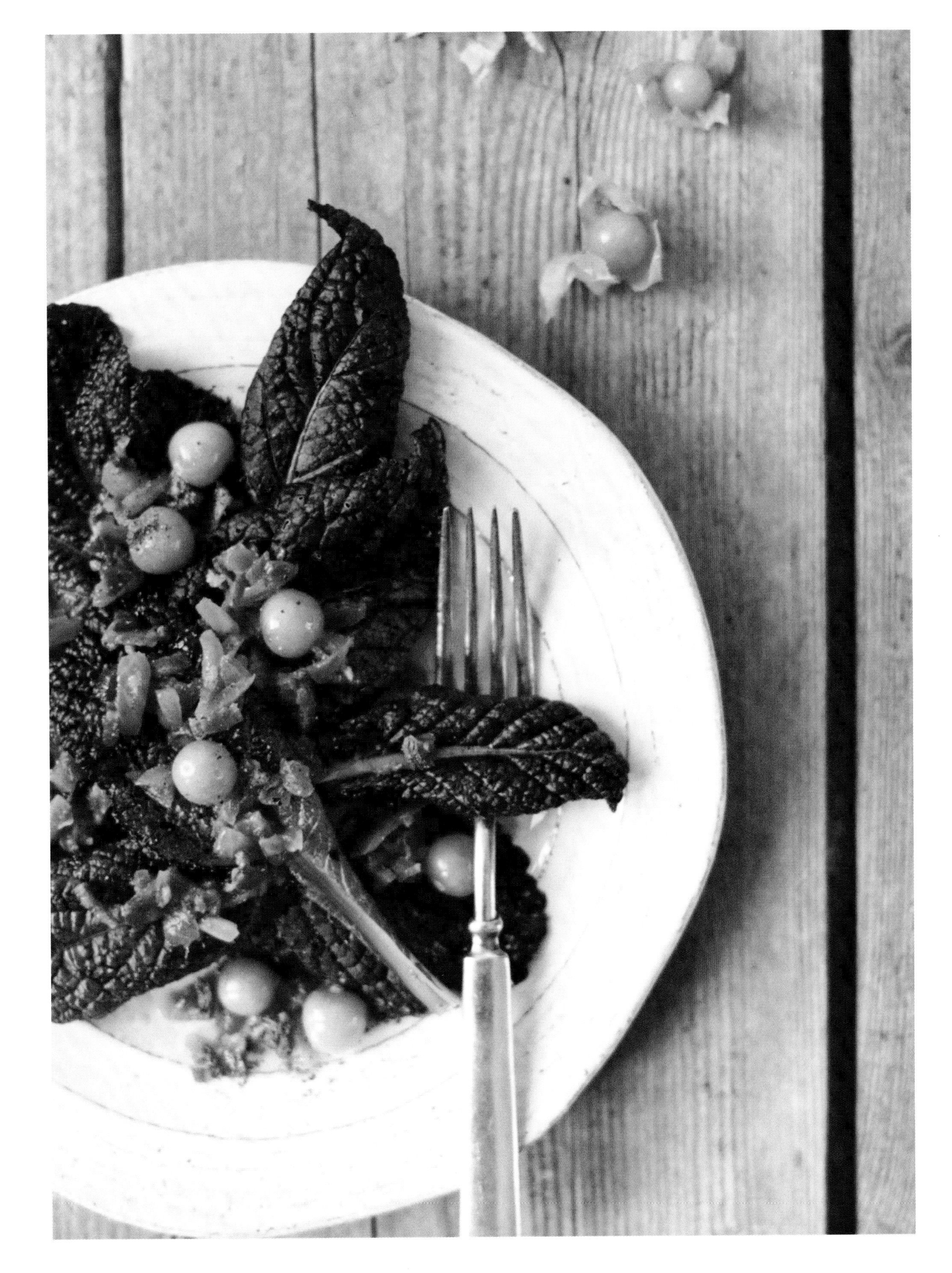

Moroccan Egg and Lamb Tagine

The flavors in this dish take me back to my trip to Morocco. I can hear the call to prayer over the loudspeakers and smell the fresh spices in the market. I love this combination of farm-fresh eggs with Moroccan spices and rich, satisfying meatballs. If you want a completely impressive brunch dish, this is it!

Serves 4 to 6

For the meatballs

- *1 cup minced yellow onion*
- *1 tablespoon minced fresh mint leaves*
- *1 tablespoon minced fresh cilantro leaves*
- *½ teaspoon grated fresh ginger*
- *1 teaspoon ground coriander*
- *1 teaspoon ground cumin*
- *½ teaspoon ground black pepper*
- *½ teaspoon sea salt*
- *1 pound ground lamb*

For the sauce

- *1 teaspoon coconut oil or cooking fat of choice*
- *1 medium yellow onion, diced*
- *3 cloves garlic, minced*
- *1 cup chopped roasted red bell pepper (about 1 large pepper)*
- *2 (14½-ounce) cans diced tomatoes or 5 cups diced fresh tomatoes*
- *½ teaspoon ground cumin*
- *⅛ teaspoon ground cinnamon*

- *4 to 6 eggs (1 per person)*
- *2 tablespoons minced fresh parsley leaves, for garnish*

1. Make the meatballs: Combine the onion, mint, cilantro, ginger, spices, and salt in a large bowl.
2. Add the ground lamb and mix well with your hands. Form into about 16 golf ball–sized meatballs.
3. In a skillet over medium heat, working in batches, brown the meatballs on all sides. You don't have to cook them through, as they will cook more in the sauce. Set aside.
4. Make the sauce: Over medium heat, warm the coconut oil in a large, heatproof clay tagine or sauté pan with deep sides. Sauté the onion for a few minutes, until soft.
5. Add the garlic, bell pepper, tomatoes, cumin, and cinnamon. Simmer for 10 minutes, or until the pepper is soft.
6. Add the meatballs and cover the dish. Cook for 10 minutes to finish cooking the meatballs and allow the flavors to meld.
7. Add the eggs in between the meatballs by carefully cracking each egg into the sauce. Cover again and cook for 5 minutes, until the eggs are set but still runny. Garnish with fresh parsley.

NOTES: *Don't like lamb? Use ground beef or pork instead.*

Whole30	Yes
Nut-free	Yes
Egg-free	Omit the eggs.
AIP	No

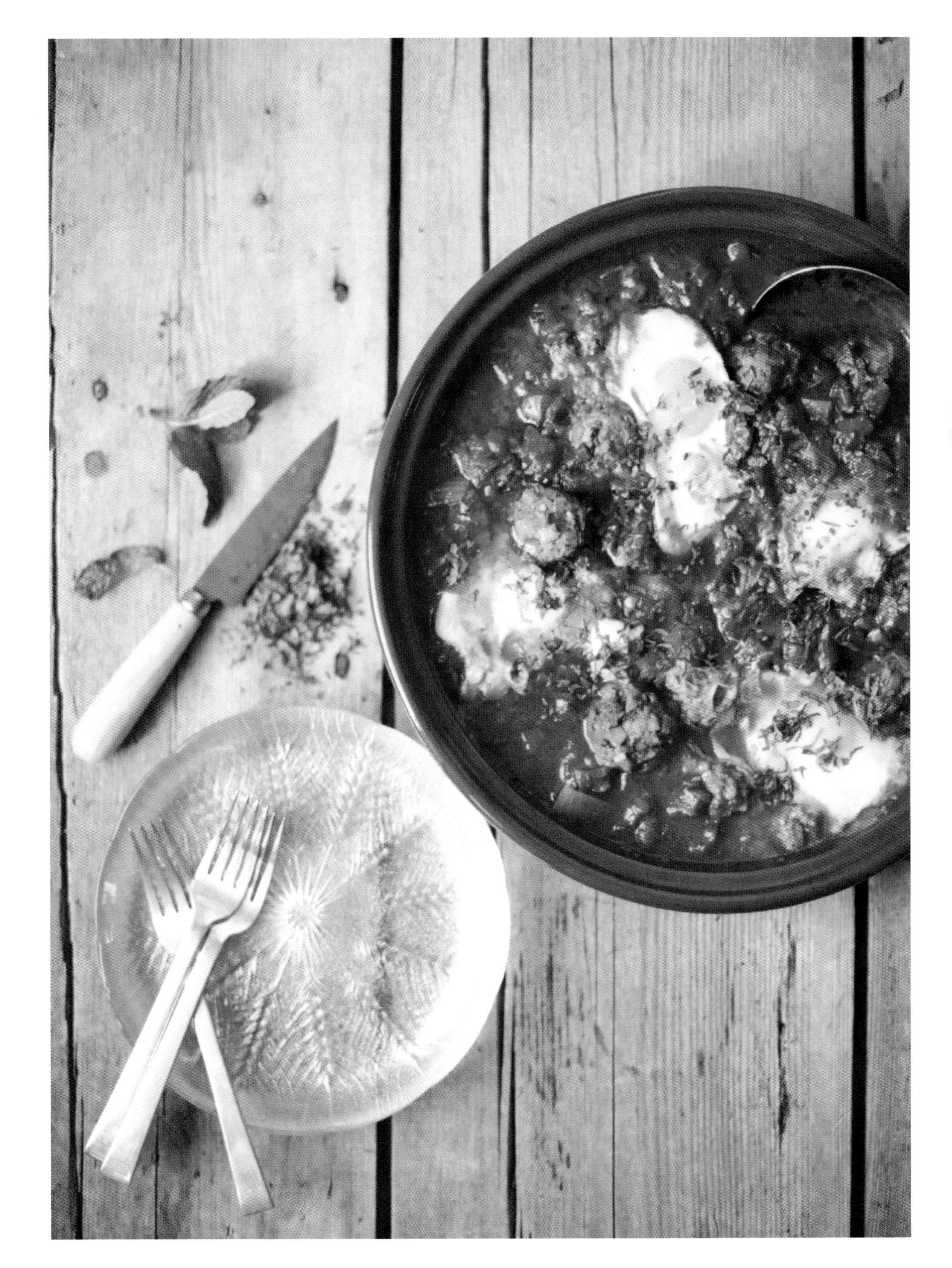

Curry Hash

My husband is not a huge fan of eggs; he much prefers to start his day with a big bowl of meat and vegetables. This spicy hash is one of his favorite breakfasts. The curry of potatoes, lamb, and onion is great for powering you through a long morning. Feel free to top with a fried or poached egg, if you wish.

Serves 4

- *1 pound Yukon Gold or other waxy potatoes (about 2 medium-sized potatoes), peeled and diced or cut into thin coins*
- *1 tablespoon bacon fat, ghee (page 347), or coconut oil*
- *1 cup diced yellow onions*
- *2 teaspoons madras curry powder*
- *Pinch of red pepper flakes*
- *1 pound ground lamb*
- *2 cups chopped tatsoi, spinach, kale, chard, or other greens*
- *Sea salt and ground black pepper*
- *2 tablespoons chopped fresh cilantro leaves, for garnish*

1. In a pot with a little water and a steamer, or in a microwave, steam the potatoes until fork-tender, about 10 minutes.
2. In a large skillet, warm the bacon fat over medium heat. Add the potatoes and sauté for a few minutes, until light brown.
3. Add the onions, curry powder, and red pepper flakes and combine well.
4. Add the lamb and cook until the lamb is no longer pink, about 5 minutes.
5. Add the greens and cook for just a few minutes, until wilted.
6. Season to taste with salt and pepper, and garnish with the cilantro.

NOTES: *Other ground meats also work great in this recipe. If you can't find madras curry powder, you can use regular curry powder.*

Whole30	Yes
Nut-free	Yes
Egg-free	Yes
AIP	No

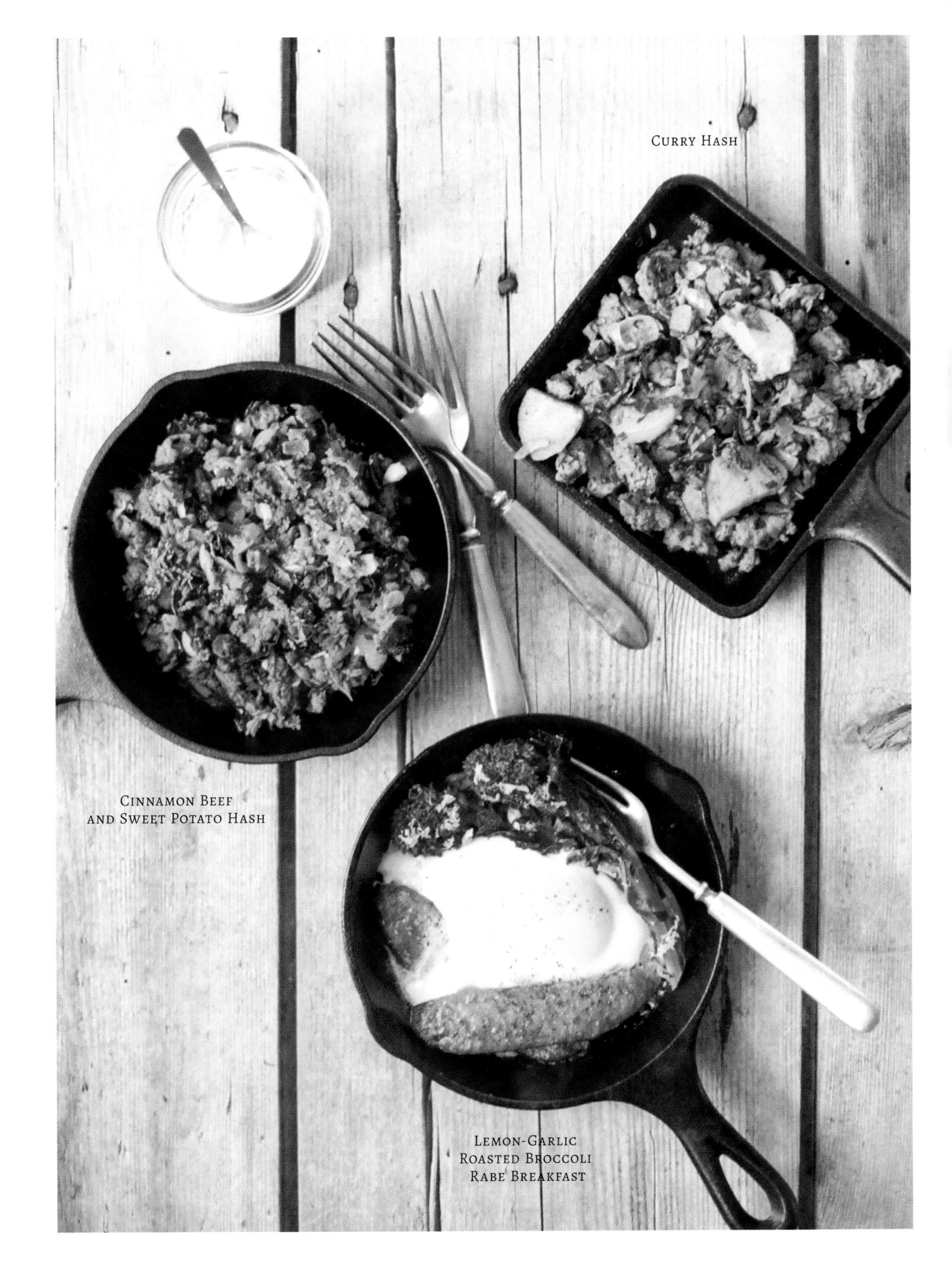
Curry Hash
Cinnamon Beef and Sweet Potato Hash
Lemon-Garlic Roasted Broccoli Rabe Breakfast

Cinnamon Beef and Sweet Potato Hash

I've been making this dish for years and find it to be much more satiating than eggs for breakfast. If you're trying to break an addiction to sweet foods, cinnamon is a sweet, warm spice that can satisfy a sugar craving. Feel free to substitute pork for the beef and spinach or chard for the kale.

Serves 4

- *1 tablespoon ghee (page 347)*
- *1 medium sweet potato, peeled and shredded (about 2½ cups)*
- *1 pound ground beef*
- *1 medium yellow onion, chopped*
- *3 cloves garlic, minced*
- *½ teaspoon ground cinnamon*
- *½ teaspoon ground cloves*
- *1 teaspoon ground cumin*
- *½ teaspoon ground coriander*
- *Pinch of red pepper flakes*
- *1 roasted red bell pepper, diced*
- *4 cups chopped kale*
- *1 tablespoon coconut aminos or wheat-free tamari*
- *Sea salt and ground black pepper*
- *2 tablespoons chopped fresh cilantro leaves, for garnish*

1. In a large skillet, warm the ghee over medium heat. Add the shredded sweet potato and sauté for 10 minutes.
2. Add the beef, onion, garlic, cinnamon, cloves, cumin, coriander, and red pepper flakes. Sauté until the beef is cooked, about 10 minutes.
3. Add the red bell pepper, kale, and coconut aminos. Sauté until the kale is wilted, about 3 minutes.
4. Season to taste with salt and pepper and garnish with the cilantro.

See photo on page 269.

NOTES: *Other ground meats work well in this recipe.*

Whole30	Yes
Nut-free	Yes
Egg-free	Yes
AIP	No

Lemon-Garlic Roasted Broccoli Rabe Breakfast

Broccoli rabe is amazing with lemon and garlic, and blanching and then roasting it with lemon removes some of the bitterness. This simple dish goes great with sausage and eggs in the morning. If you like spicy food, try it with an all-natural chorizo. If you can't handle that much heat in the morning, try kielbasa. I love making this recipe in little individual-sized skillets, but it can also be made in one large cast-iron skillet or a well-greased casserole dish.

Serves 4

- *8 to 12 stalks broccoli rabe*
- *1 teaspoon cold-pressed, extra-virgin olive oil*
- *2 tablespoons grated lemon zest*
- *1 tablespoon minced garlic*
- *4 chorizo sausage links or other cured/precooked sausage of your choice, halved*
- *1 tablespoon butter (page 348) or ghee (page 347)*
- *4 eggs*

1. Preheat the oven to 400°F.
2. Fill a medium saucepan halfway with water and bring to a boil.
3. Drop in the broccoli rabe and blanch for 2 minutes.
4. Divide the broccoli rabe among 4 small cast-iron skillets, or place it all in one large skillet or well-greased casserole dish. Drizzle with the olive oil, lemon zest, and garlic. Add the sausage to the pan(s) and drizzle with a touch of olive oil.
5. Roast for 8 to 10 minutes.
6. Remove the pan(s) from the oven. Create a well in the center of each small skillet, or create 4 wells in the large skillet or casserole dish. Coat the bottom of each well with a pat of butter or ghee. Crack the eggs into the wells and then place the pan(s) back in the oven.
7. Roast for another 10 minutes, or until the eggs are set to your liking.

See photo on page 269.

Whole30	Yes
Nut-free	Yes
Egg-free	No
AIP	No

Butternut Stew with Pork and Spinach

This warm and comforting dish is perfect to come home to on a cold night. It's got just the right amount of smoky heat from the red pepper flakes and paprika. It is also packed with nutrients: Butternut squash is a nutrient-dense source of starch, a fantastic source of vitamin A (it has more than 400 percent of the daily value per cup), and a very good source of vitamin C, potassium, and manganese. Add spinach to the mix, and now you've got vitamin K, folate, and lots of minerals. I look forward to the cooler months so I can make rich, soothing foods like this to nourish my family. I even make it for our farm crew for a hearty midday lunch.

Serves 6

- *1 pound ground pork*
- *1 medium yellow onion, diced*
- *4 cloves garlic, minced*
- *1 teaspoon minced fresh ginger*
- *½ teaspoon red pepper flakes*
- *½ teaspoon smoked sweet paprika*
- *½ teaspoon ground cumin*
- *½ teaspoon ground cinnamon*
- *1 teaspoon ground fennel*
- *½ teaspoon ground white pepper*
- *⅛ teaspoon ground cloves*
- *¼ teaspoon sea salt*
- *1 medium-sized butternut squash, peeled, seeded, and cut into 1½-inch cubes*
- *1 (14½-ounce) can diced tomatoes*
- *1 quart homemade chicken stock (page 338)*
- *2 heaping tablespoons tomato paste (½ of a 6-ounce can)*
- *2 quarts chopped spinach (about 6 ounces spinach leaves)*
- *3 tablespoons minced fresh mint leaves, for garnish*
- *3 tablespoons minced fresh cilantro leaves, for garnish*
- *3 tablespoons minced fresh basil leaves, for garnish*

1. In a large soup pot over medium heat, brown the pork, breaking it up into small pieces with a spatula as you go. Drain off the fat.
2. Add the onion, garlic, ginger, spices, and salt and cook for about 10 minutes, until the onion is soft.
3. Add the squash, tomatoes, chicken stock, and tomato paste and simmer, uncovered, for about 1 hour on low heat. This will reduce the stock and make the soupy mixture more like a stew.
4. Remove from the heat and stir in the spinach. As soon as the spinach has wilted, ladle the stew into bowls and serve garnished with the fresh herbs.

NOTES: *Feel free to substitute any winter squash for the butternut and ground turkey, lamb, or beef for the pork.*

Whole30	Yes
Nut-free	Yes
Egg-free	Yes
AIP	No

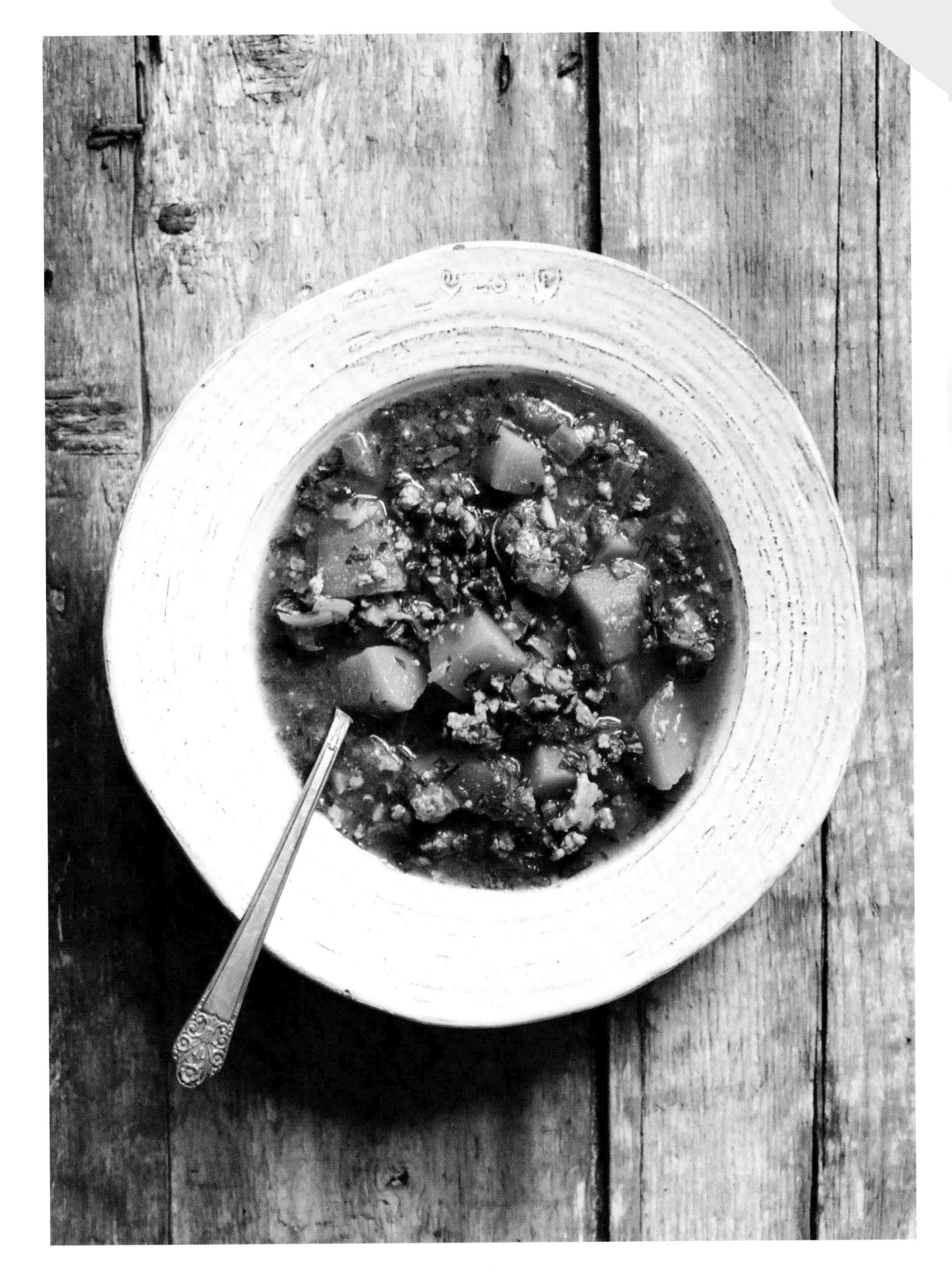

Late-Season Vegetable Soup with Pesto

In September, as the summer winds down and the nights get cooler, this silky and beautiful soup will warm you up. It's bursting with fresh vegetables, perfectly in season. My kids really love it, possibly because it's a puree, so they can't tell how many different nutritious veggies are packed in there. Serve it garnished with pesto and fennel fronds and with a side of dinner sausages for an easy meal that will please everyone. It's also lovely with a big pat of Sea Salted Herb Butter (page 348) on top, in addition to or in place of the pesto.

Serves 6

- *1 tablespoon ghee (page 347)*
- *1 medium yellow onion, diced*
- *2 stalks celery, diced*
- *2 cups diced carrots*
- *1 small bulb fennel, diced*
- *1 large kohlrabi, diced (about 2½ cups)*
- *2 tablespoons minced garlic*
- *2 quarts homemade chicken stock (page 338)*
- *1 medium zucchini, peeled and diced*
- *Sea salt and ground black pepper*
- *1 tablespoon pesto, for garnish*
- *6 pieces fresh fennel fronds, for garnish (optional)*

Whole30	Yes
Nut-free	Yes
Egg-free	Yes
AIP	Substitute coconut oil for the ghee. Omit the black pepper.

1. In a large soup pot over medium heat, melt the ghee.
2. Add the onion, celery, carrots, fennel, and kohlrabi and sauté for 10 minutes.
3. Add the garlic and continue to cook for another 5 minutes.
4. Add the chicken stock and bring to a simmer. Gently simmer, covered, for 1 hour, or until the kohlrabi and carrots are soft.
5. Add the zucchini and simmer for another 10 minutes, or until the zucchini is soft.
6. With an immersion blender, puree the soup well.
7. Season with salt and pepper to taste.
8. Ladle into bowls. Garnish each bowl with ½ teaspoon of pesto and a fennel frond, if you wish.

NOTES: *No kohlrabi? Use broccoli stems or hakurei turnips. I also love to add sautéed chopped fennel bulb to this soup.*

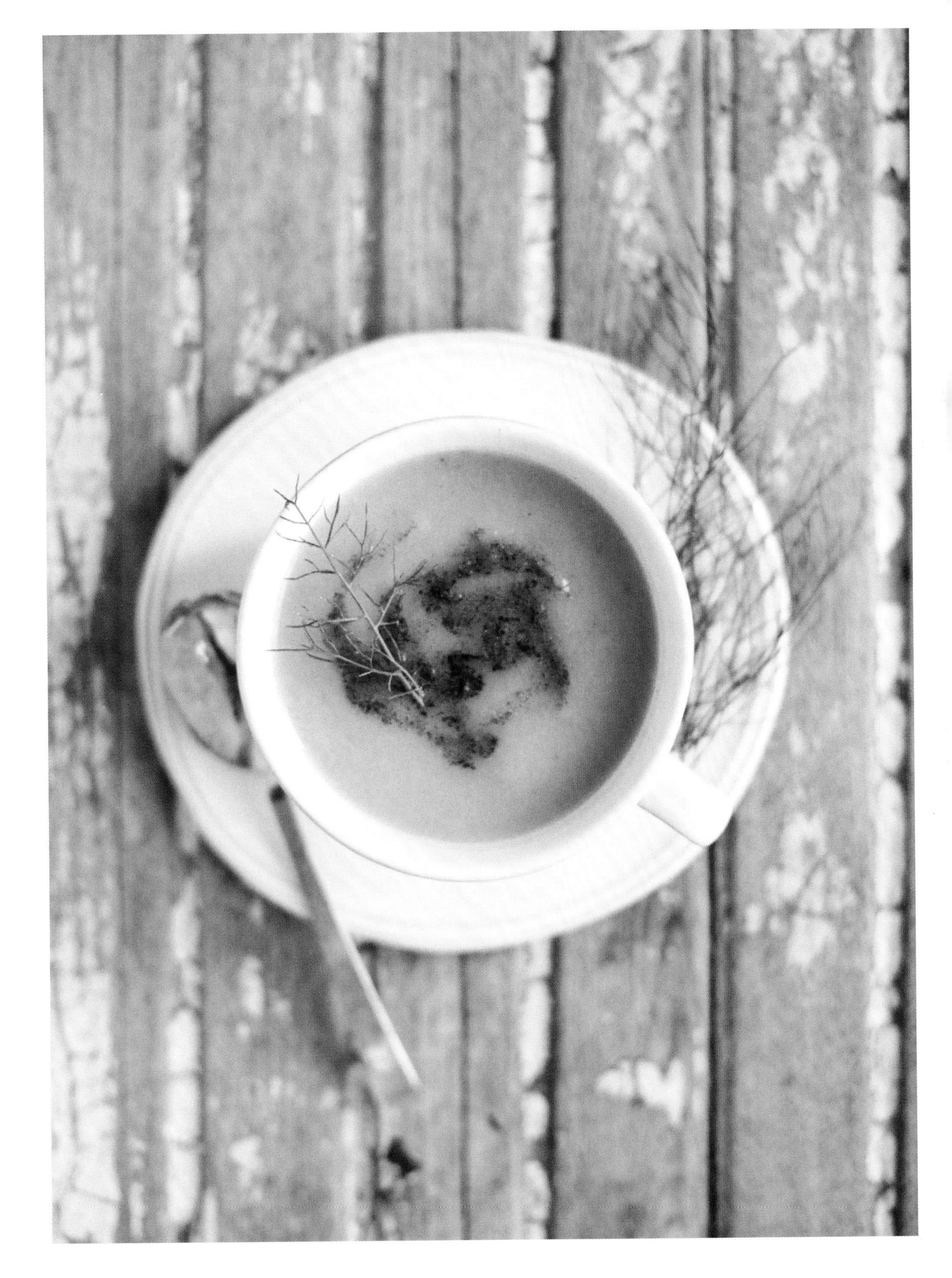

Hard Cider 101

Making your own hard cider is easy and fun. You just need a few pieces of special equipment, and you're off and running. There are millions of resources out there on how to make cider, and entire books on the subject. This is how I do it, and it always turns out great.

Makes about nine 12-ounce bottles

- *1 gallon preservative-free, fresh cider (see Notes)*
- *1 cup white sugar*
- *1 cup brown sugar (plus ¼ cup for fizzy cider)*
- *1 (5-gram) package champagne yeast*

Special equipment

- *1-gallon glass carboy, sterilized*
- *Vapor lock*
- *Funnel*
- *3-foot-long plastic tube or rubber hose*
- *9 (12-ounce) beer bottles*
- *Rubber- or silicone-tipped tongs*
- *Bottle caps and capper*

NOTES: *It's crucial to use preservative-free cider. Preservatives kill the yeast and the cider will not ferment. In a pinch, you can use all-natural apple juice, but cider is best. If you have a juicer, you can make your own juice: 1 bushel = 42 pounds of apples = 3 gallons of juice. It takes 10 to 15 pounds of apples to make 1 gallon of juice. I like Granny Smith for cider making. White wine yeast also works, but I prefer the results with champagne yeast.*

Whole30	No (all alcohol should be avoided)
Nut-free	Yes
Egg-free	Yes
AIP	I suggest avoiding alcohol on AIP.

1. Wash the carboy and finish with a rinse of very hot water.
2. Pour the cider into a large soup pot and set it over medium heat. Heat the cider for 45 minutes, keeping it just below a simmer at all times. Stir with a plastic or metal spoon (not wood).
3. Add the white sugar and 1 cup of the brown sugar and stir well.
4. Allow to cool to room temperature.
5. Add three-quarters of the yeast packet and stir well.
6. Using a funnel, carefully ladle or pour the cider into the sterilized carboy.
7. Fill the vapor lock with water and cap the cider.
8. Allow to sit at room temperature in an undisturbed place without major fluctuations in heat (not near a heater, cool window, or super-sunny spot) for 1 to 2 weeks.
9. Check the frequency of bubbles in the airlock. At first, you should see a constant stream of bubbles, which means that the cider is fermenting. After a week or two, the frequency will reduce to about one bubble per minute. When it reaches this point, proceed to the next step.

Continued on page 278.

SOURCING BREWING SUPPLIES

Champagne yeast, glass carboys, vapor locks, bottles, bottle caps, and the capper can all be purchased at a brewing supply company. The food-safe plastic tube or rubber hose used to siphon off the cider can be purchased at a hardware store. You can also save and repurpose cool old bottles from other beverages. See Resources (page 398) for brewing suppliers.

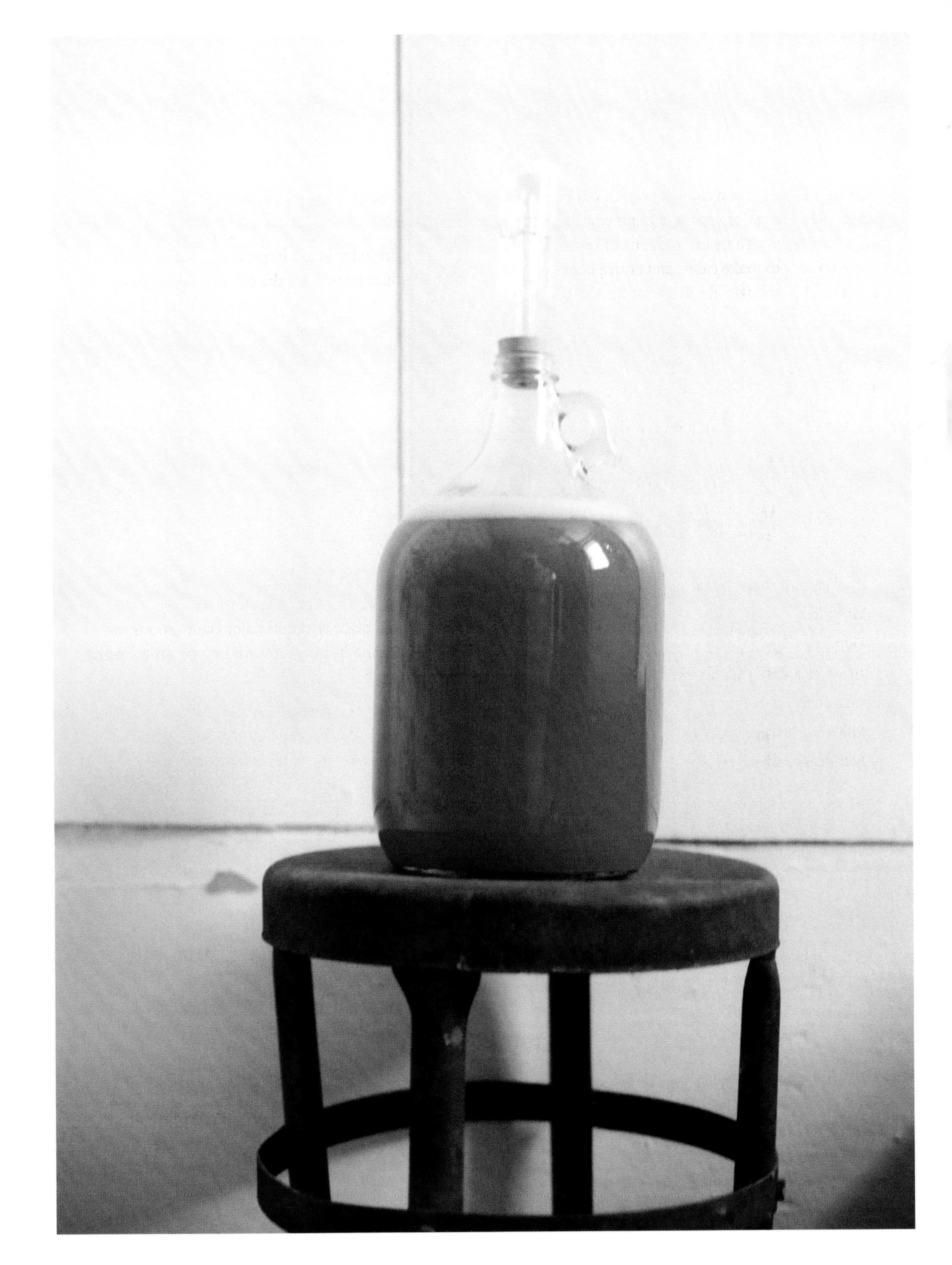

10. When the airlock shows just one bubble per minute, it's time to "rack" the cider. This process makes for a better-tasting brew and allows the cider to clarify. Remove the top and siphon the cider into a pot, being careful not to disturb any of the yeast at the bottom of the carboy. That's what you're trying to remove from the cider. Rinse out the carboy and put the cider back in the clean carboy. Allow the cider to sit for 1 more week. No fermentation will happen during this time.

11. Now you're ready to bottle the cider. If you'd like fizzy cider, this is the time to add more sugar, which will make a little more fermentation happen right in the bottles. Dissolve ¼ cup of brown sugar in ½ cup of warm water and allow to cool to room temperature.

12. While the sugar water cools, sterilize the bottles by carefully submerging them in boiling water for 5 minutes. Remove them with rubber- or silicone-tipped tongs and allow them to air-dry. Get out the capper and caps.

13. If making fizzy cider, add the sugar to the cider and stir well.

14. Using a funnel, carefully ladle the cider into the bottles, leaving about 1½ inches of space at the top. Cap the bottles and place them in a cabinet for a week. If you added too much sugar or something goes wrong, the bottle can explode, so please don't leave them out on the counter where kids could get a face full of glass. Be safe here.

15. How quickly the cider is done depends on the temperature of your house and what's going on inside the bottles. Try opening one of the bottles after a week. It should have a little "pop." If you've got a geyser, it's done! Put all of the bottles in the fridge to stop the fermentation process immediately.

16. If you had a little "pop," you can recap the bottle and let the cider sit for another week or longer, checking on it periodically. I tend to make cider in early October (when the house is about 67 degrees on average), and it takes a week or so to ferment, a week to clarify, and about 2 weeks in the bottles before I place it in the fridge.

17. Drink your cider. Better yet, throw a pig roast (page 383) and share it with friends and family!

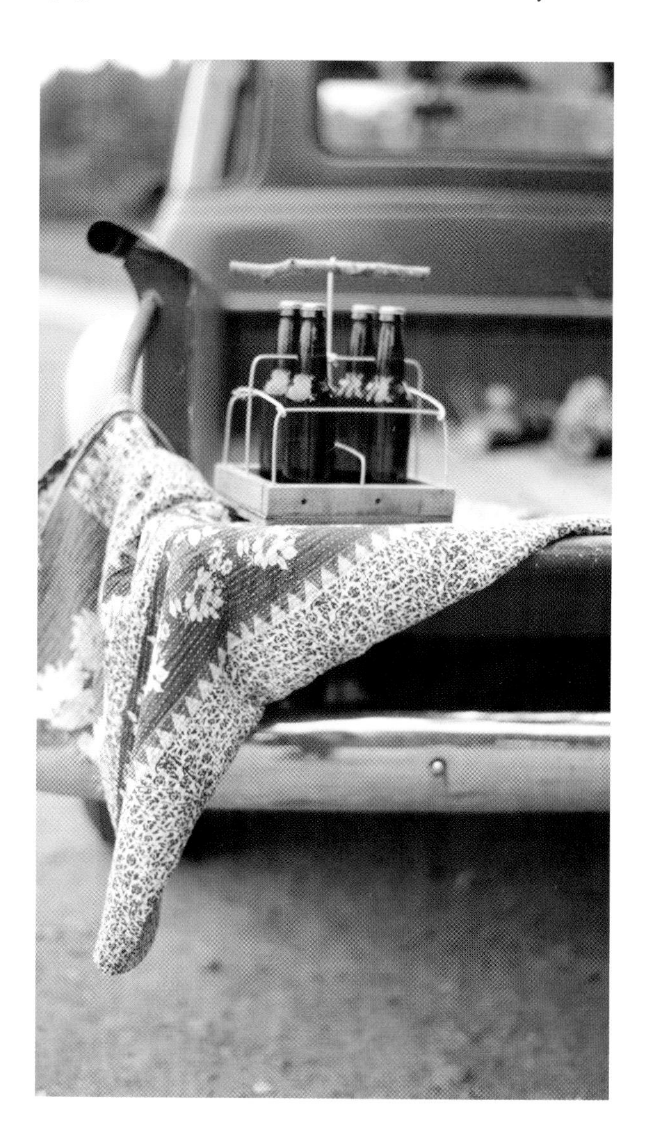

Hot Mulled Cider

There's something so comforting and lovely about hot cider on a chilly day.

Makes 1 gallon

- *1 gallon apple cider*
- *1 orange, sliced*
- *2 cinnamon sticks*
- *10 cardamom pods*
- *10 whole cloves*
- *5 allspice berries*
- *½ teaspoon ground nutmeg*

Whole30	Yes
Nut-free	Yes
Egg-free	Yes
AIP	Use an additional stick of cinnamon and omit the other spices.

1. Place all of the ingredients in a pot and simmer for about 20 minutes. Strain into mugs and serve.

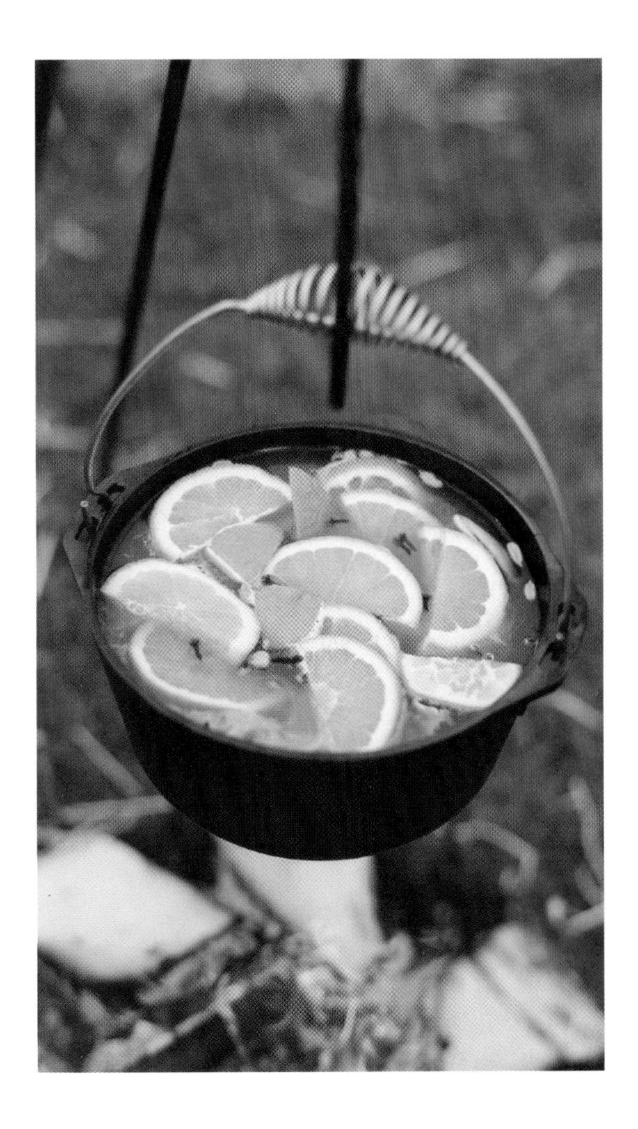

Spicy Red Cabbage Slaw

This dish is fantastic with grilled fish or chicken, or to dress up a boring burger. The acidity also cuts the fat of a dish like pulled pork really well. This slaw has a kick and gets even better as it sits in the fridge overnight. I really love it on a hot summer evening. It's very easy to make, but you do need to plan ahead to give the cabbage 3 hours to drain excess moisture.

Serves 6 to 8

- *½ head red cabbage, shredded (about 3 cups)*
- *2 teaspoons sea salt*
- *1 cup peeled and grated carrots*
- *1 cup apple cider vinegar*
- *⅔ cup chopped fresh cilantro leaves*
- *2 tablespoons grated fresh ginger*
- *2 tablespoons honey*
- *1 tablespoon cold-pressed sesame oil*
- *¼ teaspoon red pepper flakes*

1. Place the cabbage in a colander and toss it with the salt. Place a plate over the cabbage and then top it with a heavy book, brick, or something else to weigh it down. Let it sit for 3 hours.
2. Remove the weight and the plate. Rinse the cabbage in a salad spinner and spin dry, or rinse in a colander and pat dry.
3. Combine the cabbage with the other ingredients in a large bowl and mix well.
4. Serve immediately or allow to sit—it gets better with time!

NOTES: *You can substitute green cabbage if you like.*

Whole30	Omit the honey.
Nut-free	Yes
Egg-free	Yes
AIP	Omit the sesame oil and red pepper flakes.

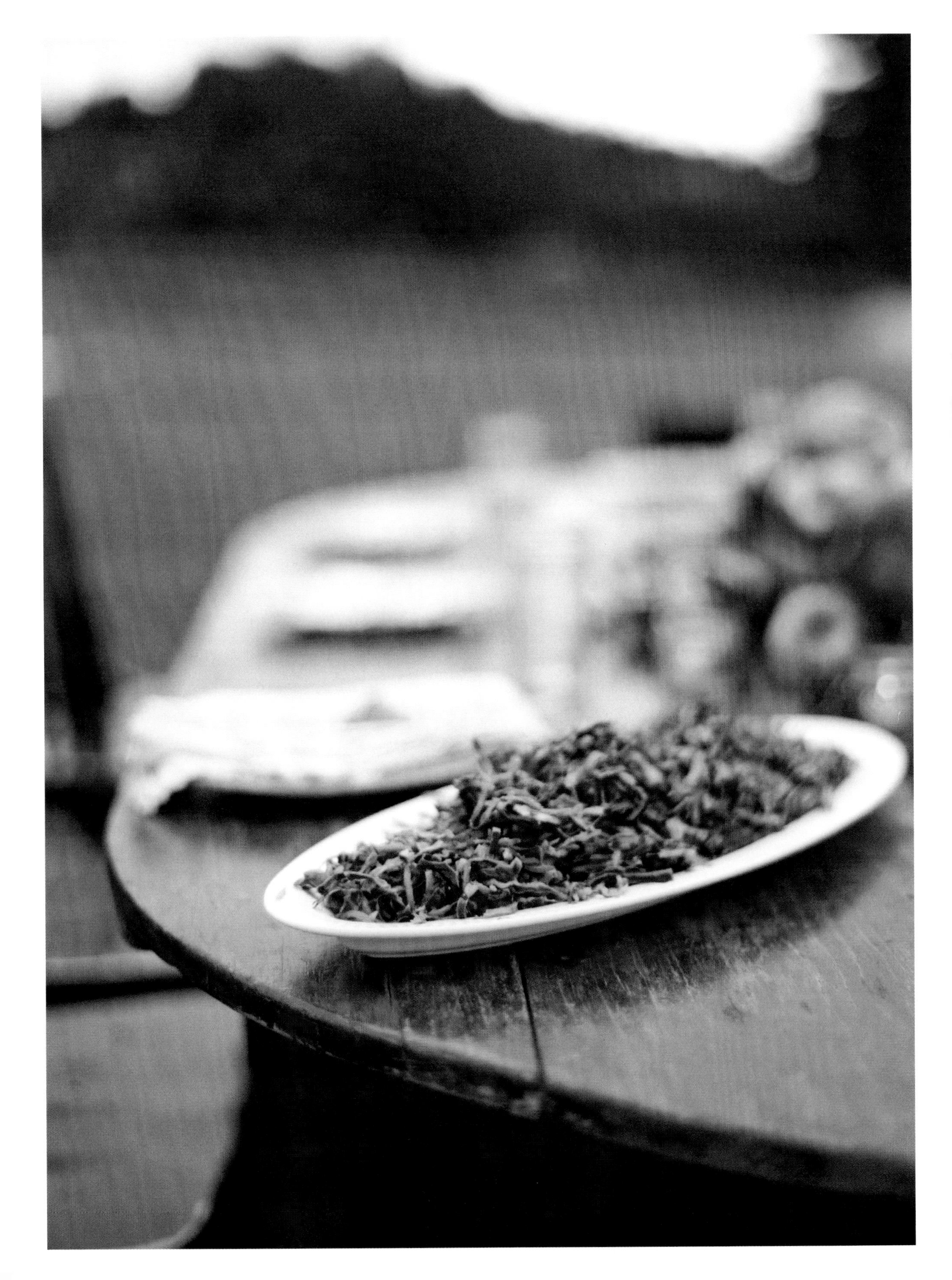

Roasted Sweet Potatoes with Sweet and Savory Toppings

My guests love being able to choose their own toppings for roasted sweet potatoes. It's an easy side dish to serve at a pig roast or any party. Be creative and invent your own toppings, or serve the ones listed below, which were all hits. My favorite combo is figs, crème fraîche, chopped pecans, and shredded coconut. Just set out a half cup of each topping and let your guests help themselves!

Serves 12

- *6 large sweet potatoes*

For the sweet toppings

- *Shredded unsweetened coconut*
- *Roasted, unsalted pecans, chopped*
- *Crème fraîche (page 347)*
- *Warm Cinnamon Pears (page 283)*
- *Diced fresh figs*
- *Dried cherries*

For the savory toppings

- *Goat cheese*
- *Sliced scallions*
- *Chopped sundried tomatoes*
- *Roasted pepitas*
- *Diced red onion*
- *Minced fresh cilantro leaves*

Whole30	Omit the crème fraîche and goat cheese.
Nut-free	Omit the nuts.
Egg-free	Yes
AIP	Omit the nuts, crème fraîche, and pepitas.

1. Preheat the oven to 350°F.
2. Poke each sweet potato 3 times with a fork.
3. Place the sweet potatoes on a rimmed baking sheet and roast for 1 hour, or until you can easily insert a knife into the center of the potatoes.
4. Remove from the oven and cut each sweet potato in half lengthwise.
5. Place the halved sweet potatoes on a platter and allow folks to help themselves to the toppings.

See photo on page 285.

NOTES: *You can wrap the sweet potatoes in aluminum foil for softer skin, if you like.*

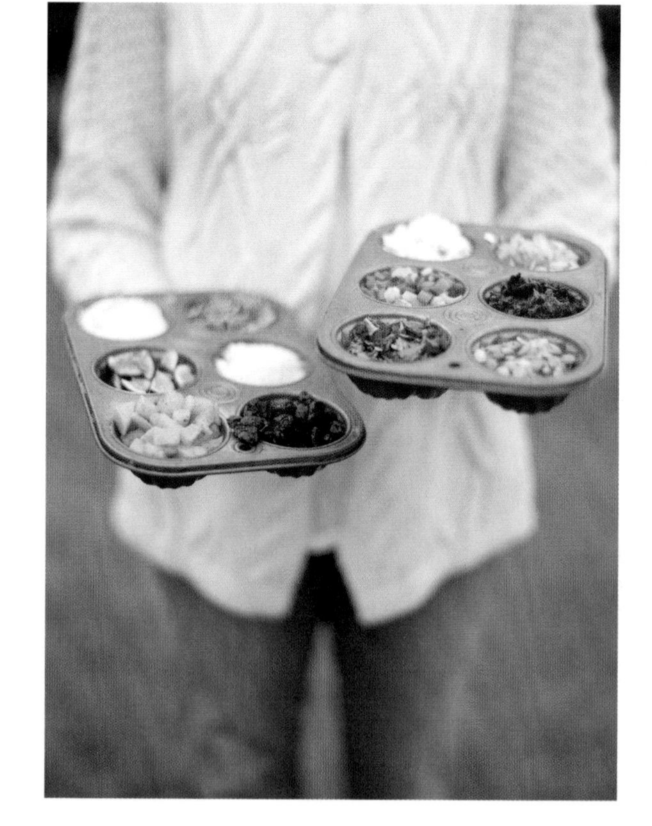

Warm Cinnamon Pears

This quick and easy side dish is lovely over Roasted Sweet Potatoes (page 282), alongside sausages in the morning, or even eaten as a dessert with whole-milk yogurt or ice cream. It's also fantastic with Lemon Crêpes (page 258). You'll swear there is sugar in this recipe, but it's all healthy, natural sweetness.

Makes about 2½ cups

- *2 tablespoons unsalted butter (page 348)*
- *5 pears, peeled and diced*
- *¼ teaspoon ground cinnamon*

1. Melt the butter in a saucepan over medium-low heat.

2. Add the diced pears and cinnamon. Cook for 10 minutes, stirring often. Serve warm.

NOTES: *This recipe also works great with apples.*

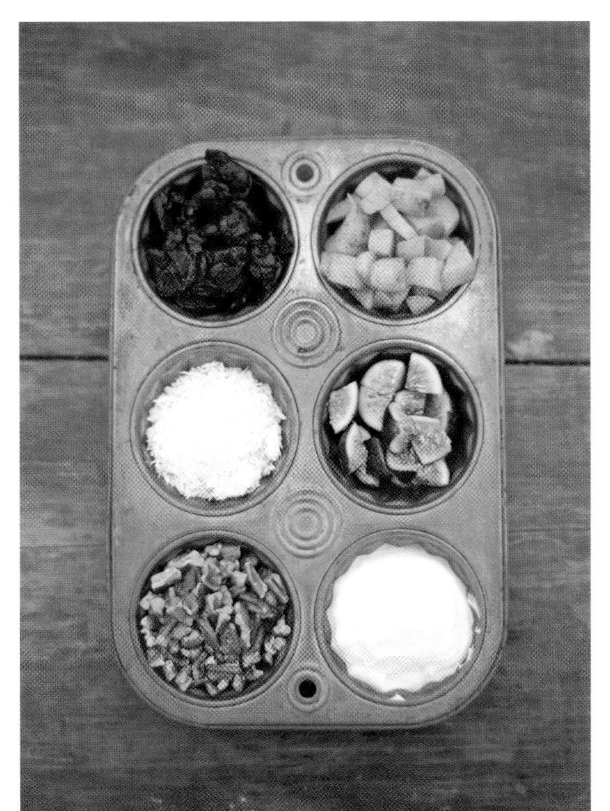

DRIED CHERRIES

WARM CINNAMON PEARS

SHREDDED COCONUT

FRESH FIGS

CHOPPED PECANS

CRÈME FRAÎCHE

Whole30	Substitute ghee for the butter.
Nut-free	Yes
Egg-free	Yes
AIP	Substitute coconut oil for the butter.

Apple Cider and Cinnamon Pulled Pork

Apples and pork are a perfect match for the fall season. If you can't hold an old-fashioned pig roast (page 383), this pulled pork is the next best thing. It's sweet and a little salty, and just wonderful with Brussels sprouts, cabbage, or other greens. You can use leftovers to make Apple Curry Pork Cakes with Brussels Sprouts (page 286).

Serves 4 to 6

- *3 tablespoons sea salt*
- *3 tablespoons ground cumin*
- *1 tablespoon ground cinnamon*
- *2 tablespoons minced garlic*
- *1 teaspoon grated fresh ginger*
- *4 pounds boneless pork butt (shoulder meat), with some of the excess fat trimmed*
- *2 cups apple cider or apple juice*
- *2 medium apples, any variety, peeled and cut into large pieces*

1. Preheat the oven to 350°F.
2. In a small bowl, mix together the salt, spices, garlic, and ginger.
3. Season the pork with the spice mixture and place it in a braising pan. Add the apple cider and apples.
4. Place in the oven and roast for 4 hours.
5. Remove from the oven and discard the liquid. Allow to cool for 30 minutes.
6. Remove any extra fat and, using 2 forks, shred the meat, mashing the soft apples and mixing them in.

Shown with Spicy Red Cabbage Slaw (page 280) and Roasted Sweet Potatoes with Sweet and Savory Toppings (page 282).

NOTES: *You can also use pears in place of the apples.*

Whole30	Yes
Nut-free	Yes
Egg-free	Yes
AIP	Omit the cumin.

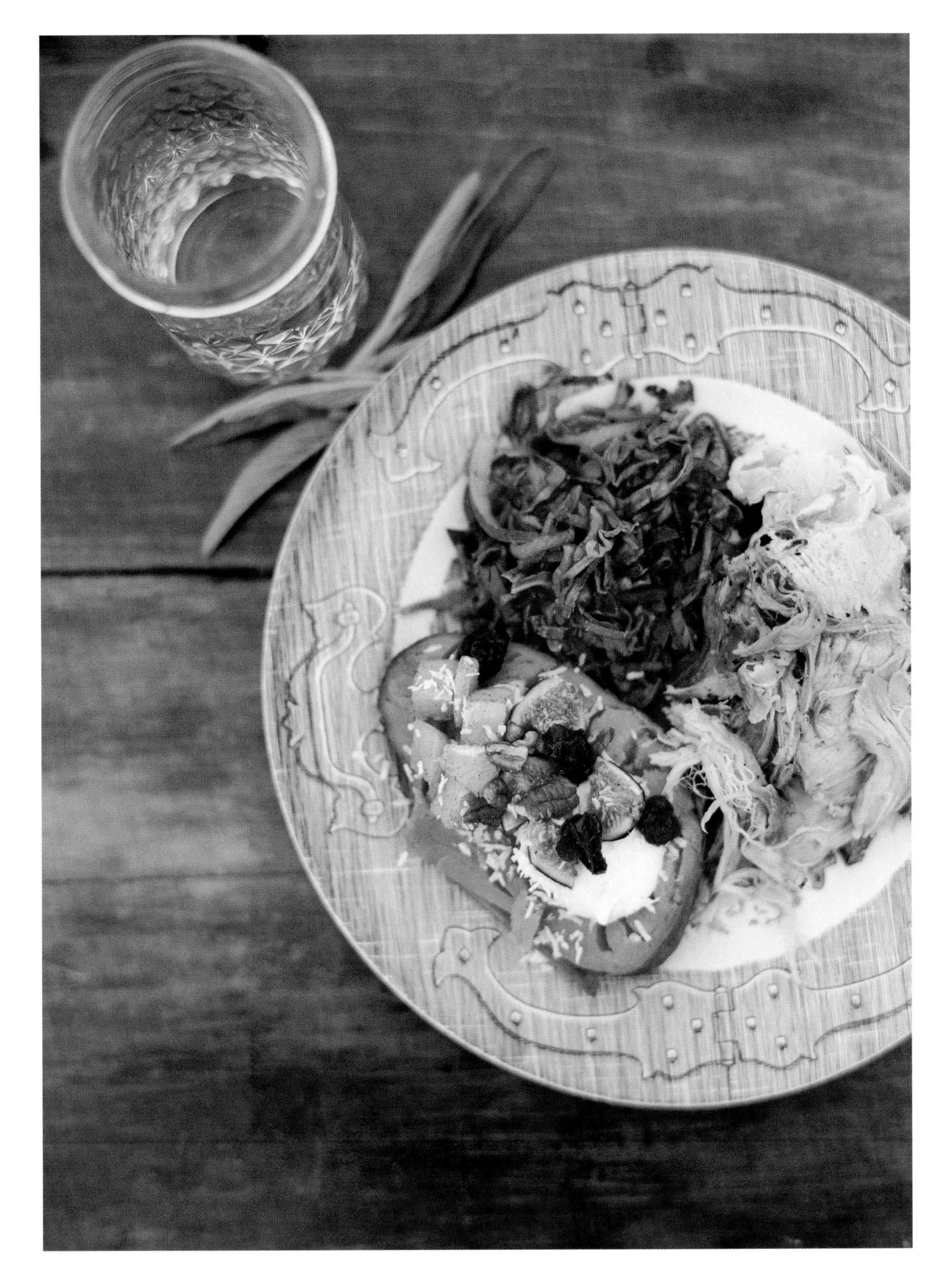

Apple Curry Pork Cakes with Brussels Sprouts

These cakes are to die for. They're sweet from the apples and have a warm curry flavor, with a little crunch from the Brussels sprouts. It takes a little time to make them, so plan on filling your house with the sweet smell of cider on a chilly Sunday afternoon. My husband likes to eat them with spicy kimchee on the side. A crunchy and tart salad would also be great with these, and leftovers are amazing for breakfast with a fried egg on top.

Makes about 16 small cakes, serving 4 to 8

- *4 cups Apple Cider and Cinnamon Pulled Pork (page 284)*
- *2 cups shredded Brussels sprouts*
- *¼ cup minced red onion*
- *½ cup chopped fresh cilantro leaves*
- *3 eggs*
- *½ cup potato starch*
- *2 teaspoons curry powder*
- *⅛ teaspoon sea salt*
- *Pinch of ground cinnamon*
- *1 tablespoon coconut oil, plus more as needed*

1. In a large bowl, combine the pork with the Brussels sprouts, onion, and cilantro.
2. In a separate bowl, whisk together the eggs, potato starch, curry powder, salt, and cinnamon.
3. Add the egg mixture to the pork mixture and mix until thoroughly combined.
4. Warm a skillet over medium heat. Melt 1 tablespoon of coconut oil in the pan.
5. While the oil is heating up, use your hands to form the mixture into small cakes about 4 inches in diameter and 1½ inches thick.
6. Fry the cakes in batches, 4 at a time, until brown on the bottom, about 5 minutes. Then flip, flatten with a spatula, and cook for another 3 minutes, until browned on both sides.
7. Repeat with the remainder of the cakes until you have cooked the entire batch. Add more coconut oil to the pan between batches if needed.
8. Serve with a fried egg on top or with a green salad.

NOTES: *You can substitute cabbage for the Brussels sprouts.*

Whole30	Yes
Nut-free	Yes
Egg-free	No
AIP	No

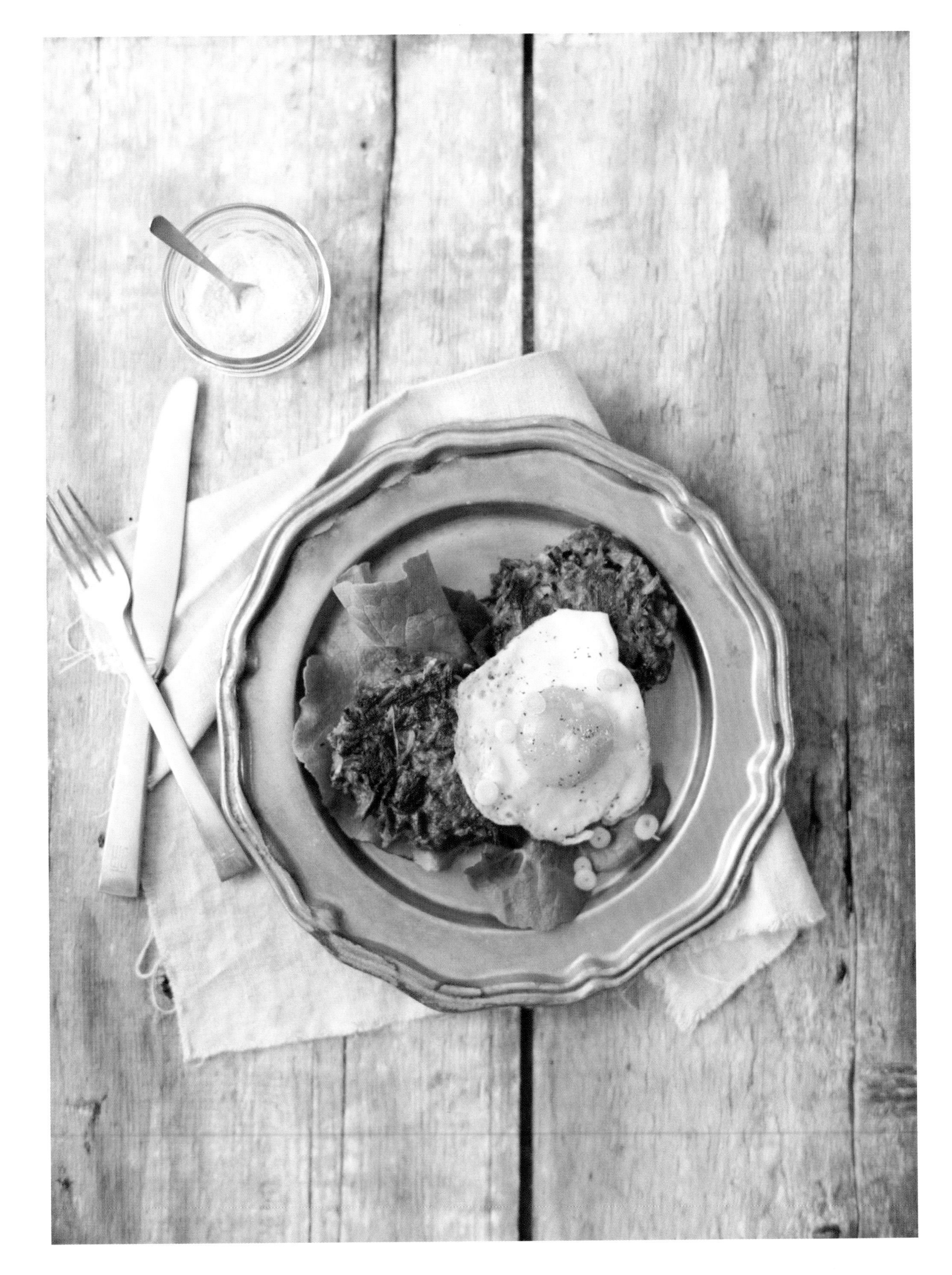

Cajun Rabbit Stew with Andouille Sausage and Mushrooms

As this Cajun-inspired dish bubbles away, the amazing scent filling your home will really get your mouth watering. Don't be scared at the thought of eating rabbit. It tastes just like dark chicken meat—in fact, if I didn't know better, I would have sworn these rabbit legs came from a bird. Even better, rabbit scores much higher than chicken legs in niacin and vitamins B6 and B12. Rabbit also has more iron, more protein, fewer calories, and less omega-6 fatty acids than chicken. I say rabbit is a winner! The best part is, my whole family loves it. Try it with Quick and Dirty Cauliflower Rice (page 299), as shown.

Serves 4

- *4 rabbit legs or 1 whole rabbit, cut into parts*
- *1 tablespoon ghee (page 347)*
- *1 medium yellow onion, diced*
- *4 stalks celery, diced*
- *4 large carrots, peeled and diced*
- *2 cups diced green and red bell peppers*
- *1 jalapeño pepper, seeded and minced*
- *Pinch to ⅛ teaspoon cayenne pepper*
- *¼ teaspoon ground black pepper*
- *1 tablespoon minced garlic*
- *½ pound andouille sausage, diced*
- *2 cups mushrooms (assorted varieties), chopped or halved*
- *2 cups homemade chicken stock (page 338) or water (see Note)*
- *3 tablespoons arrowroot starch*
- *3 tablespoons cold water*
- *2 tablespoons minced fresh cilantro leaves, for garnish*

1. Bring the rabbit to room temperature. Set aside.
2. In a Dutch oven or large soup pot, warm the ghee over medium-high heat.
3. Working in batches, fry the rabbit legs on both sides until brown. Remove to a plate.
4. Turn the heat down to medium and add the onion, celery, carrots, bell peppers, jalapeño, cayenne pepper, black pepper, and garlic. Sauté for 10 minutes, or until soft.
5. Add the sausage, mushrooms, and chicken stock. Stir to combine, and place the rabbit parts on top of the mixture.
6. Cover and simmer for 1 hour.
7. After 1 hour, remove the rabbit to a plate. Increase the heat slightly and maintain a rapid simmer for 20 minutes, uncovered, to help reduce the liquid.
8. Mix the arrowroot starch with the cold water in a small bowl. Turn off the heat and stir in the arrowroot slurry to thicken the stew. Remove the stew from the heat. If you continue to cook it after adding the arrowroot slurry, it will lose its thickness.
9. Taste and adjust the seasoning, if needed (though the sausage is pretty salty, so it's unlikely you'll need more salt). Garnish with the cilantro and serve.

NOTES: *Store-bought chicken stock will make this stew too salty, so if you don't have any homemade stock, just use water. If you don't have access to rabbit, substitute 3 pounds of chicken or duck legs, skin removed.*

Whole30	Yes
Nut-free	Yes
Egg-free	Yes
AIP	Omit the bell peppers, cayenne pepper, and black pepper. Use a sausage that does not have added pepper or fennel. Substitute bacon fat for the ghee.

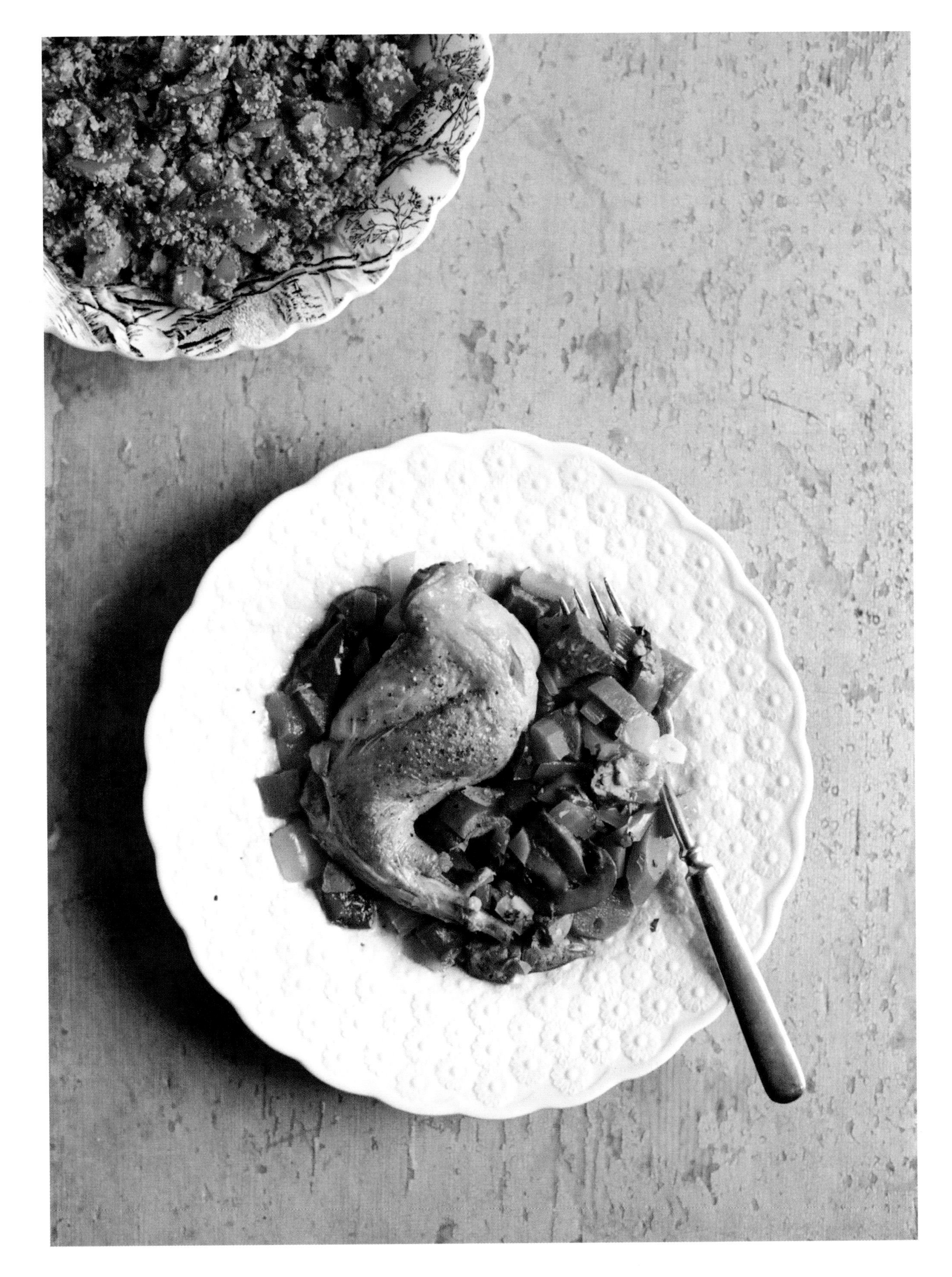

Indian Lamb Stew with Spinach

Also called Indian or vine spinach, Malabar spinach is a succulent type of vine-growing spinach that is easy to grow. It's widely used in India and Africa in soups and stews. I love to use it in this stew, but if you can't find it, the recipe also works with standard spinach, or even chard or kale. Sometimes, greens can get lost in a stew, so sautéing them with a little garlic and adding them at the end, when they are still bright and flavorful, is a fun twist. This curry-style stew is lovely with a dollop of whole-milk yogurt on top. It's a perfect dish for a cool fall night.

Serves 4 to 6

- *2 tablespoons ghee (page 347)*
- *2 pounds lamb or goat stew meat*
- *2 cups diced white or yellow onions*
- *3 cloves garlic, minced*
- *3 tablespoons grated ginger*
- *1½ cups diced tomatoes (or canned, if tomato season has passed)*
- *2 teaspoons red chili powder*
- *2 teaspoons sea salt*
- *½ teaspoon turmeric*
- *1 jalapeño pepper, seeded and diced*

For the topping

- *½ pound Malabar spinach or regular spinach*
- *1 tablespoon ghee (page 347)*
- *1 clove garlic, minced*
- *Juice of ½ lime*
- *4 to 6 tablespoons whole-milk yogurt or crème fraîche (page 347), for garnish (optional)*

1. Preheat the oven to 275°F.
2. In a large Dutch oven, warm the ghee over medium heat.
3. Add the lamb and sauté until browned on all sides.
4. Add the onions, garlic, ginger, tomatoes, chili powder, salt, turmeric, and jalapeño and continue cooking for 10 minutes, until the onions are soft.
5. Add enough water to just cover the meat.
6. Cover the pot and place in the oven for 3 hours.
7. Remove from the oven and adjust the seasoning, if needed. Set aside.
8. To make the topping, slice the spinach into ¼-inch-wide strips.
9. Heat the ghee in a skillet over medium heat. Add the garlic and spinach and sauté for just a few minutes, until bright green. Remove from the heat and stir in the lime juice.
10. To serve, ladle a serving of the stew into a bowl. Top each bowl with some of the sautéed greens and, if you wish, a tablespoon of yogurt.

NOTES: *You can substitute beef stew meat for the lamb, if you wish.*

Whole30	Omit the yogurt and crème fraîche.
Nut-free	Yes
Egg-free	Yes
AIP	Substitute the same amount of canned pumpkin for the tomatoes and omit the chili powder and jalapeño. Substitute coconut oil for the ghee. Omit the yogurt and crème fraîche.

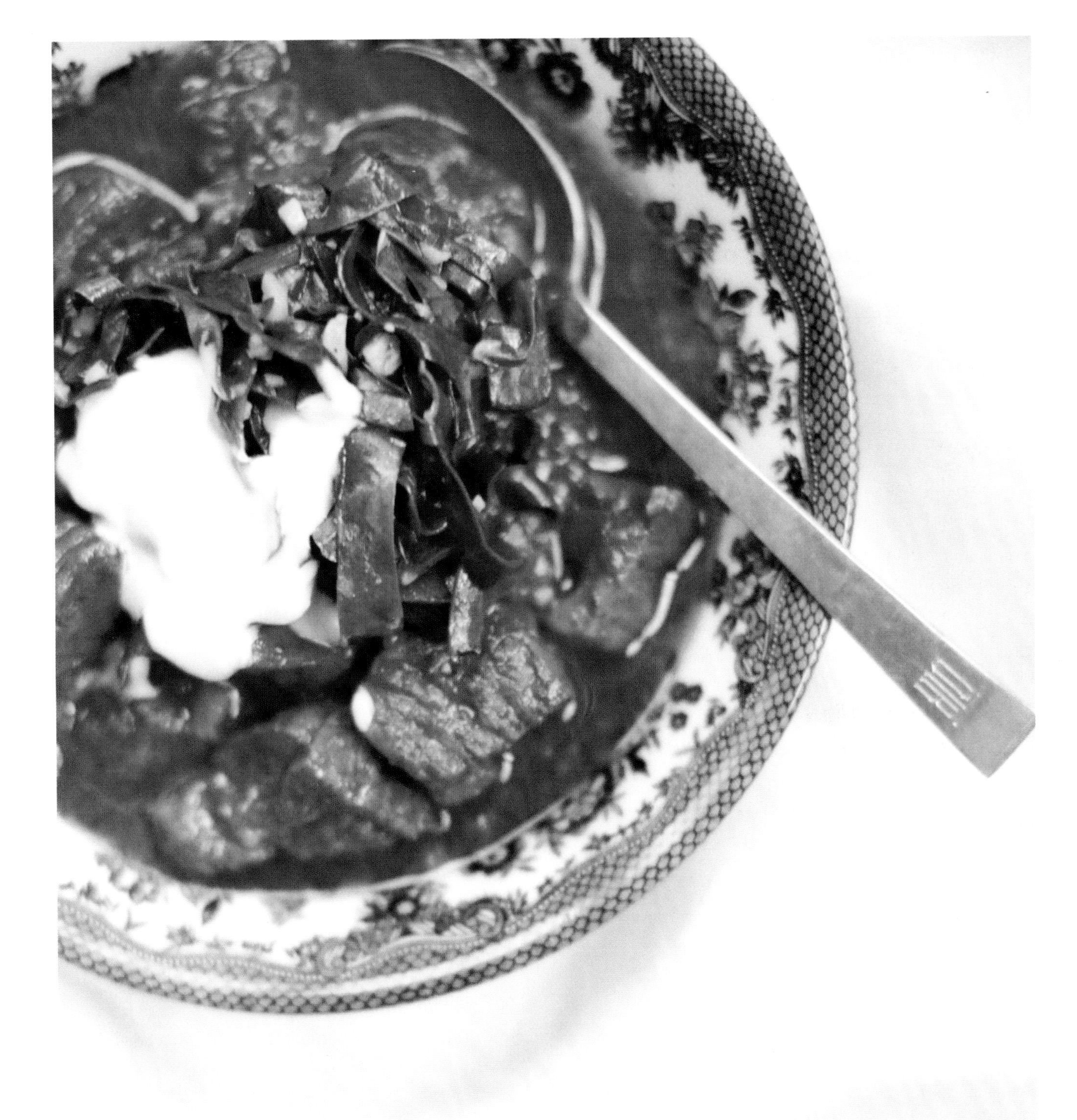

Rosemary Potato Stacks

My family absolutely loves potatoes Anna. The classic French dish is basically layers of thin potato coins cooked in butter in a large cast-iron skillet. I thought it would be interesting to try making individual servings, stacking the potatoes in a muffin tin and roasting them until crisp. The result is crunchy, buttery, and delicious. Serve it alongside any roasted meat.

Serves 4 to 6

- *2 pounds Yukon Gold or other waxy potatoes*
- *⅔ cup unsalted butter (page 348) or ghee (page 347)*
- *1 tablespoon minced garlic*
- *Juice of 1 lemon*
- *1 tablespoon minced fresh rosemary leaves*
- *1 teaspoon sea salt, plus a bit more for topping*
- *½ teaspoon ground black pepper*

1. Peel the potatoes and slice on a mandoline to 1/16 inch thick. Place the potatoes in a bowl.
2. Preheat the oven to 350°F.
3. Melt the butter in a small saucepan. Add the garlic and lemon juice.
4. Brush the cups of a muffin tin with the butter mixture. Cut out small circles of parchment paper and place in the bottoms of the greased muffin cups.
5. Divide the rosemary among the muffin cups, placing it on top of the parchment paper.
6. Pour about ½ teaspoon of the melted butter into each muffin cup, on top of the rosemary.
7. Pour the rest of the butter mixture over the potatoes and add the salt and pepper. Mix well.
8. Divide the potato slices among the muffin cups. Press down when done. Cover with parchment paper.
9. Place in the oven and bake for 30 minutes.
10. Remove from the oven and turn the heat up to 425°F.
11. Line a rimmed baking sheet with parchment paper.
12. With a spoon, carefully remove each potato stack and invert it onto the baking sheet, removing the round of parchment paper that is now on top. Adjust the stacks to stand straight if needed.
13. Sprinkle generously with salt.
14. Return to the oven and roast for another 20 minutes, or until golden brown.

Whole30	Use ghee, not butter.
Nut-free	Yes
Egg-free	Yes
AIP	Make this recipe with sweet potatoes or turnips. Substitute bacon fat for the butter. Omit the black pepper.

NOTES: *Instead of rosemary, try using fresh oregano or basil.*

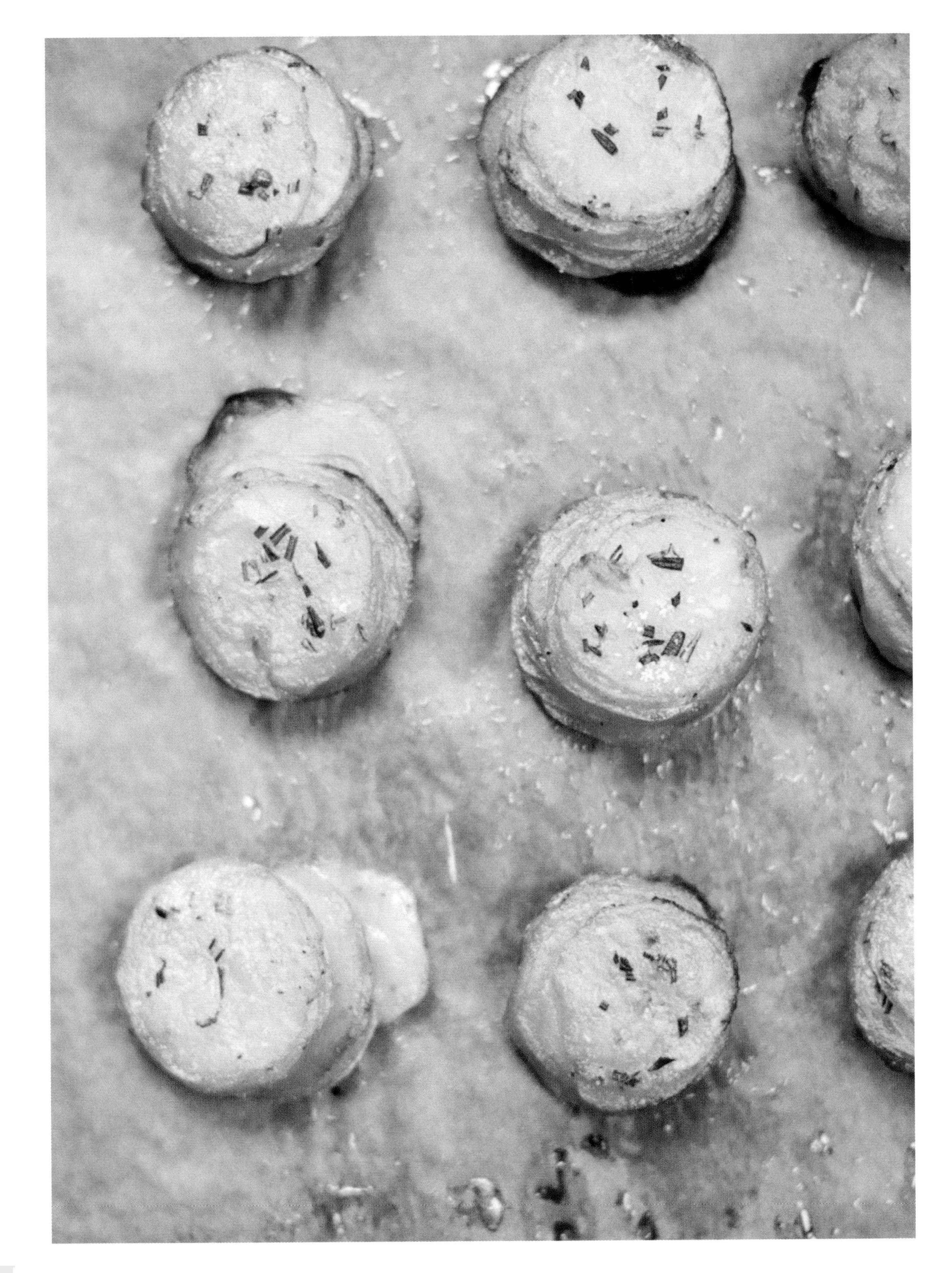

Roasted Marrowbones with Parsley-Fennel Salad

Marrowbones are one of my son's favorite things to eat. They cook very quickly and are full of nutrient-dense goodness. They are also very rich, so this tart parsley-fennel salad is a great side. I also like to serve these with briny cornichons and Salted Herb Crackers (page 298). Give marrow a try—it couldn't be easier to prepare, and it's one of the best primal foods there is! You can ask your butcher to slice the bones down the middle, which makes them a bit easier to eat, and when you're done, add the bones to a broth to infuse it with more minerals.

Serves 6 as a rich appetizer

- *3 marrowbones, sliced lengthwise down the middle by your butcher*
- *Sea salt and ground black pepper*

For the salad

- *1 cup thinly sliced fennel bulb*
- *½ cup finely diced yellow onions*
- *2 tablespoons capers with juice*
- *1 cup chopped fresh parsley leaves*
- *Juice of 1 lemon*
- *6 sprigs fresh thyme, for garnish*

Accompaniments

- *30 cornichons*
- *Salted Herb Crackers (page 298)*

Whole30	Omit the crackers.
Nut-free	Yes
Egg-free	Yes
AIP	Omit the black pepper and cornichons, and serve on cucumbers instead of crackers.

1. Preheat the oven to 425°F. Line a rimmed baking sheet with parchment paper.

2. Place the marrowbones, cut side up, on the baking sheet. Sprinkle with salt and pepper.

3. Roast for about 12 minutes.

4. While the bones are roasting, combine the fennel, onions, capers, parsley, and lemon juice in a bowl.

5. Remove the bones from the oven and place one on each plate. Serve with the parsley salad, cornichons, and crackers, and garnish with a sprig of fresh thyme.

NOTES: *Marrow is best eaten with a slender spoon or spread onto crackers with a little knife.*

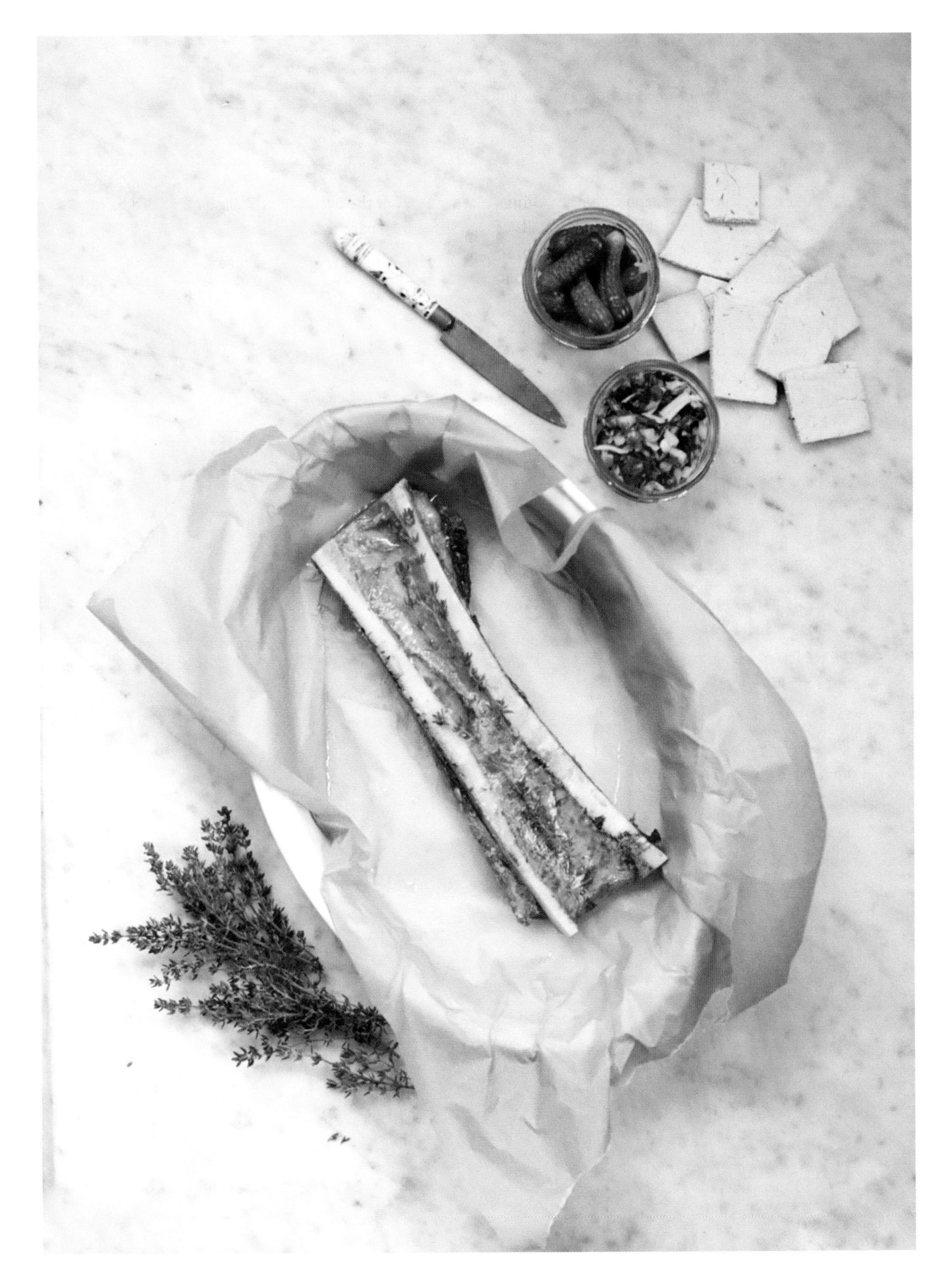

Bagna Cauda

My husband and I were lucky enough to travel to the Piedmont region of northern Italy a few years back, when we were U.S. delegates to the Slow Food International conference. This lovely hot dip is traditionally served as an appetizer there. It's a simple dish with many variations based on the town or family. *Bagna cauda* literally translates as "hot bath," and it's usually served as part of a celebration and is meant to be shared.

Serves 6

- *6 tablespoons unsalted butter (page 348)*
- *8 cloves garlic, minced*
- *⅓ cup cold-pressed, extra-virgin olive oil*
- *1 (2-ounce) tin anchovies, chopped*
- *⅛ teaspoon red pepper flakes*
- *1 tablespoon minced fresh parsley leaves*

- *Assorted seasonal vegetables, raw or blanched, for dipping (see suggestions at right)*

1. In a small saucepan, melt the butter over medium heat.
2. Add the garlic and sauté for a few minutes; do not brown.
3. Add the olive oil, anchovies, and red pepper flakes and bring to a simmer. Cook for 5 minutes.
4. Right before serving, add the parsley.
5. Serve warm with vegetables for dipping. If you want to stay true to tradition, serve it in a small fondue pot to keep it warm.

VEGETABLE SUGGESTIONS

Steamed cauliflower and broccoli florets
Blanched string beans
Boiled potatoes, sliced or quartered
Sliced bell peppers
Sliced cabbage
Sliced cucumbers
Sliced fennel bulb
Sliced leeks
Sliced radishes
Sliced zucchini or summer squash
Endives, radicchio, or other bitter, firm greens

NOTES: *Don't be afraid of anchovies—you won't know you're eating little fish!*

Whole30	Substitute ghee for the butter.
Nut-free	Yes
Egg-free	Yes
AIP	Substitute chicken stock for the butter and omit the red pepper flakes. Do not include potatoes or peppers among the assorted seasonal vegetables.

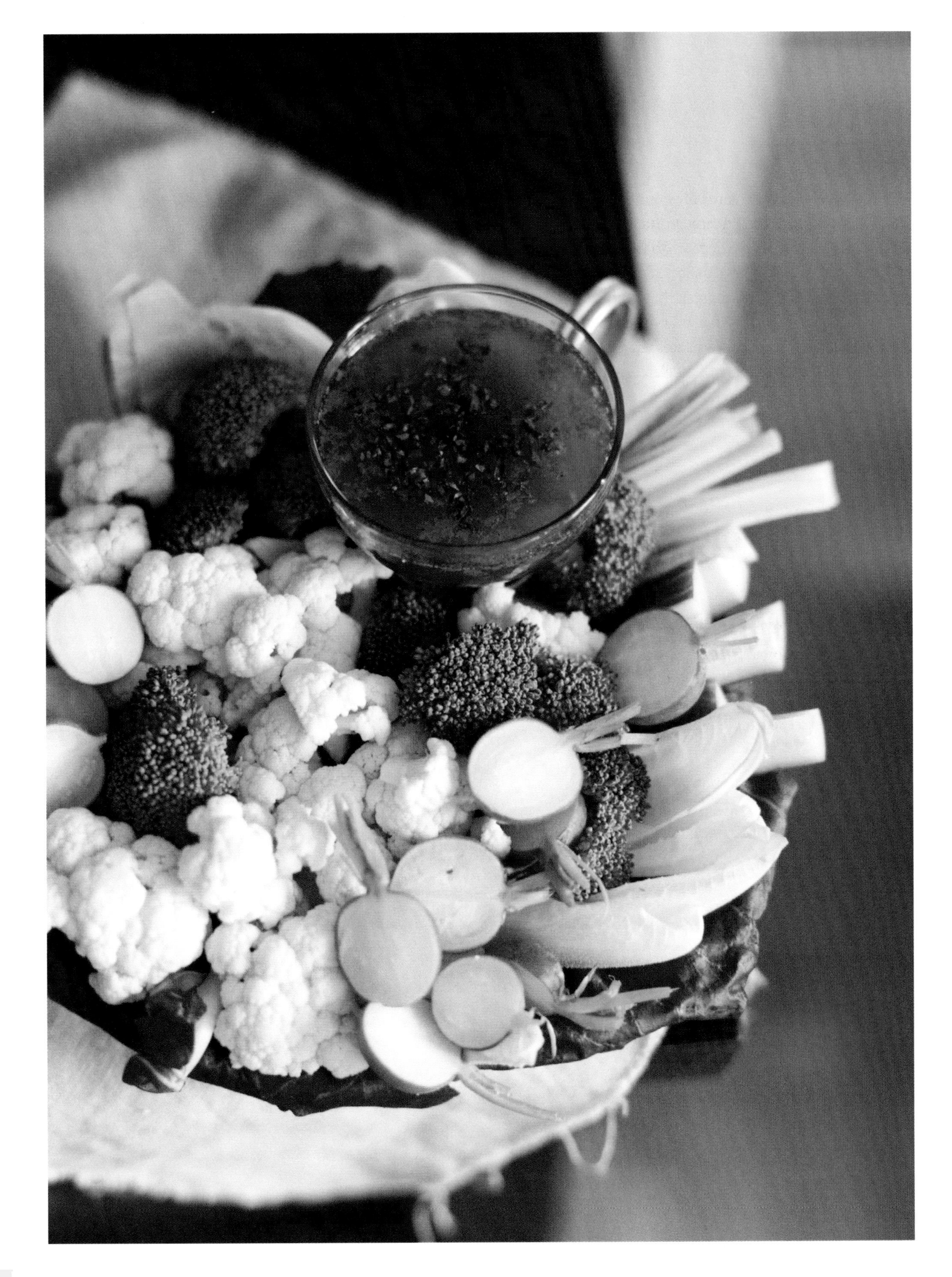

Salted Herb Crackers

These crackers are to die for—crunchy, salty, and extremely flavorful. Feel free to play around with the herbs to come up with your own creation. Fresh basil, mint, tarragon, or thyme would also work well, and a tablespoon of minced sundried tomatoes is a wonderful addition. These are excellent with my Primal Crostini Neri (page 300), and they're excellent with chicken liver pâté. Make sure you roll out the dough very thin, to get the right texture and crunch.

Makes about 20 crackers

- *1 cup tapioca starch*
- *½ cup coconut flour*
- *½ teaspoon sea salt, plus more to sprinkle on top*
- *½ teaspoon ground black pepper*
- *1 tablespoon chopped fresh rosemary, thyme, or sage leaves*
- *1 tablespoon minced fresh chives*
- *½ teaspoon garlic powder*
- *½ teaspoon onion powder*
- *2 eggs, beaten*
- *2 tablespoons melted ghee (page 347)*
- *2 tablespoons water*

1. Preheat the oven to 350°F. Line a baking sheet with parchment paper.

2. In a medium-sized bowl, combine the tapioca starch, coconut flour, salt, pepper, herbs, garlic powder, and onion powder and mix well.

3. Add the eggs, ghee, and water and mix with your hands to form a dough ball. It will be very dry at first, but keep working it and a ball will form.

4. Place the dough ball on the baking sheet and flatten it with your hands to about ½ inch thick.

5. Cover with parchment paper and, using a rolling pin, roll out the dough until it is very thin, about 1/8 inch thick. Sprinkle with a small amount of salt, if desired.

6. With a sharp knife, score the dough into 2-by-2-inch squares.

7. Bake for approximately 15 to 20 minutes, until lightly browned. You may have to remove some of the thinner, outer crackers early to prevent burning. Once cool, store them in an airtight container and eat within a few days (if you don't eat them all in 2 minutes!).

See photo on page 301.

Whole30	No
Nut-free	Yes
Egg-free	No
AIP	No

Quick and Dirty Cauliflower Rice

I know lots of folks who don't eat nutrient-dense organ meats on a regular basis. That's a shame, because even if you don't like the flavor, there are many ways to incorporate it into your diet—often completely undetected. "Dirty rice" is traditionally made with sautéed chicken livers and gizzards, but if you're not used to cooking with liver, using desiccated liver powder—as I do here—is a great way to incorporate liver into your diet without even having to touch it! I also hide a sprinkle of desiccated liver powder in burgers, meatballs, and other dishes. Serve this side with my Cajun Rabbit Stew with Andouille Sausage and Mushrooms (page 288). You'll never know you're eating liver!

Serves 4

- *1 medium to large head cauliflower*
- *1 tablespoon bacon fat*
- *2 cups diced yellow onions*
- *2 cups diced celery*
- *1 teaspoon dried oregano leaves*
- *1 teaspoon dried thyme leaves*
- *1 teaspoon minced garlic*
- *1 cup diced green bell peppers*
- *1½ tablespoons desiccated liver powder or ¼ cup cooked and minced chicken livers (see Notes)*
- *½ teaspoon paprika (if you want it a bit spicy, use hot smoked paprika)*
- *Sea salt and ground black pepper*

Whole30	Yes
Nut-free	Yes
Egg-free	Yes
AIP	Omit the bell peppers, paprika, and black pepper.

1. Break the cauliflower into florets.
2. In a food processor, pulse the cauliflower into small pieces. You will need to work in batches; it won't all fit at once.
3. In a large skillet with deep sides, warm the bacon fat over medium heat.
4. Sauté the onions, celery, oregano, thyme, garlic, and bell peppers for 10 minutes, or until the onions are soft.
5. Add the cauliflower and continue to sauté for another 5 minutes.
6. Add the liver powder and paprika and stir well.
7. Season with salt and pepper to taste.

See photo on page 289.

NOTES: *For desiccated liver powder, I like the brand Radiant Life (for where to buy, see Resources, page 398). If the idea of eating liver freaks you out, you can omit it altogether.*

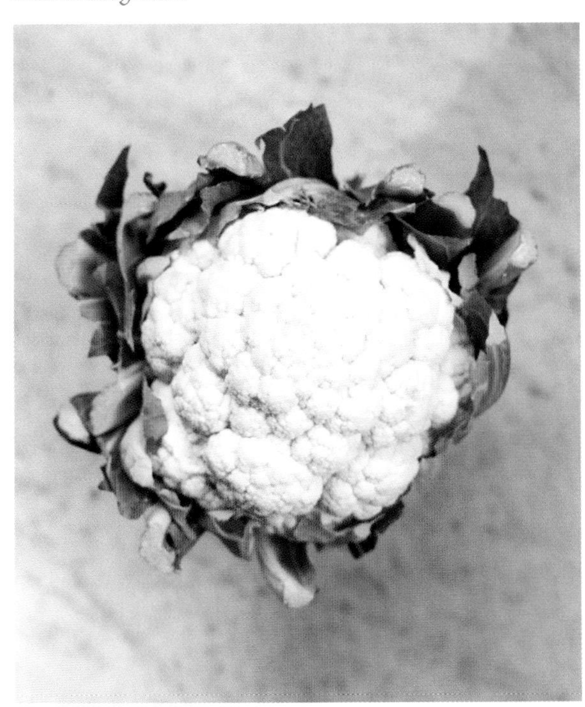

Primal Crostini Neri

If you think you don't like liver, give this pâté a shot. I still have a bit of a hard time with organ meats, which is why I keep desiccated liver powder on hand and add it to meatballs and stews. This pâté, however, will change your mind about chicken liver. It's got chunky carrots and lots of herbs mixed in, and it's wonderful served on Salted Herb Crackers (page 298). The inspiration for this recipe came from a friend of mine who lives in northern Italy; it's her favorite way to eat liver.

Makes about 3 cups of pâté, serving 8

- *½ cup unsalted butter (page 348)*
- *1 pound chicken livers, rinsed*
- *½ medium red onion, diced*
- *1 medium carrot, diced small*
- *1 stalk celery, diced small*
- *3 tablespoons capers, rinsed*
- *1 tablespoon ground sage*
- *1 tablespoon chopped fresh rosemary leaves*
- *¼ cup white wine, homemade chicken stock (page 338), or water*
- *1 tablespoon anchovy paste*
- *¼ cup minced fresh parsley leaves*
- *¼ teaspoon ground black pepper (or more to taste)*
- *Sea salt (if needed)*
- *1 batch Salted Herb Crackers (page 298) or 4 to 6 apples, sliced, for serving*

1. In a large skillet, melt the butter. Add the chicken livers, onion, carrot, celery, capers, sage, and rosemary and cook for about 40 minutes, stirring occasionally.
2. Allow to cool slightly, then place in a food processor and pulse about 10 times.
3. Add the white wine and anchovy paste and pulse twice more to mix.
4. Remove the mixture to a bowl and stir in the parsley and black pepper.
5. Taste and adjust the salt and pepper as needed. The anchovy paste and capers are pretty salty, so it's unlikely you'll need more salt, but you may prefer a bit more pepper.
6. Serve with crackers or sliced apples.

Shown with Salted Herb Crackers (page 298).

NOTES: *Try to use pasture-raised, organic chicken livers. It's better for the chickens, the environment, and you!*

Whole30	No
Nut-free	Yes
Egg-free	Yes
AIP	No

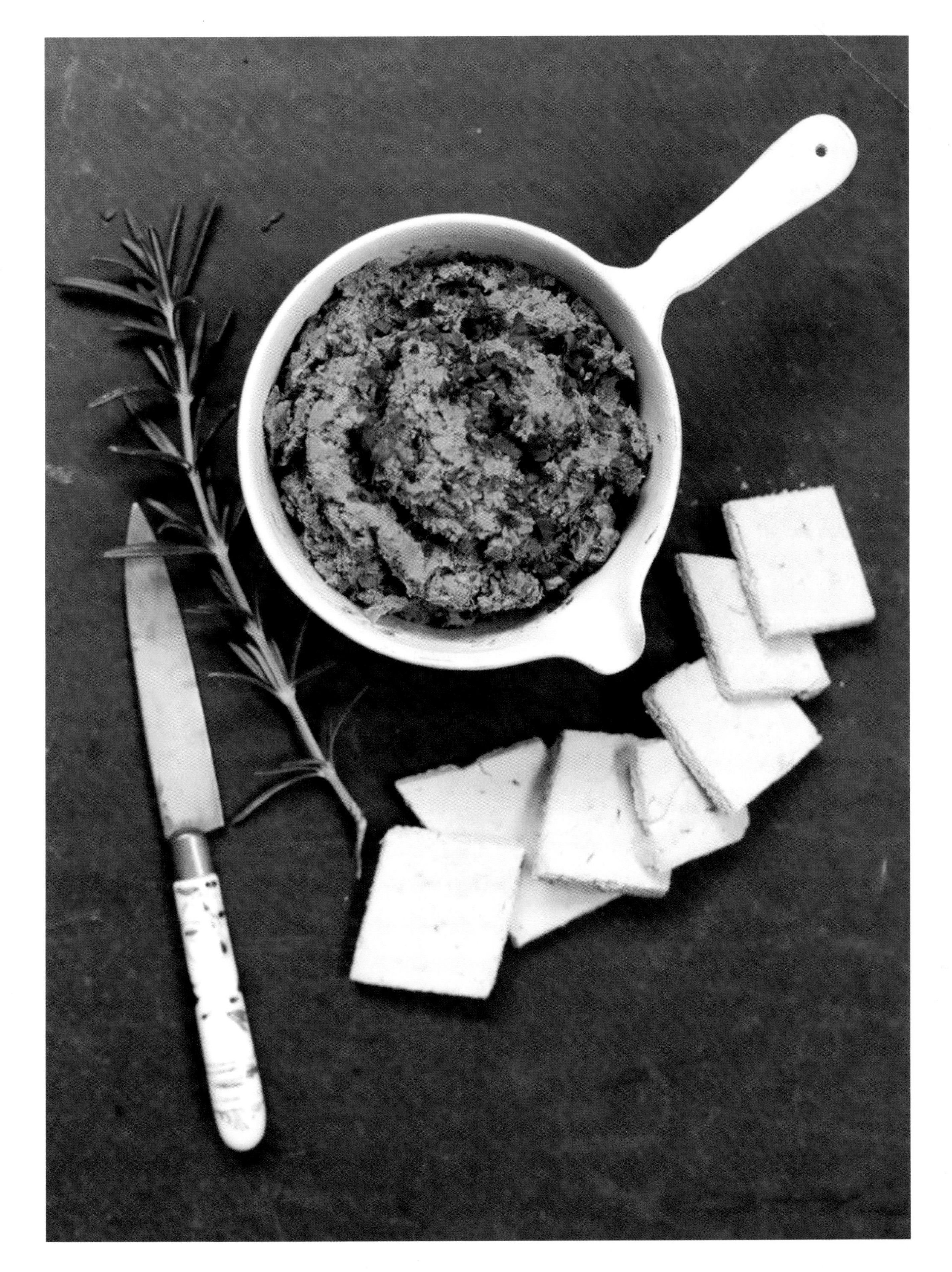

Roasted Cauliflower with Apples, Bacon, and Balsamic Vinegar

This recipe was inspired by a surprise trip to Montreal that my husband took me on for my birthday. Montreal is one of my absolute favorite cities, and it has an amazing food scene. When the restaurant Joe Beef was too crowded, we ended up at their new wine bar up the street, where we were served at picnic tables on the patio. My favorite dish was a whole roasted cauliflower covered in vinegar and served with chicken skin. When we got home, I re-created the dish, but with a few changes: I added apples, replaced the chicken skin with bacon, and used pieces of cauliflower instead of the whole head, so it takes a little less time to cook. This one is a winner!

Serves 4 to 6

- *1 head cauliflower, cut into florets*
- *2 tablespoons aged balsamic vinegar*
- *4 Granny Smith apples or other firm, tart variety, peeled and cut into thick slices*
- *4 strips bacon, chopped*
- *Sea salt and ground black pepper*

1. Marinate the cauliflower in the vinegar for 1 hour.
2. Preheat the oven to 400°F. Line a rimmed baking sheet with parchment paper.
3. Spread out the cauliflower and apple slices on the prepared baking sheet and cover with the chopped bacon and generous amounts of salt and pepper.
4. Cover the baking sheet with another piece of parchment paper and roast for 40 minutes.
5. Remove from the oven and uncover. Using a spatula, flip the cauliflower mixture.
6. Place back in the oven and roast for another 15 minutes, or until the cauliflower is tender and the bacon is crisp.

Whole30	Yes
Nut-free	Yes
Egg-free	Yes
AIP	Omit the black pepper.

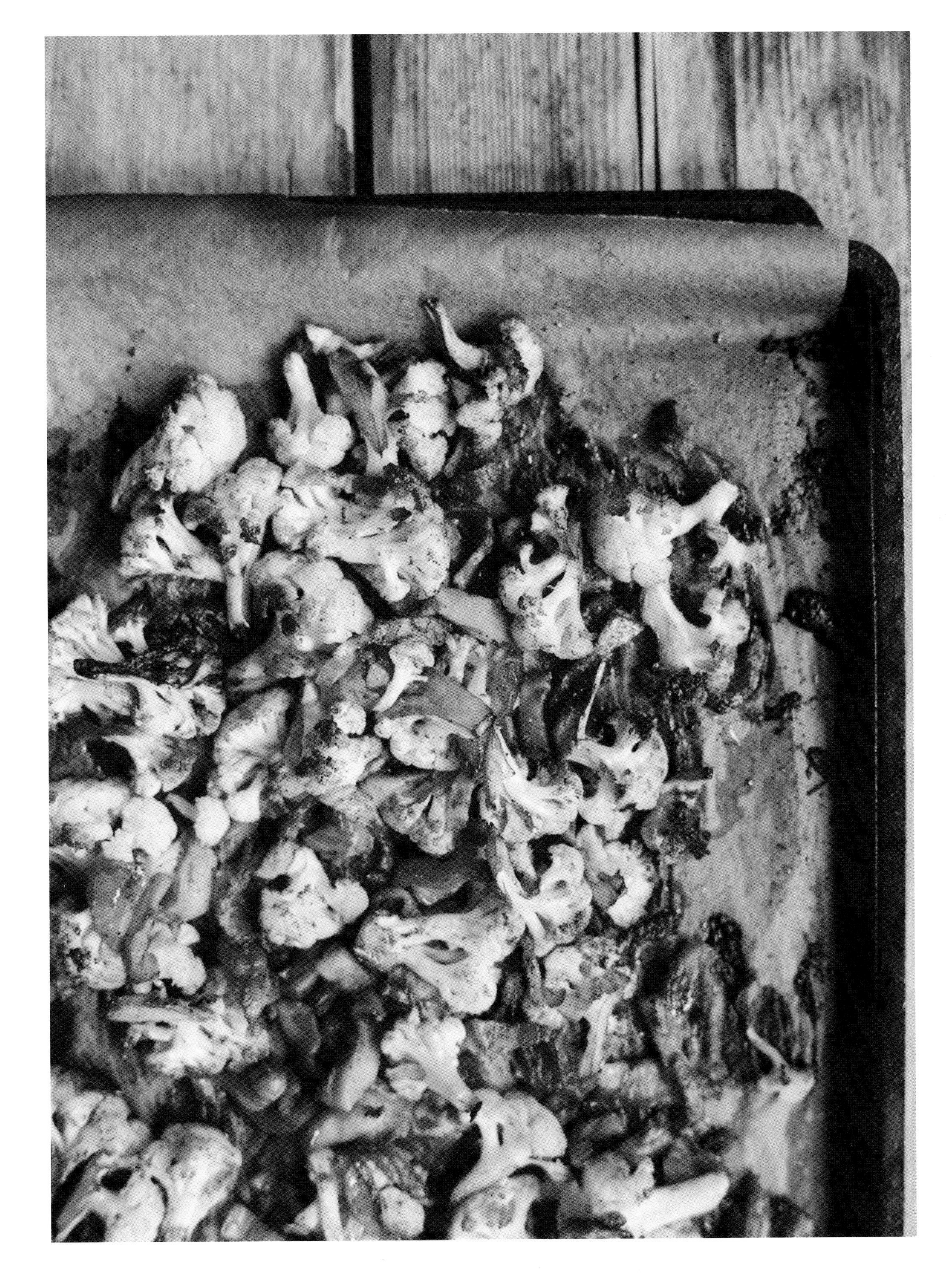

Italian Braised Lamb Shoulder Chops

This is a true homestead comfort dish. Shoulder chops are an inexpensive cut of lamb, and they're full of flavor. But they're also bony and pretty fatty, and folks often have a hard time figuring out how to cook them. I used to sear them in a pan, but the fat would shrink around the meat, making the whole piece distorted and difficult to eat. Braising it, however, takes this cut to a whole new level. With the toppings I suggest here, this is like lamb candy, sweet and fork-tender. Try it with a side of sautéed greens and served over Parsnip Celeriac Mash with Dijon (page 306). You can make this dish in a braising pot or covered casserole dish, if you have one, but a baking dish lined with unbleached parchment paper and then tightly covered with parchment will do the trick just as well, and with less cleanup.

Serves 4

- *1 tablespoon coconut oil or ghee (page 347)*
- *4 (6- to 8-ounce) lamb shoulder chops*
- *Sea salt and ground black pepper*
- *1 cup diced tomatoes*
- *2 tablespoons tomato paste*
- *1 large yellow onion, sliced thin*
- *1 teaspoon dried thyme leaves*
- *1 teaspoon dried oregano leaves*
- *1 teaspoon ground fennel*
- *1 batch Parsnip Celeriac Mash with Dijon (page 306), for serving (optional)*
- *10 sprigs fresh thyme, for garnish*

Whole30	Yes
Nut-free	Yes
Egg-free	Yes
AIP	No

1. Preheat the oven to 300°F. Have a braising pot or covered casserole dish on hand, or prepare a large baking dish by lining it with unbleached parchment paper.

2. In a skillet, heat the coconut oil over medium heat.

3. Season the chops on both sides with salt and pepper, then add them to the hot pan. Sear on both sides, working in batches if necessary to avoid overcrowding the pan. Place the seared chops in the braising pot, casserole dish, or prepared baking dish.

4. Combine the diced tomatoes and tomato paste in a bowl.

5. Cover the chops with the sliced onion and tomato mixture, then sprinkle on the thyme, oregano, and fennel.

6. Place the lid on the braising pot, casserole dish, or baking dish. If your baking dish does not have a tight-fitting lid, place another piece of parchment paper on top and tuck in the edges to create a seal. Braise in the oven for 2 hours, or until the meat is fork-tender. Serve over the parsnip mash, if you like, and garnish with the thyme sprigs.

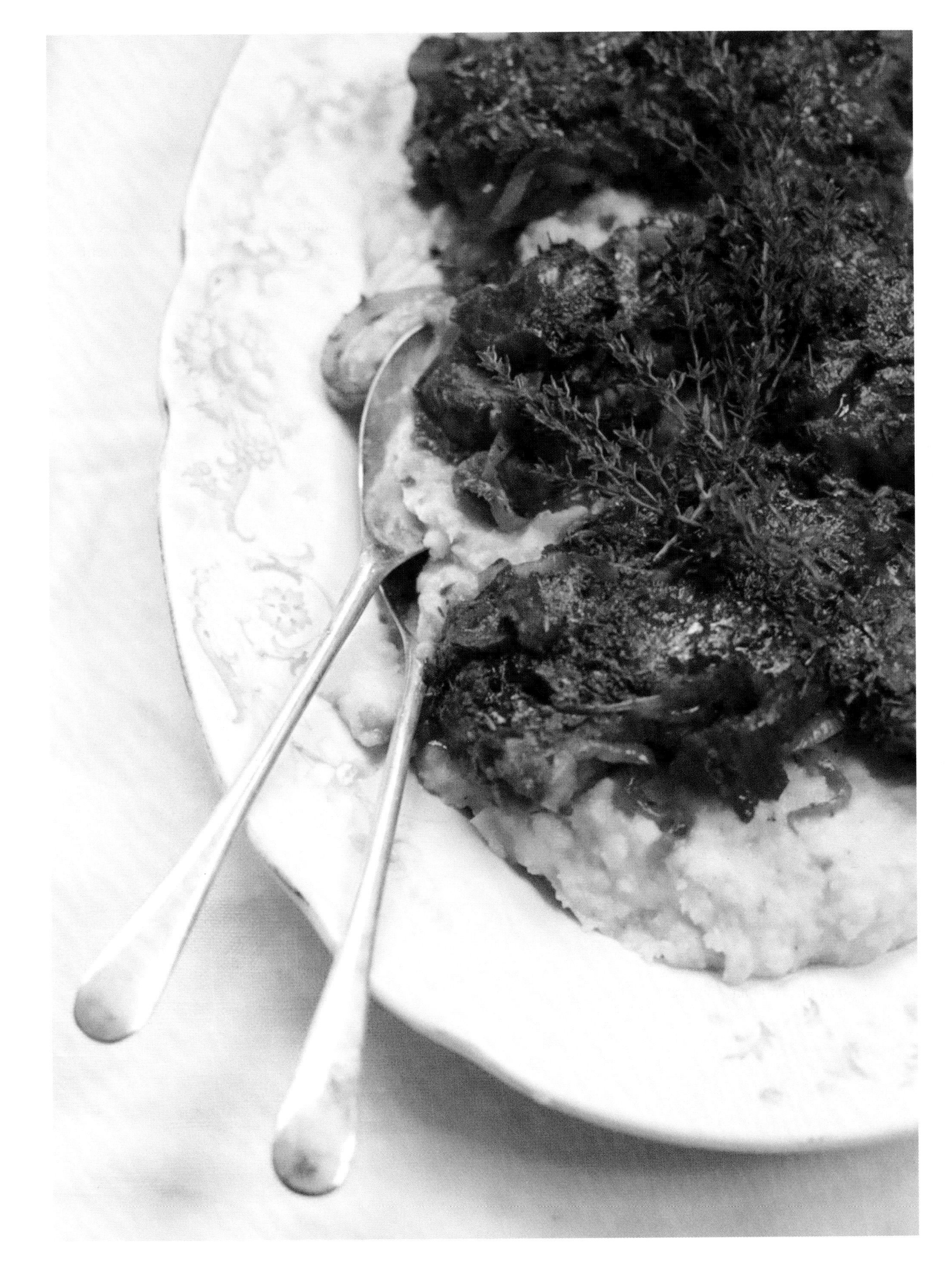

Parsnip Celeriac Mash with Dijon

This mash is a creamy, sweet, and slightly tart alternative to mashed potatoes. Serve it under Italian Braised Lamb Shoulder Chops (page 304) or with Lamb Meatballs with North African Olive Sauce (page 310). It's very easy to make and is just right for soaking up any sauce or as a side to your favorite meats.

Serves 4 to 6

- *2 pounds parsnips, peeled and cut into 1-inch pieces*
- *2 pounds celeriac, peeled and cut into 2-inch chunks*
- *3 cups homemade chicken stock (page 338)*
- *About 1 cup heavy cream or canned, full-fat coconut milk*
- *2 teaspoons Dijon mustard*
- *1 tablespoon minced fresh chives (optional), for garnish*
- *Sea salt and ground black pepper*

1. In a large pot, bring the parsnips, celeriac, and chicken stock to a simmer.
2. Cover and cook for 30 to 40 minutes, until the roots are tender.
3. Without draining the cooking liquid, add the cream and blend until smooth using an immersion blender. Depending on how much stock escaped from the roots while they cooked, you may need slightly more liquid for a smooth mixture.
4. Garnish with chives, if desired, and season with salt and pepper to taste.

See photo on page 305.

NOTES: *Kohlrabi can be used in place of the parsnips.*

Whole30	Use coconut milk, not heavy cream.
Nut-free	Yes
Egg-free	Yes
AIP	Use coconut milk, not heavy cream, and omit the mustard and black pepper.

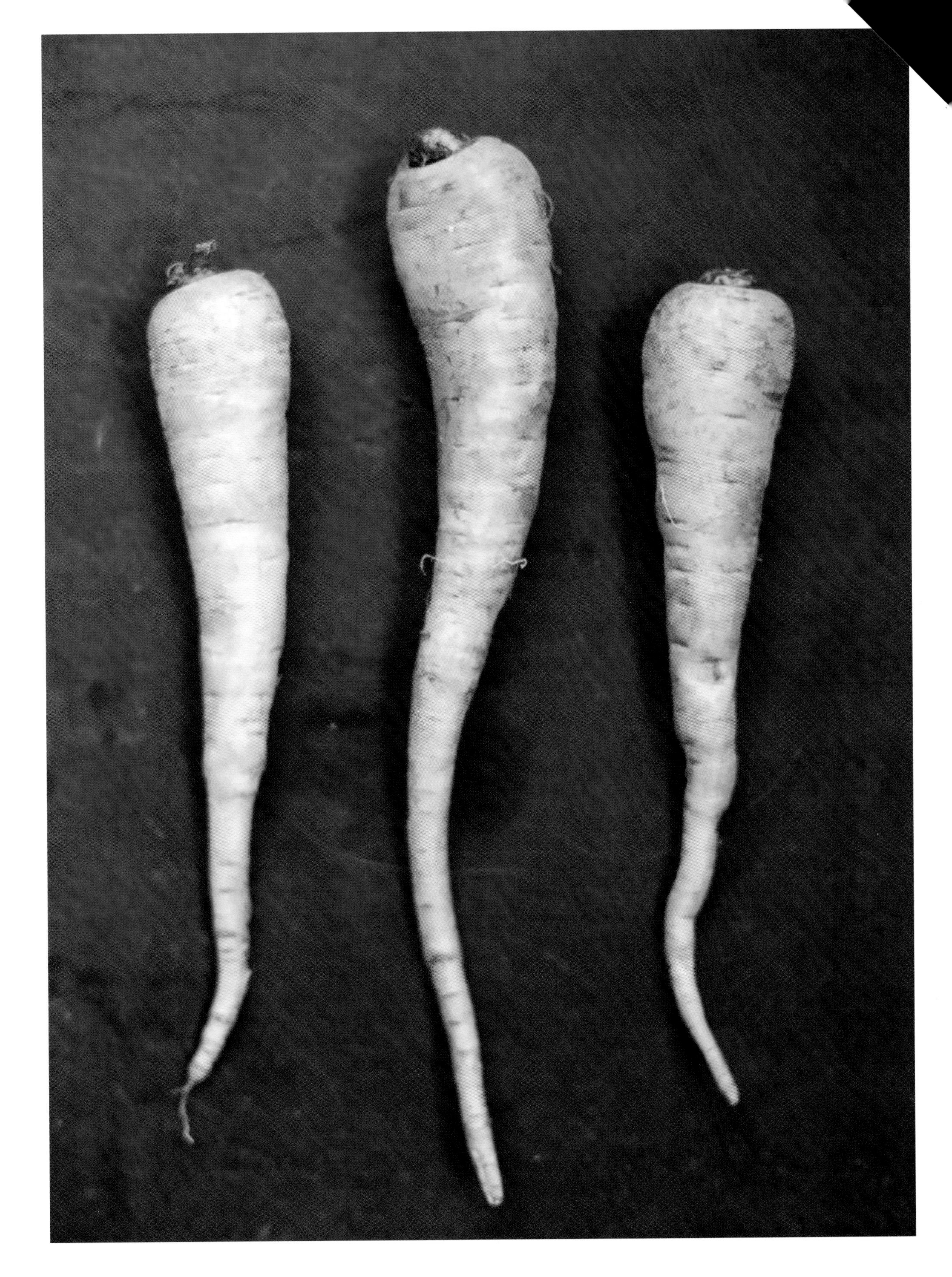

Oven-Roasted Carrots with Orange, Tarragon, and Chives

Once the first frost hits the fields, carrots really come to life and become very sweet. It's my favorite time of year to eat them. Roasted carrots can take a long time to cook if you keep them whole, but they're so strikingly beautiful. This is a fantastic side with any roasted meat. A drizzle of sour cream, yogurt, or crème fraîche is a lovely extra touch.

Serves 4 to 6

- *1½ to 2 pounds slender to medium carrots, peeled (thin ones will cook faster)*
- *⅓ cup orange juice (about 2 large oranges)*
- *2 tablespoons chopped fresh tarragon leaves*
- *1 tablespoon minced fresh chives*
- *Sea salt and ground black pepper*
- *2 tablespoons whole-milk sour cream, yogurt, or crème fraîche (page 347), for garnish (optional)*

1. Preheat the oven to 400°F.
2. In a baking dish or on a rimmed baking sheet lined with parchment paper, coat the carrots in the orange juice.
3. Sprinkle with the fresh tarragon, chives, and generous amounts of salt and pepper.
4. Cover the dish with parchment paper and roast for 30 to 45 minutes, until the carrots are tender.
5. Remove the top sheet of parchment paper, and stir the carrots and toss them in the juice a bit.
6. Place back in the oven and roast, uncovered, until the carrots are light brown and soft, another 10 to 20 minutes (depending on the thickness of the carrots).
7. Drizzle the sour cream, yogurt, or crème fraîche over the top, if you wish.

Whole30	Omit the dairy.
Nut-free	Yes
Egg-free	Yes
AIP	Omit the black pepper and dairy.

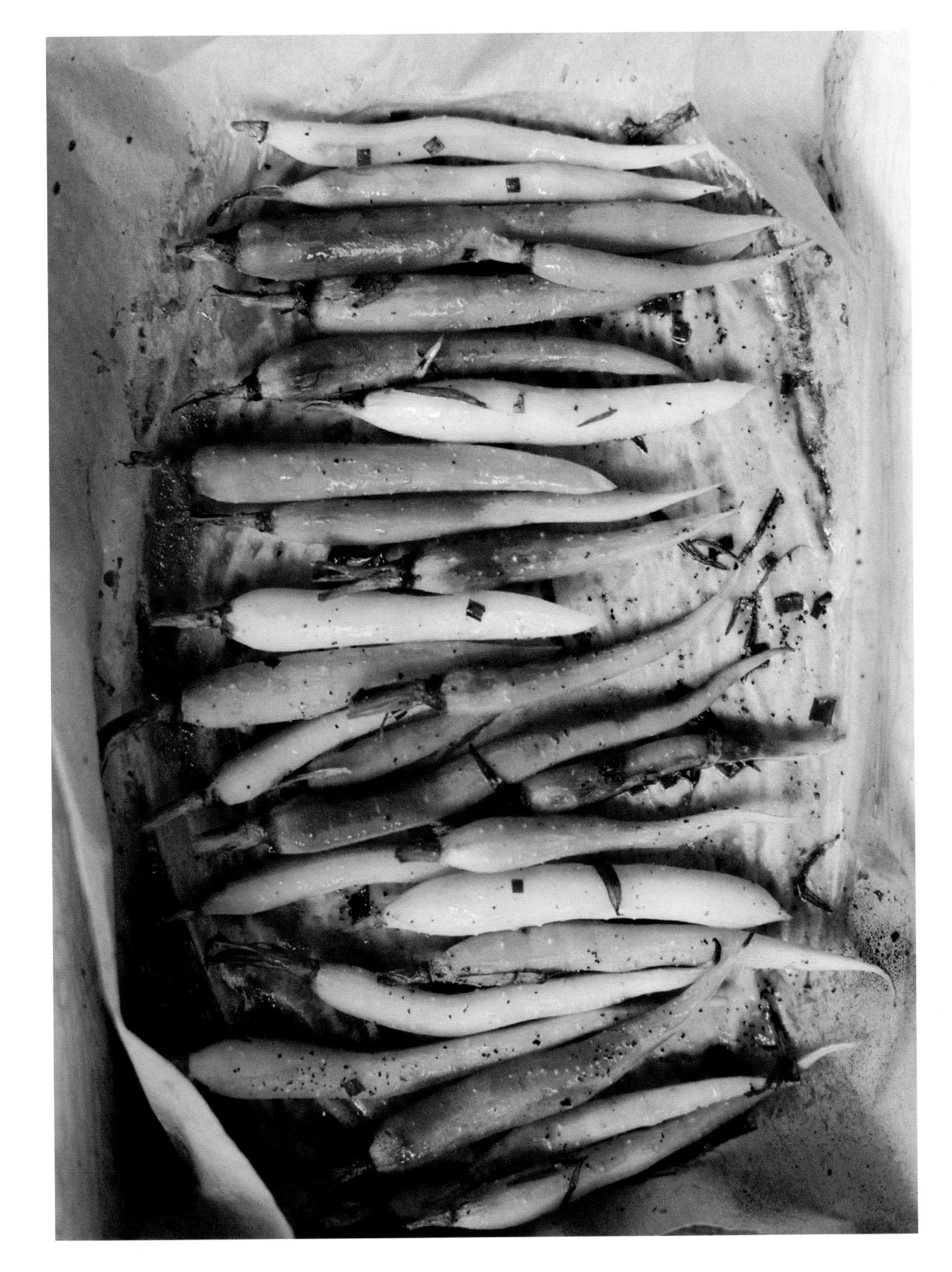

Lamb Meatballs with North African Olive Sauce

This dish is so delicious. The meatballs are moist and full of flavor, and I love the lemony olive sauce that goes along with them. Serve over pureed butternut squash or with Parsnip Celeriac Mash with Dijon (page 306).

Serves 4 to 6

For the meatballs

- *1 egg, beaten*
- *3 tablespoons tomato paste*
- *1 cup cremini mushrooms*
- *½ cup finely chopped fresh cilantro leaves*
- *2 teaspoons ground cumin*
- *1 tablespoon minced fresh ginger*
- *1 tablespoon minced garlic*
- *½ teaspoon sea salt*
- *½ teaspoon ground black pepper*
- *2 pounds ground lamb*

For the sauce

- *2 tablespoons unsalted butter (page 348) or ghee (page 347)*
- *2 cups diced white onion*
- *4 cloves garlic, minced*
- *¼ teaspoon red pepper flakes*
- *1 tablespoon grated lemon zest (about 2 lemons)*
- *¾ cup sliced green olives*
- *1 cup white wine*
- *½ cup homemade chicken stock (page 338)*
- *2 cups diced tomatoes*
- *1 tablespoon tomato paste*
- *⅛ teaspoon ground cinnamon*
- *¼ teaspoon ground black pepper*

1. Preheat the oven to 450°F. Line a rimmed baking sheet with parchment paper.
2. Make the meatballs: In a large bowl, mix together all of the ingredients except the lamb, then add the lamb and mix just until combined. Do not overmix.
3. Using your hands, form the mixture into about 20 to 25 golf ball–sized meatballs and place them on the prepared baking sheet.
4. Bake for 15 minutes, or until browned. When done, place on a wire rack set over a rimmed baking sheet.
5. While the meatballs are cooking, begin the sauce: In a large saucepan, heat the butter and sauté the onions until soft.
6. Add the garlic, red pepper flakes, lemon zest, and olives and cook for another minute.
7. Add the white wine and simmer for about 5 minutes.
8. Add the chicken stock, tomatoes, tomato paste, cinnamon, and black pepper and simmer for 10 minutes.
9. To serve, ladle the sauce over the meatballs.

NOTES: *Feel free to substitute another ground meat if you don't have lamb.*

Whole30	Use ghee, not butter. Omit the wine and increase the total amount of chicken stock to 1½ cups.
Nut-free	Yes
Egg-free	No
AIP	No

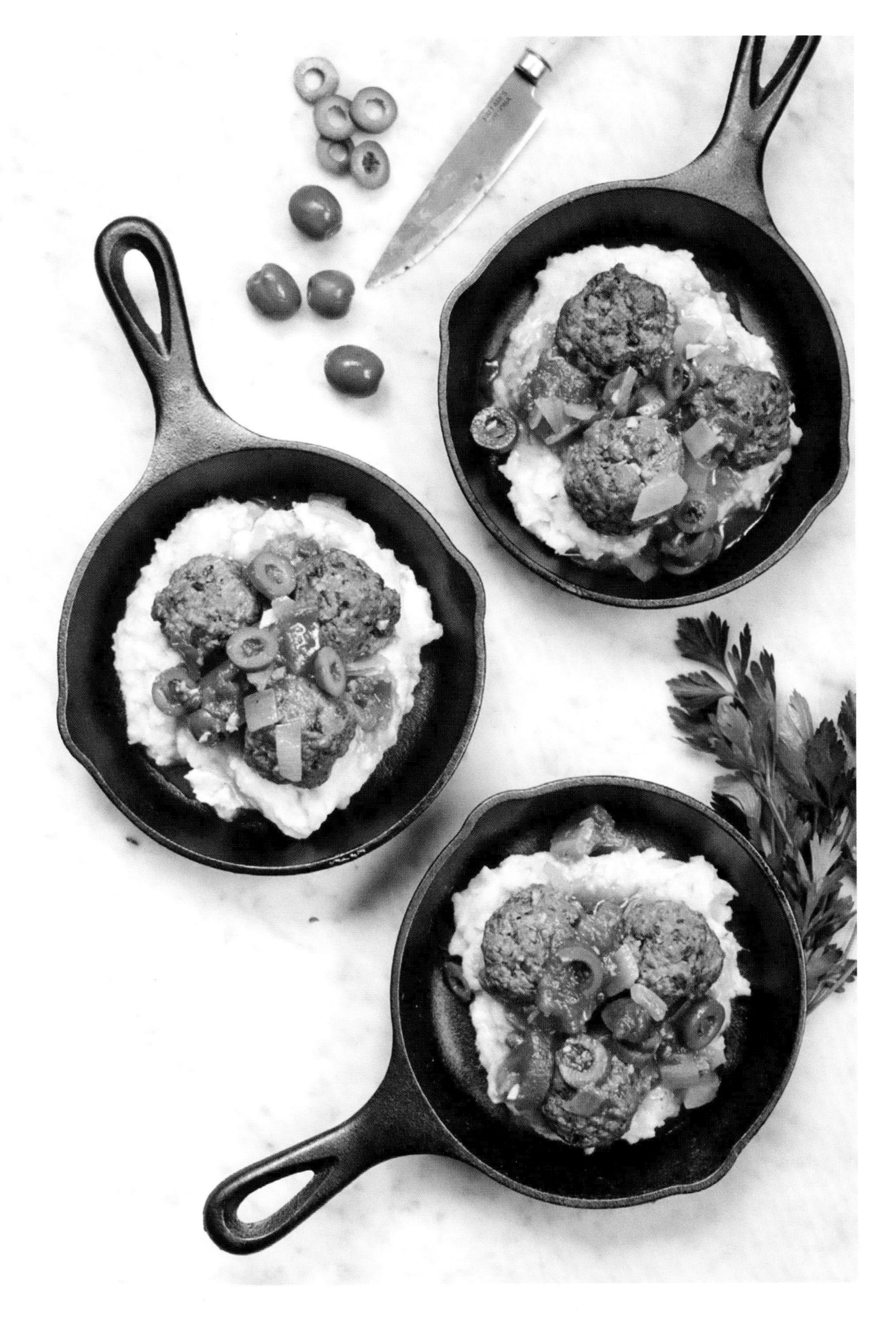

Venison Stew with Orange and Cranberries

Last fall, I visited Plimoth Plantation in Plymouth, Massachusetts, with my children. We were fascinated by the living reenactment of the Wampanoag tribe. They were boiling a stew of cranberries and venison over an open flame, and that inspired me to create this dish, which has become a family favorite. I love making this easy stew on a chilly, windy Sunday. In the winter, we eat a lot of venison, and stews are an easy way to make a lot of nutrient-dense food in one batch. This dish is sweet and really highlights the flavor of the meat. Serve with freshly sautéed vegetables like broccoli or cabbage to brighten it up, if you wish.

Serves 6

- *2½ to 3 pounds venison stew meat, cut into bite-sized pieces*
- *Sea salt and ground black pepper*
- *1 tablespoon bacon fat, ghee (page 347), or coconut oil*
- *1 large yellow onion, diced*
- *4 cloves garlic, minced*
- *2 teaspoons minced fresh ginger*
- *Pinch of dry mustard*
- *Pinch of ground cinnamon*
- *Pinch of ground cloves*
- *Pinch of red pepper flakes*
- *½ cup ruby port*
- *1 orange, rind cut into long strips and flesh diced*
- *½ cup dried cranberries*
- *4 medium carrots, peeled and cut into chunks*
- *2 to 3 purple-top turnips, peeled and cut into chunks*
- *1 cup homemade beef or lamb stock (page 340)*
- *2 tablespoons minced fresh mint leaves, for garnish*

1. Preheat the oven to 325°F.
2. Sprinkle the meat with salt and pepper.
3. In a large Dutch oven or other ovenproof pot with a lid, warm the bacon fat over medium-high heat. Brown the meat in batches.
4. When you've finished the last batch, return all of the meat to the pan. Add the onion, garlic, ginger, and spices and cook for 5 minutes.
5. Add the port and deglaze the pot with a spatula, scraping up all the pieces of venison that are stuck to the pan. Simmer for a few minutes to reduce.
6. Add the orange rind and flesh, cranberries, carrots, turnips, and beef stock. Cover the pot and place in the oven for 2 hours.
7. Remove from the oven. Discard the orange rind and season the stew with salt and pepper to taste. Garnish with fresh mint.

NOTES: *Goat, beef, or lamb stew meat also works well if you can't find venison. Purple-top turnips are the most common type of white-fleshed turnip, easily found at farmers markets and grocery stores.*

Whole30	Use apple juice instead of port.
Nut-free	Yes
Egg-free	Yes
AIP	Use apple juice instead of port. Omit the black pepper, mustard, ground cloves, and red pepper flakes.

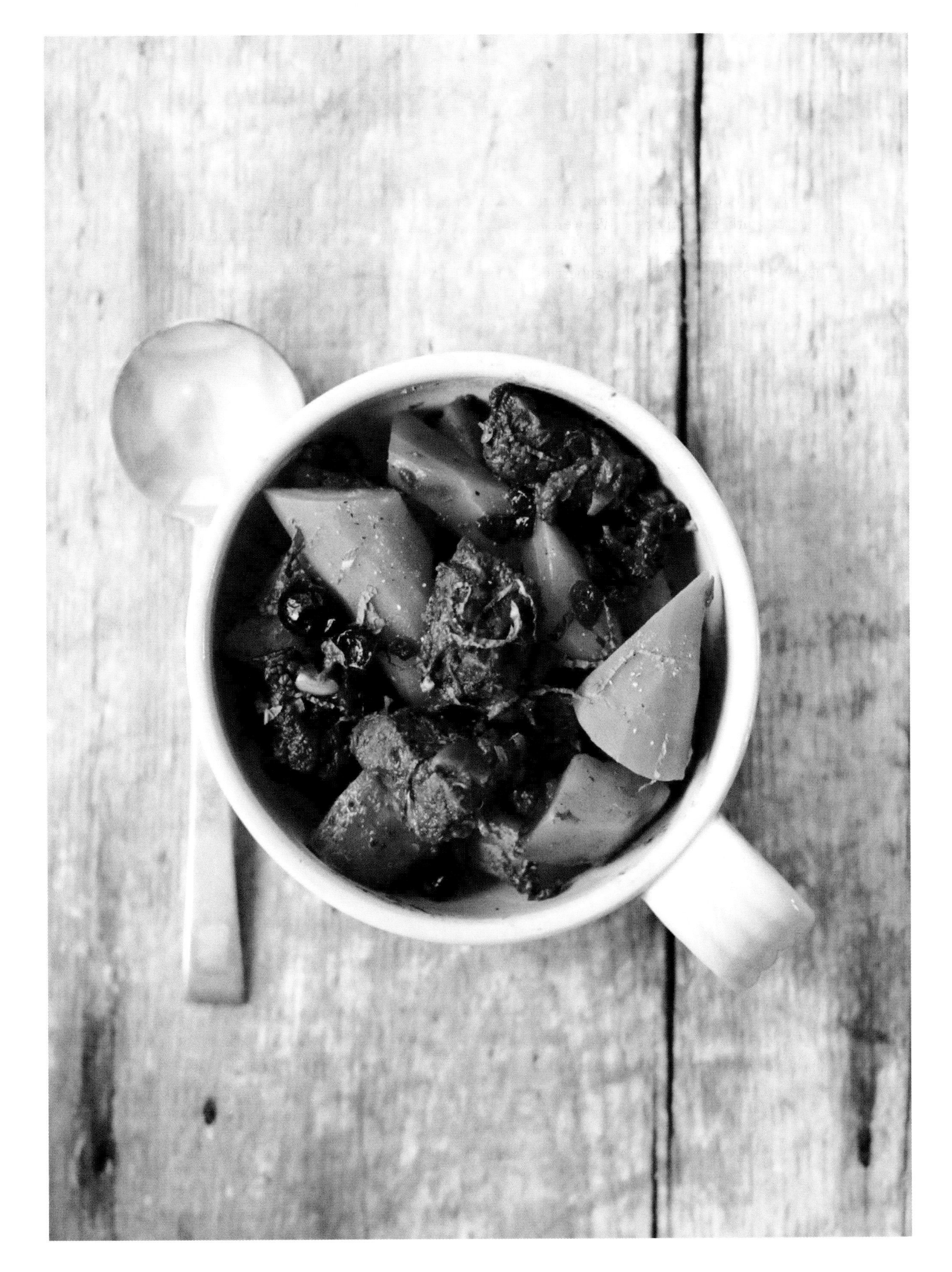

Winter Mushroom Soup

This silky soup is very indulgent, especially when drunk from a mug by the fire. It's a regular dish in my winter rotation. I just can't get enough of it.

Serves 4 to 6

- *½ cup dried porcini mushrooms*
- *1 cup warm water*
- *5 tablespoons unsalted butter (page 348), divided*
- *1½ pounds yellow onions, sliced thin*
- *1 teaspoon dried thyme leaves*
- *1 pound portobello mushrooms, sliced thin*
- *1 quart homemade chicken stock (page 338)*
- *2 ounces high-quality dry sherry (optional)*
- *Sea salt and ground black pepper*
- *4 ounces chanterelles, morels, or cremini mushrooms, sliced, for garnish*
- *½ cup minced fresh parsley leaves, for garnish*
- *Truffle oil, for garnish (optional)*

1. Soak the porcini mushrooms in the warm water while you prepare the rest of the dish.
2. Melt 4 tablespoons of the butter in a heavy soup pot over medium heat.
3. Add the onions and thyme and cook (don't brown) for 5 minutes, lowering the heat if needed.
4. Add the portobello mushrooms and cook for another 5 minutes.
5. Add the porcini and their soaking water and raise the heat to a rapid simmer to reduce the liquid for 5 minutes.
6. Add the chicken stock and simmer for 1 hour.
7. Remove the pot from the heat and puree the soup with an immersion blender.
8. Add the sherry, if using, and salt and pepper to taste.
9. In a separate saucepan, heat the remaining tablespoon of butter over medium-high heat. Sear the 4 ounces of fresh mushrooms in the butter for a few minutes per side.
10. To serve, ladle out the soup and garnish with the parsley and a few of the seared mushrooms. Add a drizzle of truffle oil, if you wish!

Whole30	Omit the sherry. Substitute ghee for the butter.
Nut-free	Yes
Egg-free	Yes
AIP	Substitute coconut oil for the butter. Omit the sherry and black pepper.

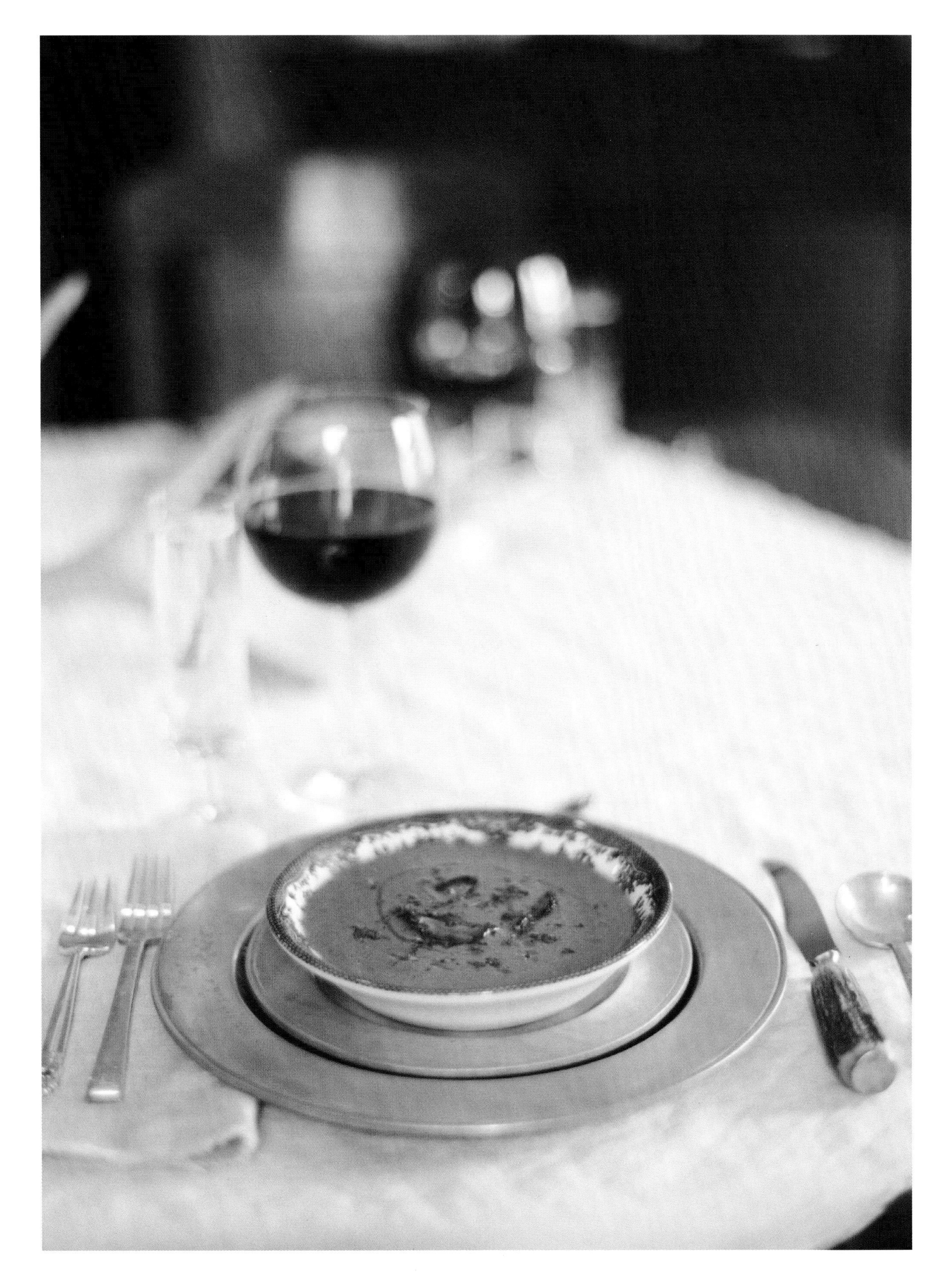

Venison with Red Currant Sauce

This classic sauce, which is also called Cumberland sauce, is sweet and savory and really easy to make. It's excellent with all kinds of game, including duck, goose, elk, or any other rich meat, but we really love it with the fresh venison we receive from friends every fall.

Serves 4 to 6

- *1 (3-pound) venison rib roast (backstrap), in one piece (see Notes)*
- *Sea salt and ground black pepper*
- *1 tablespoon bacon fat, coconut oil, or ghee (page 347)*

For the sauce

- *1 tablespoon unsalted butter (page 348) or ghee (page 347)*
- *1 shallot, minced*
- *½ cup ruby port*
- *½ cup homemade chicken stock (page 338)*
- *Grated zest of 1 orange*
- *Grated zest of 1 lemon*
- *¼ cup red currant jelly (not jam; no sugar added)*
- *⅛ teaspoon grated fresh ginger*
- *⅛ teaspoon ground black pepper*
- *Pinch of ground cinnamon*
- *Pinch of dry mustard*
- *Pinch of cayenne pepper*

Whole30	Use ghee in the sauce, not butter. Substitute apple juice for the port.
Nut-free	Yes
Egg-free	Yes
AIP	Substitute coconut oil for the butter or ghee in the sauce. Substitute apple juice for the port. Omit the black pepper, mustard, and cayenne..

1. Allow the meat to sit on the counter for about 30 minutes to come to room temperature.

2. Season the meat generously with salt and pepper.

3. In a heavy skillet, warm the cooking fat over medium-high heat. Sear the venison on all sides.

4. Reduce the heat to low and cover with a lid. Cook, rotating occasionally, until the internal temperature reaches 135°F. Depending on the thickness of the meat, this could take about 45 minutes. I usually stick in a digital meat thermometer after 20 minutes and leave it there for easy temperature checks.

5. Remove the meat to a cutting board and allow it to rest while you make the sauce.

6. In the same pan, melt the butter over medium-low heat and cook the shallot until soft (do not brown).

7. Add the port and deglaze the pan with a spatula, scraping up all the pieces of venison that are stuck to the pan.

8. Add the rest of the sauce ingredients and allow to simmer for 10 minutes.

9. To serve, slice the meat into ¾-inch-thick pieces and coat with the sauce.

Shown with Mashed Turnips with Potatoes, Leeks, and Apples (page 318) and Lemony Brussels Sprouts with Pancetta and Oyster Mushrooms (page 319).

NOTES: *If you can't find a venison rib roast, you can use two tenderloins; just tie the pieces together with twine so they cook evenly. If you can't get your hands on venison rib roast or tenderloin, feel free to substitute pork or beef tenderloin.*

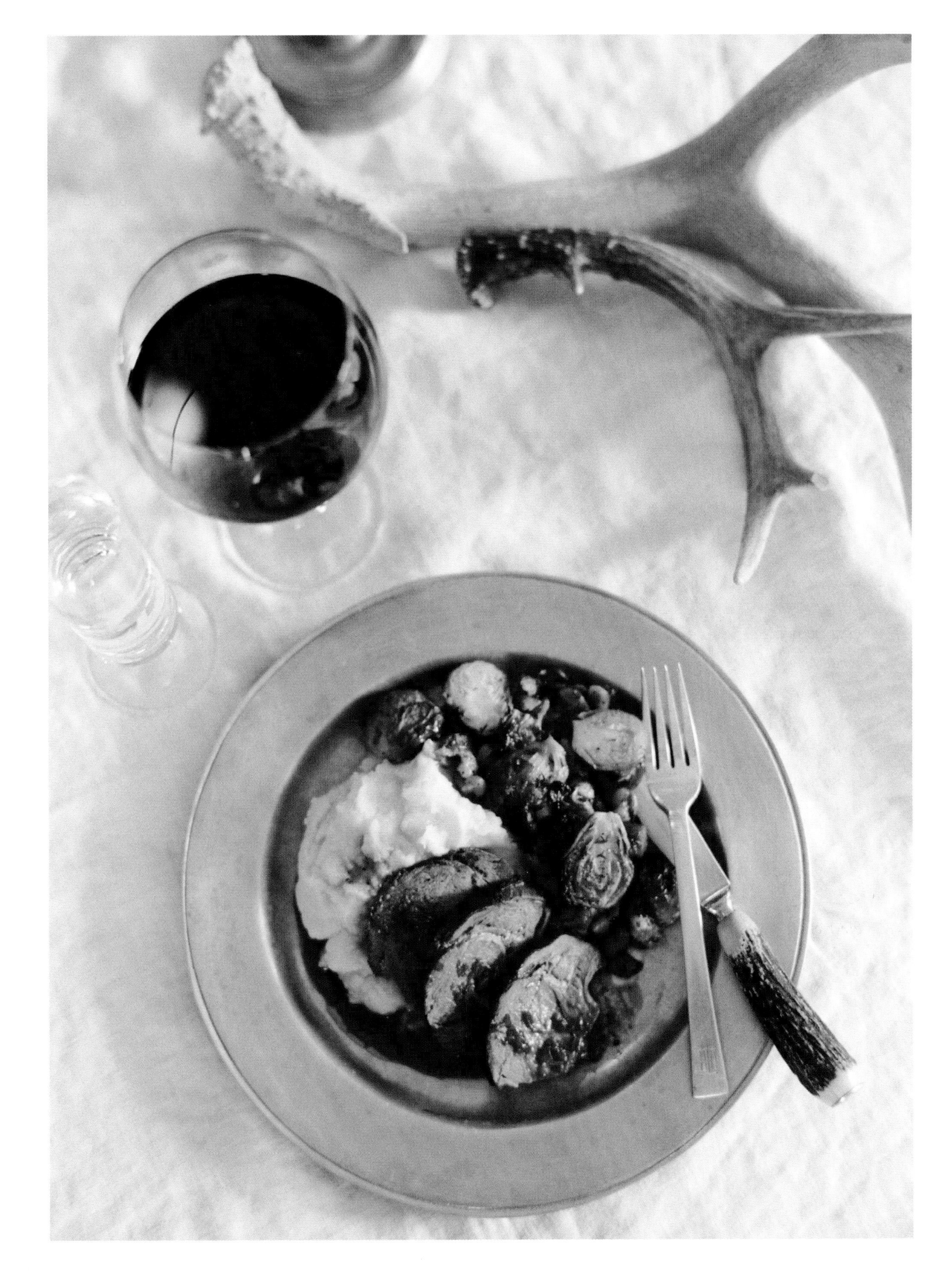

Mashed Turnips with Potatoes, Leeks, and Apples

A new fall classic! This creamy white side is sweet, tart, and surprisingly light. I have to admit that ubiquitous purple-top turnips are not my favorite vegetable, but combining them with potatoes and apples transforms them into a lovely, comforting, seasonal dish. Add this to your list of mashed potato alternatives. It is especially delicious with game.

Serves 4 to 6

- *2 pounds yellow potatoes, peeled and cut into 2-inch pieces*
- *1½ pounds purple-top turnips, peeled and cut into 2-inch pieces*
- *1 leek, white part only, thoroughly cleaned and diced*
- *1 Granny Smith apple or variety of your preference, peeled and cut into large pieces*
- *2 tablespoons unsalted butter (page 348) or ghee (page 347)*
- *Sea salt and ground black pepper*

Whole30	Use ghee, not butter.
Nut-free	Yes
Egg-free	Yes
AIP	No

1. Place the potatoes, turnips, and leek in a large pot and add water just to cover.
2. Bring to a boil and cook for 30 minutes, or until the potatoes and turnips are soft.
3. Add the apple and continue cooking for about 5 minutes, until the apple is soft.
4. Drain the water and return the vegetables and apple to the pot.
5. Add the butter and mash with a potato masher, or with an immersion blender for a smoother puree.
6. Finish with salt and pepper to taste.

See photo on page 317.

NOTES: *Purple-top turnips are the most common type of white-fleshed turnip, easily found at farmers markets and grocery stores. You can substitute rutabaga for the turnips, if you wish.*

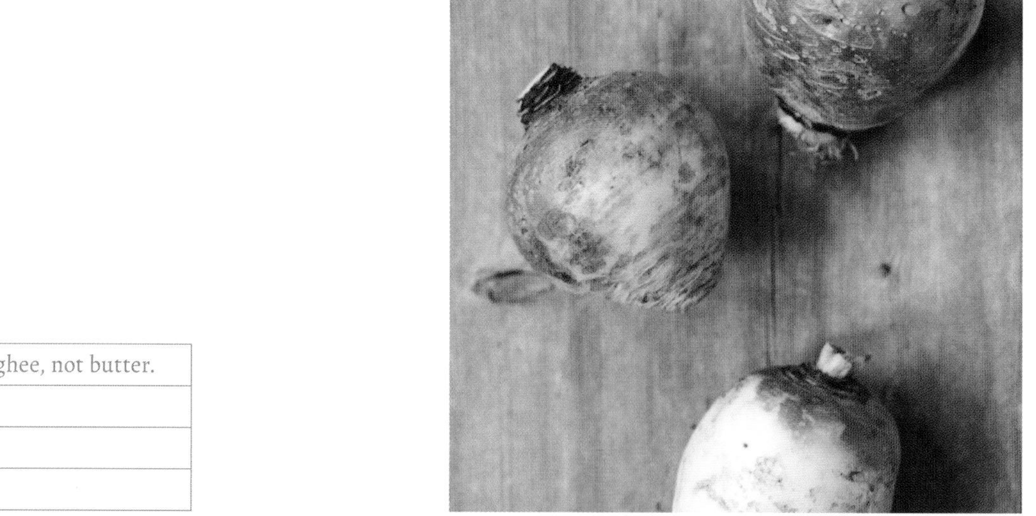

Lemony Brussels Sprouts with Pancetta and Oyster Mushrooms

I adore Brussels sprouts. I find that most folks who think they don't like them have never had them cooked this way. (Probably, they've only eaten them boiled, which I don't care for, either.) The chicken stock seeps deep into the little leaves, and when paired with pancetta, mushrooms, and a hint of lemon, they become the best side dish to any fall recipe. I often bring this dish to Thanksgiving dinner at the request of numerous family members.

Serves 4 to 6

- *1½ pounds Brussels sprouts, trimmed and halved*
- *1½ cups homemade chicken stock (page 338)*
- *½ pound oyster mushrooms, chopped*
- *½ pound pancetta, diced small*
- *1 tablespoon lemon juice*
- *1 teaspoon grated lemon zest*
- *1½ teaspoons dried thyme leaves*
- *Sea salt and ground black pepper*

Whole30	Yes
Nut-free	Yes
Egg-free	Yes
AIP	Omit the black pepper.

1. Preheat the oven to 400°F. Line a rimmed baking sheet with parchment paper.
2. Place the Brussels sprouts and chicken stock in a small pot and bring to a boil. Then reduce the heat and simmer for 5 minutes. Drain the Brussels sprouts.
3. Place the Brussels sprouts, mushrooms, and pancetta on the prepared baking sheet and arrange evenly so everything has a little space.
4. Drizzle with the lemon juice and sprinkle the lemon zest, thyme, a pinch of salt, and generous amounts of black pepper over the top. Toss to coat.
5. Roast for 10 minutes. Remove from the oven and toss the mixture with a spatula.
6. Return to the oven and roast for another 5 minutes, or until pancetta is crispy.

See photo on page 317.

NOTES: *If you can't find oyster mushrooms, substitute another type.*

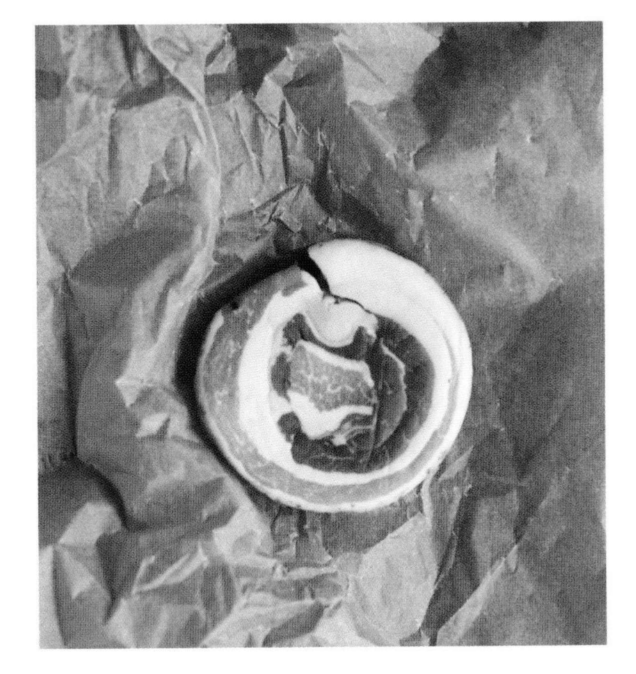

Beet and Orange Salad over Greens

Oranges and beets are a great combination. The oranges brighten and sweeten the earthier flavor of the beets. Beets are a very good source of folate and manganese, plus they're stunning on the plate, especially when paired with oranges.

Serves 6

- *4 medium beets*
- *1 tablespoon cold-pressed, extra-virgin olive oil, plus more for coating the beets*
- *1 teaspoon blood orange vinegar*
- *2 oranges*
- *Juice of ½ lemon*
- *Juice of ½ lime*
- *Sea salt and ground black pepper*
- *1 small head radicchio, torn into small pieces*
- *1 small endive, leaves separated*
- *½ cup chopped fresh parsley leaves, for garnish*

1. Preheat the oven to 350°F. Rinse the beets with water and place each one on a square of foil. Coat them lightly with olive oil and wrap them up. Roast for about 45 minutes, or until you can pierce them with a fork.

2. Remove the beets from the oven and set aside for about 10 minutes, until they are cool enough to handle but still warm. Peel and slice the beets, then place them in a large bowl and drizzle with the vinegar while they are still warm.

3. Peel the oranges. If you want to be fancy, you can section them, but there are some good nutrients in the white pith, so I usually just slice them into bite-sized pieces, leaving some pith.

4. In a small bowl, whisk together the lemon juice, lime juice, and 1 tablespoon of olive oil. Season with salt and pepper to taste.

5. Place the greens in a bowl, drizzle with the dressing, and toss to coat.

6. To serve the salad, divide the dressed greens among 6 plates. Then layer with the oranges and beets. Garnish with a bit of the parsley and a pinch of salt and pepper.

NOTES: *This salad has lots of beautiful color and pattern possibilities, depending on the types of beets and oranges you use. Try mixing it up with golden or striped beets and blood oranges.*

Whole30	Yes
Nut-free	Yes
Egg-free	Yes
AIP	Omit the black pepper.

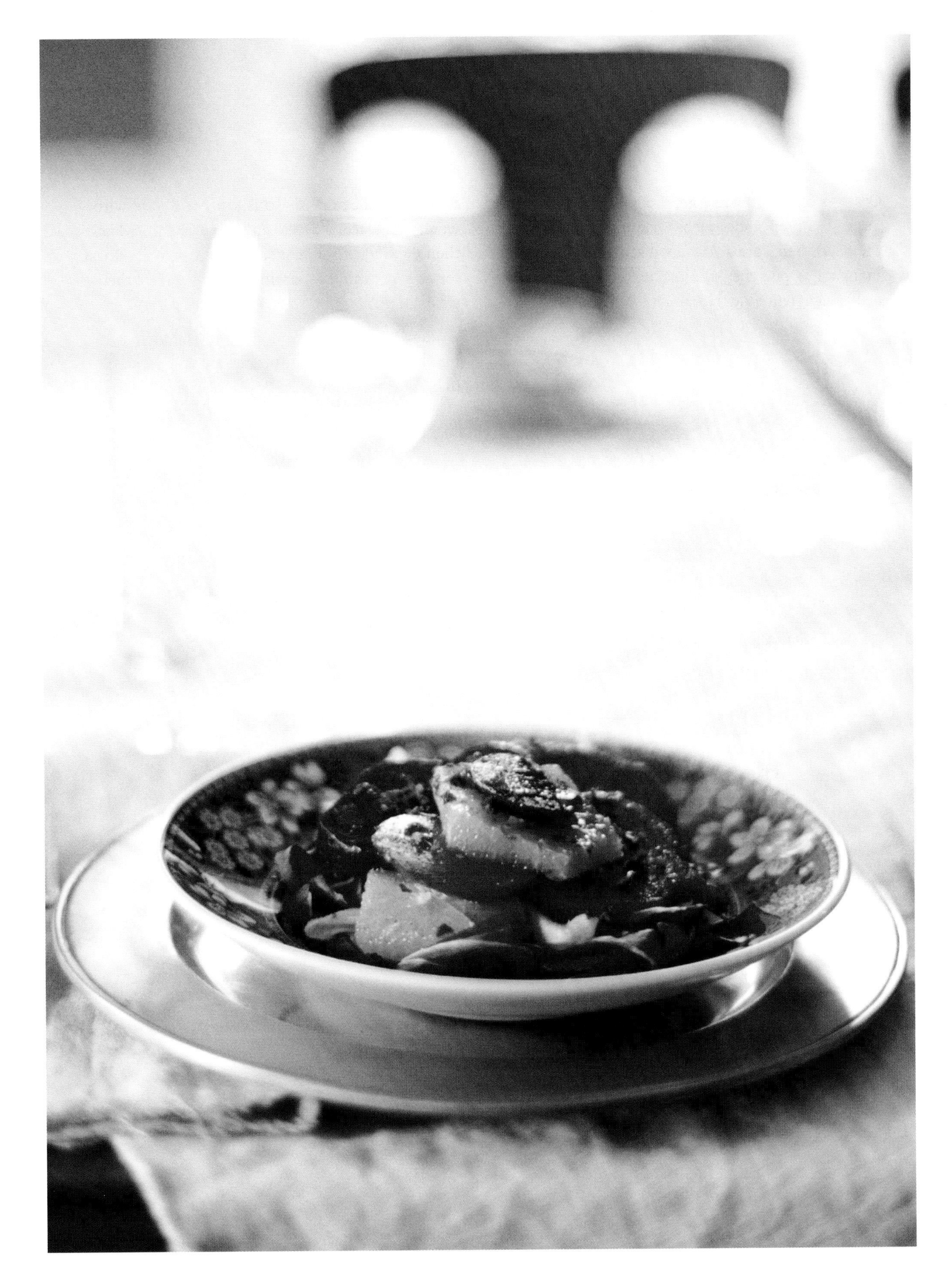

Cardamom-Ginger Pots de Crème with Coconut Whipped Cream

I don't make a lot of desserts, so when I do, they'd better be easy and delicious. This one is both. Having said that, it does take some planning and attention to process, so please follow the directions exactly to have success and super-smooth results! The first important step is to remember to set a can of coconut milk in the fridge the day before you plan to make this dessert, for the coconut whipped cream, and make sure to have a thermometer on hand when you make the pots de crème. The technique for this recipe comes from my good friend, Michelle Tam, author of *Nom Nom Paleo: Food for Humans*. She makes this dessert with ancho chili powder. I swapped out the ancho chili and added a few of my own touches to make it the perfect ending to a rich meal during the depths of winter. If you're a fan of dark chocolate, you'll absolutely love it! This is not a creamy, sweet mousse, but more like a super-dark dive into heaven. I like to garnish it with slivers of Candied Orange and Ginger (page 324).

Makes 6 (3½-ounce) servings

For the pots de crème

- *7 ounces dark chocolate (at least 70%), finely chopped (about 2 standard bars; see Notes)*
- *1 (14-ounce) can full-fat coconut milk*
- *2 egg yolks, beaten*
- *1 teaspoon ground cardamom*
- *2 teaspoons grated fresh ginger*
- *⅛ teaspoon ground cinnamon*
- *⅛ teaspoon sea salt*
- *1 tablespoon maple syrup*
- *1 tablespoon vanilla extract*

For the coconut whipped cream

- *1 (14-ounce) can full-fat coconut milk, chilled upside-down in the fridge overnight*
- *1 teaspoon maple syrup*
- *¼ teaspoon vanilla extract*

- *6 slivers Candied Orange and Ginger (page 324), for garnish (optional)*

Whole30	No
Nut-free	Yes
Egg-free	No
AIP	No

1. Make the pots de crème: Place the chocolate in a heatproof bowl and set aside.

2. In a saucepan over medium heat, slowly warm the coconut milk, egg yolks, cardamom, ginger, cinnamon, and salt, stirring constantly. Do not allow it to come to a simmer. When the mixture reaches 175°F, remove it from the heat. This will take about 10 minutes.

3. Pour the coconut milk mixture through a fine-mesh sieve over the chocolate and set a timer for 5 minutes. Walk away from the bowl and do not disturb it for the full 5 minutes.

4. After the timer goes off, very slowly stir the mixture until it is completely smooth. This will take a few minutes. If you stir it too fast, you'll get grainy results, so stir slowly!

5. Stir in the maple syrup and vanilla and pour into 6 teacups or small ramekins.

NOTES: *The chocolate industry has some major social justice issues—in particular, child slavery is a huge problem among many African cacao farms. It's critical to seek out fair-trade chocolate, especially if the beans come from West Africa. See the note on fair trade on page 27 for more information.*

6. Allow to cool to room temperature, then cover and chill in the fridge for at least 4 hours.

7. Make the coconut whipped cream: Keeping the chilled can upside down, open it and scoop out the cream that has risen to the top. Place the cream in a bowl and whip until soft peaks form. Add the maple syrup and vanilla and whip to incorporate. This can be made several hours ahead and kept in the fridge until needed.

8. To serve, place a dollop of the whipped coconut cream on each pot de crème and garnish with a sliver of candied orange and ginger, if desired. There you have it! Sinfully delicious.

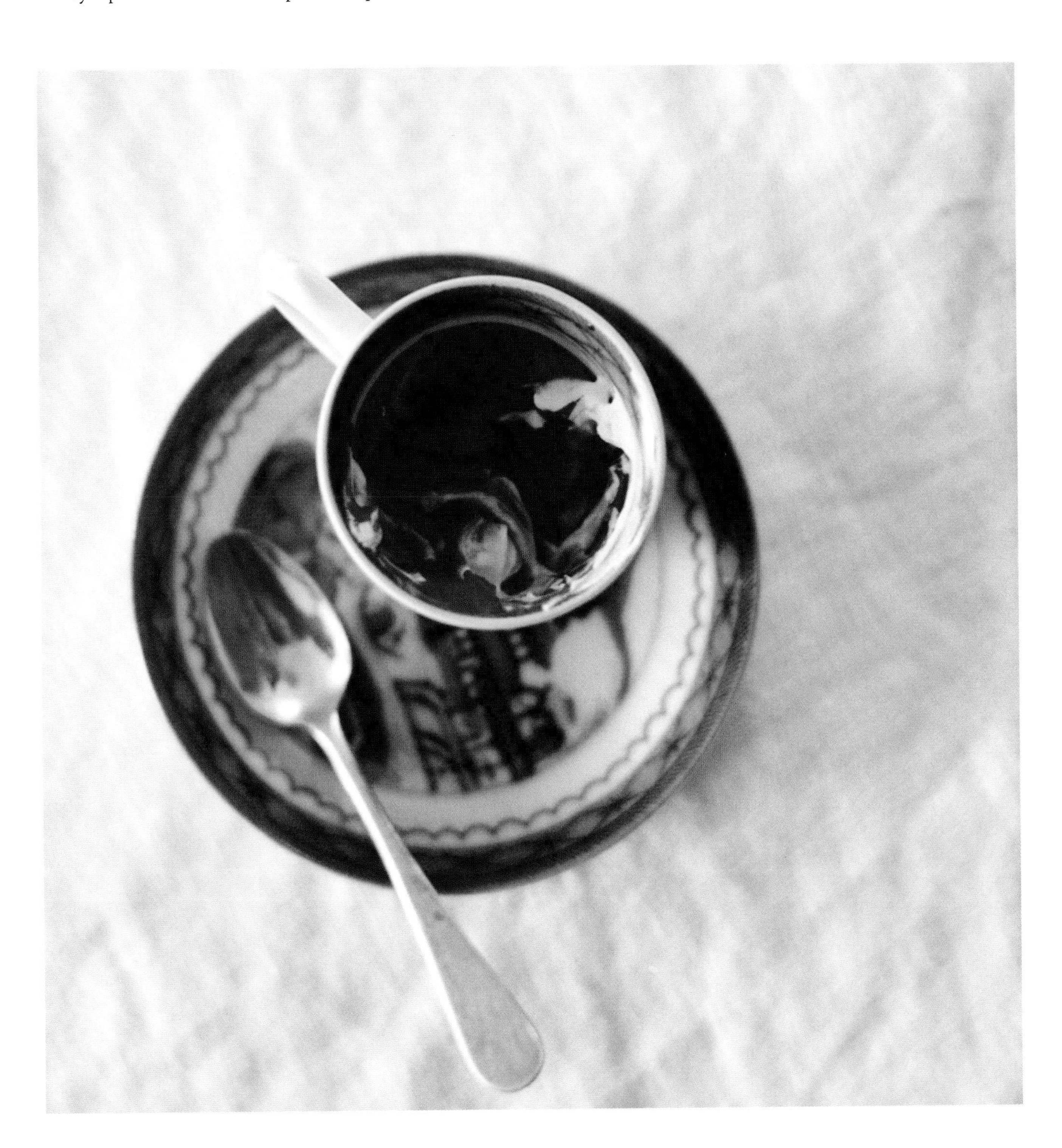

Candied Orange and Ginger

I like to make these candied ginger and orange stripes on special occasions, as a treat alongside squares of rich dark chocolate or to serve with the Cardamom-Ginger Pots de Crème (page 322), as shown. The method isn't too tricky, and the results are amazing. The ginger infuses the orange and vice versa. They taste like sweet little bites of orangey gingerness and have a wonderful gummy texture.

Makes about 2 cups

- *4 oranges*
- *1 (5-inch) piece of ginger*
- *⅓ cup honey*
- *¾ cup water*
- *½ teaspoon vanilla extract*
- *1½ cups unsweetened, finely shredded coconut*

Whole30	No
Nut-free	Yes
Egg-free	Yes
AIP	Yes

1. With a sharp knife, remove the skins of the oranges, outer colored portions only, being careful not to get too much of the white pith, which will make these little candies taste bitter. If you mess up, you can also use the knife to remove the pith from the peel (try shaving it extra close to the surface). Slice the orange peels into matchsticks. Reserve the orange flesh for another use (like my Beet and Orange Salad over Greens, page 320).

2. Peel the ginger. Using a mandoline or sharp knife, slice the ginger lengthwise into long thin pieces, then into matchsticks.

3. Place the orange peel and ginger in a saucepan and cover with water. Boil for 30 minutes. Drain the water and keep the orange peels and ginger in the pot.

4. Add the honey and ¾ cup of water to the pot and bring to a simmer. Simmer over medium-low heat for about 30 minutes, stirring occasionally. Keep a watchful eye on the mixture toward the end, as it can burn if the water evaporates. If the water seems to be evaporating too quickly, lower the heat and add a tablespoon of water. After about 30 minutes, you should have a syrupy coating on the orange peels and ginger, with no water remaining—just a sticky mess.

5. Add the vanilla to the orange and ginger mixture and stir.

6. Pour the coconut onto a large plate. Line a rimmed baking sheet with parchment paper.

7. Transfer the orange peel and ginger to the plate with the coconut and mix until all of the pieces are well coated in the coconut. Transfer the pieces to the prepared baking sheet and allow to cool and set for a few hours. Serve alone or with the pots de crème on page 322.

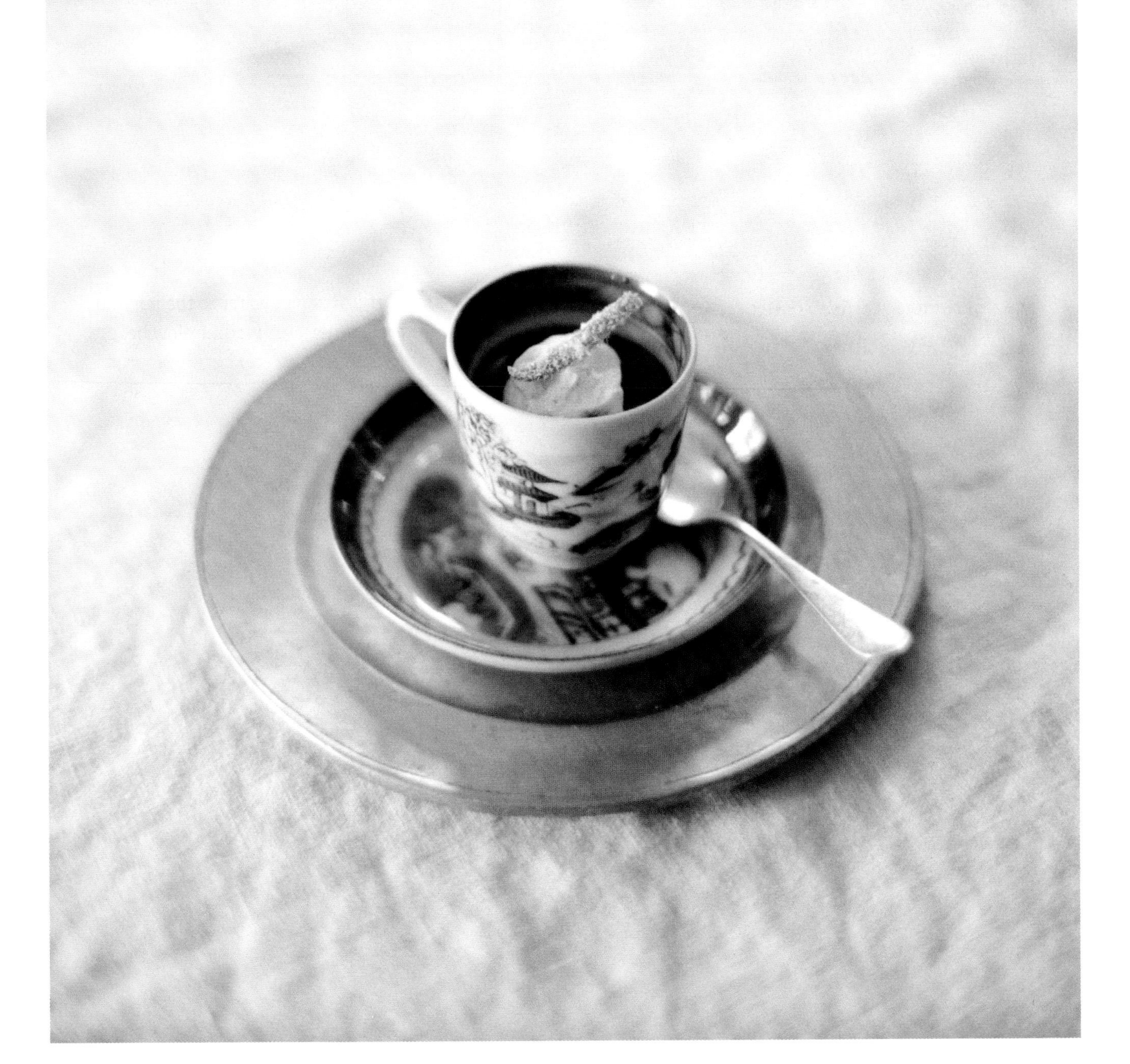

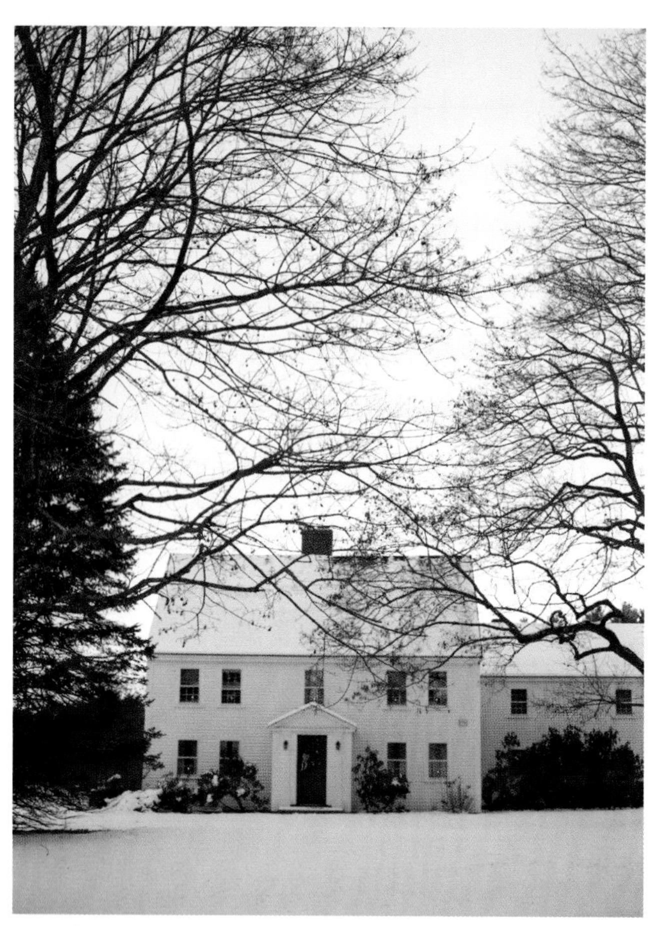
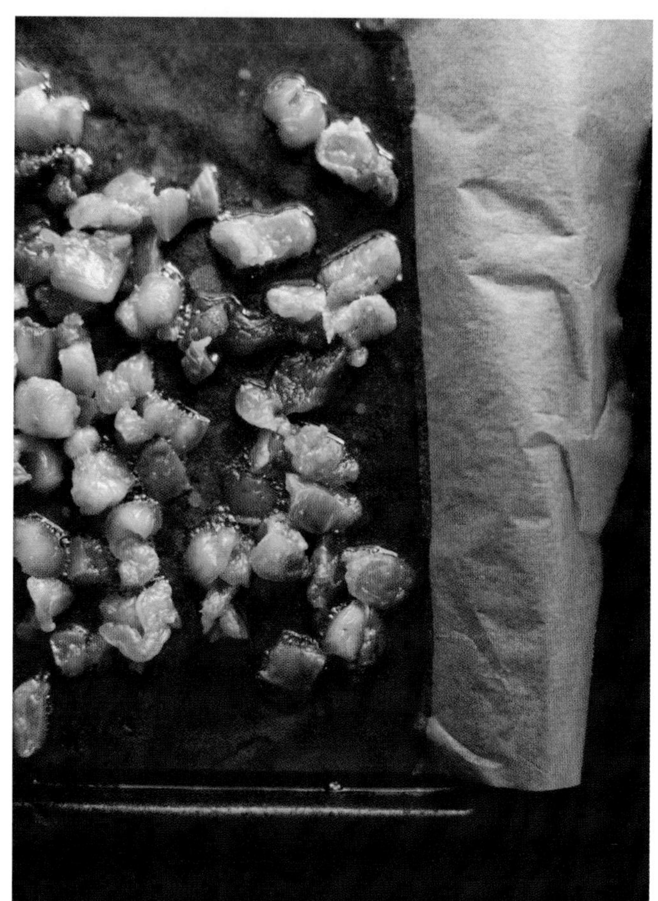
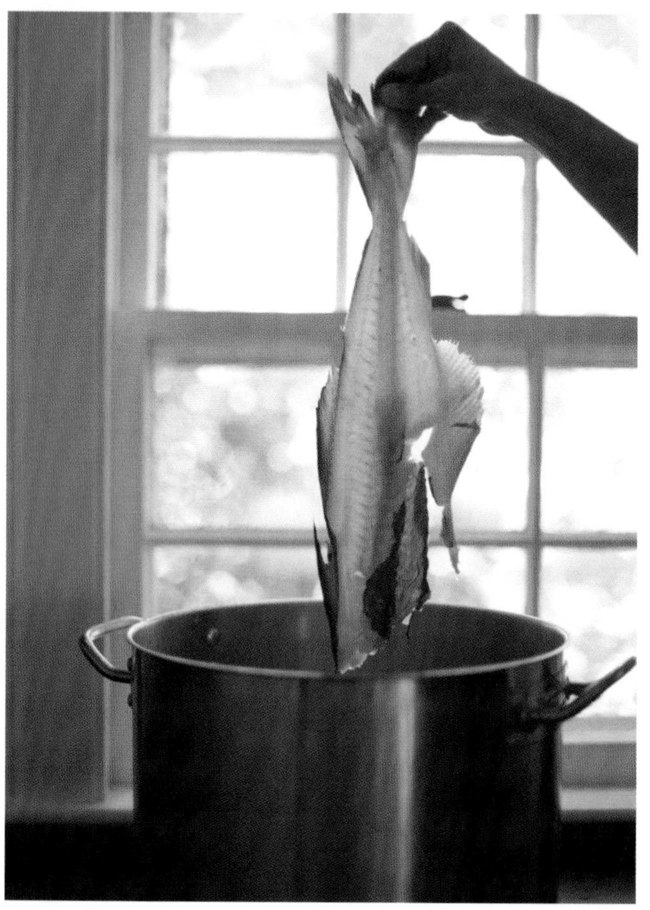
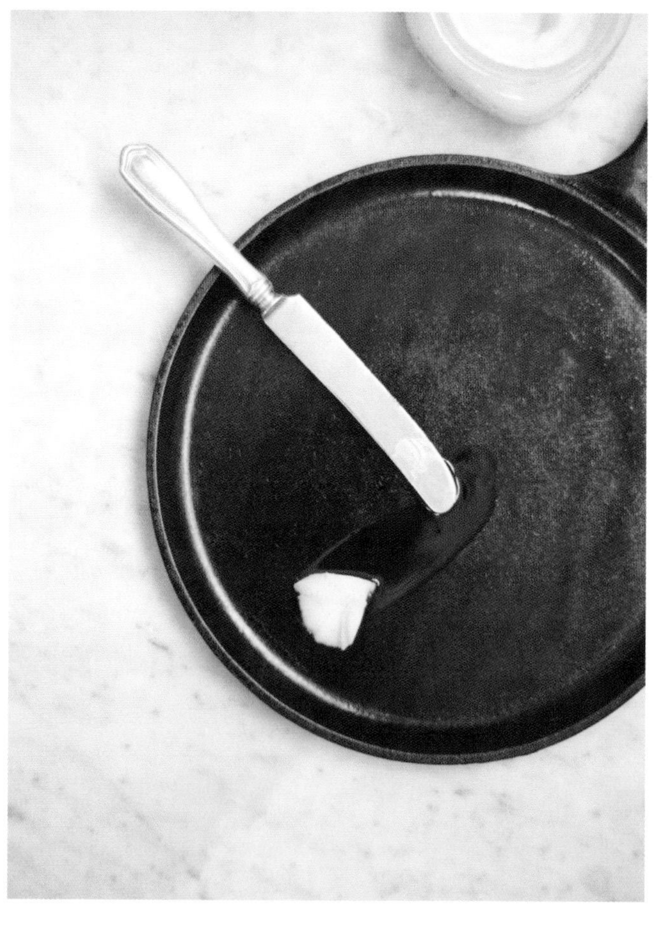

Basic Cooking Methods and Recipes

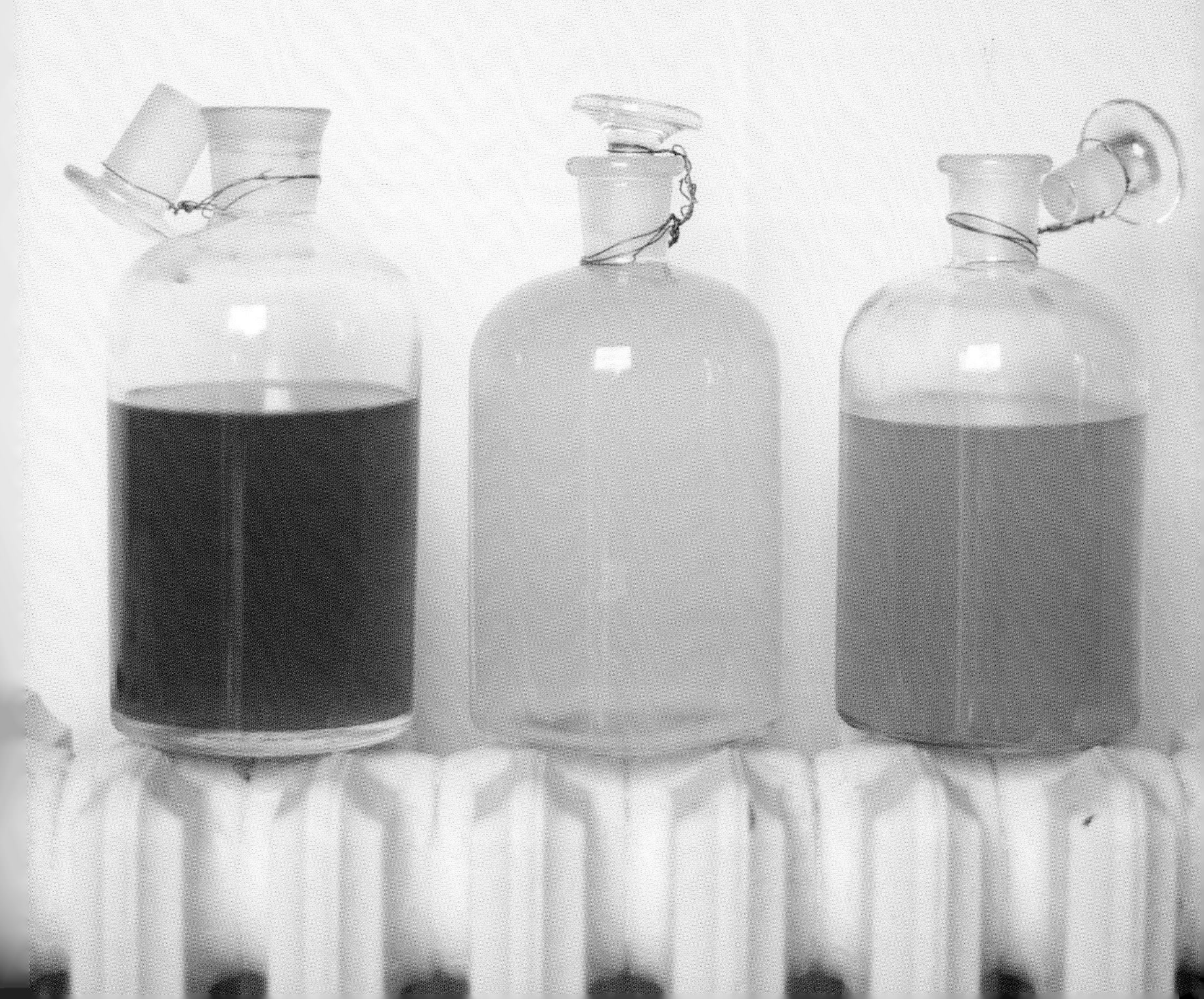

Spicy Kale and Carrot Kraut

Numerous ancient cultures have used lacto-fermentation to preserve food and improve its digestibility and nutrient density. When I was first trying to get used to fermented vegetables, I preferred the sweeter taste of ginger carrots made by a small Massachusetts company called Real Pickles. Now that I'm more used to the sour taste of fermented veggies and am comfortable making my own fermented concoctions, I love this spicy and gingery kale and carrot mixture, which makes a great condiment for any meal. I usually make more than our family can consume, so I repackage it into smaller jars and give some away as gifts, which are always welcomed. If you like more heat, add more red pepper flakes.

Makes about 2 quarts

- *2 bunches red Russian kale, chopped*
- *1 cup diced red cabbage (about ¼ small head)*
- *3 medium carrots, peeled and grated*
- *¼ cup minced fresh cilantro leaves*
- *¼ cup minced fresh mint leaves*
- *¼ cup minced fresh basil leaves*
- *1 tablespoon grated fresh ginger*
- *½ teaspoon red pepper flakes*
- *1 clove garlic, minced*
- *¼ cup minced red onion*
- *2 tablespoons sea salt*

Special equipment

- *½ gallon glass jar, sterilized*
- *Sauerkraut pounder (helpful but not necessary)*
- *Cheesecloth or towel*

1. In a large bowl, combine all of the ingredients for the kraut. Working with your hands, massage well for about 5 to 10 minutes, until the mixture starts to release liquid.

2. Pack the mixture into a sterilized ½-gallon jar. Using your fist, a kraut pounder, or a wooden spoon, tamp down the mixture to remove any air bubbles and fully submerge the vegetables in the liquid. If you need to add more liquid, mix 1 cup of water with 2 teaspoons of salt, then pour on top of the vegetables.

3. Cover tightly with several layers of cheesecloth or a towel and secure with string or a rubber band. Allow to ferment at room temperature for about 1 week.

4. Taste the mixture. In the heat of summer, 1 week of fermenting produces a nice kraut. You may prefer the taste of a longer ferment. The warmer it is, the quicker the fermentation.

5. When the kraut has the sour flavor you like, store it in the refrigerator.

Whole30	Yes
Nut-free	Yes
Egg-free	Yes
AIP	Omit the red pepper flakes.

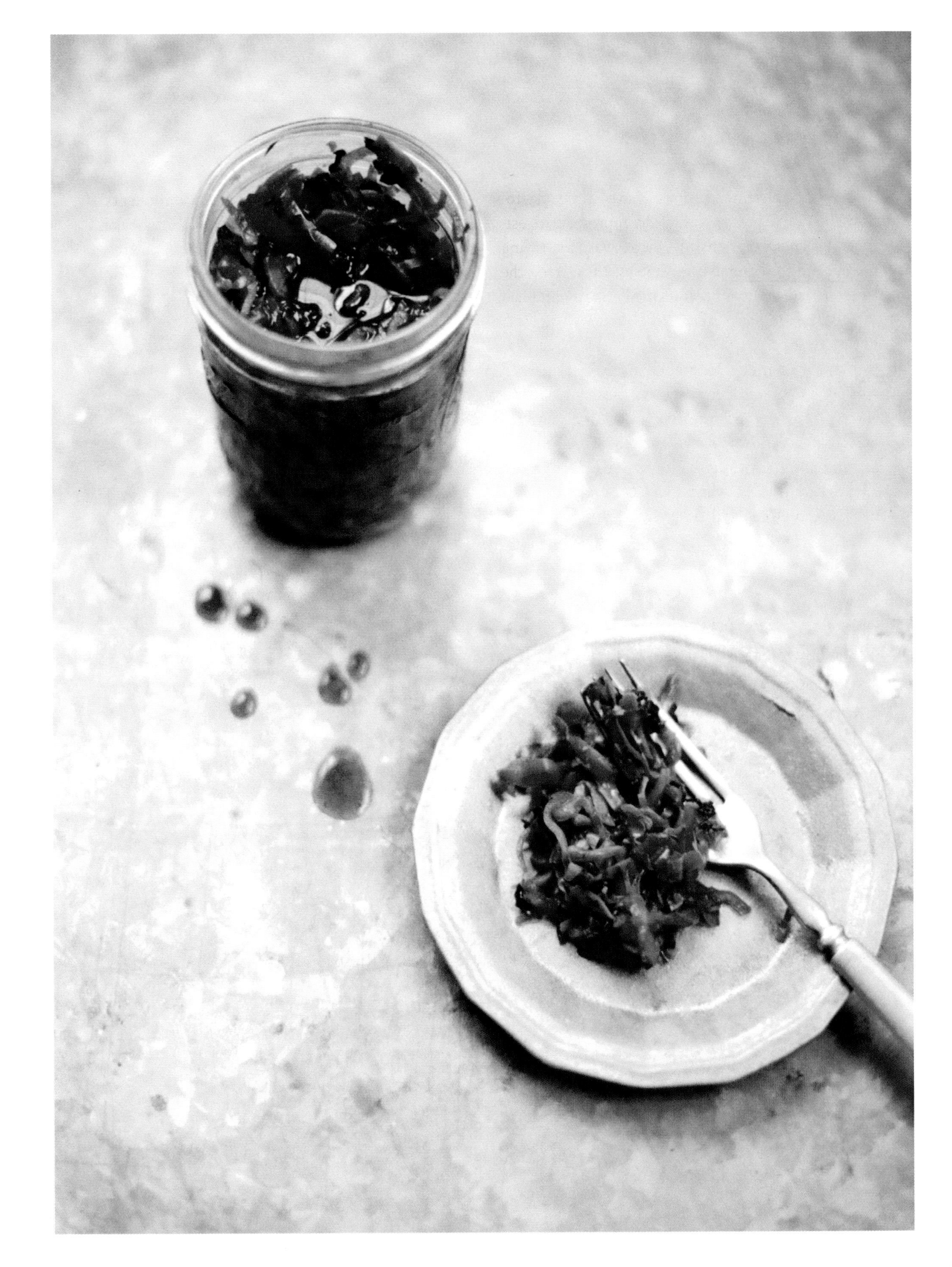

Kombucha

Kombucha is a fermented tea and should be consumed as a digestive aid, though Andrew seems to down it like a Big Gulp. Making kombucha is much easier than you think and will save you tons of money. Our local health food store sells a pint for almost $4.50. Yikes! To make kombucha, you'll need to obtain a SCOBY, which stands for "symbiotic colony of bacteria and yeast," though other folks refer to it as a "mushroom," even though it is not a fungus, or "mother," because it can make little baby SCOBYs batch after batch. That's why the easiest way to obtain a SCOBY is to get one from a friend who makes kombucha. People usually are dying to give away their baby SCOBYs because it feels sort of wrong to toss them in the compost. If you don't have any kombucha-making friends, you can order a dehydrated SCOBY online (see Resources, page 398). The SCOBY feeds on a sweet black or green tea blended with sugar, and after five to thirty days produces a slightly carbonated and acidic beverage that is packed with B vitamins.

Makes three 16-ounce bottles

- *6 cups filtered water, divided*
- *4 organic black or oolong tea bags*
- *½ cup evaporated cane juice or unprocessed cane sugar*
- *1 cup kombucha from a previous batch or distilled white vinegar (5% or higher acidity)*
- *Grated fresh ginger (optional)*

Special equipment

- *1 kombucha SCOBY (see Notes)*
- *1 (½-gallon or 64-ounce) canning jar*
- *Cheesecloth or towel to cover the jar while fermenting*
- *3 (16-ounce) Grolsch-type bottles*
- *Plastic strainer*
- *Small funnel*

NOTES: *If you're making kombucha for the first time and don't have some leftover from a previous batch, distilled white vinegar works fine; just don't use cider or raw vinegar.*

Whole30	Yes
Nut-free	Yes
Egg-free	Yes
AIP	Yes

IMPORTANT INFORMATION

- Never let the SCOBY touch metal, like stainless-steel spoons or cups. It's best to use glass containers and plastic strainers.
- Never consume kombucha that looks, smells, or tastes unpleasant—just toss out your batch and start a new one.
- Warmer temperatures cause kombucha to ferment faster. In the summer, I allow 1 week for it to ferment on the counter; in the winter, it can take up to 3 weeks.
- Kombucha does contain a small amount of alcohol. If you or someone you know has an alcohol issue, kombucha might not be a great beverage for daily consumption.
- If you're using a dehydrated SCOBY, you'll need to rehydrate it for 30 days. Follow the directions for rehydration that come with your SCOBY.
- Any size SCOBY can work—no need to worry about it being too small or too large.
- There's no need to worry about the sugar used to make kombucha. It's digested by the SCOBY and will not end up raising your insulin!

1. Bring 1 cup of the filtered water to a boil and pour it into a ½-gallon canning jar. Drop in the tea bags and sugar and allow to steep for 10 minutes.

2. Remove the tea bags and fill the container with the remaining 5 cups of cold filtered water.

3. Add the reserved kombucha from a previous batch. Stir well.

4. Add the SCOBY and cover with a towel or several layers of cheesecloth. You want the mixture to be able to breathe, but you don't want it to attract fruit flies. Secure with string or a rubber band.

5. You may notice another, smaller SCOBY forming on the bottom of the tea. This is normal. The SCOBY on the top may sink or float sideways in your tea, and this is okay, too.

6. After about 5 days (especially in a warmer climate), insert a straw and taste the kombucha. You may stop the process now or keep it going. The longer you allow it to ferment, the more acidic it will taste. I like to let it ferment about 7 days in the summer and about 14 to 20 days in the winter.

7. Remove the SCOBY with clean hands and store it in a jar with about 1 cup of the kombucha until you are ready to make another batch. You can keep it in the refrigerator for up to a year to halt the fermentation process.

8. With a funnel and a plastic strainer, carefully pour the kombucha into the Grolsch bottles, leaving about 1 inch between the liquid and the top of the bottle.

9. You can drink the kombucha like this, or cap and refrigerate it, or do a second ferment and add ginger for a much fizzier and tastier drink. To make the fizzy ginger version, add 1 teaspoon of grated fresh ginger to each bottle and cap it. Allow to sit out on the counter overnight if the weather is warm or for up to a few days if it's cooler. Use caution during this process—you don't want it to explode!

10. Refrigerate the kombucha until you are ready to drink it.

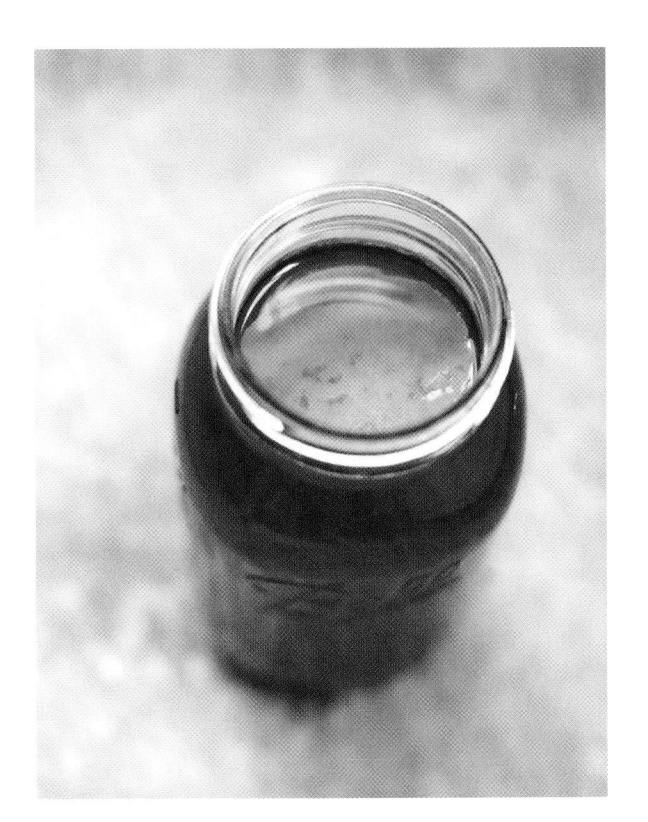

VARIATION

Fruit-Flavored Kombucha. *If ginger isn't your thing, try adding a small amount of Concord grape juice or a few small pieces of fruit, like blueberries or raspberries, instead of the ginger, and allow the second ferment to happen for a day or so. Experiment until you find the combination that you like best!*

Milk Kefir

Many traditional cultures have been fermenting dairy products like kefir for centuries. The word *kefir* comes from the Turkish word *keif*, which means "good feeling." Kefir can be made from goat's, sheep's, and cow's milk and even coconut milk. Yes, milk isn't technically Paleo, but if you do incorporate dairy into your diet, you should try making your own kefir. If you avoid dairy, try making milk kefir with coconut milk. Kefir contains high levels of thiamin, biotin, folate, vitamin B12, and vitamin K2. It's also a potent probiotic that improves the immune system, making it a superfood. You can order the "grains" online (see Resources, page 398) or get them from a friend, as they multiply as you use them. (Don't worry, Paleo friends, these are not actual grains.) There are numerous uses for kefir: you can add it to smoothies, use it to make a type of cream cheese, and drink it alone. As when working with kombucha SCOBYs and water kefir grains, do not allow the milk kefir grains to come into contact with metal. Use glass jars, plastic strainers, and wooden or plastic stirring utensils.

Makes 1 quart

- *2 teaspoons milk kefir grains (if dehydrated, plan on about 5 days to rehydrate; see Notes)*
- *1 quart whole milk, raw or pasteurized (not ultra-pasteurized)*

Special equipment

- *2 (1-pint) canning jars*
- *Cheesecloth or a towel*
- *Plastic strainer*
- *Pretty straws (optional)*

1. Divide the kefir grains between 2 glass canning jars. Add the milk and stir well with a wooden or plastic spoon (do not use metal).
2. Cover the jars with several layers of cheesecloth or a towel and secure with a rubber band.
3. Leave the jars in a warm place for 24 hours.
4. Depending on how active the fermentation is (which depends on how many grains you've added, how healthy they are, and how warm it is in your kitchen), the milk will be either slightly thickened or very thick.
5. Strain out the kefir grains using a plastic strainer. You can now refrigerate the milk kefir and drink it as is. Serve with straws if desired. It will keep in the refrigerator for 2 to 3 weeks.
6. With the leftover kefir grains, you can make a new batch. Try to talk your friends and neighbors into making milk kefir, because the grains multiply fast and you'll soon have way too many on your hands!

VARIATION

Strawberry-Vanilla Probiotic Smoothie

- *1 quart milk kefir*
- *1 cup strawberries, hulled*
- *1 teaspoon vanilla extract*

In a blender or with an immersion blender, blend the milk kefir, strawberries, and vanilla until smooth.

Whole30	Use coconut milk (see Notes).
Nut-free	Yes
Egg-free	Yes
AIP	Use coconut milk (see Notes).

NOTES: *If using coconut milk, allow the grains to culture in cow's or goat's milk for 24 hours once every few batches to revitalize them. When using dehydrated kefir grains for the first time, rehydrate them in cow's or goat's milk before using them in coconut milk. Sometimes kefir grains require an adjustment period, so the first batch of coconut milk kefir may not culture as desired. Simply use the coconut milk for cooking and place the kefir grains in new coconut milk. An adjustment period isn't uncommon whenever kefir grains are switched from one type of milk to another (cow's to goat's, pasteurized to raw, dairy to coconut).*

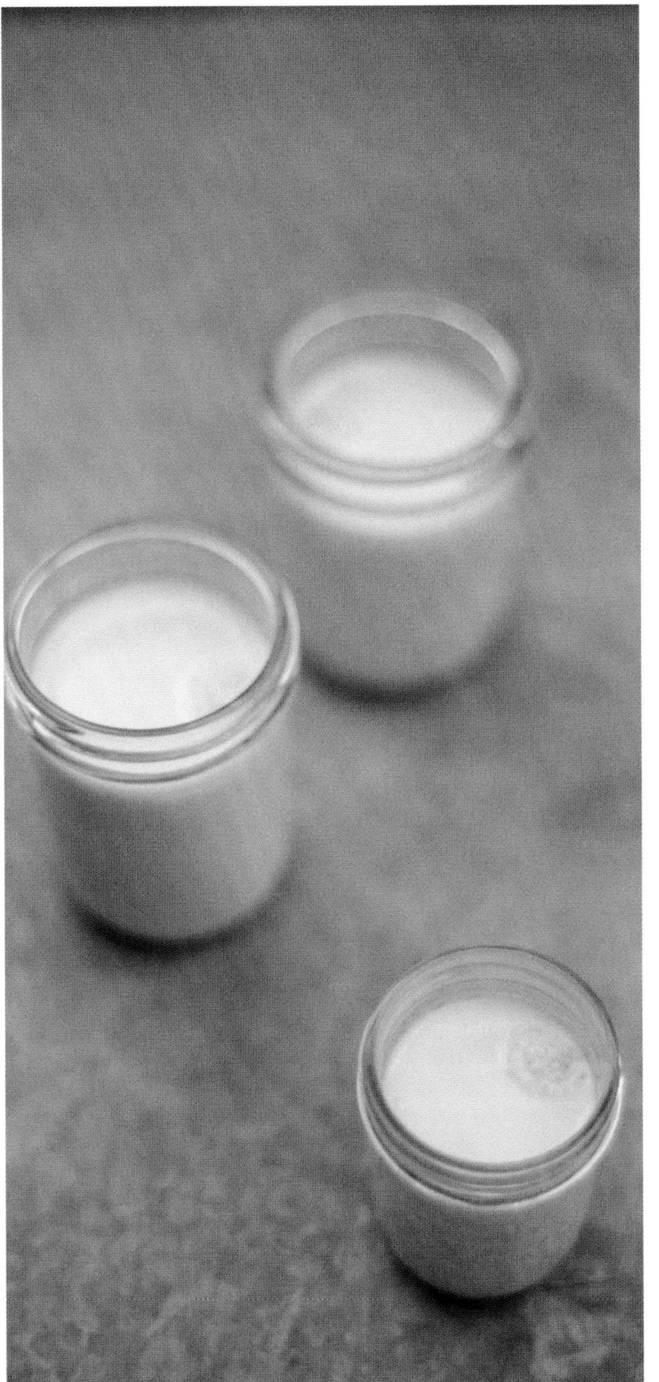

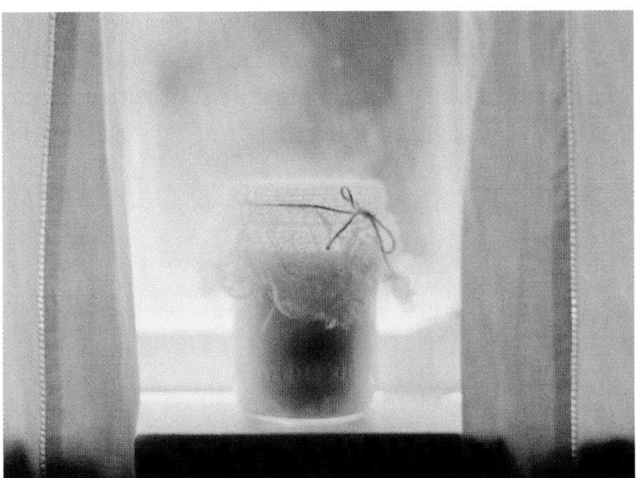

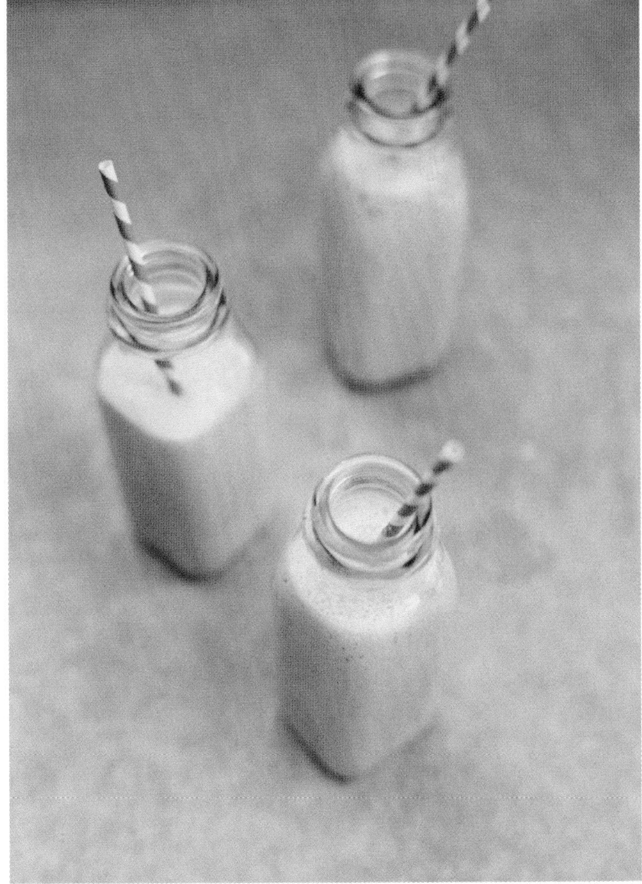

Probiotic Cream Soda (Water Kefir)

Similar to kombucha, water kefir is a refreshing fermented beverage. Water kefir grains can be made with coconut water or fruit juice. They consist of a complex polysaccharide matrix, upon which live a combination of live bacteria and yeasts. When rehydrated, they look like little chopped-up jellyfish, but harder. As with kombucha and other fermented beverages, if your kefir smells funny or looks bad, dump it and start a new batch.

Makes four 16-ounce bottles

- *About 2 quarts filtered water, divided*
- *½ cup evaporated cane juice or unprocessed cane sugar*
- *3 to 4 tablespoons water kefir grains (see Notes)*
- *2 to 4 teaspoons vanilla extract*

Special equipment

- *1 (½-gallon or 64-ounce) canning jar*
- *Cheesecloth or towel*
- *Plastic strainer*
- *Small funnel*
- *4 (16-ounce) Grolsch-type bottles*

1. Bring 1 cup of filtered water to a boil and pour it into a ½-gallon canning jar. Add the sugar and, using a wooden or plastic (not metal) spoon, stir well to dissolve.
2. Add cold filtered water to fill the jar to about 2 inches from the top. Mix well with the wooden or plastic spoon.
3. Add the water kefir grains, cover with several layers of cheesecloth or a towel, and secure with string or a rubber band.
4. Allow the mixture to ferment on the counter for 24 hours. Some people let it go for 48 hours, but I've always had success stopping the process after 1 full day.
5. Strain out the grains using a plastic strainer (they can be reused). Using a funnel, pour the water kefir into the Grolsch-type bottles, leaving 1 inch at the top.
6. To each bottle, add ½ to 1 teaspoon of vanilla extract. Cap the bottles and allow them to sit out on the counter for another 24 hours. This second ferment will yield a fizzier soda.
7. Chill and enjoy.

NOTES: *If you're using dehydrated kefir grains, plan on 4 days to rehydrate and follow the package directions. Resources for kefir grains are listed on page 398.*

Whole30	Yes
Nut-free	Yes
Egg-free	Yes
AIP	Maybe. Try a small amount first to see if it's tolerated. Water kefir can cause a reaction in some people with sensitive GI systems.

VARIATIONS

Fruit-Flavored Probiotic Cream Soda. *To each bottle, add one of the following before adding the water kefir:*

- *A few fresh raspberries or blueberries*
- *1 tablespoon finely diced fresh melon and ½ teaspoon grated fresh ginger (my favorite)*
- *½ cup fruit juice (grape is nice)*

Allow to sit on the counter for 24 hours before refrigerating.

Birch Bark–Flavored Probiotic Cream Soda. *To each bottle, add ½ cup of Birch Bark Sun Tea (page 200), then top off with the water kefir. Allow to sit on the counter for 24 hours before refrigerating.*

Herbal Probiotic Cream Soda. *To each bottle, add ½ cup of your favorite brewed herbal tea (berry and mint blends are great!), then top off with the water kefir. Allow to sit on the counter for 24 hours before refrigerating.*

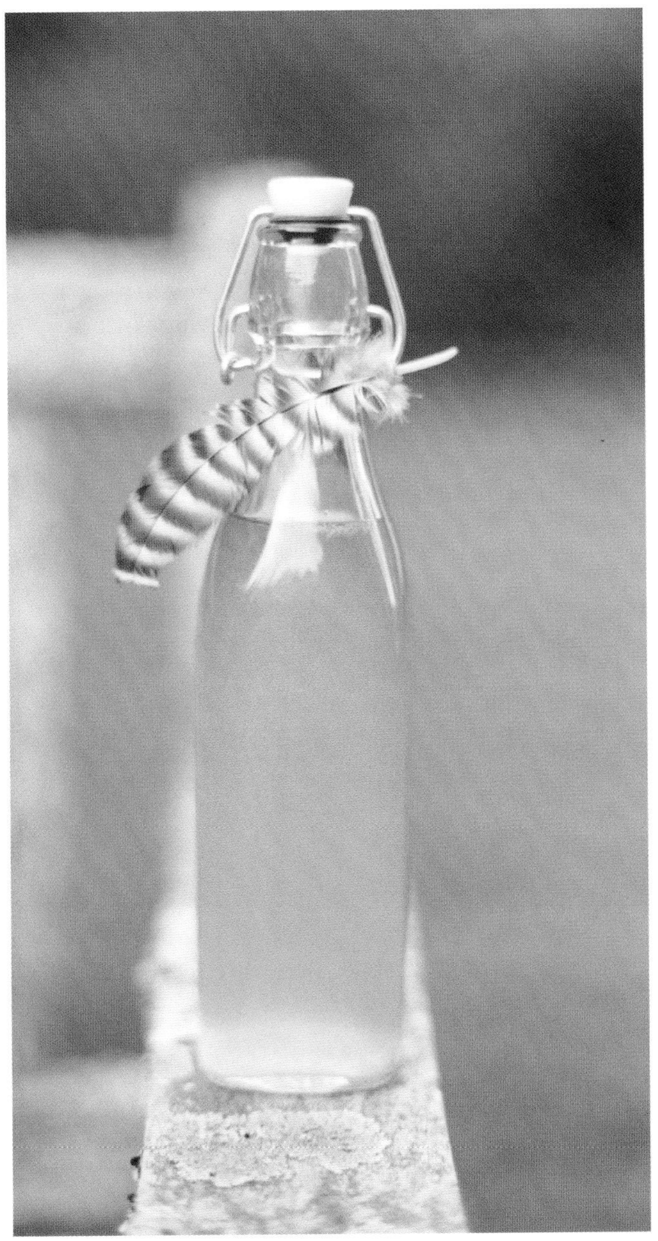

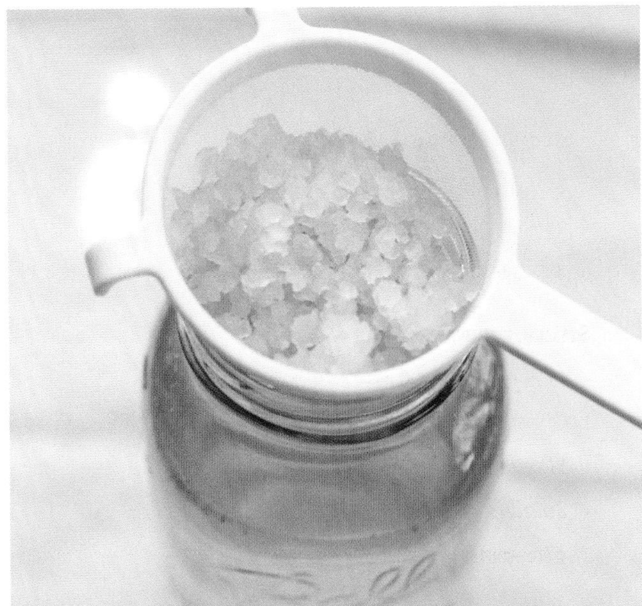

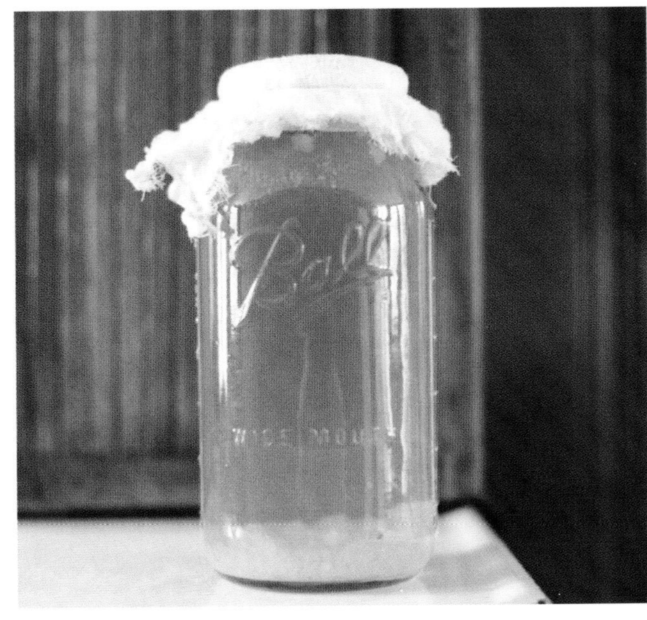

Roasted Chicken

I prefer roasting an entire chicken to buying boneless, skinless chicken breasts because I can use the rest of that chicken for making stock (see page 338). The best place to get your chickens is from a farmer, and the most sustainable chicken to purchase is one that has already had a purpose in laying eggs. However, old egg layers are not the most tender and moist birds to roast, so I save those for the stockpot. Free-range, pasture-raised chickens that are raised for meat are a little tougher than battery-raised birds and can cost about twice as much, but they produce a much better taste and are a better choice from a sustainability standpoint. (See page 14 for more information.)

Serves 4

- *1 (3- to 4-pound) roasting chicken*
- *2 tablespoons coconut oil, bacon fat, lard, or duck fat, melted*
- *2 teaspoons sea salt*
- *1 teaspoon ground black pepper*
- *½ lemon*
- *2 sprigs fresh thyme, leaves removed, or ½ teaspoon dried thyme leaves*

1. Preheat the oven to 350°F. Rinse the chicken and remove the giblets. I like to put the giblets in a bag and freeze them until I'm ready to make stock, or fry the livers in a little butter while the chicken is roasting.
2. Place the chicken in a baking dish lined with parchment paper. (You can skip the parchment paper if you prefer, but it makes cleanup much easier and can be composted.)
3. Pat the chicken dry with paper towels and rub it with the melted fat. Sprinkle with the salt and pepper and squeeze the half lemon over the top. Pop the used lemon half inside the chicken cavity along with the thyme.
4. Roast the chicken for approximately 2 hours before checking to see if it's cooked. The best tool for this is a digital instant-read thermometer. The internal temperature should be 165°F, read at the thigh, but don't let the probe touch the bones or it will throw your reading off. The ideal place to put the thermometer is right at the junction of the leg to the breast, about midway up the side of the chicken.

NOTES: *If you don't have a meat thermometer, you can try these two tricks. When you wiggle the leg, you should almost be able to pull it off of the bird easily. You can also pierce the thigh meat with a knife to see if the juices are clear (as opposed to pinkish, which indicates an undercooked bird).*

Whole30	Yes
Nut-free	Yes
Egg-free	Yes
AIP	Omit the black pepper.

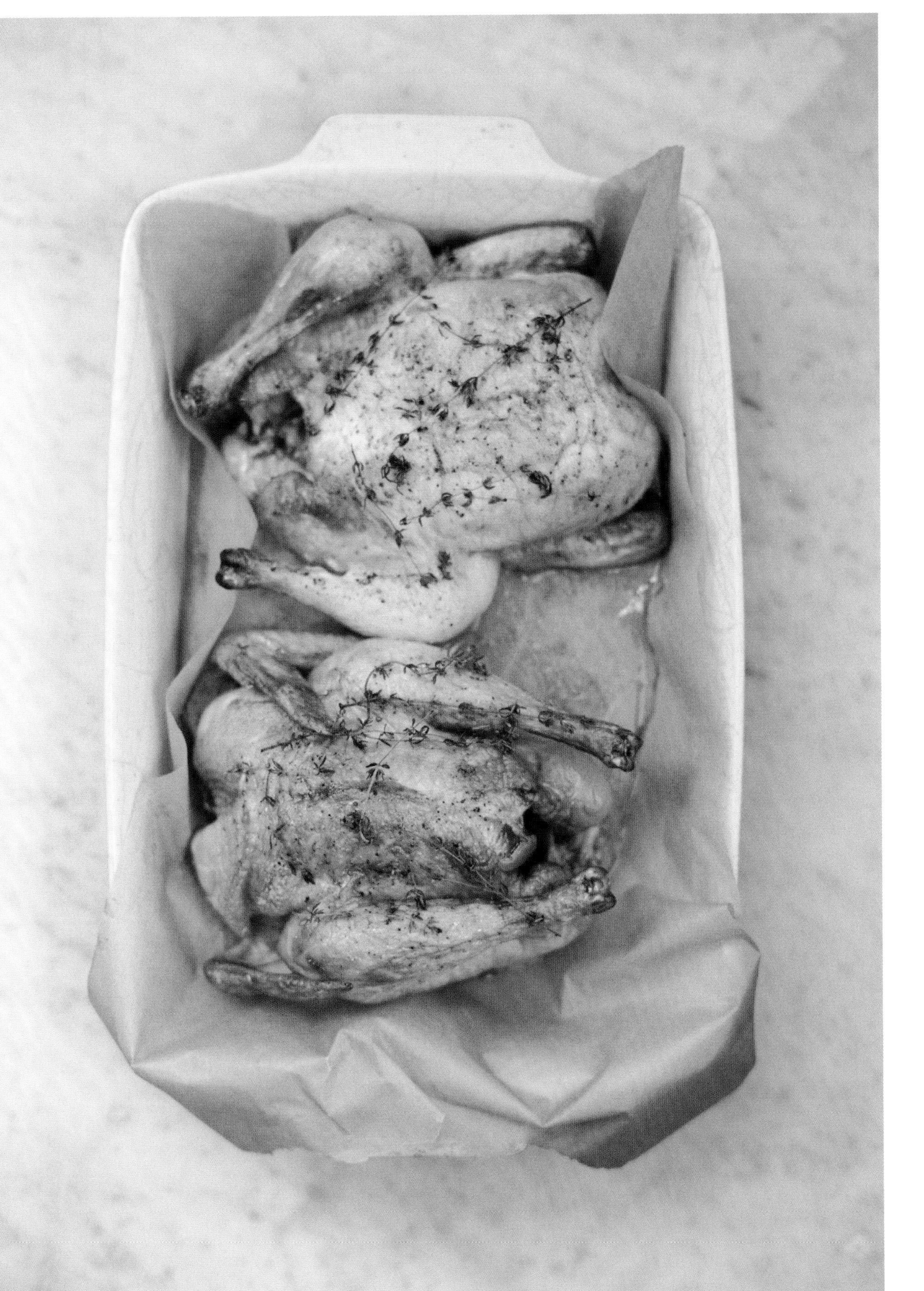

Chicken Stock

I make this magic stock a few times a month. When I'm done feeding my family the meat from a whole chicken, I place the carcass in a freezer bag and save it until I'm ready to make stock. I also save the organs and other parts, like the feet, which give the stock extra richness and gelatin.

Makes 6 to 7 quarts

- *4 to 5 quarts cold filtered water*
- *3 leftover roasted chicken carcasses, plus bonus chicken feet and/or organs*
- *¼ cup apple cider vinegar*
- *1 large yellow or white onion, halved*
- *4 medium carrots, peeled*
- *3 stalks celery*
- *1 tablespoon black peppercorns*
- *3 bay leaves*

1. Fill a large stockpot with the cold water and add the chicken carcasses and vinegar. Allow to sit for 30 minutes, then bring to a boil and skim off any scum that comes to the surface.

2. Add the onion halves, carrots, celery (no need to chop them), peppercorns, and bay leaves, reduce the heat to a very low simmer, and cover. The longer you cook the stock, the richer it will be. I usually start mine early in the morning and turn off the heat at the end of the day, before bed. After you've turned off the heat, allow it to cool on the counter for about 1 hour.

3. Strain the stock (line the strainer with cheesecloth for a clearer product) into a large bowl or separate, smaller pots and place in the refrigerator to cool (I usually do this overnight).

4. When the stock is fully cooled, skim off and discard the fat that has risen to the top. Ladle the stock into freezer-safe containers. Label, date, and store in the freezer until you're ready to use it. It will keep in the freezer for up to a year.

NOTES: *The longer you cook the stock, the more water will evaporate and the smaller the yield will be. For 6 to 7 quarts, simmer the stock for about 15 hours. You can also make stock with a whole raw chicken using this same process. I do this with older laying hens that wouldn't be very tender when roasted.*

Whole30	Yes
Nut-free	Yes
Egg-free	Yes
AIP	Omit the peppercorns.

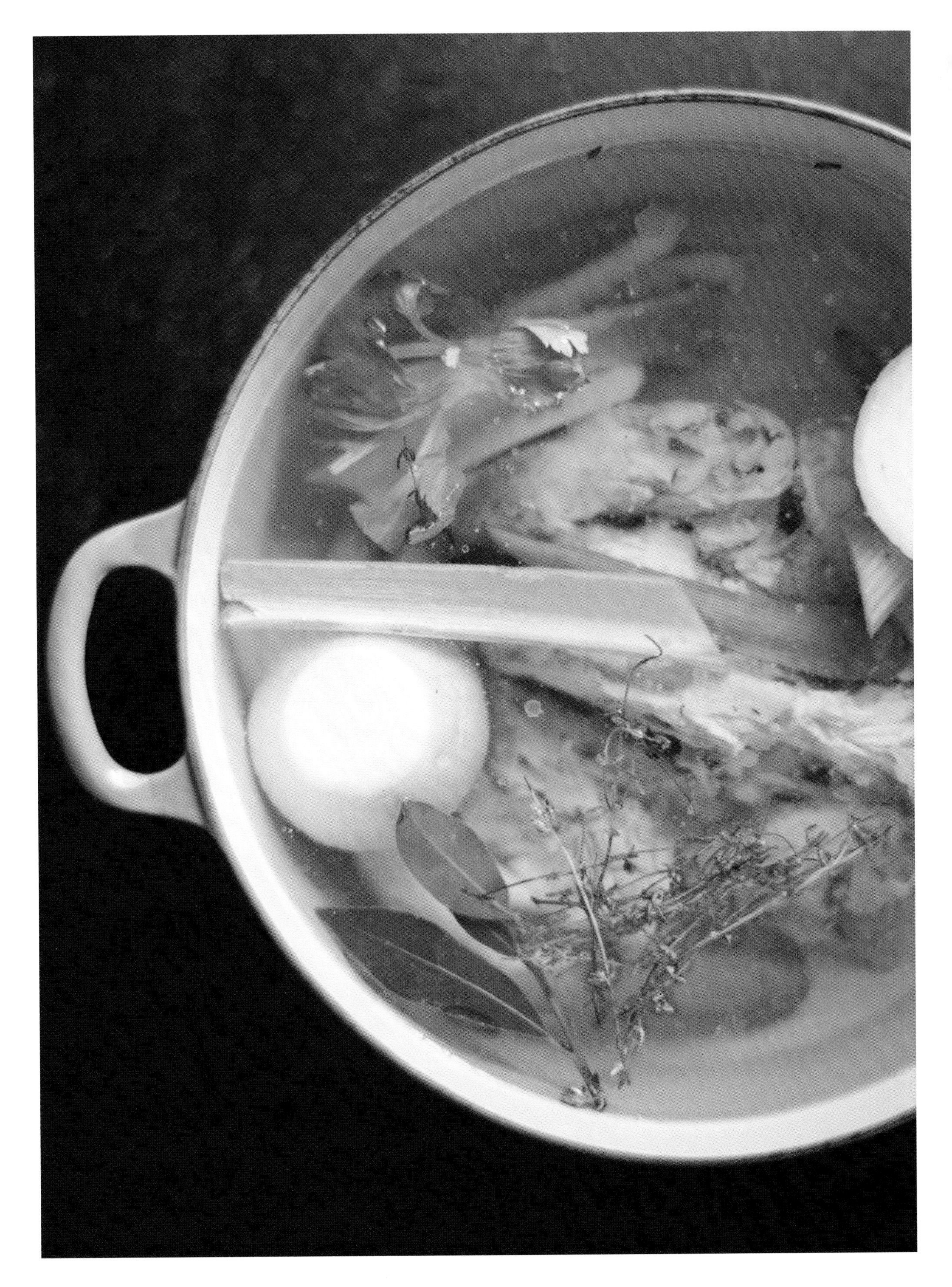

Brown Beef Stock

I've been making beef bone stock for years, but it never looked "beefy"—the way I remember the canned beef stock that my mother bought used to look. When you make a stock with just bones and no meat, or you don't roast the bones and meat first, the color ends up looking a whole lot like chicken stock. It gels well and is very nutritious, but sometimes it's nice to have a classic brown stock like this one. Adding more meat and some mushrooms not only makes the stock nice and dark, it really improves the flavor, too. It's worth it to make your own stock instead of buying it in a can or package, and it's really not difficult. Also, please don't skip the vinegar, which helps bring out more minerals from the bones.

Makes about 5 quarts

- *4 pounds meaty shanks with the bone*
- *2 pounds marrowbones*
- *5 medium carrots*
- *2 stalks celery*
- *2 medium yellow onions, halved*
- *Cold filtered water*
- *6 sprigs fresh thyme or 1 teaspoon dried thyme leaves*
- *3 bay leaves*
- *¼ cup apple cider vinegar*

1. Preheat the oven to 350°F. Line a roasting pan or rimmed baking sheet with parchment paper.
2. Spread out the meat, bones, carrots, celery, and onions on the lined pan.
3. Roast for about 45 minutes, flipping halfway through. You want it all to be nicely browned.
4. Remove from oven and place in the largest pot you own.
5. Fill the pot with cold filtered water. (Warm water ends up producing a cloudier stock.)
6. Add the thyme, bay leaves, and vinegar. Bring to a boil, then reduce to a very low simmer.
7. Skim any scum off the top. The scum forms right in the beginning.
8. Loosely cover and let the pot slowly bubble for 12 to 24 hours. I allow it to go overnight.
9. When the stock is done, turn off the heat and allow it to cool on the counter for about 1 hour.
10. Strain the stock through a cheesecloth-lined strainer (to catch any loose herbs) into a large bowl or separate, smaller pots and place in the refrigerator to cool (I usually do this overnight).
11. When the stock is fully cooled, skim off and discard any fat that has risen to the top. Ladle the stock into freezer-proof containers. Label, date, and store in the freezer until you're ready to use it. It will keep in the freezer for up to a year.

Whole30	Yes
Nut-free	Yes
Egg-free	Yes
AIP	Yes

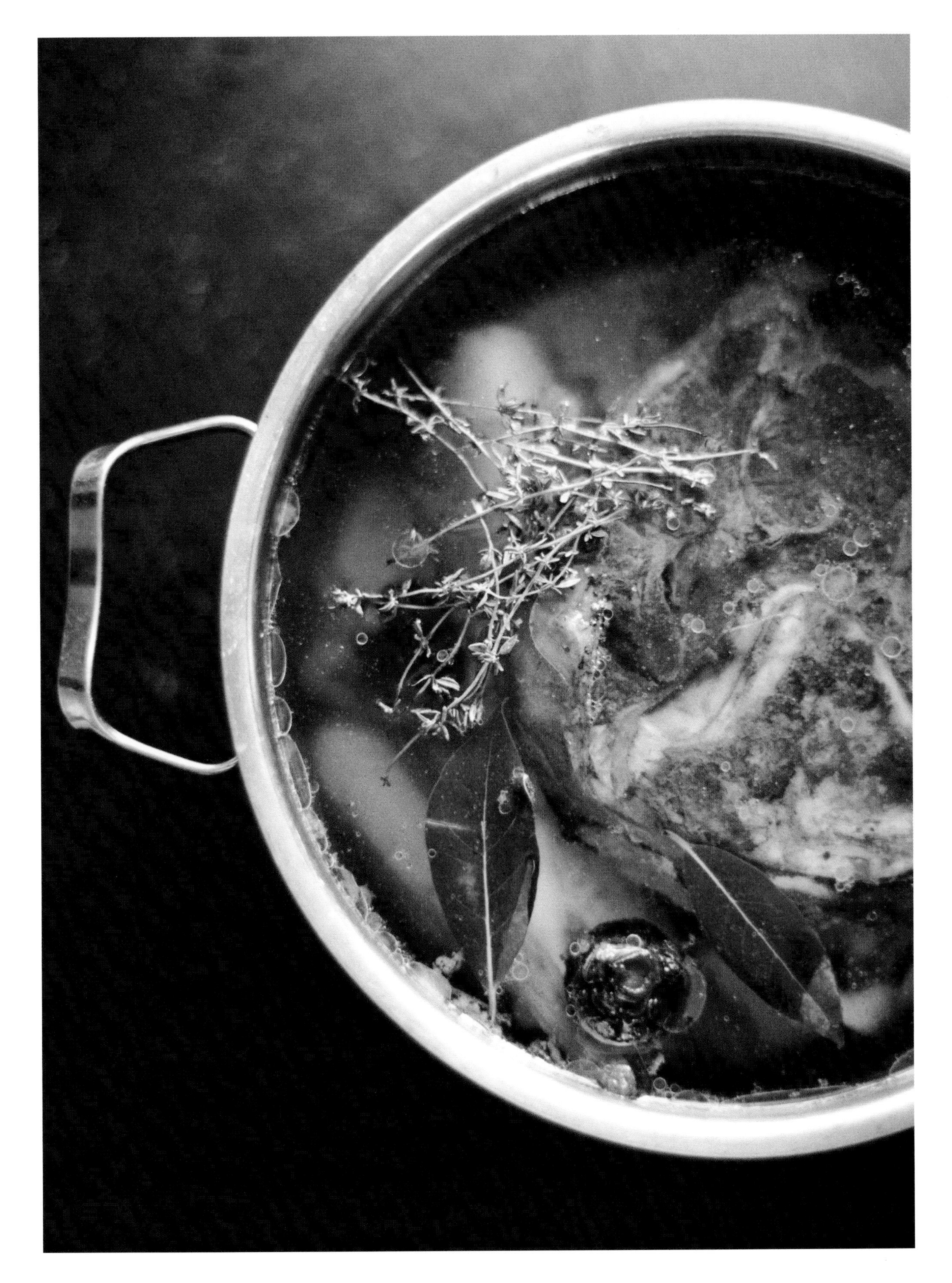

Fish Stock

Fish stock is super fast to make, and one big batch can make enough for many months of chowders and fish soups. Because fish have more delicate oils, you don't want to boil it for as long as beef or chicken stock. Half an hour to 45 minutes is all you need for a lovely, delicate flavor that is an excellent base for all kinds of soups. Ask at your local seafood store for fish "wracks," which are the carcasses of fish left over from the filleting process. I think they charged me $1.20 for 5 pounds for a recent batch of stock. It's a pretty good deal! It's important not to use an oily fish like salmon or mackerel, though, as they will produce an unpleasant stock.

Makes about 5 quarts

- *2½ to 5 pounds fish "wracks" or whole carcasses of nonoily fish, such as haddock*
- *4 sprigs fresh thyme*
- *3 bay leaves*
- *3 medium carrots*
- *1 medium yellow onion*
- *3 stalks celery*
- *Cold filtered water*

Whole30	Yes
Nut-free	Yes
Egg-free	Yes
AIP	Yes

1. Place all of the ingredients in a large stockpot and add filtered water to cover.

2. Bring to a boil and skim the scum off the top. Simmer gently for 30 to 45 minutes.

3. Remove from the heat and allow to cool on the counter for about 1 hour.

4. Strain the stock through a cheesecloth-lined strainer (to catch any loose herbs) into a large bowl or separate, smaller pots and place in the refrigerator to cool (I usually do this overnight).

5. Ladle the stock into freezer-safe containers. Label, date, and store in the freezer until you're ready to use it. It will keep in the freezer for up to a year.

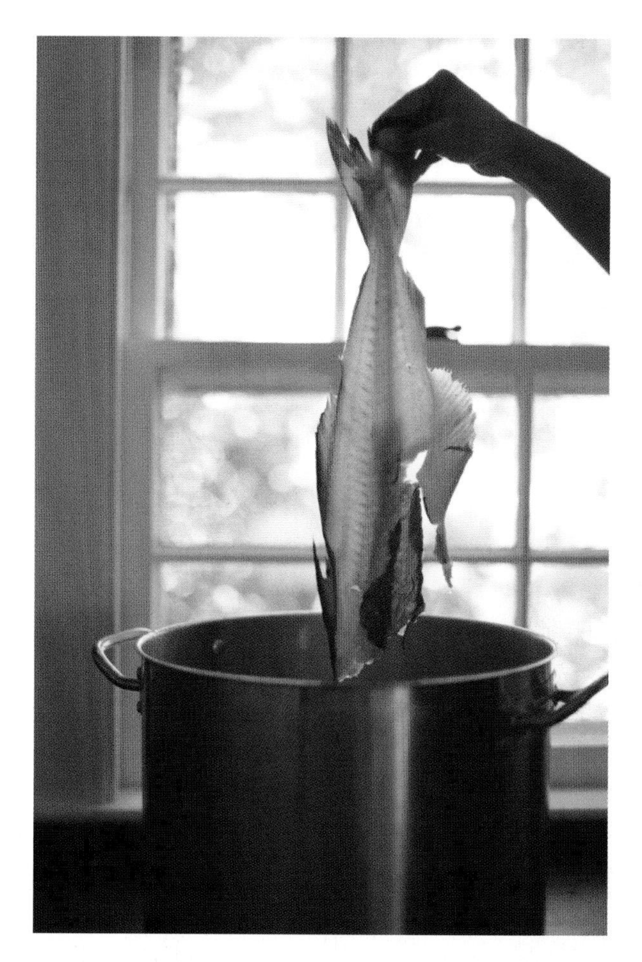

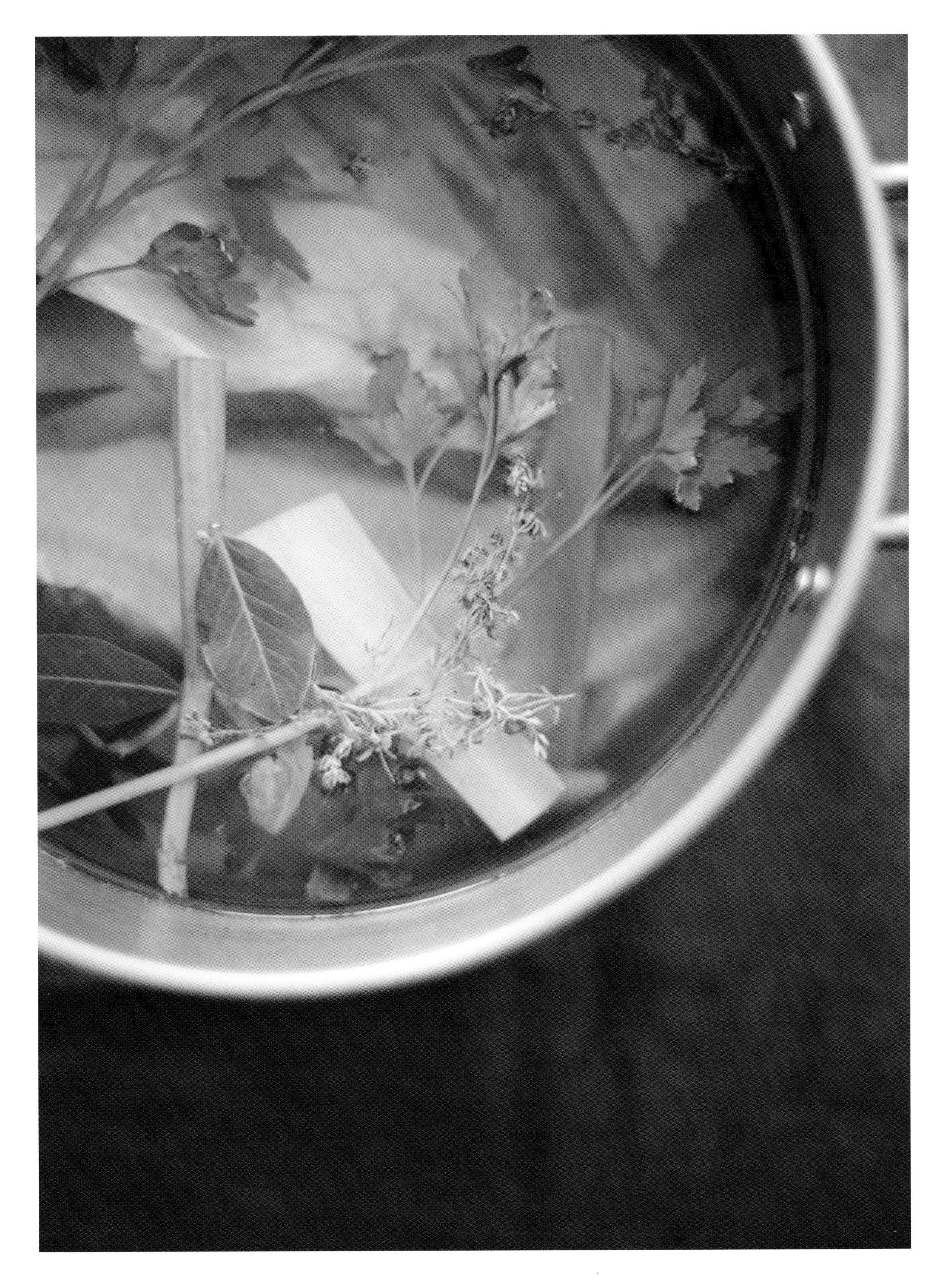

Homemade Mayonnaise

It may seem like a hassle, but once you have tried homemade mayonnaise, you'll never eat the jarred stuff again. The mayo you find at the grocery store is usually made with canola oil, which is not a good fat source because the high heat used in its processing makes it rancid. I used to have problems with my homemade mayo separating, but then I learned the secret trick: adding a teaspoon of water, which helps create a foolproof emulsion. One batch will keep in the fridge for a week, and you can make it even more flavorful by adding fresh herbs, extra lemon juice, extra mustard, or some chipotle peppers. I like to make this in a plastic quart-sized container with a handheld immersion blender, but you can use a food processor or hand whisk instead. (It will take a while with a whisk, but it will work.)

Makes about 2 cups

- *1 egg yolk*
- *1 teaspoon water*
- *1 teaspoon Dijon mustard*
- *Juice of ½ lemon*
- *1 cup light olive oil*
- *Sea salt and ground black pepper*

1. Place the egg yolk, water, mustard, and lemon juice in an immersion blender cup or a tall and narrow quart-sized container (such as a plastic storage container, canning jar, or Pyrex measuring cup). Add the olive oil and allow to settle for 15 seconds.
2. Place the immersion blender head at the bottom of the container and turn it on. When the mayo starts to form, slowly draw the head of the blender upward to the top of the container.
3. Add a pinch or two of salt and pepper to taste. It's that simple!

NOTES: *I like to use light olive oil because it has a more neutral taste than other olive oils. You can also use macadamia nut oil or avocado oil.*

Whole30	Yes
Nut-free	Yes
Egg-free	No
AIP	No

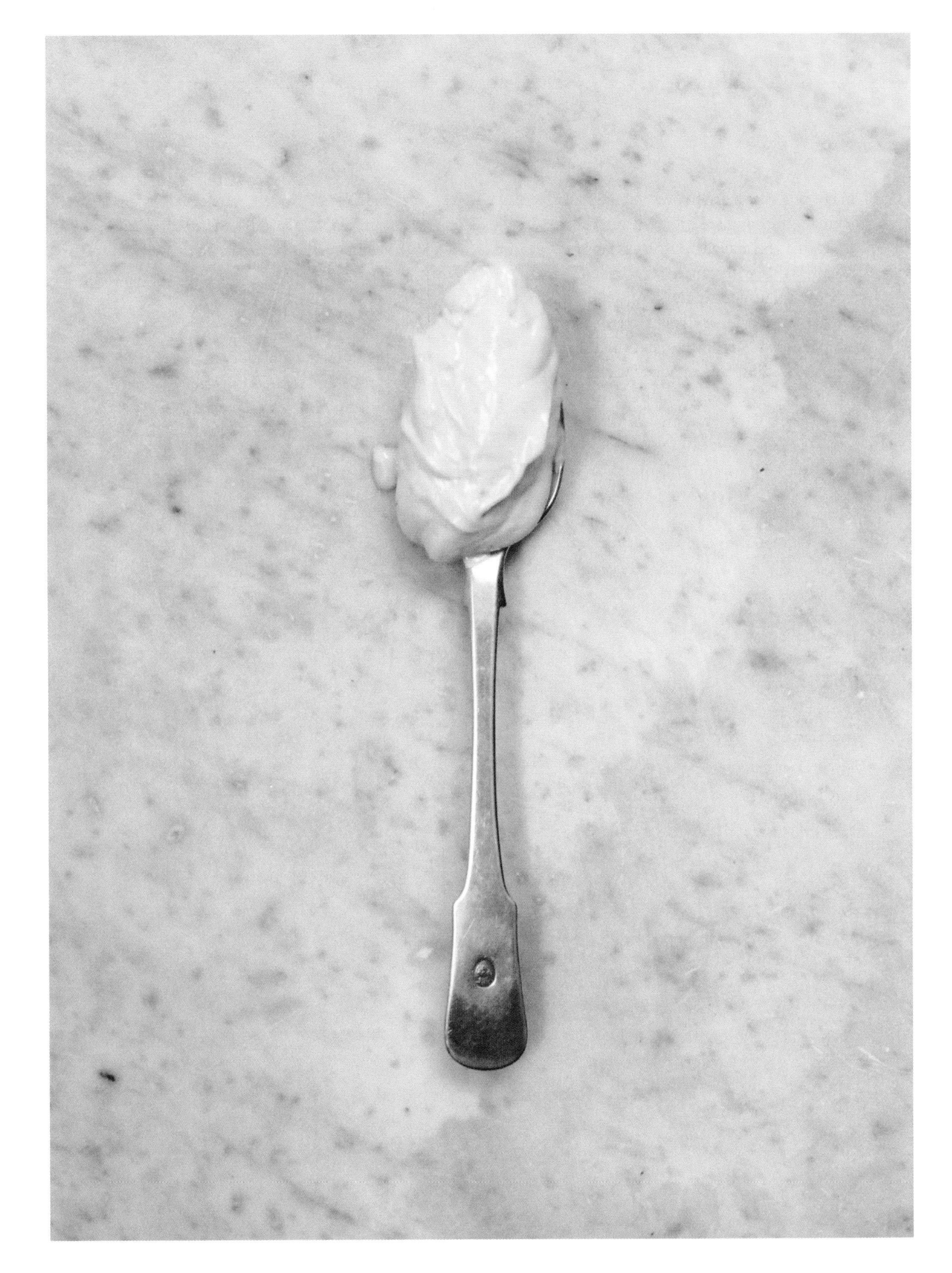

Smoky BBQ Sauce

This sauce is a mixture of all the flavors I love in other barbecue sauces. It's smoky, thick, and perfect with Frank's Hickory-Smoked Brisket (page 220) or any other grilled meat. Store-bought barbecue sauce usually contains high-fructose corn syrup or other sweeteners. This one gets a touch of sweetness from the applesauce.

Makes about 2 cups

- *1 tablespoon bacon fat or coconut oil*
- *1 cup diced yellow onions*
- *4 cloves garlic, minced*
- *2 stalks celery, diced*
- *1 (14½-ounce) can diced tomatoes and their juices, or 5 to 6 fresh Roma tomatoes*
- *½ cup apple cider vinegar*
- *¼ cup applesauce*
- *2 tablespoons tomato paste*
- *2 tablespoons paprika*
- *1 tablespoon dry mustard*
- *1 tablespoon all-natural liquid smoke*
- *2 teaspoons sea salt*
- *2 teaspoons ground black pepper*
- *⅛ teaspoon cayenne pepper*

1. In a large saucepan, warm the bacon fat over medium-low heat. Cook the onions, garlic, and celery in the bacon fat for about 10 minutes, or until soft.
2. Add the rest of the ingredients and simmer, uncovered, for 1 hour, or until thickened to the desired consistency.
3. Puree in a blender or with an immersion blender.
4. Adjust the seasoning as needed. Serve immediately, or allow to cool and place in glass storage jars for later use. The sauce will keep for 1 week in the fridge.

Whole30	Yes
Nut-free	Yes
Egg-free	Yes
AIP	No

How to Make Crème Fraîche

I love adding a touch of crème fraîche to soups. It's easy to make and has a sweet, nutty, and silky sour cream–like flavor. You'll wonder where it's been all your life.

Makes 1 cup

- *1 cup heavy cream*
- *1 tablespoon buttermilk*

Whole30	No
Nut-free	Yes
Egg-free	Yes
AIP	No

1. Combine the cream and buttermilk in a jar and cover with a towel. Place in a warm place overnight. In the morning it will be thick, like sour cream.
2. Store in the fridge for up to 3 weeks.

How to Make Ghee

Ghee is clarified butter that has a longer shelf life and is traditionally used in Indian cuisine. Browning the milk solids and straining them out lends ghee a nuttier flavor than clarified butter.

Makes about ½ cup

- *1 pound unsalted butter (page 348)*

Whole30	Yes
Nut-free	Yes
Egg-free	Yes
AIP	No

1. Gently melt the butter in a saucepan over medium-low heat. In a few minutes, the butter will separate, and you'll see a layer of foam rise to the top. With a spoon, remove the top foamy layer until all you see is clear yellow liquid.
2. Allow the melted butter to simmer for a few more minutes, but don't allow the bits at the bottom of the pan to burn.
3. Remove the pan from the heat and allow to cool slightly. Pour through a cheesecloth-lined strainer into a clean jar.
4. Allow the ghee to cool completely before sealing the jar. It can be stored at room temperature for up to 1 month.

How to Make Butter

You must try making homemade butter. It's incredible, especially if you use rich, raw, grass-fed cream, and nothing like store-bought butter. I like to add a small dab of fresh herb butter to soups or spread it on Salted Herb Crackers (page 298). It's also wonderful on top of a nice thick steak! The process is easy, too—just be sure to wear an apron or old shirt, as it can be a little messy.

Makes about 8 ounces

- *1 pint heavy cream*

VARIATIONS

Sea Salted Butter. *Mix ½ teaspoon of sea salt into the butter after you've completed Step 5. Then press into the preferred shape.*

Sea Salted Herb Butter. *Mix ½ teaspoon of sea salt and 2 tablespoons of minced fresh parsley (or fresh herb of your choice) into the butter after you've completed Step 5. Then press into the preferred shape.*

Cultured Butter. *The night before you make the butter add 2 tablespoons of plain whole-milk yogurt to the cream. Cover with a towel and allow to culture overnight. Make your butter the next day. It will have a slightly tangy taste. Add sea salt to taste, if desired.*

Kefir Butter. *The night before you make the butter, add 1 teaspoon of kefir grains to the cream, cover with a towel, and allow to ferment slightly overnight. The next morning, strain out the grains and make your butter. Add sea salt to taste, if desired.*

1. Place the cream in a large bowl. With a mixer on medium speed, beat the cream until it is whipped cream, then keep on going.

2. This is where it gets a bit messy. You'll soon notice the cream beginning to separate. There will be yellowish chunks and some watery stuff in the bowl. The water may splash a bit. Keep on beating until you're left with all chunks and water.

3. Carefully pour the mixture through a cheesecloth-lined strainer, holding the butter solids back in the bowl. Allow the buttermilk to strain through, then drop the butter solids into the cheesecloth.

4. Gather the cloth around the butter solids and squeeze hard with your fist. Do this several times to get as much buttermilk out of the butter as possible. You can save the buttermilk and make crème fraîche (page 347).

5. When you think you've gotten all of the buttermilk out of the solids, squeeze one more time. Run it under cold water and squeeze again until all you can see is the butter. You want to rinse off all of the buttermilk.

6. Press the butter into any shape you like, or package it in small mason jars and give as gifts. It will keep for 2 to 3 weeks in the refrigerator.

Whole30	No
Nut-free	Yes
Egg-free	Yes
AIP	No

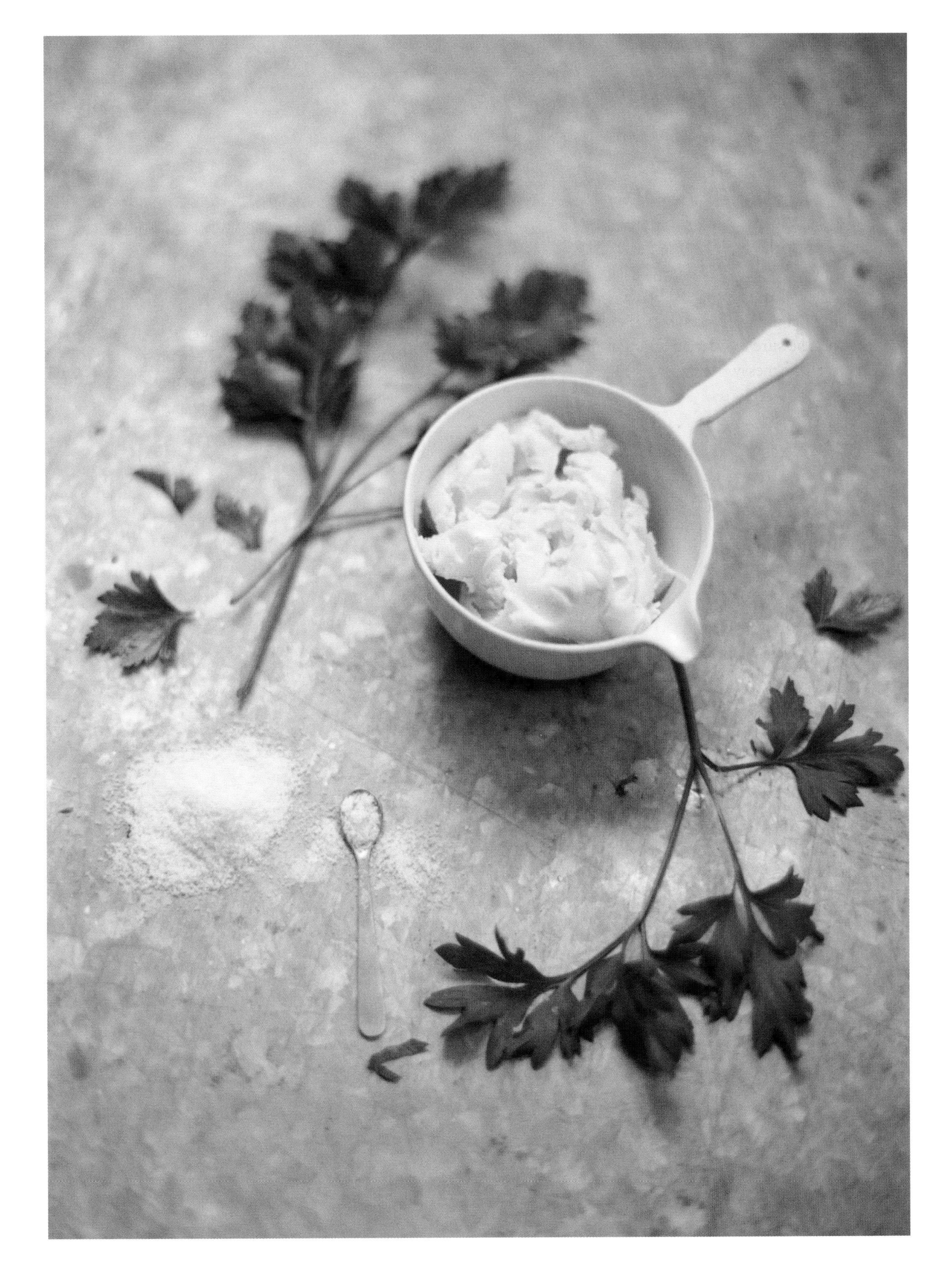

How to Render Lard

When you have a pork share or raise your own pigs, you'll end up with some fat with skin on it and, if you're lucky, some organ fat that can be made into leaf lard—the pure white kind that used to be a prized possession of housewives. It's nearly impossible to find high-quality lard in stores, and it's a fantastic cooking fat that can be used in most recipes. Plus, lard from pasture-raised pigs is high in vitamin D. Making lard is not difficult; it's just a little messy and time-consuming to cut up the fat. Some people make it on the stovetop, but I roast it on low heat.

Special equipment

- *Small canning jars or freezer-safe containers with lids*

1. Heat the oven to 275°F.
2. Chop the fat into 1- to 2-inch pieces. It's easier to cut the organ fat than the fat with the skin attached, so if you have a ton of fat, use the organ fat first. It also produces whiter and tastier lard.
3. Place the fat pieces in a roasting pan, large casserole dish, or rimmed baking sheet lined with parchment paper and place in the oven for 1 to 2 hours.
4. Check on it every once in a while, making sure the fat isn't too hot and browning. Once there are chunks floating on the top and a nice layer of liquid fat on the bottom, you can strain the larger pieces using a cheesecloth-lined strainer. These pieces are called "cracklins," and kids love them sprinkled with a little salt.
5. Strain the rest of the liquid through a cheesecloth into canning jars or freezer-safe containers. Store in the fridge for up to 1 month or freezer for up to 6 months.

NOTES: *If you have a meat grinder, you can grind the fat. It's easier on your body (chopping all that fat can be tiring!), and you'll have more rendered lard at the end of the process. For ground fat, use a casserole dish with deep sides.*

Whole30	Yes
Nut-free	Yes
Egg-free	Yes
AIP	Yes

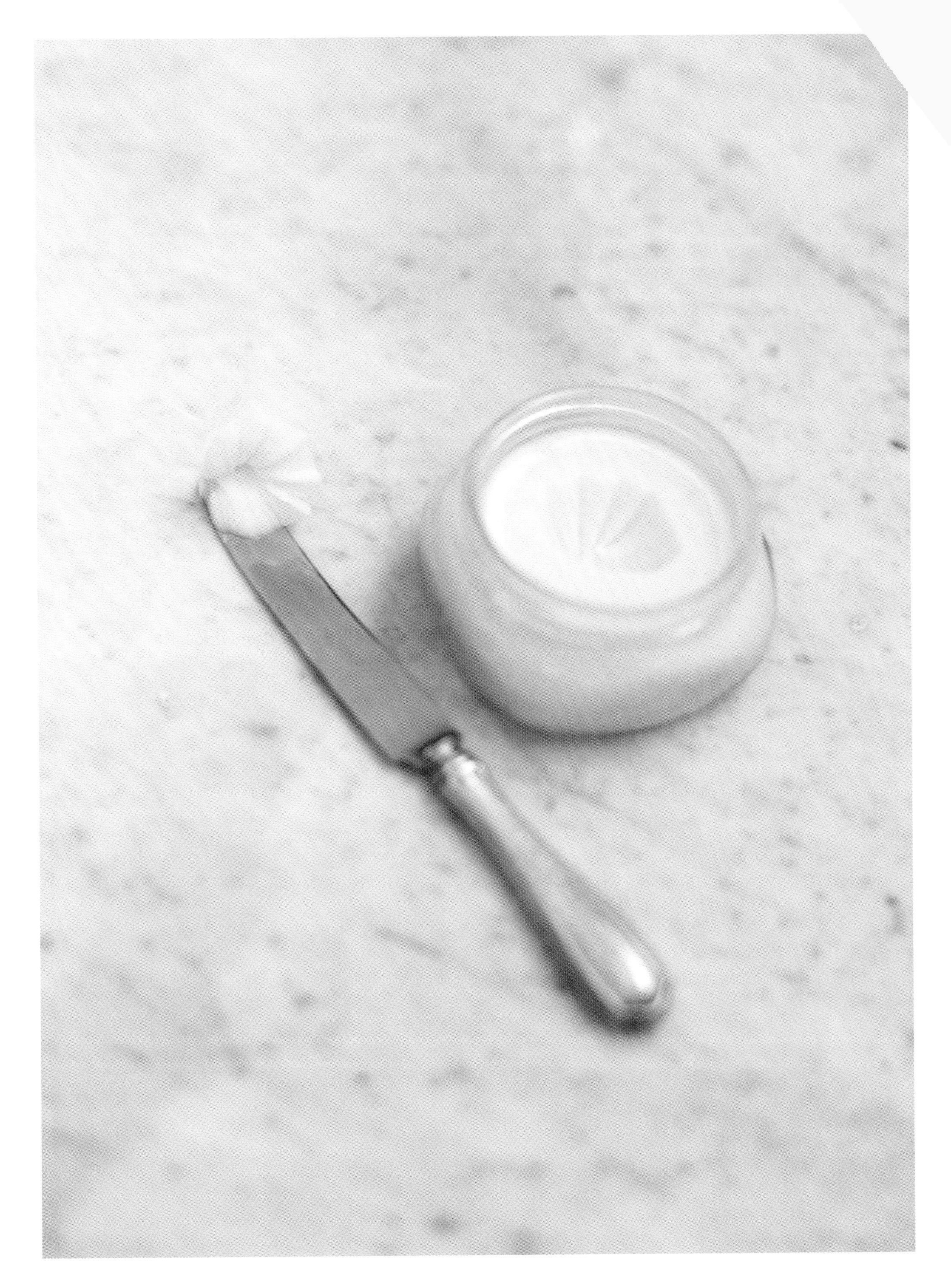

How to Freeze Greens

Swiss chard, kale, spinach, mustard, beet greens, turnip greens, and all of the many other garden greens can be frozen so that you can enjoy them during the winter months. All you need is some ice cube trays. I use these cubes when I want to add greens to soups or stews. I like to drop in whole cubes, but you can also thaw and drain them before using. With just a little extra work in the summer, you'll save money and have greens during the cold months.

Makes about 12 cubes of frozen greens

- *1 large bunch of greens, stems removed*

1. Bring a large pot of water to a boil. Have ready a bowl full of ice water and a slotted spoon.
2. Plunk the greens in the boiling water and blanch them for 2 to 3 minutes; they will brighten in color.
3. Using the slotted spoon, remove the greens from the boiling water and place them in the ice bath.
4. Roughly chop the greens.
5. Evenly distribute the greens among the little ice cube slots.
6. Cover the greens with water, tamping down any that stick up.
7. Place in the freezer overnight.
8. Remove the cubes from the trays and place in a freezer-proof container.

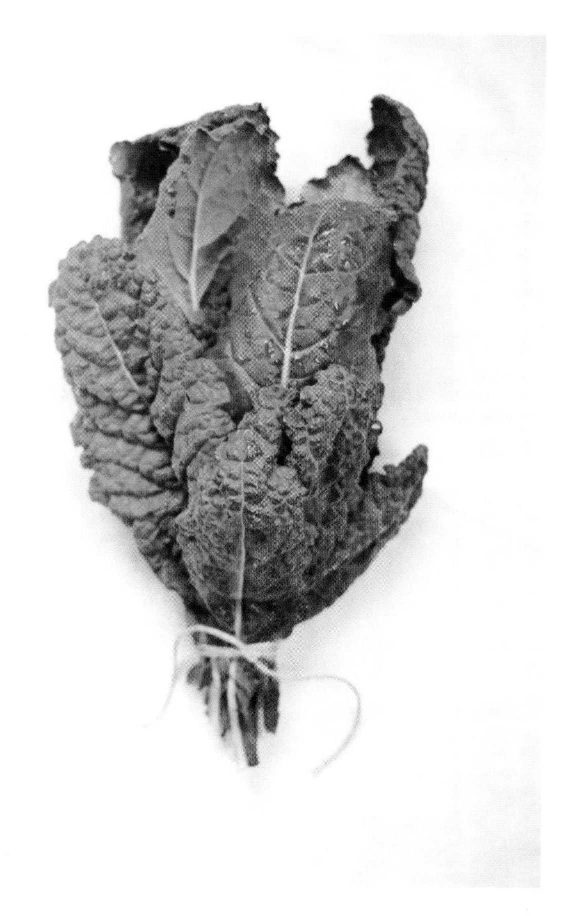

Whole30	Yes
Nut-free	Yes
Egg-free	Yes
AIP	Yes

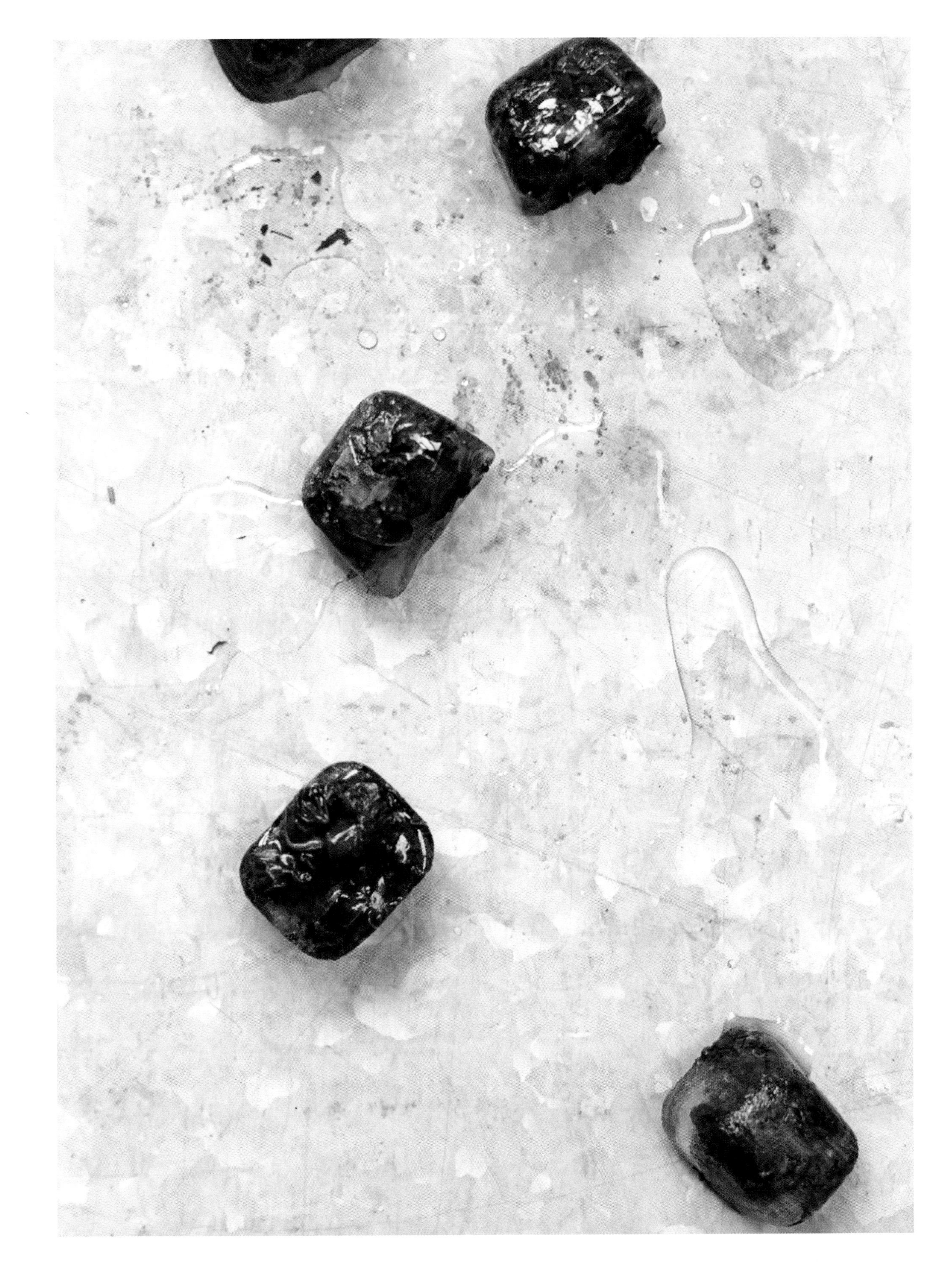

How to Can Tomatoes

Canning is easier than you think! Canned tomatoes in particular are a must for my pantry. It's important to use fresh, firm, high-acid tomatoes for canning, so it's best to stay away from sweet yellow heirlooms or overly ripe tomatoes, which lose their acidity as they become wrinkled and soft. I use standard Italian paste tomatoes. It's hard to judge how many tomatoes you'll need to fill your jars—it all depends on how large, ripe, and dense your tomatoes are. Be flexible and just experiment. For this process, make sure you use a water bath canner, not a pressure canner.

Makes about 10 pints

- *About 20 pounds paste tomatoes*

Special equipment

- *Canning tongs*
- *Water bath canner*
- *Funnel (not necessary, but makes putting the tomatoes in the jars much easier)*
- *10 pint-sized canning jars (I prefer wide-mouth jars)*
- *10 lids and screw bands*
- *Metal jar rack*

Whole30	Yes
Nut-free	Yes
Egg-free	Yes
AIP	No

1. Inspect the jars for cracks or chips and wash them with soapy water. Place the jars and lids in a saucepan filled with boiling water and sterilize for 5 minutes or so, then use the canning tongs to remove them to a clean surface and allow to air-dry.

2. Fill a water bath canner two-thirds full of water and heat it over medium heat (do not bring it to a boil). Fill another large pot two-thirds full of water and bring it to a boil.

3. Wash the tomatoes. Cut out the core and make an X in the bottom of each tomato.

4. Prepare a bowl of ice water.

5. Working in batches, place the tomatoes in the boiling water for about 30 seconds, then remove to the bowl of ice water. Continue until all of the tomatoes are blanched and in the ice bath.

6. It's now really easy to remove the skins from the tomatoes. Peel all the tomatoes and compost the skins.

7. Dice the peeled tomatoes and place them in another bowl. You'll soon have a big sloppy mess of diced tomatoes in the bowl.

8. Fill the jars with the diced tomatoes, stopping ½ inch from the top. Use the handle of a wooden spoon to press down the tomatoes and remove any air bubbles. It's important not to use metallic utensils during this process.

9. Once all of the jars are filled, wipe off any extra liquid from the tops of the jars and place the lids on the jars. Screw the bands down evenly and tightly.

10. Place the jars on the jar rack. Using the canning tongs, gently lower the rack into the hot (not boiling) water in the water bath canner. The water should cover the jars by 1 to 2 inches. Add more water if necessary.

11. Put the lid on the water bath canner and bring the water to a boil. Process the pints for 35 minutes (45 minutes for quart-sized jars) at a gentle but steady boil.

12. Use the tongs to remove the jars and stand them several inches apart. Allow to cool overnight. Test the seals, but do not overtighten the bands. If any jars did not seal properly, place them in the refrigerator and use the tomatoes with a week. Store the sealed jars in a cool, dark pantry or cabinet for 12 to 18 months. Once opened, eat within a week.

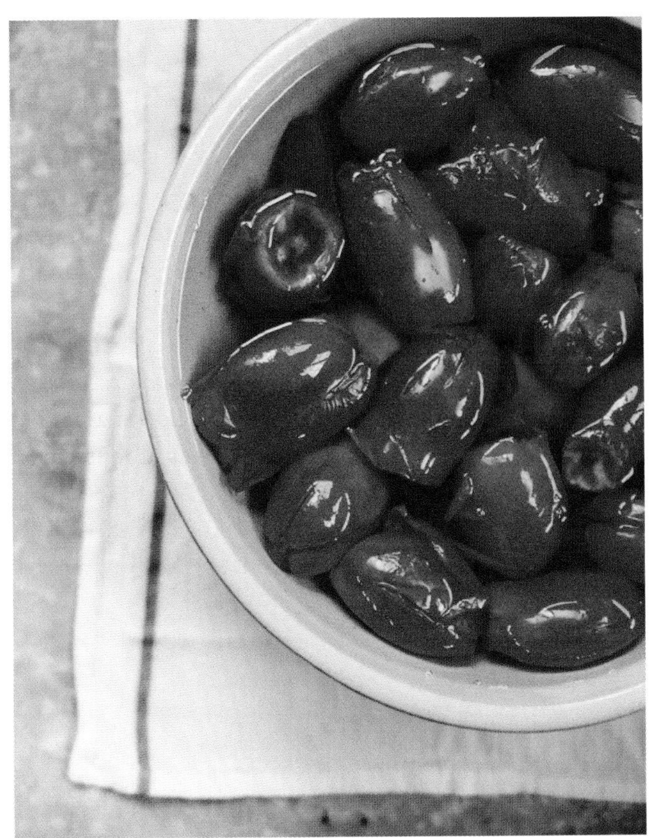

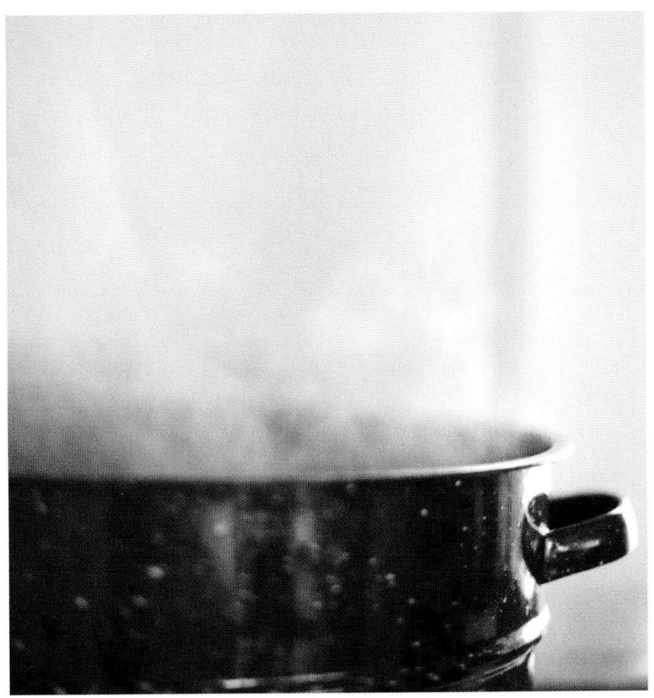

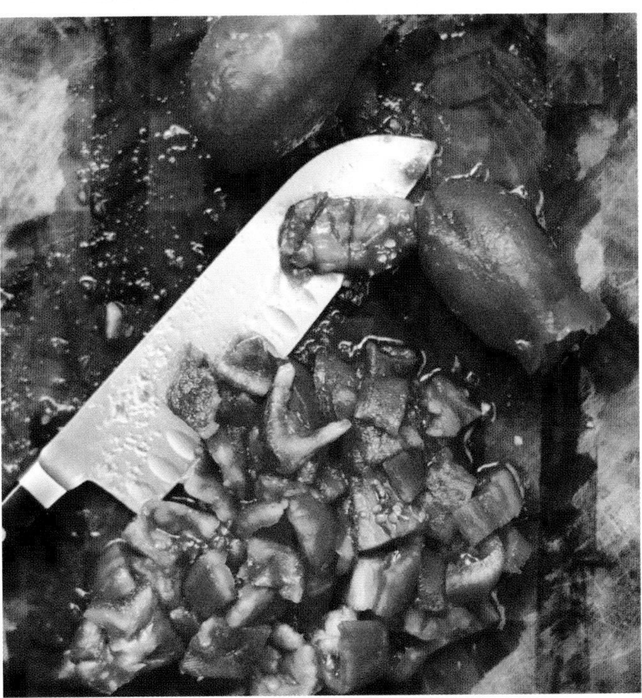

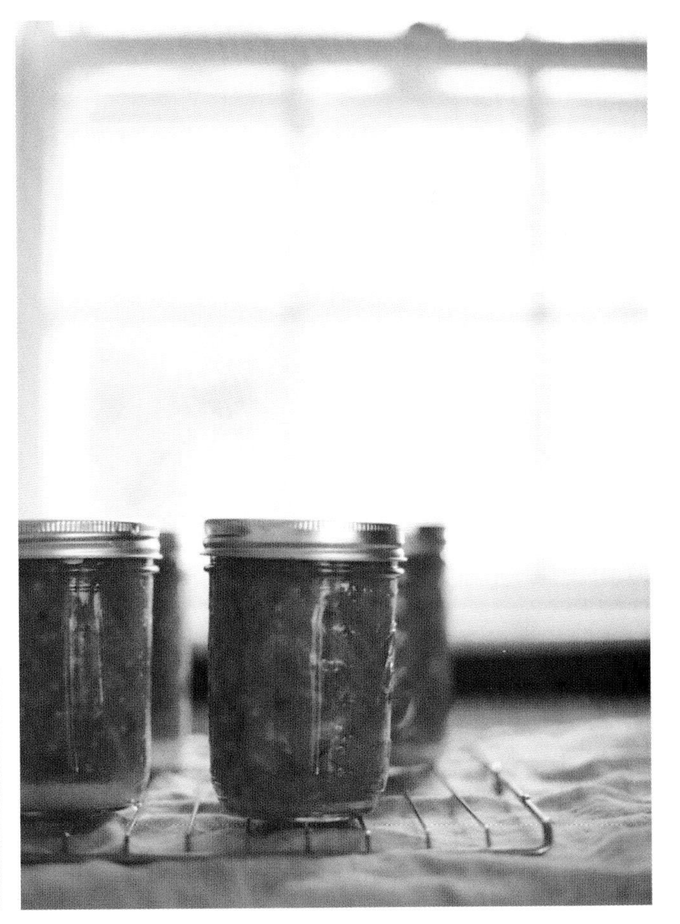

How to Refrigerate Stocks, Soups, and Stews Properly

From a food safety standpoint, it's a good idea to know how to cool and store stocks, soups, and stews. If you cook a nice big batch of chili in an enameled cast-iron Dutch oven, put the lid on it while it's still hot, and pop the whole thing in the fridge, you could be asking for some serious GI distress. That chili is not likely to come down to a safe cold temperature in a timely manner; in fact, it could still be warm in the center tomorrow morning. To avoid getting sick from your favorite soup or stew, follow these easy tips.

- Allow the food to cool for about an hour, stirring occasionally to let out some steam. However, don't allow it to sit at room temperature for much longer than an hour, because it's the ideal growing medium for bacteria.
- Place the food in smaller glass or metal containers (no hot foods in plastic!) so that it will cool more quickly in the fridge. (I prefer Pyrex or stainless-steel containers with plastic lids.)
- Place the containers in the fridge. Do not stack multiple items of hot food on top of each other.
- If you intend to freeze your food, chill it in the fridge first, then transfer it to the freezer the next day. It will be easier for it to come to the proper temperature this way. Never put hot food in the freezer, as it will raise the temperature of all of your frozen foods.
- Use caution when storing canning jars in the freezer, as they can easily crack.

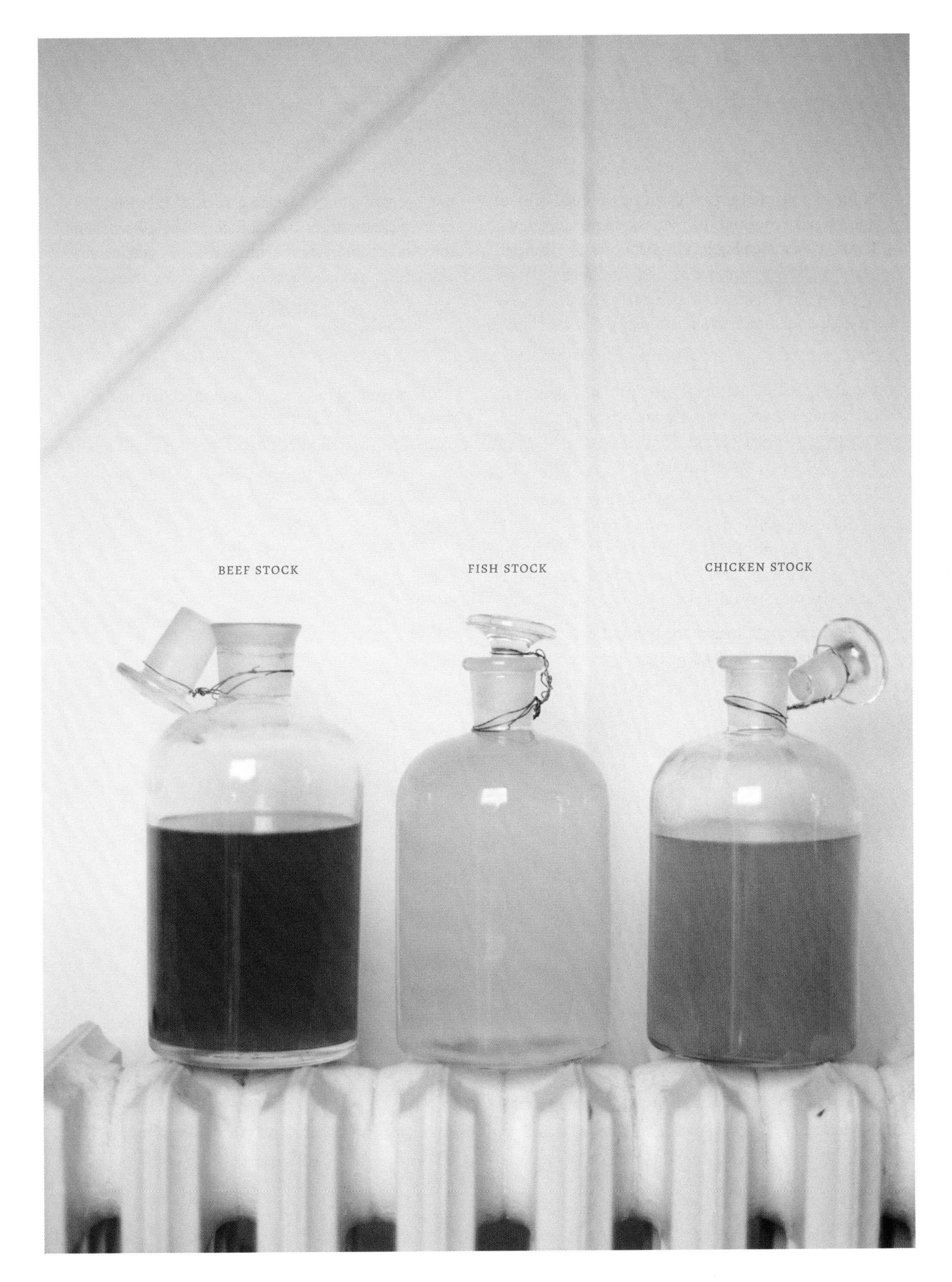
BEEF STOCK
FISH STOCK
CHICKEN STOCK

How to Thaw Meat Quickly

Each week, I take a bunch of meat from our freezer and place it in a bowl inside our refrigerator. When it's time to cook dinner, I just look to see what meat is thawed and ready to go. As someone who is certified in safe food handling, I can tell you that this slow refrigerator method is the safest way to thaw meat, since bacteria grows most quickly between 41°F and 135°F. With the slow-thaw method, the meat also has more time to reabsorb the ice crystals that formed between the fibers, which gives it a better texture.

Sometimes, however, I am stuck with no thawed meat and need some fast. To quickly thaw meat, place the wrapped meat in a large bowl in the sink. Place it under cool running water for 15 to 20 minutes. This process works great for 1-pound packages of ground meat or steaks, but it isn't great for a whole chicken or a big hunk of ham—I highly recommend that you use the slow-thaw refrigerator method for larger cuts of meat.

Just in case I need to thaw it quickly, I prefer to get our meat sealed in plastic rather than wrapped in butcher paper. Butcher paper allows water to leak in when the meat is quick-thawed, resulting in soggy meat. Also, with the see-through plastic, I can see if there is any freezer burn before unwrapping it.

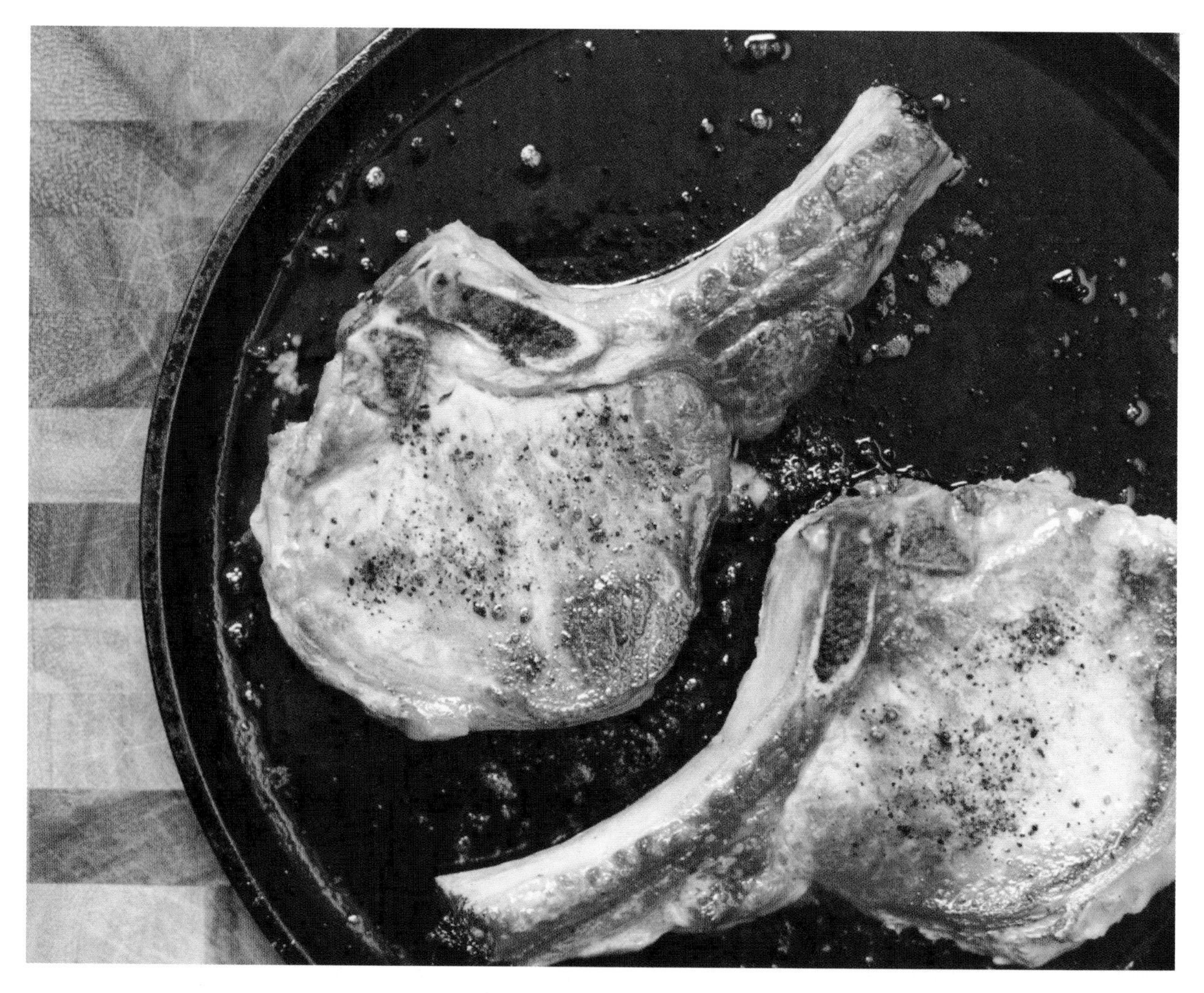

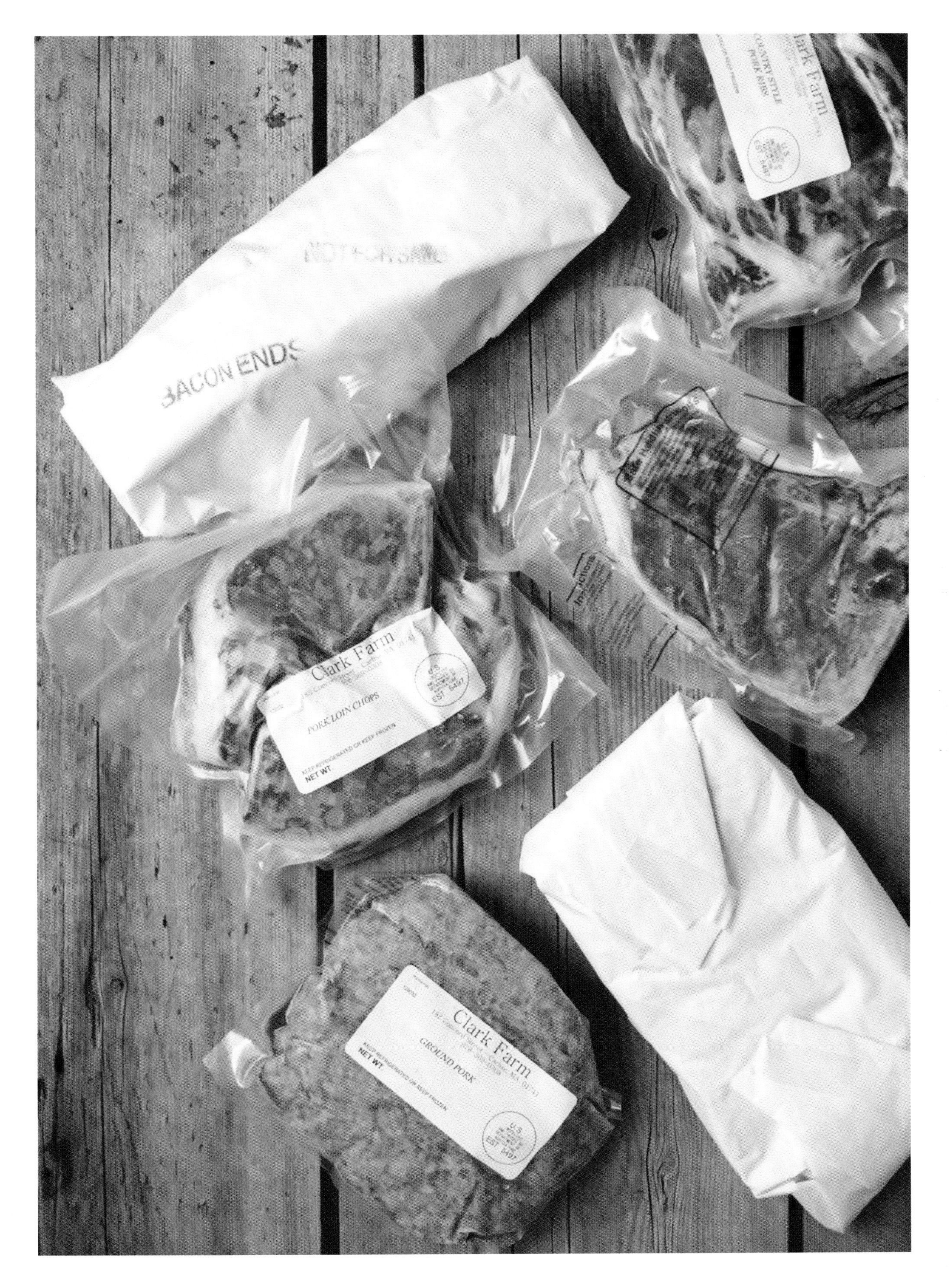
BACON ENDS
Clark Farm
PORK LOIN CHOPS
KEEP REFRIGERATED OR KEEP FROZEN
NET WT.
EST. 5497
Clark Farm
GROUND PORK
KEEP REFRIGERATED OR KEEP FROZEN
NET WT.
EST. 5497
Clark Farm
COUNTRY STYLE
PORK RIBS
EST. 5497

Meat Cooking Tips

If you're going to invest your money in good meat, you might as well treat it right! Here are several tips.

- Allow the meat to come to room temperature before cooking it.
- Use the right cooking method for the type and cut of meat you're using. Leaner cuts of grass-fed meat and pastured poultry can become tough when cooked in a hot pan on the stovetop, so for these cuts, low and slow cooking methods, such as braising, stewing, and making soup, are ideal.
- Cook the meat for the right about of time (see the chart at right).
- Use a digital meat thermometer to avoid overcooking or undercooking meat. With a digital meat thermometer, you will have no doubt when your meat is ready to eat.
- Let the meat rest after cooking it. When it's done cooking, place it on a cutting board for at least 5 minutes before cutting into it. (Larger cuts of meat require longer resting times; see the chart at right.)

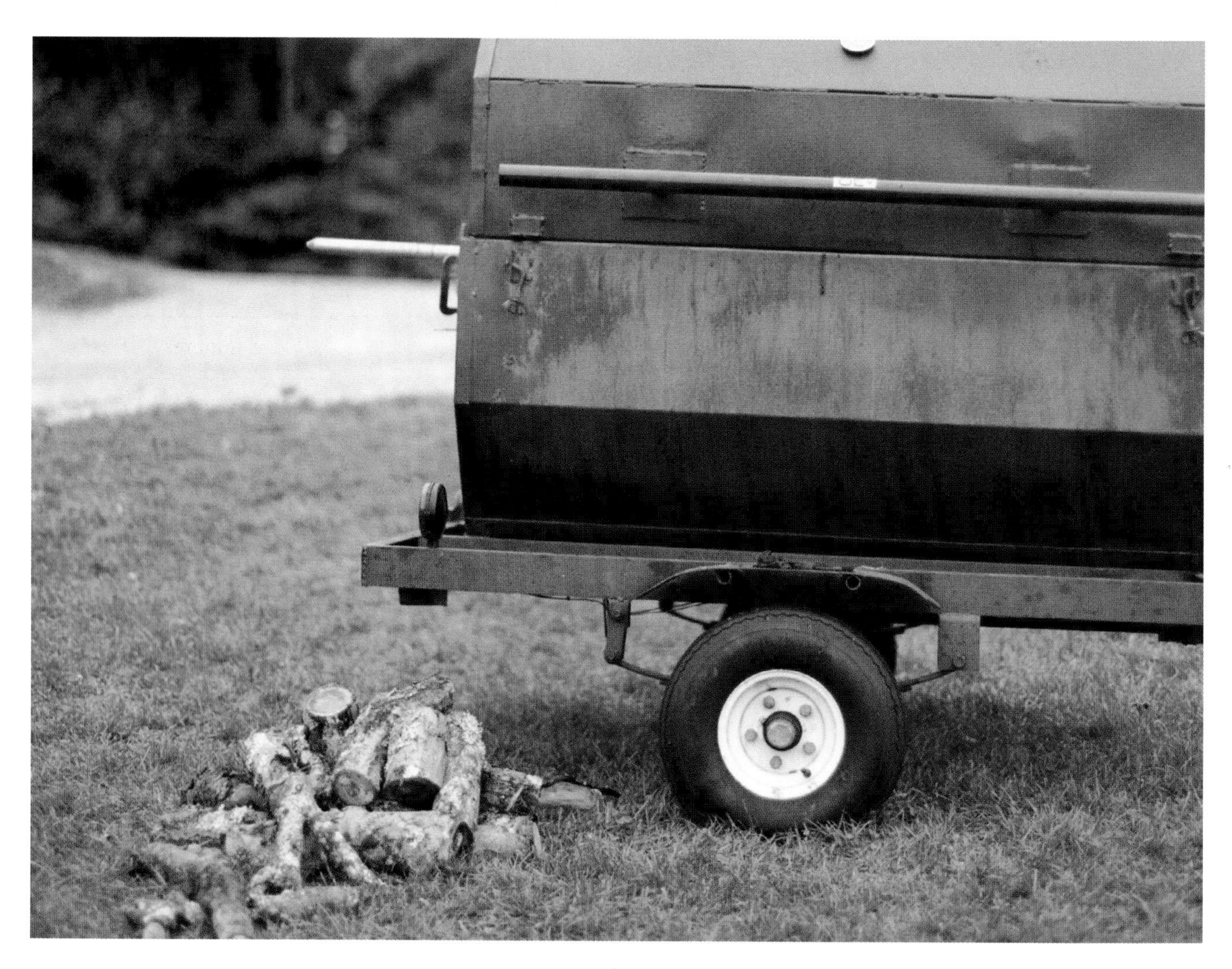

Meat Doneness Charts

Here's a handy chart on when to remove your meat from the heat source. This is not based on the USDA's guidelines, which I find tend to result in overcooked meat.

Poultry

	REMOVE	IDEAL INTERNAL TEMPERATURE	RESTING TIME
Whole Chicken, Roasted	165°F–170°F	170°F–175°F	15 minutes
Whole Turkey, Roasted	160°F–175°F	Breast meat: 165°F Dark meat: 175°F	20–60 minutes, depending on size*

**A turkey weighing over 20 pounds can take 60 minutes to rest, with a temperature increase of 20°F or more.*

Red Meat

	RARE		MEDIUM-RARE		MEDIUM		MEDIUM-WELL		RESTING TIME
	Remove	Ideal	Remove	Ideal	Remove	Ideal	Remove	Ideal	
Beef Steak	125°F	130°F	130°F	135°F	140°F	145°F	155°F	160°F	5 minutes
Beef Roast	120°F	125°F	125°F	130°F	135°F	140°F	140°F	155°F	20 minutes
Lamb Chop	125°F	130°F	130°F	135°F	140°F	145°F	155°F	160°F	5 minutes
Lamb Roast	120°F	130°F	125°F	130°F	135°F	140°F	140°F	155°F	20 minutes
Pork Chop	—	—	—	—	135°F–140°F	140°F–145°F	145°F	150°F	5 minutes
Pork Roast	—	—	—	—	140°F	150°F	150°F	160°F	20 minutes
Venison Steak	125°F	130°F	130°F	135°F	140°F	145°F	155°F	160°F	5 minutes
Venison Roast	120°F	130°F	125°F	130°F	135°F	140°F	140°F	155°F	20 minutes

How to Use a Charcoal Grill

Kicking it old school with a real grill is much more fun than standing around a gas-fueled grill that you start with the push of a button. The meat tastes better, and using natural wood charcoal for your heat source instead of propane is more sustainable.

Firing It Up

1. Place the chimney starter on the grill grates or on some bricks off to the side.
2. Roll a few sheets of newspaper into a tube and place it in the underside of the chimney, in a circle.
3. Turn the chimney over and fill it with the amount of charcoal you will need.
4. With matches or a lighter, set the newspaper on fire in a few locations. Soon you'll start to see smoke coming from the top of the chimney.
5. After about 10 minutes, you will see an orange color deep inside the chimney and some flames coming up. This is the perfect time to carefully dump the contents of the chimney into your grill. If you wait until all of the coals at the top are ash-colored, the coals at the bottom will already be spent and useless. Use a heatproof glove, as the handle will be hot.

Grilling with Indirect Heat. With indirect heat, the heat rises, reflects off the lid and interior surfaces of the grill, and slowly cooks the food evenly on all sides. The heat circulates around the food, so there's no need to flip the meat. This method is great for cooking roasts, whole chickens, and other large cuts of meat, as well as delicate fish. To grill with indirect heat, arrange the coals on one side of the grill and place a drip pan on the other side, directly below where you will place the meat. You can add water to the pan for moisture, to prevent larger cuts of meat from drying out. Place the meat on the grill grate and close the lid, lifting it only to baste the meat or to test for doneness at the end of the recommended cooking time.

Grilling with Direct Heat. This is similar to using your broiler, except the heat source is under the food instead of above it. The coals are spread evenly across your grill, and the food is cooked directly over the coals. This method is perfect for searing meats and creating those nice grill marks. To grill with direct heat, place the food on the grill grate and close the lid, lifting the lid only to turn the food or to test for doneness at the end of the recommended cooking time.

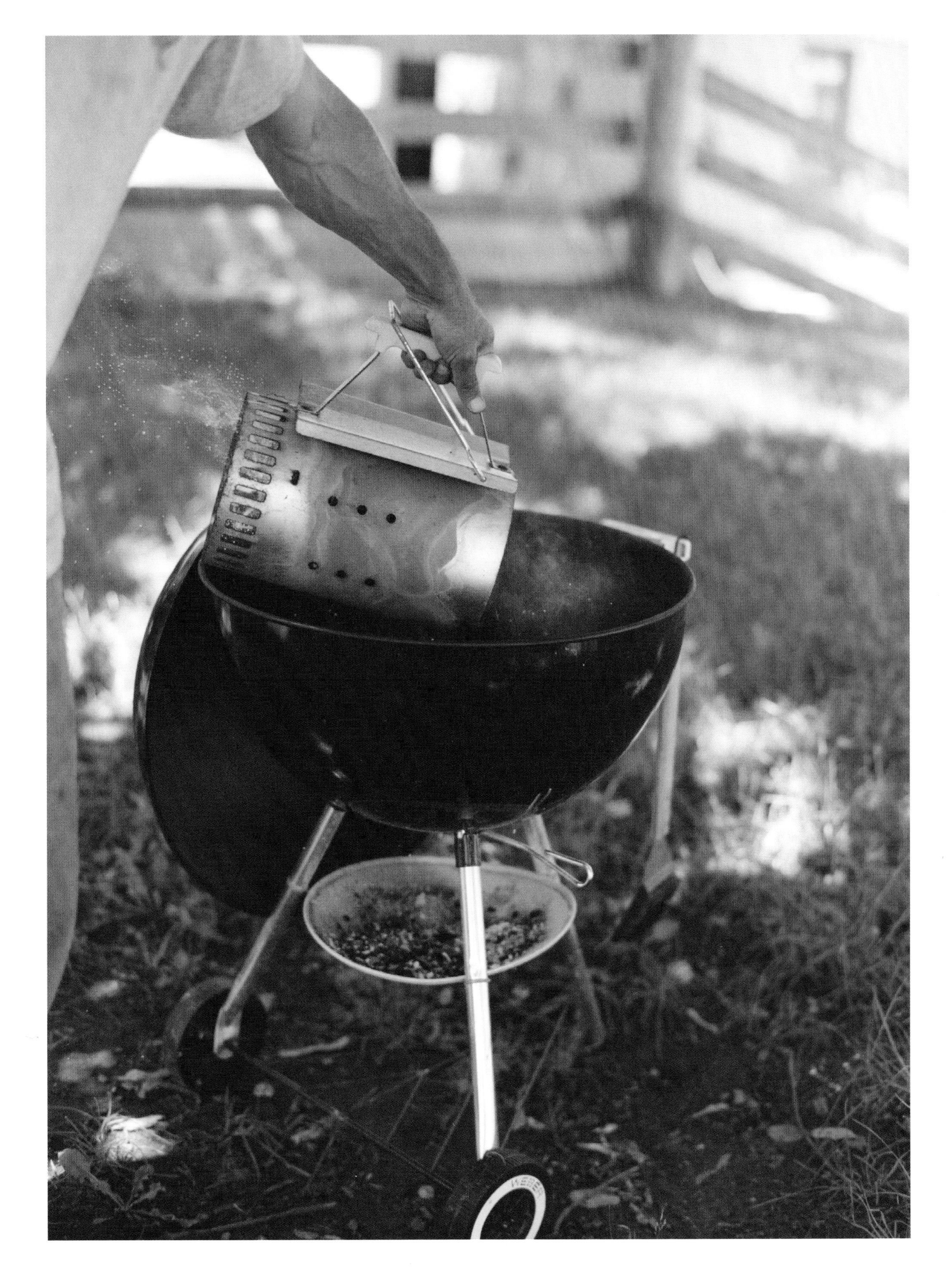

How to Care for Cast-Iron Skillets and Pots

I love using cast-iron skillets and enameled Dutch ovens for cooking. Preseasoned cast-iron skillets are a much healthier, nontoxic alternative to nonstick cookware.

Seasoning Cast Iron. If you find an old cast-iron pan at a yard sale that needs to be reseasoned, or you notice a dull, gray color on your cast iron, follow this seasoning process:

1. Wash the cookware with hot, soapy water and a stiff brush. (It's okay to use soap this time because you are preparing to reseason the cookware.) Rinse and dry completely.
2. Apply a very thin, even coating of melted coconut oil, bacon fat, or lard to the cookware inside and out. Too much oil will result in a sticky finish.
3. Place aluminum foil on the bottom rack of the oven (not directly on the bottom of the oven) to catch any drips.
4. Preheat the oven to 400°F.
5. Place the cookware upside down on the top rack of the oven to prevent pooling. Bake for at least 1 hour. After 1 hour, turn the oven off and let the cookware cool in the oven. When cooled, store it, uncovered, in a dry place. Repeat as necessary.

Caring for Cast Iron. Hand-wash with warm water only. Never use soap. Dry immediately—even before the first use. Rub with a light coat of oil, lard, or bacon fat after every wash, enough to restore the sheen without being sticky. This will help keep the iron seasoned and protected from moisture, which can cause it to rust.

What If It Gets Rusty? Without a layer of protective seasoning, cast iron can rust. It's easy to fix, however. Scour off the rust, rinse the pan, dry it, and rub it with a little coconut oil, bacon fat, or lard. If the problem persists, you will need to thoroughly remove all of the rust with a stiff wire brush and follow the seasoning instructions.

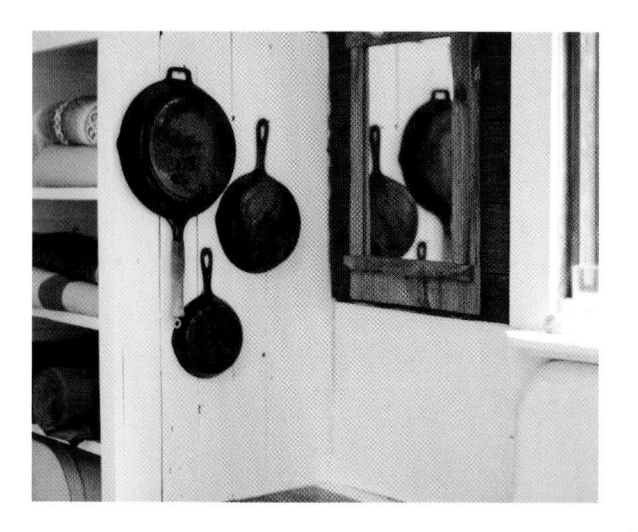

How to Care for Enameled Cast Iron

Enameled cast iron can be used on the stovetop and transferred to the oven, then to the refrigerator. When cast iron is enameled, its surface becomes nonreactive, allowing you to store food in it, even acidic foods like chili. Never use metal utensils with enamel cast iron. Wash with warm soapy water and dry with a towel. To store, place a dish towel in the pot and drape the edge of the towel over one side so that when covered by the lid, some air is able to circulate inside the pot.

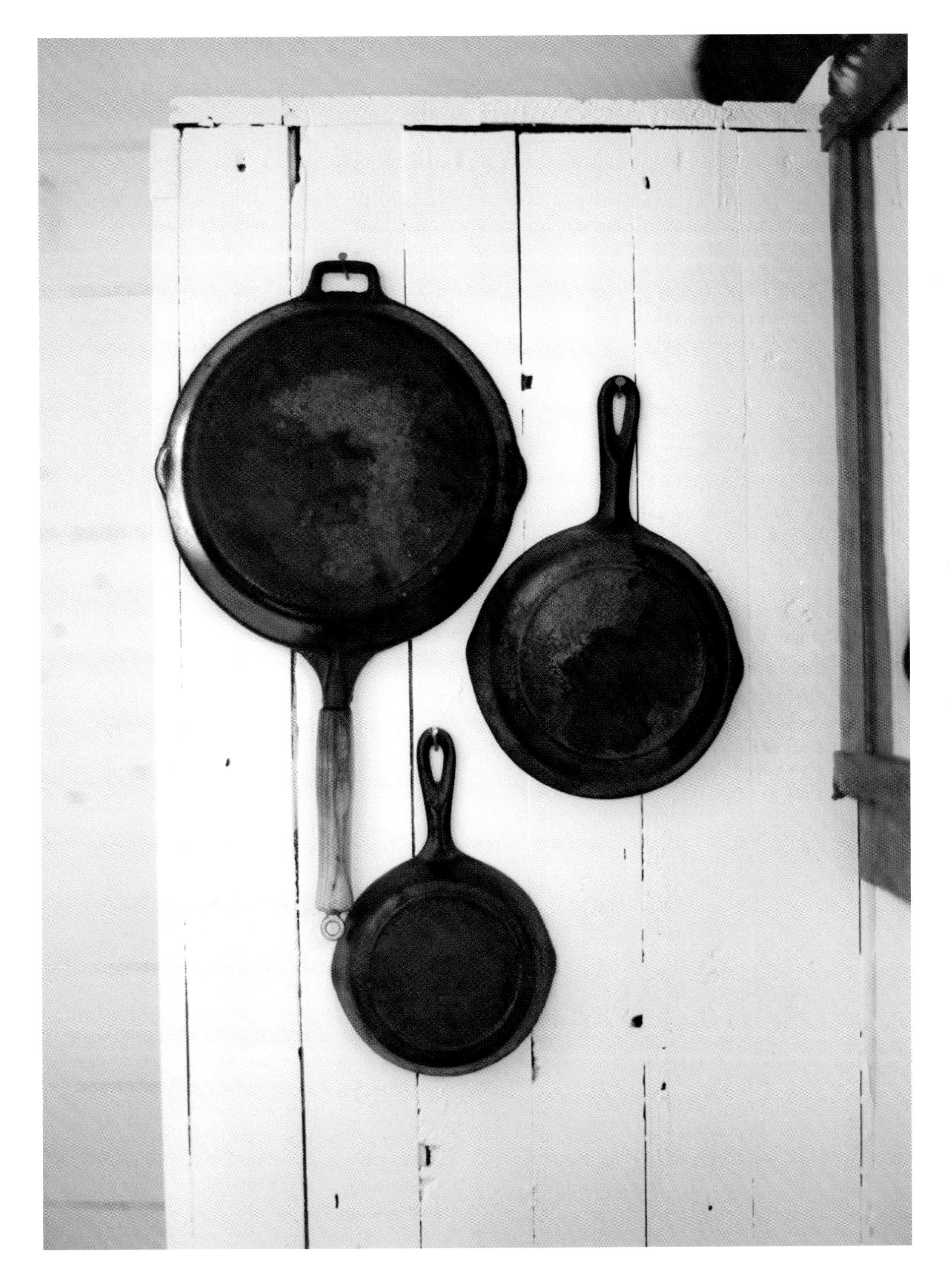

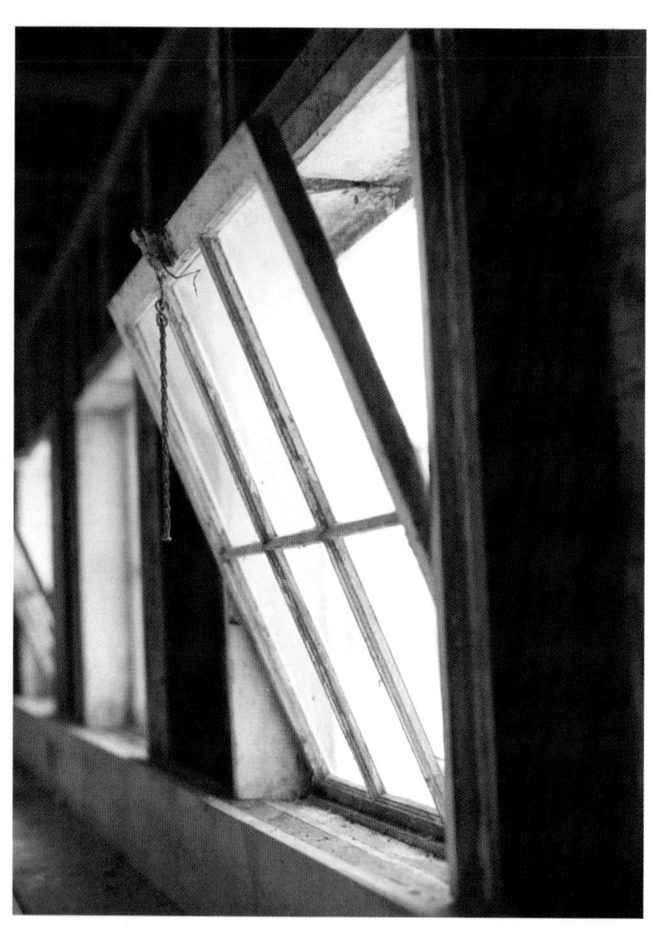

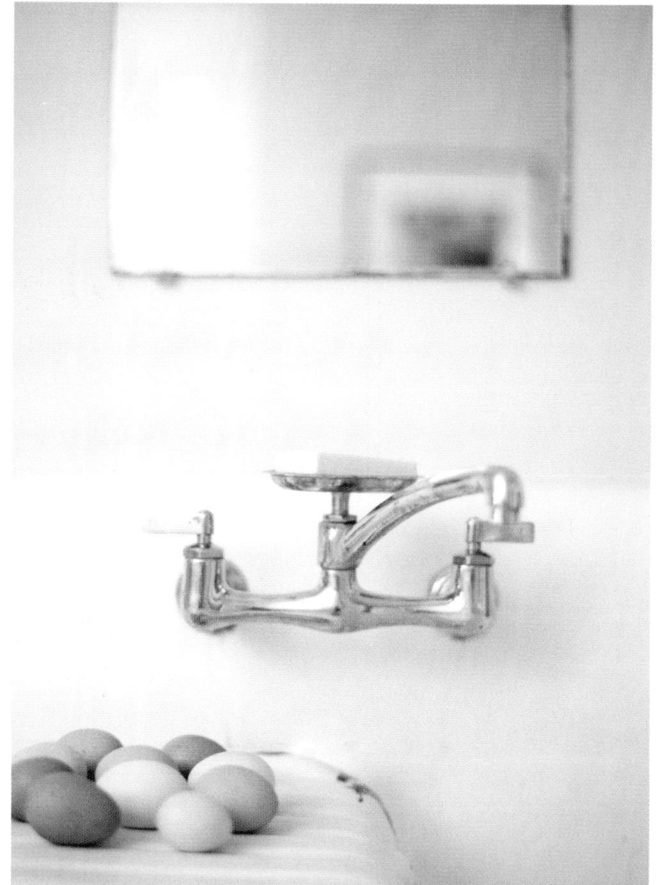

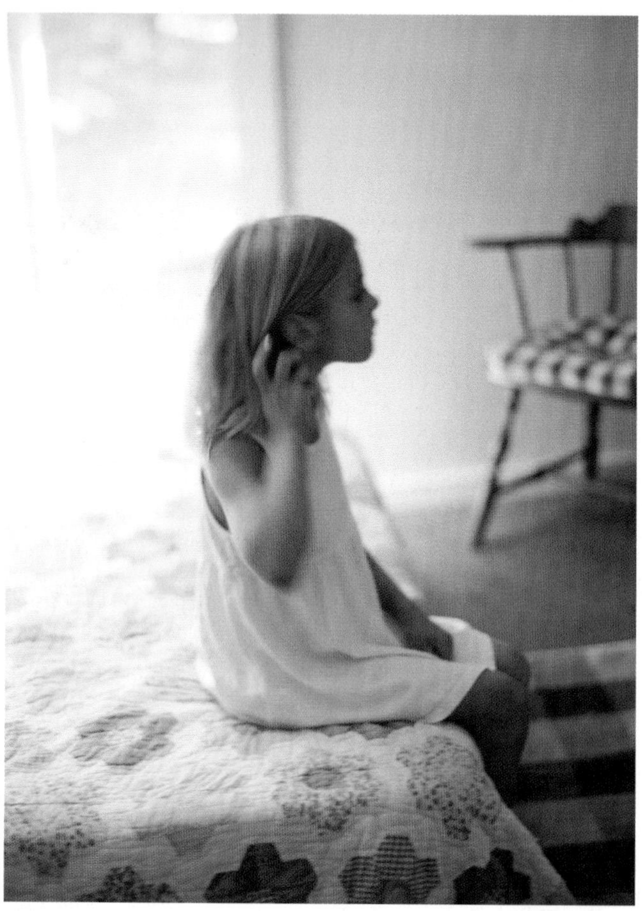

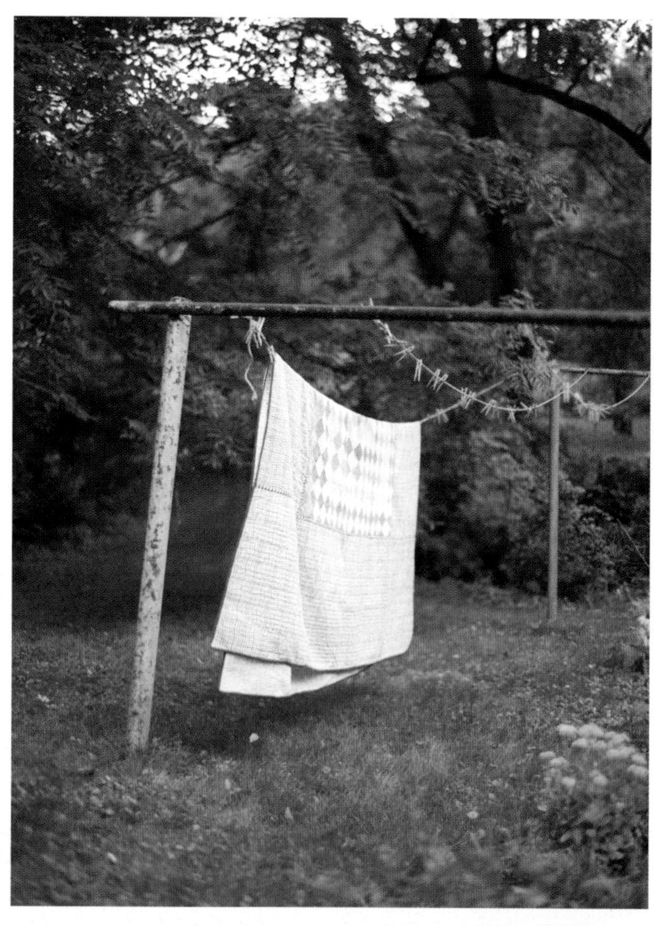

Living

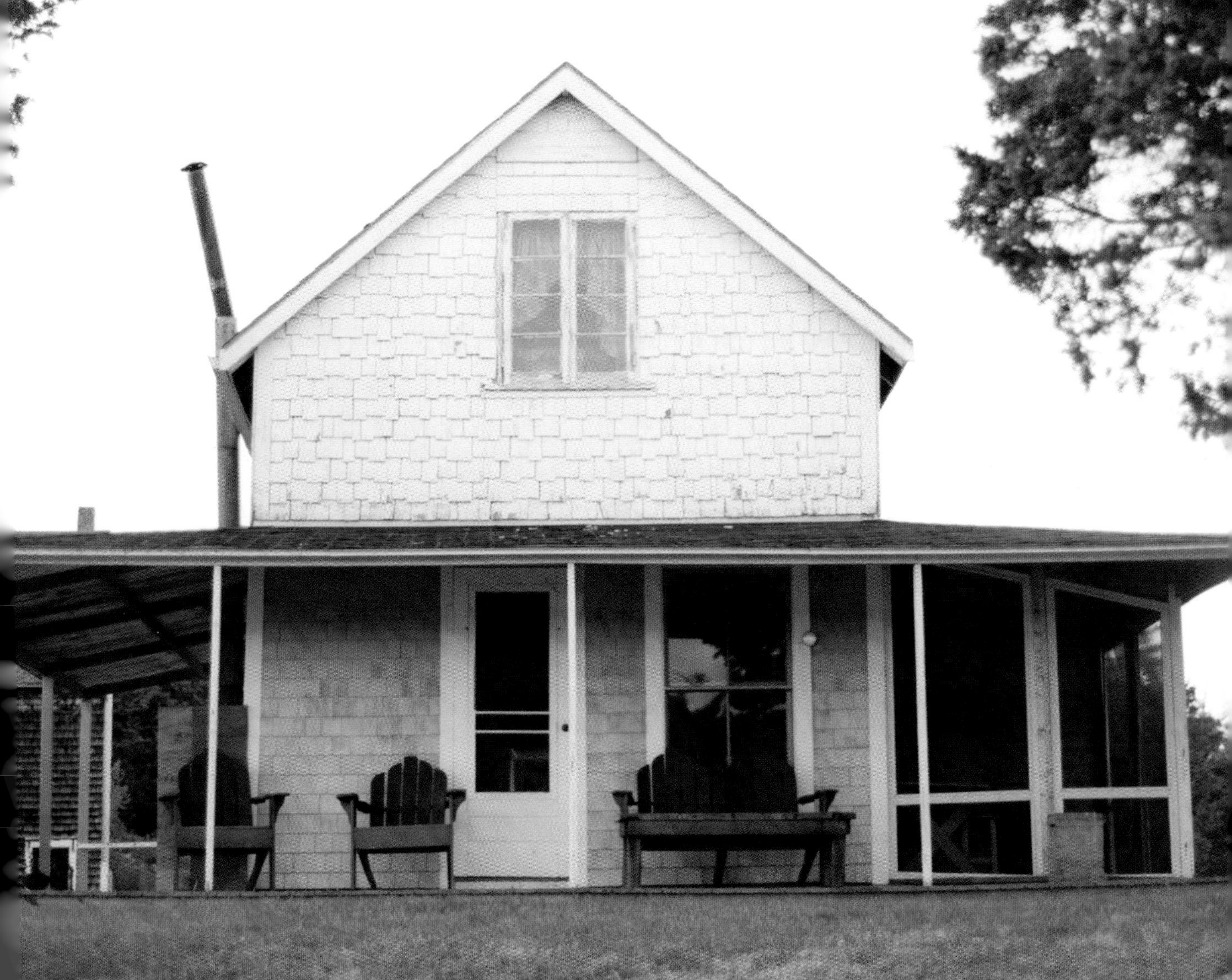

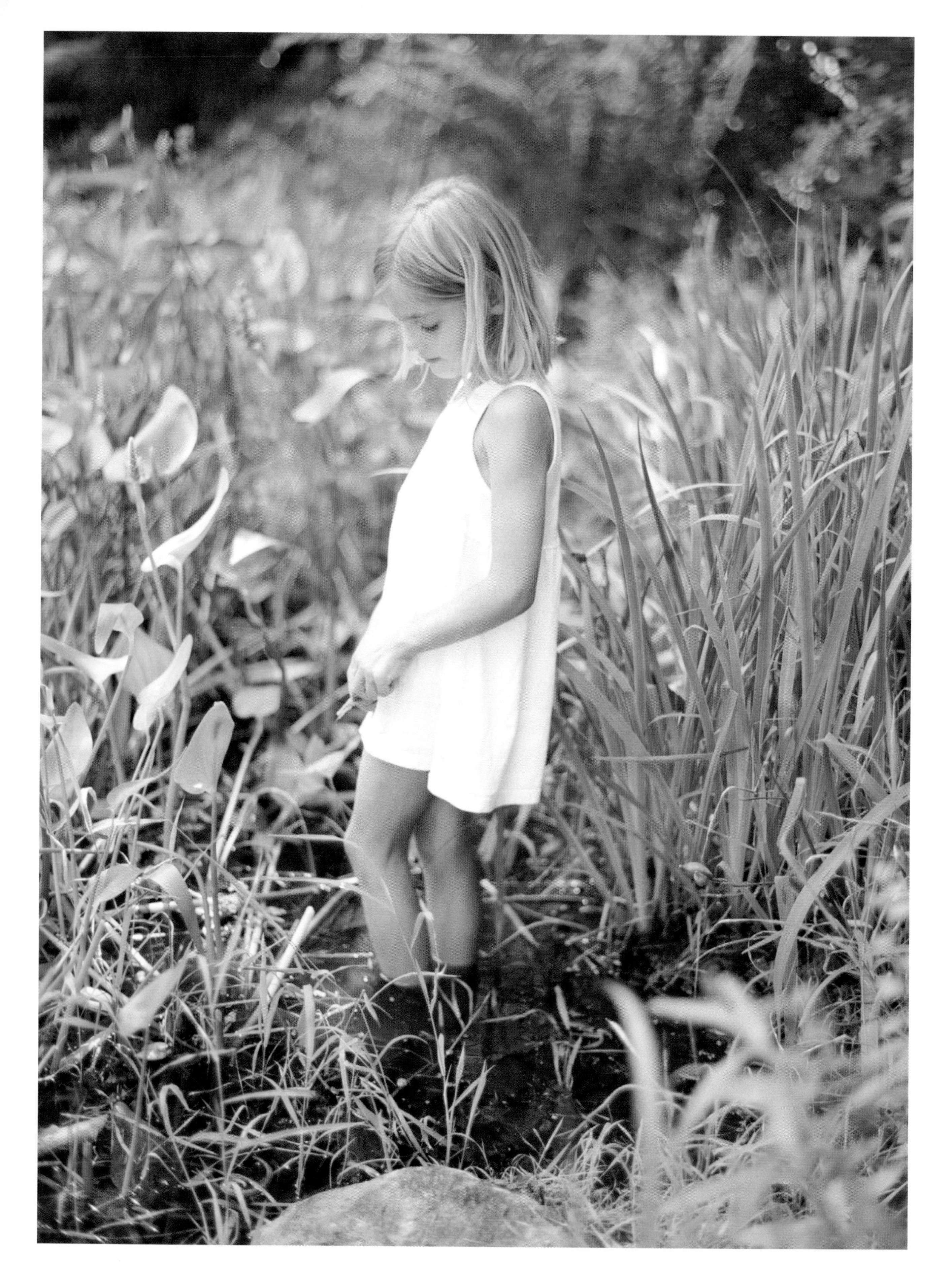

Beyond Food: Having a Healthy Lifestyle

When I meet with a new nutrition client, I actually don't start off talking about food. Instead, I let them tell me what's going on in their life and try to get a sense of what might be holding them back from optimal health.

I ask about lifestyle issues—how much sleep they get, how often they exercise, how much coffee they need to get them going, how many hours they work each day—and try to get a sense of what their support system is like. Working sixty hours a week, hitting a hard workout at 5 a.m. five times a week, and parenting three kids, all while managing a thyroid condition, does not make for a balanced life. I often see clients living this way who want me to tell them how they can eat "more Paleo," usually assuming I'll tell them to go even lower in carbs or suggest magic supplements to help them "lean out." But sometimes food is the last thing that needs to be addressed. It's important to consider your lifestyle, too, in order to improve your health for the long term—and to simply become a happier person.

Stay Active

For many people today, being thin is the hallmark of health. For others, especially those in the fitness world, six-pack abs are the true marker. But it can be difficult to attain these ideal bodies without seriously compromising other parts of your life. If your only goal is to look good naked and your workout routine is getting in the way of your home life or making you unhappy, then it's time to rethink your goal. Being healthy is much more important than getting that six-pack.

On the flip side, it's really not possible to be healthy unless you move—diet alone is not going to save you. The best exercise routine is whatever gets you to move your body on a regular basis without overly stressing yourself and causing harm. Do what you can. Lifting weights, exploring nature, and doing yoga can all be part of a healthy workout routine.

Get Enough Rest

Resting and getting enough sleep are critical to health, so going to bed late and waking up early for a workout is not ideal. According to sleep researcher Daniel Pardi, getting insufficient sleep on a regular basis—as so many people do, especially during the workweek—compromises mental function and mood. It also affects your body: sleep has a profound effect on the regulation of food intake. Studies have shown that when we don't sleep well, we tend to crave junk food and have a harder time making smart decisions about what we eat. In addition, getting enough sleep lowers our levels of cortisol, which is a hormone that can trigger weight gain, especially around the midsection.

Although you may need a little more or a little less, eight hours of sleep a night is a good goal for most people. To determine how much sleep you need, evaluate how you feel during the day. If you regularly need a pot of coffee to power you through the day, it's time to rethink your sleep habits. Try hitting the sack a little earlier and aim to wake up naturally, without an alarm, and aim to be consistent in your bedtime and wake time.

You also don't have to hit the gym seven days a week. Work out smarter, not harder. For most people, a couple of days of lifting combined with some bodyweight workouts, such as sit-ups, push-ups, and squats, are enough to stay in good shape.

Enjoy Nature and Free Play

Getting outside and having a relationship with the natural world is critical to being a healthy human. This doesn't have to mean living in the mountains or northern Canada. I go for hikes a couple of times a week and make sure my kids are playing outside in an unstructured way, and we all enjoy outdoor activities like kayaking, fishing, and exploring. As a kid, I spent hours in the woods and on the beach, and it fostered in me a love for nature that I still have today.

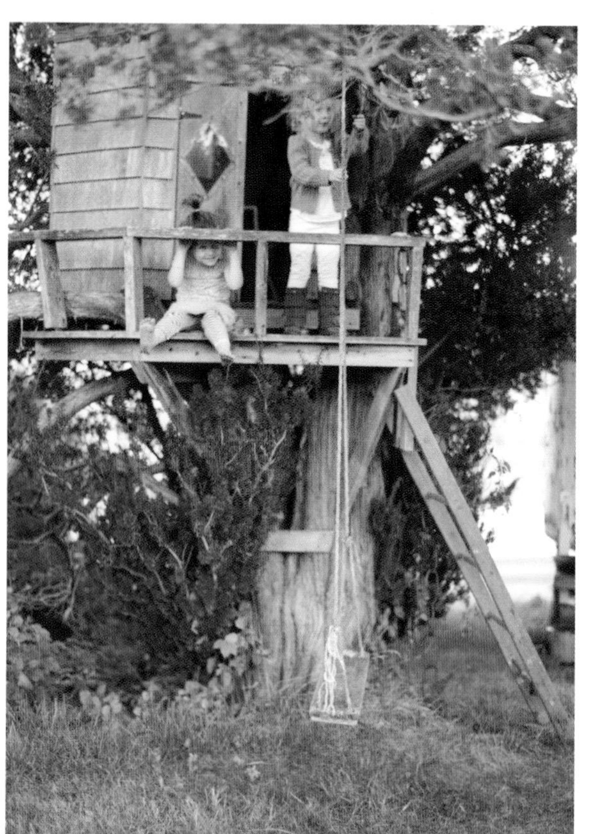

"FREE PLAY ALLOWS CHILDREN TO DEVELOP THE FLEXIBILITY NEEDED TO ADAPT TO CHANGING CIRCUMSTANCES AND ENVIRONMENTS—AN ABILITY THAT COMES IN VERY HANDY WHEN LIFE BECOMES UNPREDICTABLE AS AN ADULT."

—From a study titled "Does Playing Pay?: The Fitness Effect of Free Play During Childhood," in *Evolutionary Psychology*

There have been numerous studies showing that children receive many mental and physical health benefits from nature-based play, including reduced stress, improved mental focus, higher confidence and self-discipline, and decreased likelihood of being overweight. Not surprisingly, adults also benefit from being out in nature. One famous study looked at the effects of the Japanese practice of shinrin-yoku—"forest bathing"—and found that being in a forest reduces cortisol, a stress hormone, and lowers the heart rate and blood pressure.

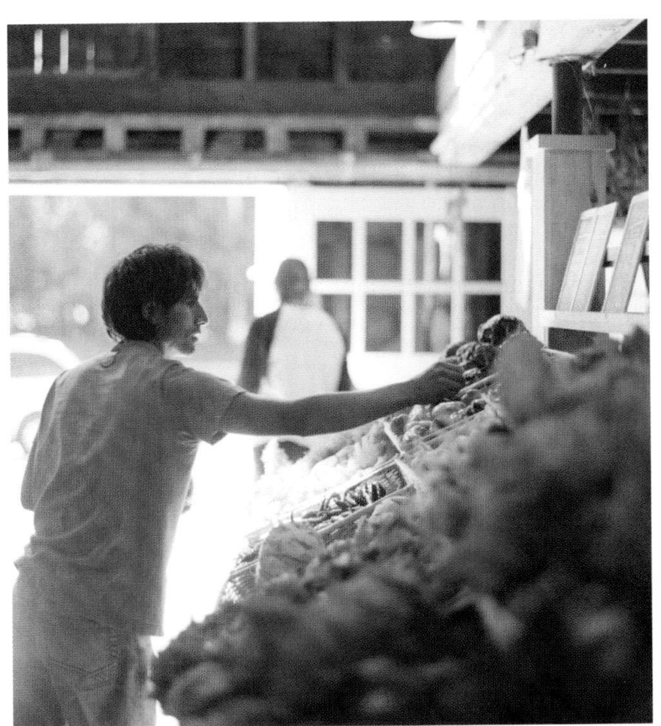

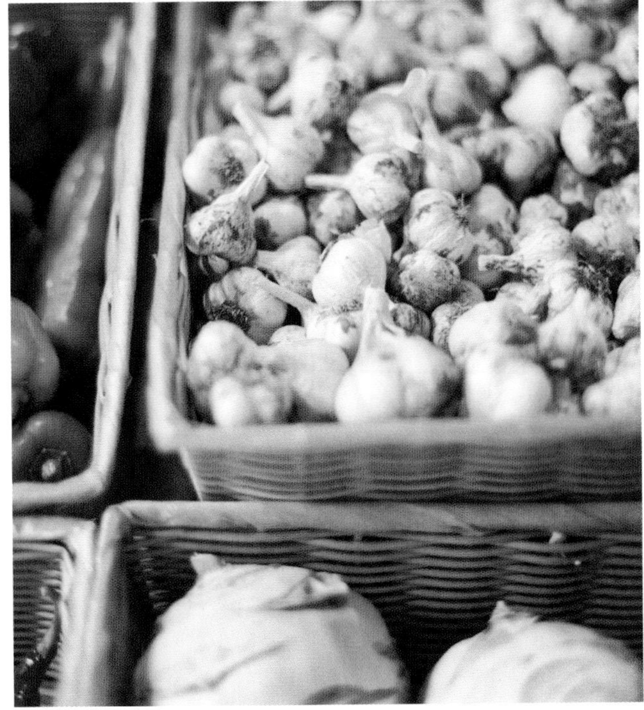

Spend Money Wisely

I get that eating healthy can be expensive. When people ask me how I afford it, the first thing I say is that it's important to reframe your thinking. Food isn't just fuel; it can either improve or damage your health. It's true that 100 calories of Twinkies are less expensive than 100 calories of grass-fed beef, but what else are you getting when you buy those Twinkies? The harmful effects of our industrial food system on our health (and on the environment) aren't factored into the cost of processed food, making it seem cheaper, but investing in nutrient-dense food is cheaper in the long run when you consider what you'll save on doctor visits, hospital stays, and medication for chronic illnesses like diabetes and heart disease—not to mention how much better you'll feel right away.

"YOU, AS A FOOD BUYER, HAVE THE DISTINCT PRIVILEGE OF PROACTIVELY PARTICIPATING IN SHAPING THE WORLD YOUR CHILDREN WILL INHERIT."

–Joel Salatin

That being said, there are certainly ways to make the Paleo lifestyle more affordable. By carefully planning out your meals, using less-expensive cuts of high-quality meat, and growing whatever food you can at home, you can really cut down on your grocery expenses. You'll also find that you tend to eat out less on Paleo, which saves money. I can have a fantastic restaurant-like experience at home for a much lower price tag, and unlike at a restaurant, I can be sure that I'm eating grass-fed, humanely raised meat; fresh, locally grown vegetables; and healthy oils. In the 1920s, less than 20 percent of each dollar spent on food was spent on "away-from-home" food. Today, that figure is almost 50 percent.

MONEY SPENT ON FOOD

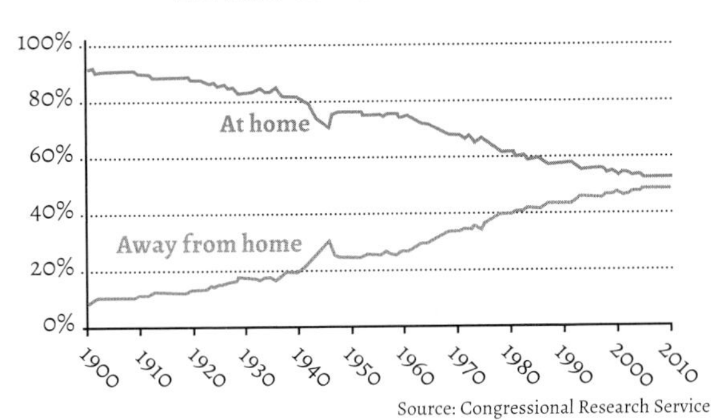

Source: Congressional Research Service

HOW TO SAVE MONEY AND STILL EAT GREAT

Have a plan

Menu planning is a lost art. If you figure out ahead of time what you'll be eating when, it's much easier to economize and save money on your grocery bill.

Cook and buy in bulk

It's just as easy to roast multiple chickens as one, and with the oven already on, it's simple to toss in a bunch of sweet potatoes. Is there a sale on your favorite olive oil? Stock up and save!

Make your own stock

It's the ultimate way to recycle a roast chicken or leg of lamb. See the recipes on pages 338 and 340.

Grow your own food

While having your own chickens might cost more, the quality of the eggs far surpasses what you'll get at the grocery store, and a veggie patch is a great way to save money. Live in a city? Maybe you can have container vegetables on the rooftop or fire escape, or you could tend a plot at a community garden.

Preserve the harvest

Freeze greens, can tomatoes, and make some sauerkraut. Not only will you save money, you'll get to enjoy garden-grown produce in the middle of winter.

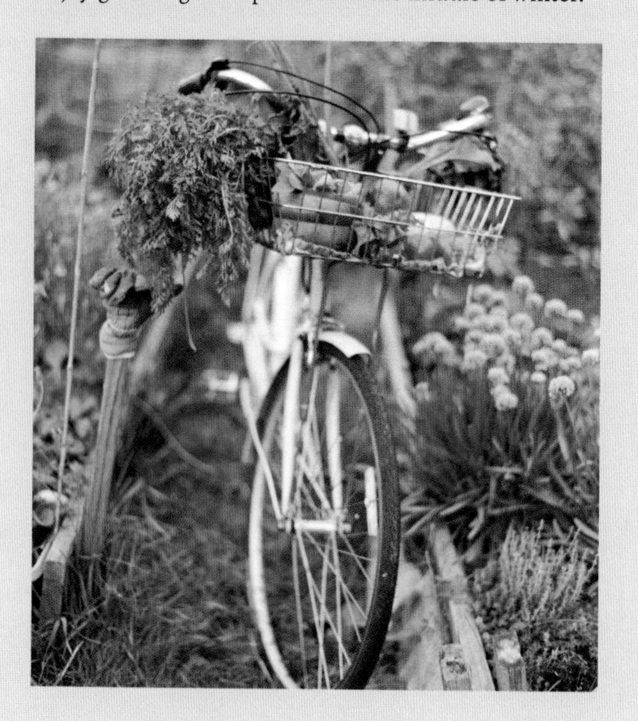

Dine in

Once you gain some confidence in the kitchen and get used to eating fantastic home-cooked food, you'll think twice before spending your money on junky takeout or a mediocre steak at the local pub. Stay in and spend half of what you would have at the restaurant on your own home cooking. Don't have much time? Scrambled eggs take less than five minutes. That's faster and cheaper than ordering a pizza!

Buy local and in season

Local, seasonal produce is fresher than what you get at a supermarket and will last longer in your fridge. Instead of going to a farmers market and only picking out the most beautiful tomatoes, consider focusing your shopping trip on what is at its peak. Is it June? Strawberries and greens are what's on the menu in New England. Is it January? Get some local cabbage, potatoes, carrots, and onions for a warm and satisfying stew. It's much more sustainable and economical to build your weekly menu around what's local and in season, and not whatever fancy recipe you crave at the moment.

Buy meat in bulk

If you have the space, invest in a chest or upright freezer so you can save money by buying meat in bulk. Look for sales on meat at the market and add it to your stash. Not only is buying a whole animal or half of one more economical, it also lets you use more varied cuts than if you just purchase boneless, skinless chicken breasts or specialty steaks—so it's a great way to explore different cuts of meat.

Seek out less-expensive ingredients

Ground meat, organ meats, trash fish—fish that aren'tgenerally eaten in a particular region, such as carp in America—and unsexy vegetables like cabbage are better bets if you're on a budget. At the farmers market, ask if they have "seconds"—vegetables that are blemished and not pretty enough for display. You could be canning extra tomatoes with a barrelful of tomato seconds at half price.

IN 1984, THE AVERAGE U.S. HOUSEHOLD SPENT 16.8 PERCENT OF ITS ANNUAL POST-TAX INCOME ON FOOD. BY 2011, AMERICANS SPENT ONLY 11.2 PERCENT. THE U.S. DEVOTES LESS OF ITS INCOME TO FOOD THAN ANY OTHER COUNTRY—HALF AS MUCH AS HOUSEHOLDS IN FRANCE AND ONE-FOURTH OF THOSE IN INDIA.

—From "America's Shrinking Grocery Bill," *Businessweek*

It's also important to spend on our food money on real food. In a typical American grocery store, practically every aisle in the center of the store is filled with processed garbage that we don't need to be eating. Cut back on packaged food and spend on whole ingredients instead.

There's a bigger picture to think about here, too. To me, living within your means is part of a sustainable lifestyle. Do you really need that expensive car loan, the latest high-tech gadget, or those regular manicures? Are you working extra hours just to pay off that luxury vacation from two years ago? Managing your finances well makes it possible to live a more balanced, healthier lifestyle.

Before you buy something, ask yourself the questions below—I like to call it the "anti-shopping list":

1. Do I really need it?
2. If it's to replace something that's broken, can I fix it instead?
3. Can I do without?
4. Can I barter for it?
5. Can I make it myself?
6. Can I grow it?
7. Can I repurpose something else instead?
8. Who am I supporting when I make this purchase (a small family, a multibillion-dollar company)?
9. Is there a way to purchase this from a local small business?
10. Is there a more sustainable option? For instance, is there an option that's fair trade, organic, or made of recycled or sustainably grown or harvested materials?

Find Personal Fulfillment

Are you so busy earning a living that you're not really living? Maybe it's not possible for you to love your job (although if that's the case, I encourage you to make a plan to change jobs or careers!), but there are other ways to feel fulfilled. Maybe for you it's volunteering for a local organization a few hours a week, or taking a class in something you've always wanted to learn, or going for a hike and getting out into nature on a regular basis. Seek out things that will make you a happier person. The most fulfilled people I know either love their jobs, have hobbies that they strongly enjoy, or find balance in their life through spiritual and personal growth.

Having close, meaningful relationships and being part of a community are also important for your overall health. Happy people tend to have strong friendships and make time for themselves and for their families.

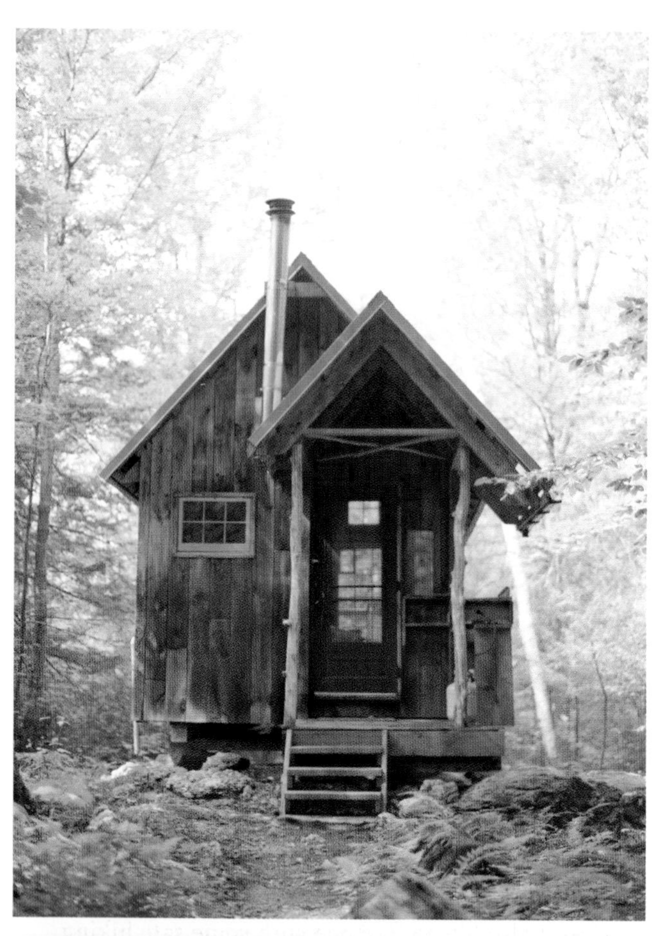

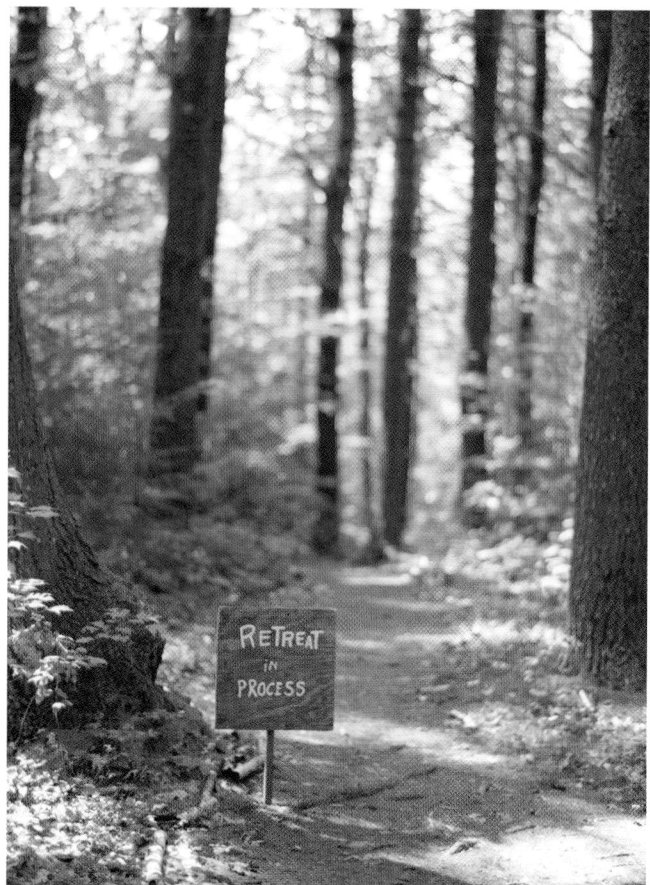
RETREAT
in
PROCESS

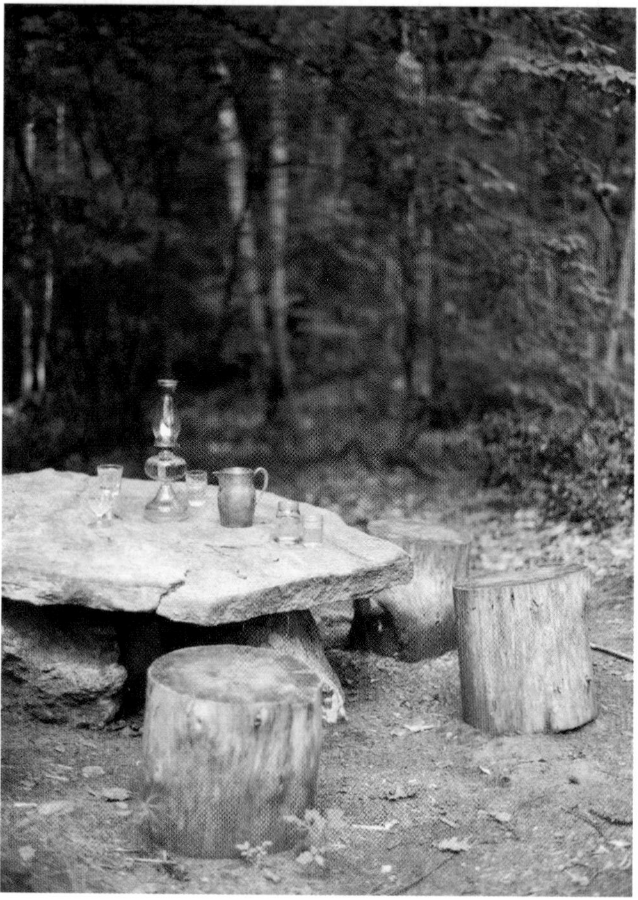

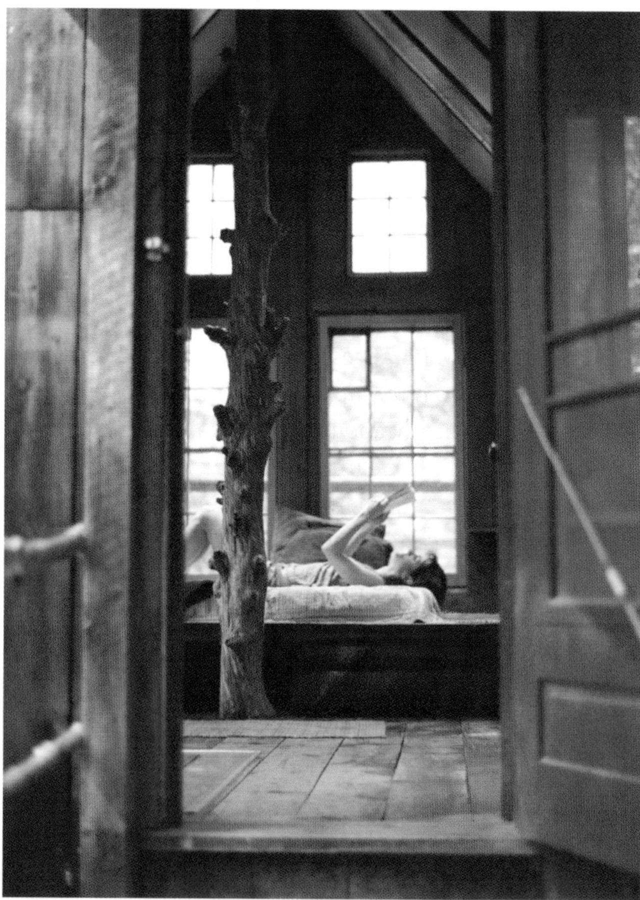

Getting Away from It All

In late summer, things slow down a bit on the farm. The major planting is done and most of the vegetables are taller than the weeds, so our main job is harvesting for our CSA and taking care of the animals. It's a good time to round up the kids and escape for a long weekend.

Last year, we took advantage of one of those late summer lulls to visit Temenos, a magical place in the mountains of western Massachusetts. The Greek word *temenos* refers to a sacred space, and with seventy-eight acres of forest preserve and mineral-rich springs, the site has become a wonderful retreat for us, a place to get away from our daily routines and enjoy time in nature.

Setting aside time each year to get away from home and responsibilities is so important for health and well-being. While everyone has a different vacation preference—the beach, the mountains, cities, ranches in the countryside—I strongly recommend spending at least one week a year in a natural setting such as a forest or national park. Getting out into nature, without electricity and many of the creature comforts of home, really fits into the Paleo lifestyle because it can remind us of what life is really all about. It's also a great bonding experience for families and creates amazing memories. Plus, it can help your kids imagine what life might have been like for our ancestors, which is an excellent way to get them to appreciate what they have and yet think critically about how much we really need all the "stuff" we accumulate in our lives.

On our trip to Temenos, the kids loved romping through the woods and listening to the sounds of the night animals, amplified by the absence of electrical appliances. We went swimming in the cold, spring-fed pond, built fairy houses (see page 377 for instructions on building your own), and of course, cooked great food, on both an open fire and a woodstove.

Tent camping is great, but I personally prefer staying in simple cabins: it's far less claustrophobic, and it's more comfortable to sleep on a futon than on the hard ground. And because cabins are usually appointed with gear for cooking, you don't need to pack as much gear to take with you. If you're planning on camping with kids, here are some other tips for making the most of the experience.

- **Pick the right campground.** Because I love canoeing, kayaking, and fishing, I like to look for a campground that is near water, whether a lake, ocean, or a river. I also like to find one with some safe hiking options. Seek out parks that are family-friendly and have quiet hours. State parks can be a good choice because they do not allow alcohol, which means there's less of a chance of late-night partiers wrecking your sleep. If it's your first time camping, consider finding a campground with yurts or cabins, which can be more comfortable than tents.

- **Do a dry run.** Try camping out in the backyard or someplace very close to home for your first night. It's a good way to get comfortable setting up your tent before you're fumbling with it in the dark, hours away from home, and it helps you figure out what you'll really need on your trip and what you won't. If a dry run isn't possible, try spending an evening without electric lights or electronics. We live in an area where the power goes out regularly, and my kids get really excited to spend the night running around with flashlights and watching the fire.

- **Go during the off season.** Camping in the middle of summer can mean lots of heat, bugs, and crowds. Go earlier or later in the season for lovely weather and a better experience.

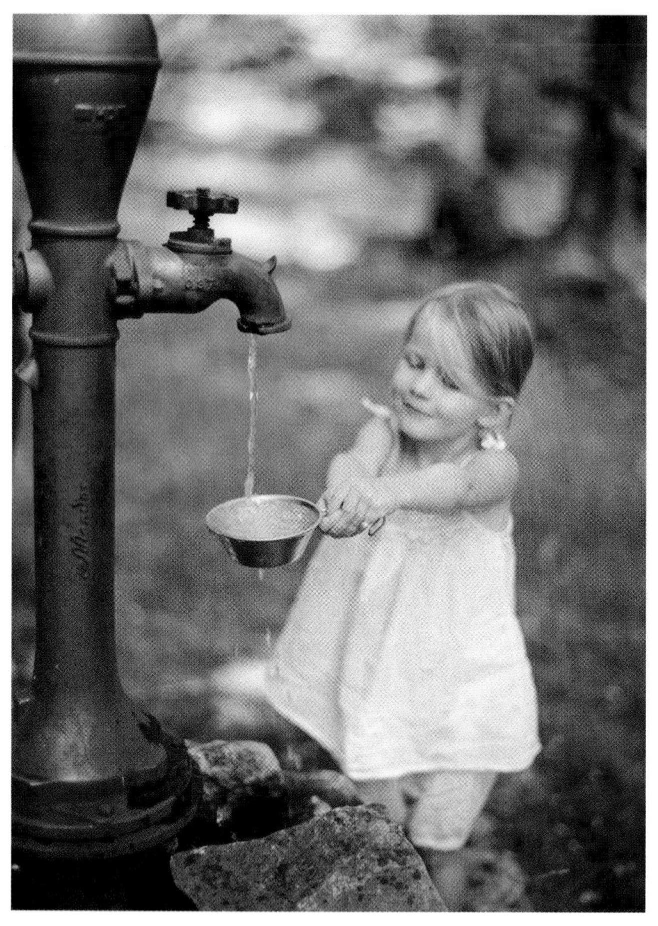

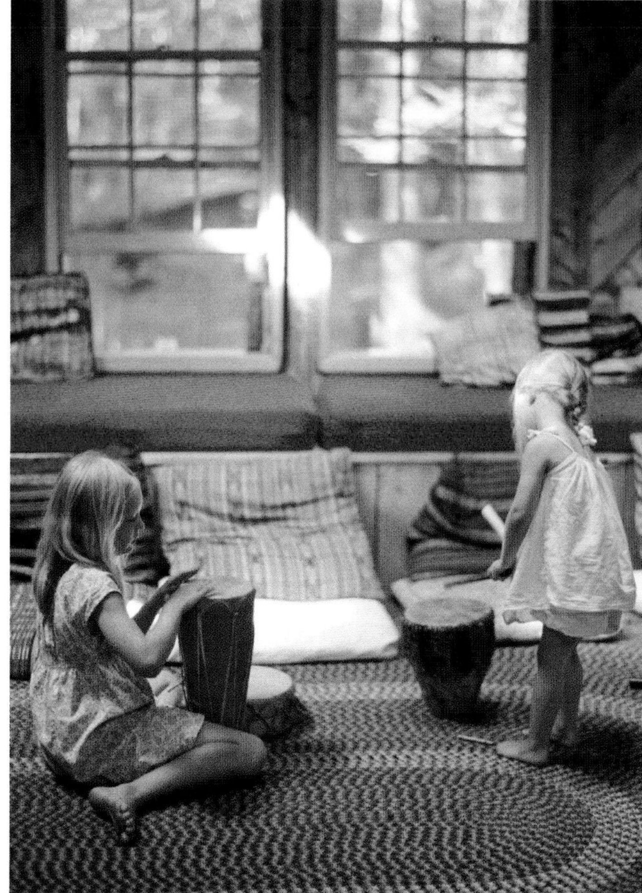

- **Make it short.** For your first time camping with kids, don't plan a weeklong adventure. Two nights is a great introduction to camping. Save the longer trips in remote wilderness for later, when everyone is more experienced and knows what to expect.

- **Go with friends.** Your kids may have more fun if they can hang with their buddies, and by splitting the cooking and childcare duties with other parents, you'll have more fun, too!

- **Rent before you buy.** Camping equipment can be expensive to buy, but sporting goods store often rent out basic equipment, such as tents, stoves, and sleeping bags. Renting is also a good way to test equipment to find out what you like.

- **Keep the food simple.** Don't plan elaborate meals with long cooking times and a daunting spice list. Pack jerky, nuts, some sausage to cook on a stick, and simple chopped veggies that can be eaten raw. If you want to make a particular dish, prep the ingredients ahead of time and bring them with you in packets, ready to hit the pan. There's no need to get complicated.

- **Have the kids help pack.** Making the kids responsible for their own packing can help them get really excited about the trip. Give them a checklist with essentials such as a flashlight, toothbrush, sleeping bag, favorite board game, and so on. Frisbees and playing cards are helpful when the kids get bored. Of course, make sure you check their work!

- **Arrive early and explain the rules.** Get to your campsite early enough to set up and learn the lay of the land well before it gets dark, and explain the ground rules to the kids right away. Show them where their boundaries are and establish what is off-limits. Consider giving each kid a whistle and using the buddy system to make sure they're safe.

- **Play.** Take the opportunity to teach your kids about what to avoid in the woods, like poison ivy, but don't forget to have fun! Do a scavenger hunt for leaves, bugs, and other wildlife. Catch frogs, go swimming, build a fairy house, and don't be afraid to get dirty!

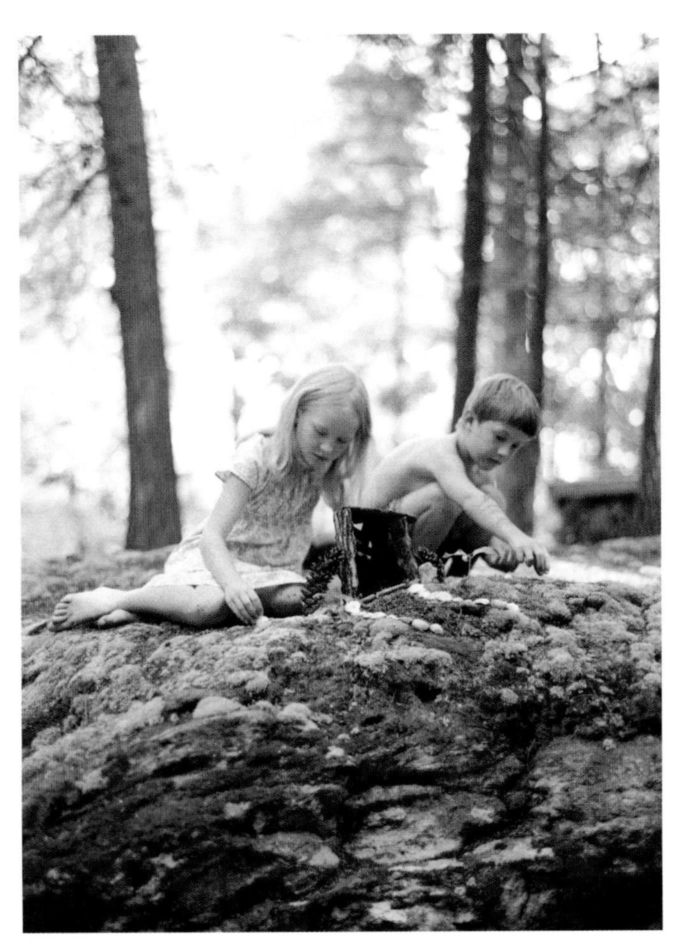

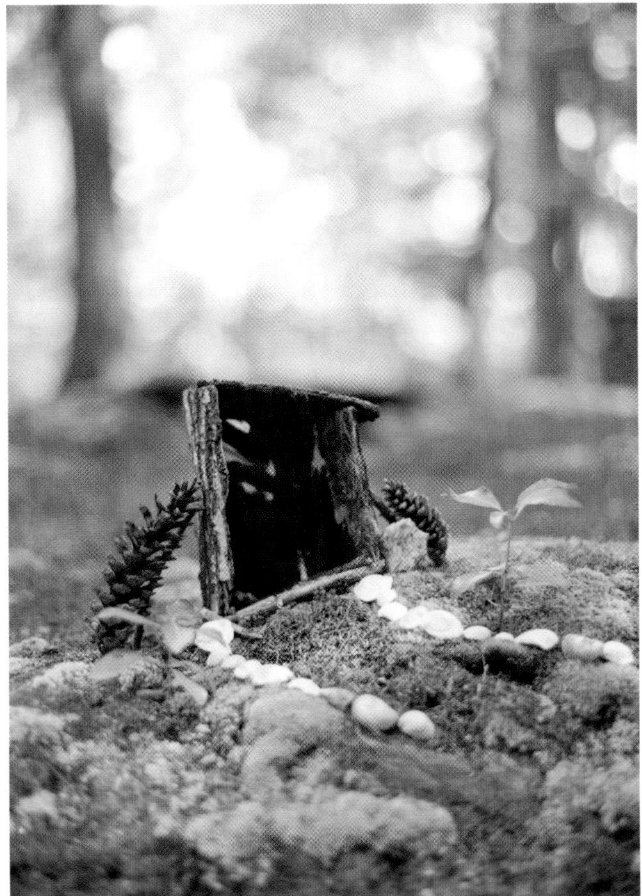

Building a Fairy House

Teaching kids to think outside the box and use their imagination is often sadly lost in today's era of standardized testing and benchmarks. Building a fairy house—a small structure made of natural materials for magical, tiny beings to inhabit once you're gone—is one way to help them rediscover creative, imaginative play, and it's a great way to get kids to spend time outdoors. Once when I was leading a workshop on building a fairy house, a three-year-old boy pointed to his fairy house and, thinking I was the queen of the fairies, told me to make myself small and get in. He'd created such a charming story around his experience of building a fairy house!

This activity isn't about bringing home something to hang on the wall. It's not about coloring neatly inside the lines. It's about inspiring kids to spend quiet, unstructured time in nature. They build a little structure of natural materials, imagine what creatures might come and visit it, and then they visit it later to see how it's doing. Building a fairy house is also a great activity to teach kids the difference between what comes from nature and what is manmade.

Although building a fairy house is all about imagination and creativity, I have found that a few basic ground rules make for the best experience.

- Don't use anything living to make your house.
- Don't strip bark from a tree or pull up flowers to decorate it.
- Use only what is already on the ground and what you can find in nature.
- A fairy house can be as big or small as you like.

Starting a Fire

Building a fire is a lost art these days, but it's a skill everyone should have. There's nothing like a blazing fire in a fireplace during a storm, and fires are essential for enjoying camping (page 375), pig roasts (page 383), and clambakes (page 380).

You will need:

- *Matches or a lighter*
- *Tinder (small bits of bark, tiny sticks, paper, moss—basically anything that is dry and small)*
- *Kindling (dry twigs and small wood pieces)*
- *Dry logs (a hardwood like oak or maple burns longer and more slowly than a softwood like pine, but it also takes longer to catch)*
- *A shovel*
- *Rocks to edge the fire ring. Don't use river rocks, as they can explode if they get hot enough. (If you don't have any rocks, you can dig a hole to contain the fire.)*
- *A bucket of water, just in case things get a little out of control*

1. Set up the area. Find a safe place and build a ring of rocks, or dig a pit several inches deep.

2. Place the kindling loosely in the center of the fire pit.

3. Place the tinder on the kindling and light the tinder.

4. Gradually add more kindling until you've got a good flame going.

5. Arrange some of the larger pieces of kindling in a cone shape to form a tepee. Good air circulation should help them catch fire quickly.

6. Once the fire is rolling along, add logs as needed to keep it going.

7. When it's time to put out the fire, extinguish it completely with water or, if you plan to light another fire with the same wood soon, with dirt or sand.

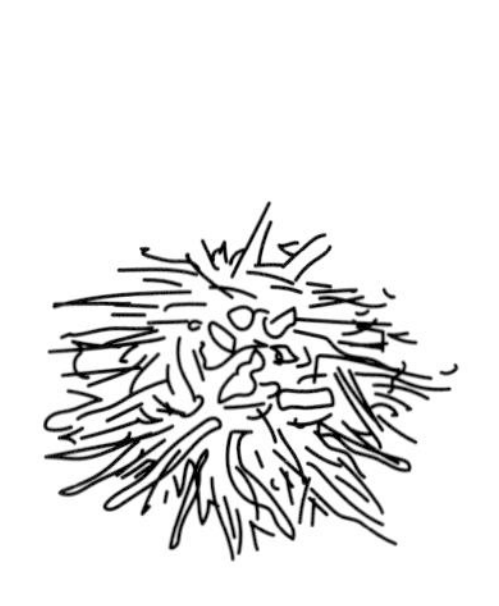

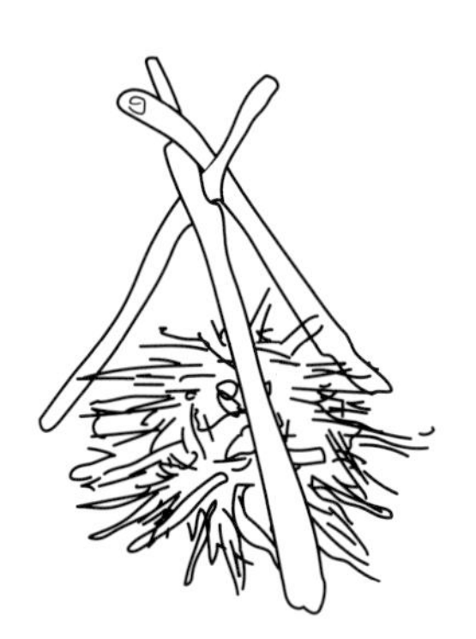

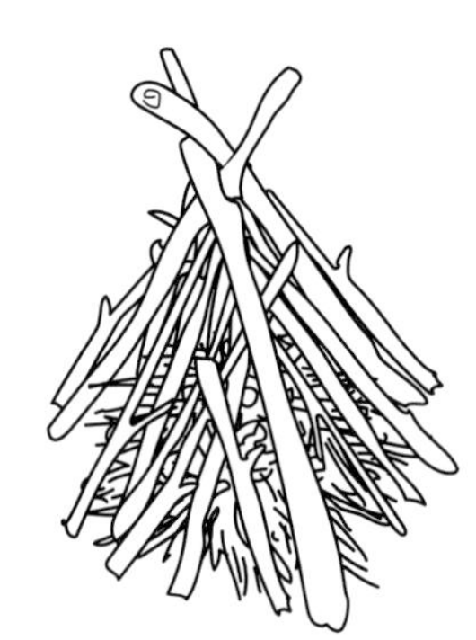

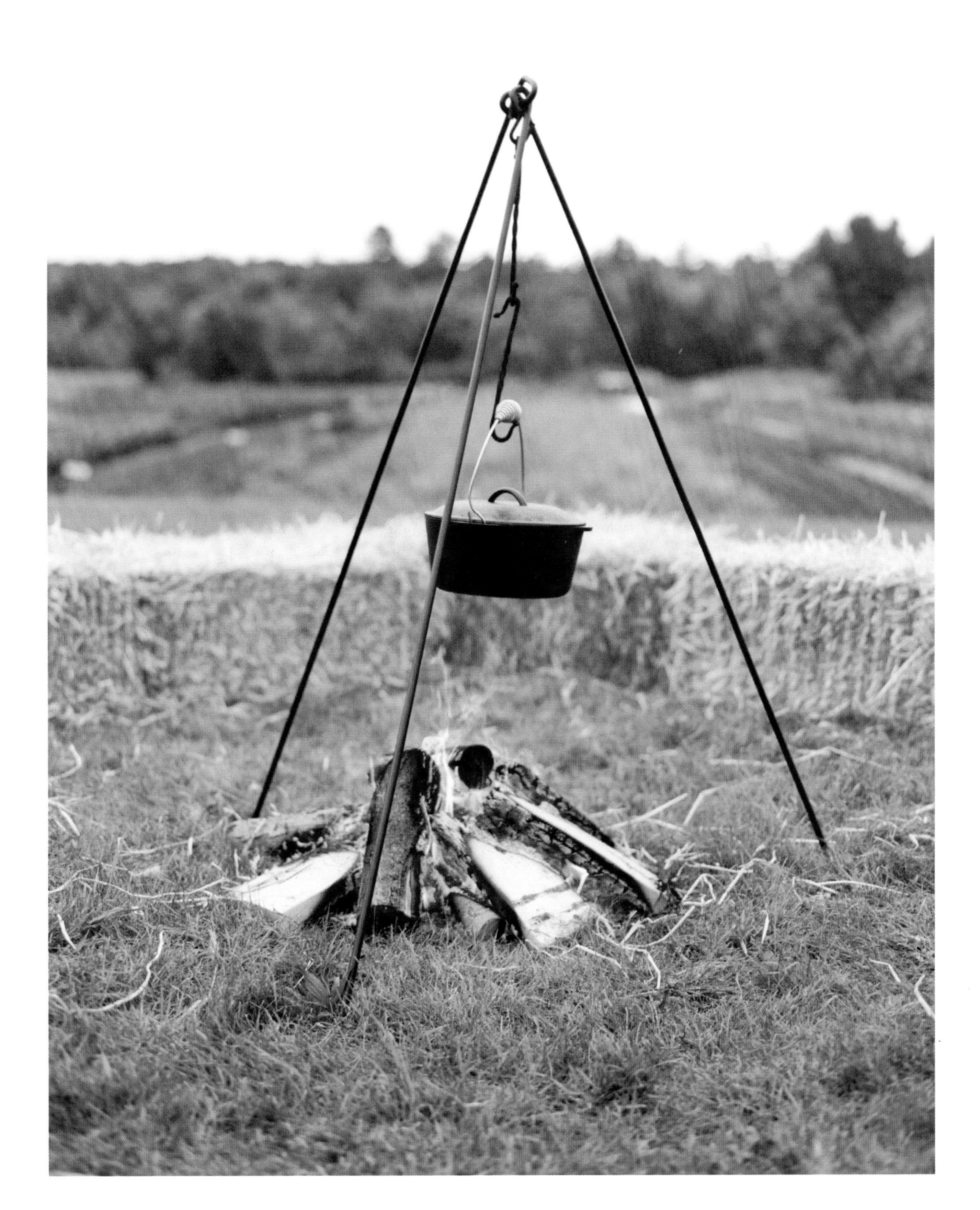

Hosting a Clambake

When I was a little kid, my dad would take me to the beach to dig clams and we would roast them right there on the sand. It's one of my fondest memories from childhood. I loved feeling the salt air and sand on my tan skin. I would pretend I was a Native American child from ages past, gathering food for my next meal. My sister, on the other hand, with her fair skin, blue eyes, and red hair, claims these times were among her worst experiences growing up. She would get sunburned and eaten by bugs, and she hated the gritty feeling of the sand on her skin. It's funny how two kids from the same parents can interpret the same event so differently. Luckily, my kids think that having a clambake is pretty cool. But if you're like my sister and would rather skip the clambake and cook lobsters and steamers at home, instructions are on page 238.

I recommend holding off on indulging in an adult beverage until the food is off the fire. It's critical that everything cooks through—you really don't want to serve raw lobster or clams to your guests!—so please pay attention until the food is done, then start partying.

To host a clambake for 12 people, you will need:

- *A fire permit*
- *A shovel*
- *About 8 to 10 rocks the size of grapefruit*
- *Firewood (don't forget the tinder and kindling)*
- *Matches or lighter*
- *20 pounds seaweed*
- *8 pounds littleneck clams, wrapped in cheesecloth*
- *12 lobsters*
- *A canvas tarp*
- *A bucket, for putting out the fire*
- *Lobster crackers or nutcrackers*
- *6 lemons, sliced*
- *1 cup butter, melted*
- *Sea salt and ground black pepper*

1. Pick a night when there is a full moon—the light makes it easier to clean up. Be aware of the tide schedule, so the water doesn't come up and drown your fire. Be aware of the local bug schedule, too. For example, greenhead flies are terrible at certain beaches in New England in the month of July. Ask folks who live near the beach when the bugs are most tolerable. Usually the last full-moon tide of August takes care of marsh bugs, and you're safe to have your clambake in comfort later in August or in September.

2. Plan on building a fire around noon if you want to eat around 6 p.m. First, you need a great big hole in the ground to contain the fire. Above the high tide line, dig a hole about 4 feet across and 2 feet deep, and make sure you don't end up with a puddle at the bottom of it from the water table. Line the fire pit with rocks.

3. Now you're ready to light a fire to get those rocks super hot—see page 378 for instructions. You want the fire to burn for about four hours before you start cooking, and I cannot stress enough that the fire needs to be huge and hot, and that it needs to burn for a good long while. This is a make-or-break situation for your party.

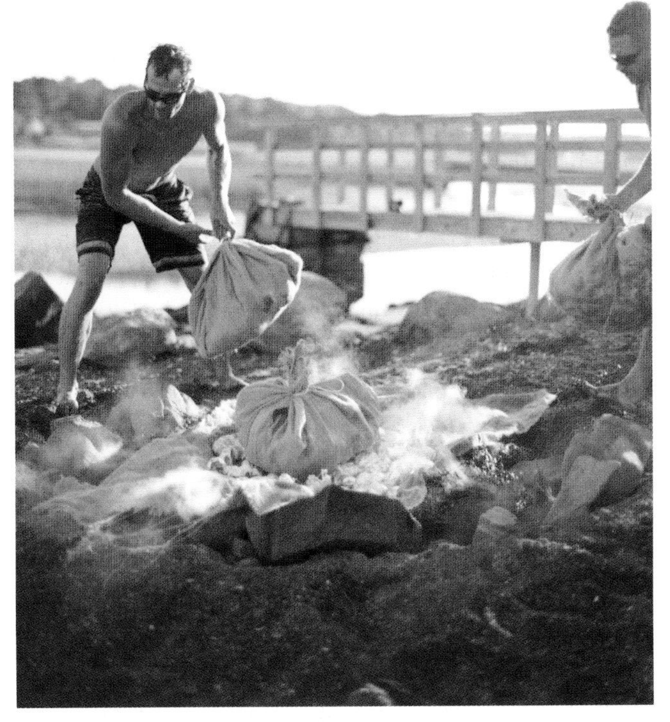

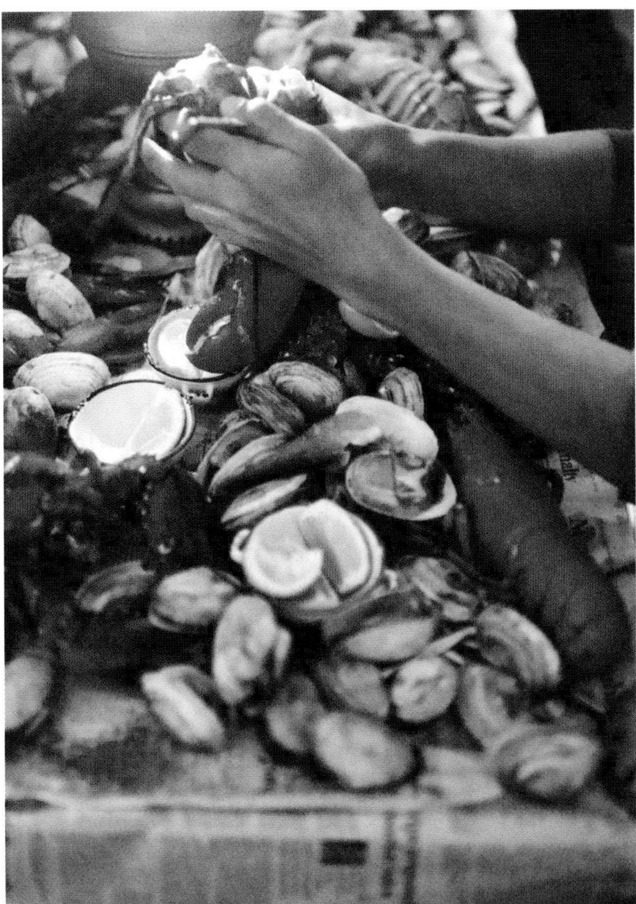

4. After the fire is blazing, gather about 20 pounds of seaweed. (You could also buy some from your fishmonger, but where's the fun in that?) The best type is rockweed, which has tiny little air pockets. Douse the seaweed well with seawater to make sure it's nice and wet.

5. When you've got a nice layer of coals and the rocks lining the fire pit are very hot, about 400°F, it's time to cover the fire with wet seaweed. Push aside some of the logs so that there's just one layer of coals over the rocks, then spread a thick layer of seaweed, about half of what you've gathered, over the entire fire. The wet seaweed will smother the fire, crackle, and create lots of smoke.

6. Place the lobsters and clams on top of the seaweed, and then cover them with another layer of seaweed. Finally, cover the entire fire pit with a damp canvas tarp, anchor the tarp on all sides with rocks, and shovel some sand on top of the tarp. You've just made a beach oven to cook your food!

7. The seafood will take about 1 to 2 hours to cook, but start checking on it after 45 minutes. When the clams are open and the lobsters are bright red, remove them from the pit and serve with sliced lemons and melted butter. Put out the fire with the bucket of water once you are done cooking. Some great side dishes are Provençal Seafood Chowder with Fennel and Tarragon (page 240), Bacon Chive Biscuits (page 242), and Summer Garden Salad with Seaweed and Lemon-Ginger Dressing (page 246).

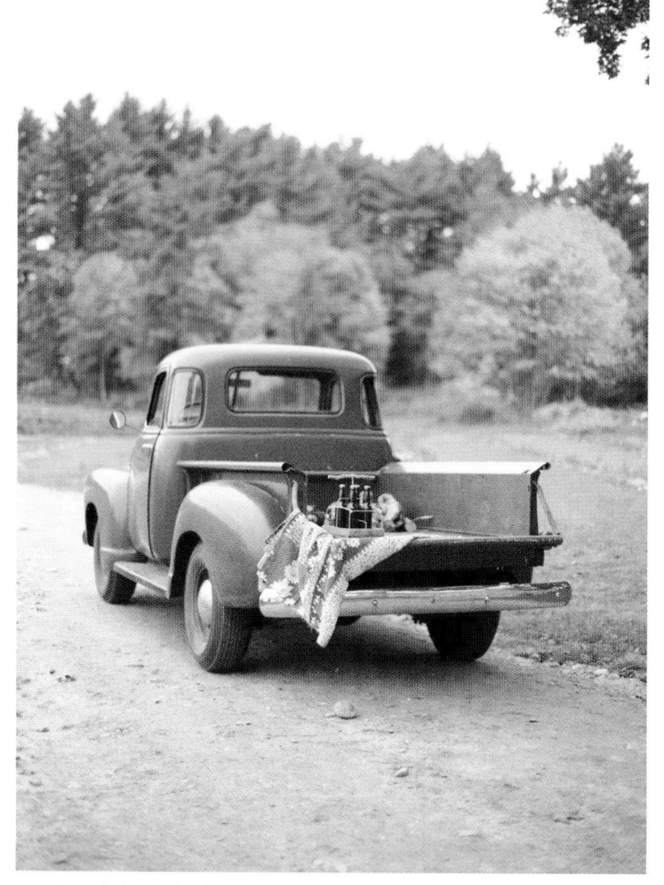

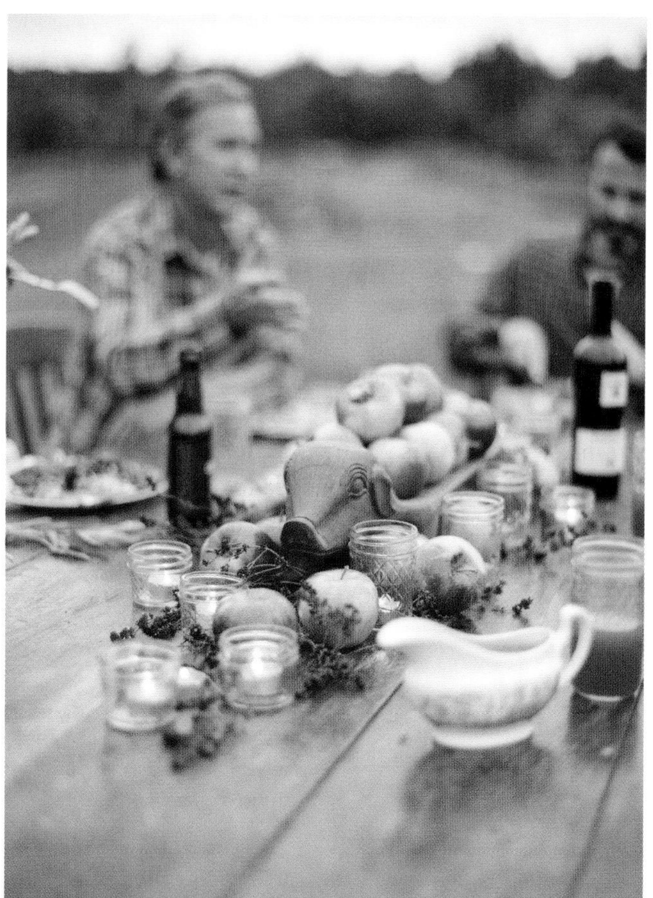

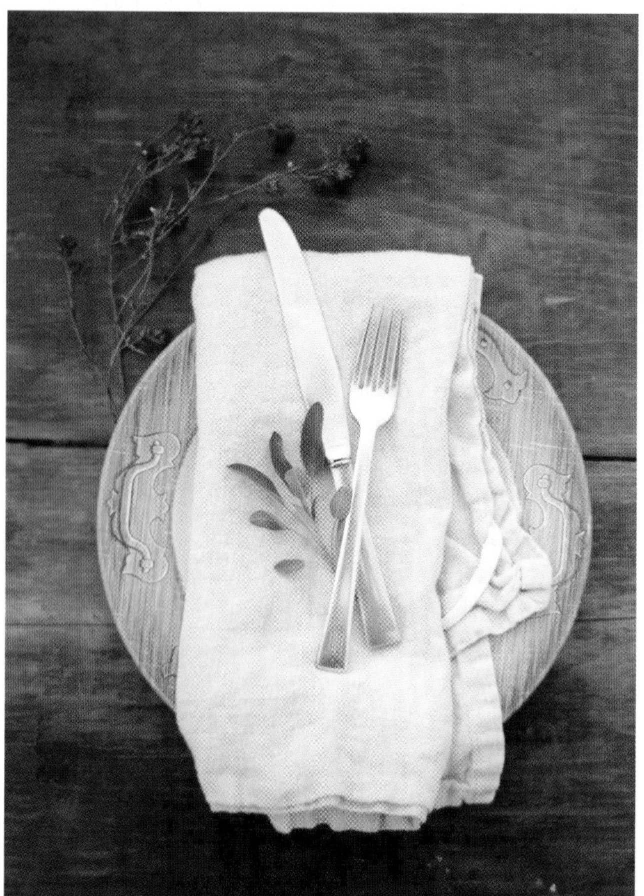

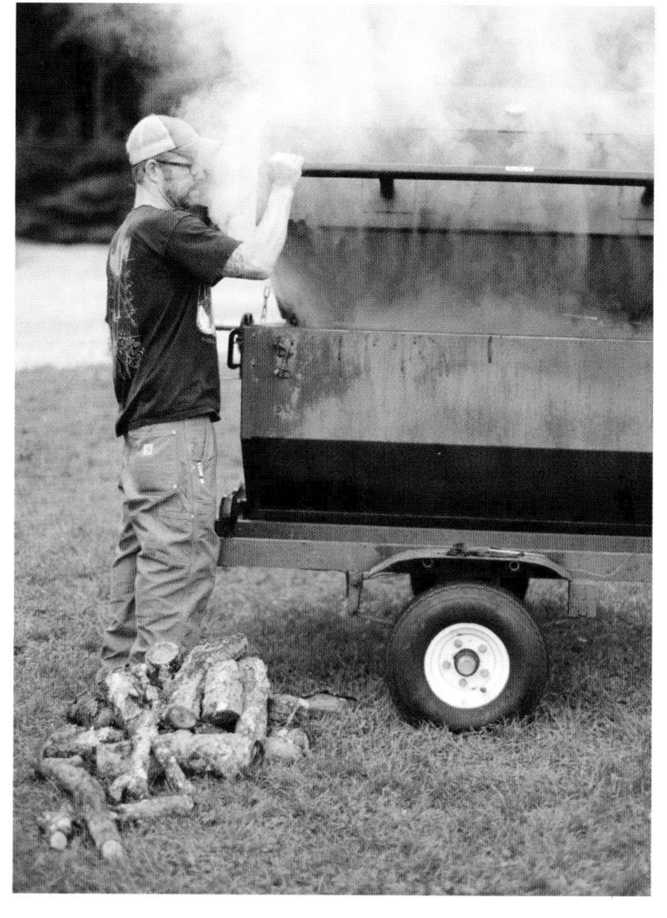

Roasting a Pig

Pig roasts are among my favorite gatherings. We love to host one every year to celebrate our community and the coming of fall. While the kids run free around the farm, their parents get to relax and sit by the fire. It's a memorable event, and one that's not as hard to pull off as you might think.

At the party, it's a good idea to designate one person as the "pig man" (or woman, as the case may be). This person is in charge of starting up the grill and keeping it at the right temperature, removing the pig from the spit once it's done, and carving it up. Your life will be much easier with one person assigned to these tasks—and don't let him or her have any hard cider until the pig is off the spit!

Have on hand some homemade hard cider (page 276) and someone to play music. A fire pit is a great addition—if you're having the pig roast in the fall, I'd almost call it mandatory—and games for the kids, like Capture the Flag (page 384) and Chicken Shit Bingo (page 385), add a lot to the party. Have fun!

You will need:

- *A pig (see the table for size, based on the number of people)*
- *Rotisserie grill*
- *Firewood*
- *A few bags of charcoal*
- *A carving knife*
- *Several large platters*
- *Cider Glaze, for serving (recipe follows)*

HOG SIZE	NUMBER OF PEOPLE	COOKING TIME
40–60 lbs	20	5–6 hours
60–80 lbs	30	5–6 hours
80–100 lbs	40–50	5–6 hours
100–120 lbs	70	6–8 hours
120–140 lbs	80	8 hours
140–160 lbs	100	8 hours
160+ lbs	120+	10 hours

Cider Glaze

- *¼ cup maple syrup*
- *2 tablespoons Dijon mustard*
- *⅛ teaspoon cayenne pepper*
- *1 cup apple cider vinegar or white vinegar*
- *1 gallon apple cider*

In a large soup pot over medium heat, combine the maple syrup, Dijon mustard, and cayenne and stir well. Add the vinegar and cider. Simmer for 45 minutes, uncovered. Pour over pork before serving.

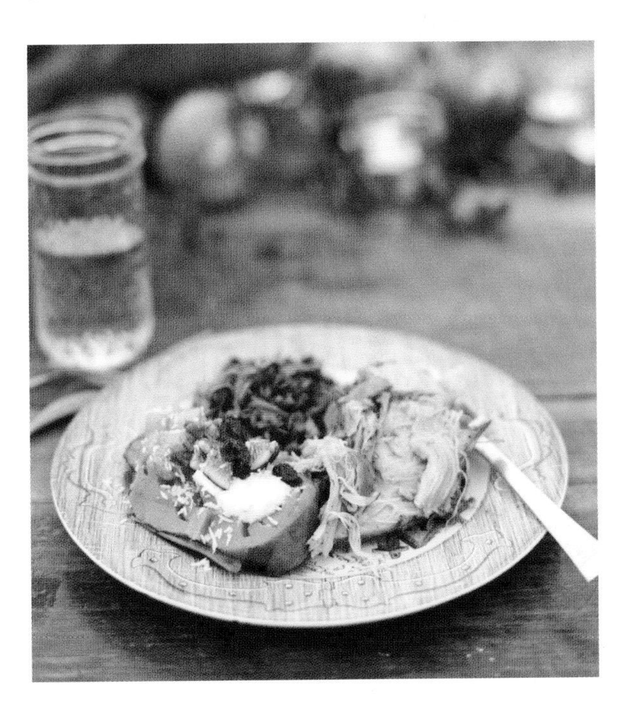

1. Plan the day based around when you want to serve the pig, taking the time the sun sets into account. You don't want to be cleaning up after dark, and you also need the light to make sure the pig is cooked through. I can't tell you how many pig roasts I've attended where the pig is served at 9 p.m. in the dark and we're all wondering if it's safe to eat. If the sun sets at 6:30 p.m., it's a good idea to aim to serve the pig at 5:00 p.m., which means it should be taken off the spit at around 4:00 p.m. A pig roast is an all-day affair, and you may need to start your pig at dawn to get it cooked in time for your party—see the table on page 383 for a guide to cooking times.

2. The easiest way to roast a pig is to rent a rotisserie grill and buy a pig already on the spit from a small slaughterhouse. Make sure you have a truck with the right trailer hitch on it when you pick up the grill and the pig. It's not easy to drive on a highway while towing a roaster, so I suggest taking the back roads.

3. Once you have the fire started and the grill heated up, maintain the temperature of the grill at about 250°F. Cool it as needed by closing the grates at the bottom, or open them to raise the temperature. For more flavorful pork, put some apple wood on the fire. It adds to the flavor of the smoke, and you'll taste it in the meat.

4. Remove the pig from the grill when its internal temperature reaches 155°F to 160°F. Place it on a large, clean table and cover it with foil to allow it to keep cooking a bit longer.

5. After allowing the pig to rest for 20 minutes or so, carve it and place it on platters. Pour Cider Glaze over the pork before serving. Sweet potatoes and a good slaw (page 217) make excellent side dishes.

Playing Capture the Flag

Remember this game from when you were a kid? Whenever we have a barbecue, pig roast, or potluck on the farm, capture the flag is the game of choice. You run hard and laugh even harder, and it's so much fun to play with a mix of adults and kids. Try it at your next outdoor gathering. You'll get a good workout and have a blast at the same time.

TIPS

It's a good idea to assign some players to defend your territory and others to go after the other team's flag. Decoys can be very effective: send some players in one direction to distract opponents while others sneak around the back way, undetected.

The Setup

Break the group into two teams and divide the playing area into two territories, one for each team. Each team gets a flag (bandanna, kitchen towel, whatever—get creative!) and hides it within their territory. Each team also picks a location on their territory for "jail."

The Rules

The object of the game is to capture your opponent's flag. To capture the flag, players must enter the opposing team's territory, take the flag, and bring it back to their territory without being tagged by the opposing team. If players are tagged in the opponent's territory, they are taken to "jail." They can only escape jail if one of their teammates is able to elude defenders and reach the jail safely. When this happens, all the jailed teammates are freed. If a player is tagged in their opponent's territory with the flag, the flag is dropped where it is and the player is taken to jail.

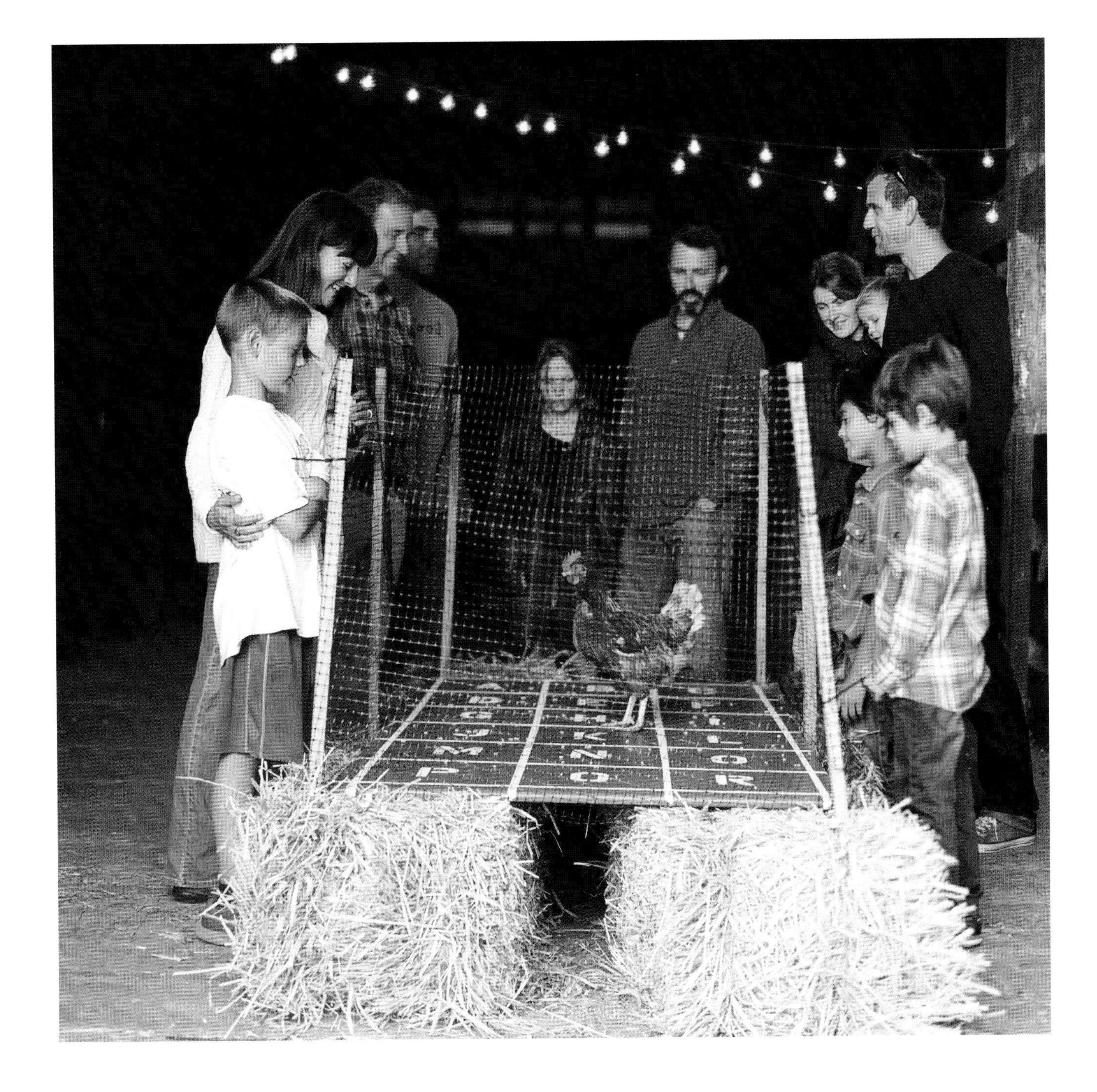

Playing Chicken Shit Bingo

If you have backyard chickens, this game is hilariously entertaining for both kids and adults. Find a piece of scrap plywood about the size of a Ping-Pong table and paint a grid of numbers or letters on it. Fence it off so that when you place the chicken inside, it can't fly out—chicken wire works well. We stick tomato stakes in hay bales and place them around the board, then zip tie deer netting to the stakes, and this works well, too.

Folks choose a square, and then everyone waits to see where the chicken poops first. For more action, place bets on which square will win, add some hard cider, and include a second chicken!

Coloring Easter Eggs

These naturally beautiful pastel eggs are so much lovelier than the sparkly neon eggs made from the kits that flood drugstores around Easter. These eggs turn out speckled and sometimes have odd spots or blotches, and each one is unique and gorgeous. There is an important lesson to be learned here: there is beauty in the imperfect. My kids were particularly surprised to see how red cabbage leaves made the eggs beautifully blue. Who needs jelly beans and cheap chocolate bunnies when you can color eggs at home with common kitchen items?

You will need:

- *White eggs*
- *1 tablespoon white vinegar*
- *1 tablespoon sea salt*
- *3 cups water*
- *A medium saucepan*
- *A needle or small nail (optional)*

For the colors:

- *Speckled pink: 1 cup raspberries*
- *Deep blue: 1 cup blueberries*
- *Deep golden yellow: 3 tablespoons turmeric*
- *Olive green: 1 big handful grass*
- *Light grey: 1 cup cherries*
- *Robin's-egg blue: 5 leaves red cabbage*
- *Brownish red: 3 red beets (see Notes)*
- *Pale orange: 4 yellow onion skins*

1. If you want to eat the eggs after you color them, boil them in a medium saucepan for 1 minute, remove from heat, then cover and let sit for 10 to 12 minutes. Then run the eggs under cold water or cool in an ice bath for 5 minutes.

   Alternatively, you can boil the eggs right in the pot with the colorant, which imparts a texture on the eggs (grass did this particularly well) and produces a deeper color.

2. Combine the vinegar, salt, water, and desired colorant in a medium saucepan and boil for 10 minutes.

3. If you aren't boiling the eggs with the colorant, after 10 minutes, strain out the colorant and let the liquid cool, then add the eggs.

4. Once you're happy with the color of the eggs, remove them from the liquid. If you haven't hard-boiled your eggs, blow out the centers so that they will keep longer: poke a hole in each end of the egg with a needle or small nail, insert the needle or nail to mix together the yolk and white, and then blow out the center. This process yields a paler color, but you'll be able to collect the eggs from year to year.

5. Coat the dyed eggs in coconut oil if you'd like to give them a slight shine. It's really a fun process!

NOTES: *If you're using beets as the colorant, leave the eggs in the dye for about 1 hour for a light red color. The longer you leave them in, the deeper brown they turn.*

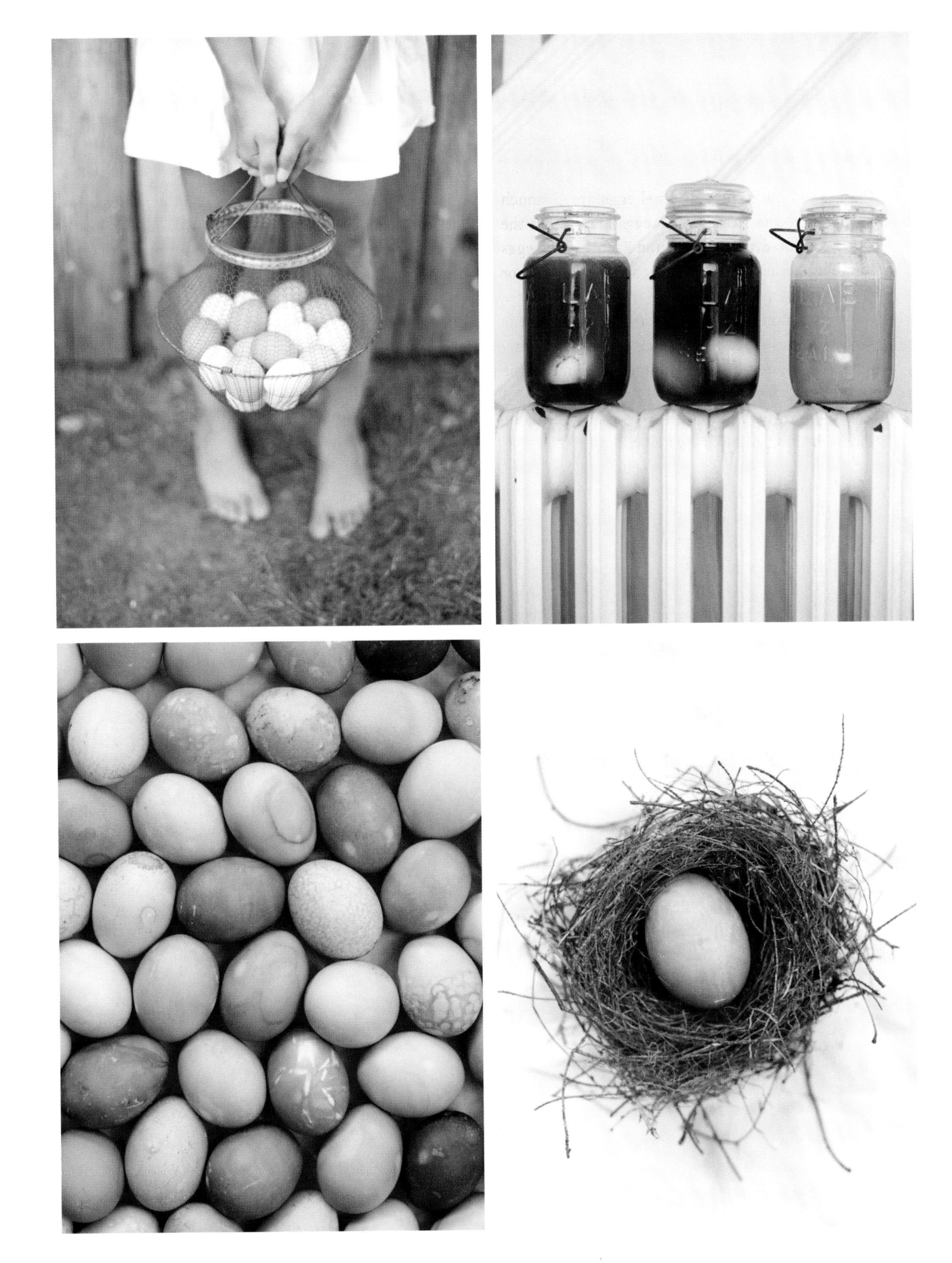

Making Beeswax Candles

Beeswax candles burn much cleaner than those made from paraffin wax. They also don't drip, they burn for a very long time, and they give off the most lovely honey scent. Plus, working with beeswax is a great introduction to candlemaking because if the candle doesn't turn out the way you wanted, you can simply melt it and start over.

Candlemaking suppliers offer a large variety of rubber molds for candles, but you can also use mason jars or other heat-safe glass containers. The more intricate the mold, the more difficult it is to remove the candle in one piece, so it's best to start with relatively simple molds, such as cylinders or molds without intricate designs. (For where to buy candlemaking supplies, see page 397.)

You will need:

- *Beeswax*
- *A double boiler (or dedicated slow cooker, or any heat-safe container placed inside a pot of hot water; just make sure the container is only used for wax)*
- *A thermometer*
- *Candle mold(s) or containers*
- *Wicks (one per candle)*
- *Scotch or masking tape*
- *Popsicle sticks*
- *Bobby pins*
- *Rubber bands*
- *Nonstick silicone spray*
- *Scissors*

1. To help the beeswax melt more quickly and evenly, cut it into pieces about 1 inch square or smaller.
2. Melt the wax in a double boiler until it reaches about 145°F. Be careful that it does not exceed 170°F.
3. While the wax is melting, prepare the wick. Insert it through the wicking hole in the bottom of the candle mold or tape it to the bottom center of your container. Secure the top of the wick in the center of the mold or container with a bobby pin held up by two popsicle sticks.
4. If using a mold, secure it with a handful of rubber bands. You might want to spray it first with nonstick silicone spray, to make removing the candle easier later on.
5. Once the wax is completely melted, carefully pour it into the mold or container.
6. If using a mold, wait about 10 to 20 minutes for the beeswax to harden—the exact amount of time will vary depending on the size of the candle and the mold—and carefully pull apart the mold to remove the candle. Be sure to remove the candle from the mold before it stiffens completely, so that it comes out in one piece.
7. Remove the bobby pin and popsicle sticks and trim the wick to ½ inch.

One pound of beeswax yields about 20 ounces of melted wax. To figure out how much beeswax you need, multiply the number of candles you're making by the amount of wax each container or mold will hold, and then divide the result by 20. For example, if you want to make thirty 8-ounce candles, the math would be: 30 (containers) x 8 (ounces per container) = 240 ounces total / 20 (ounces per pound of beeswax) = 12 pounds of beeswax.

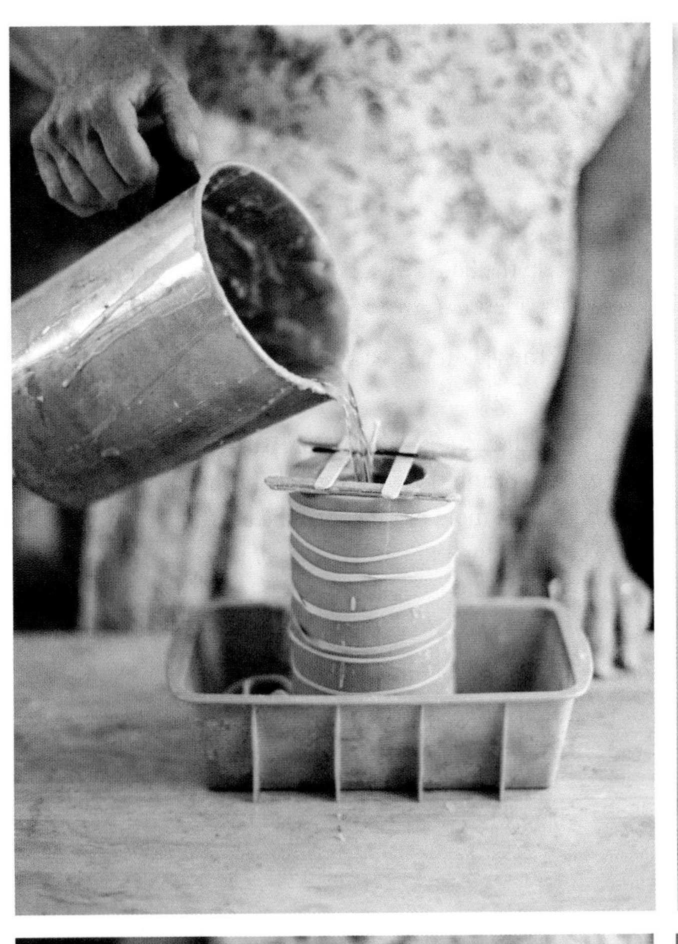
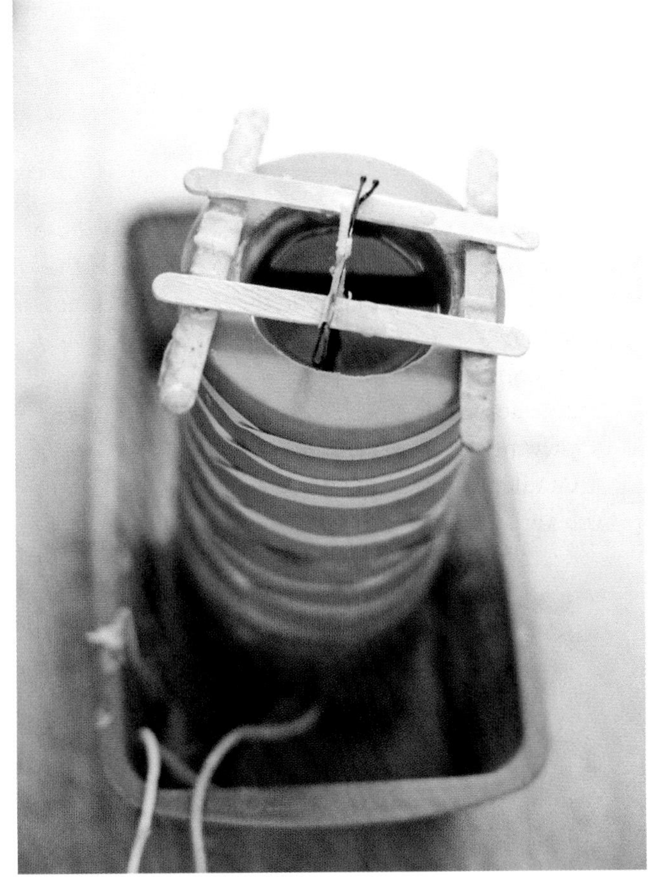
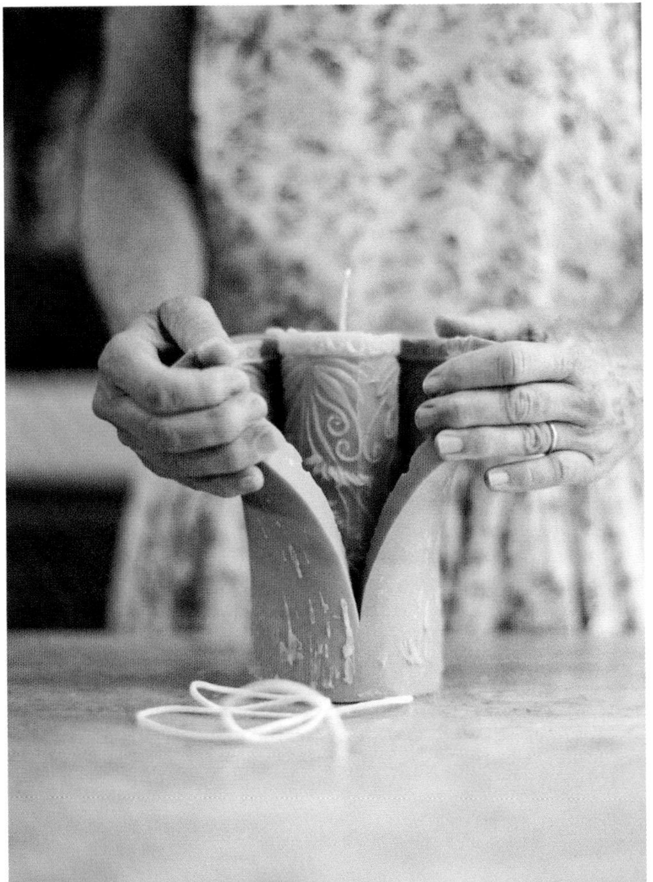
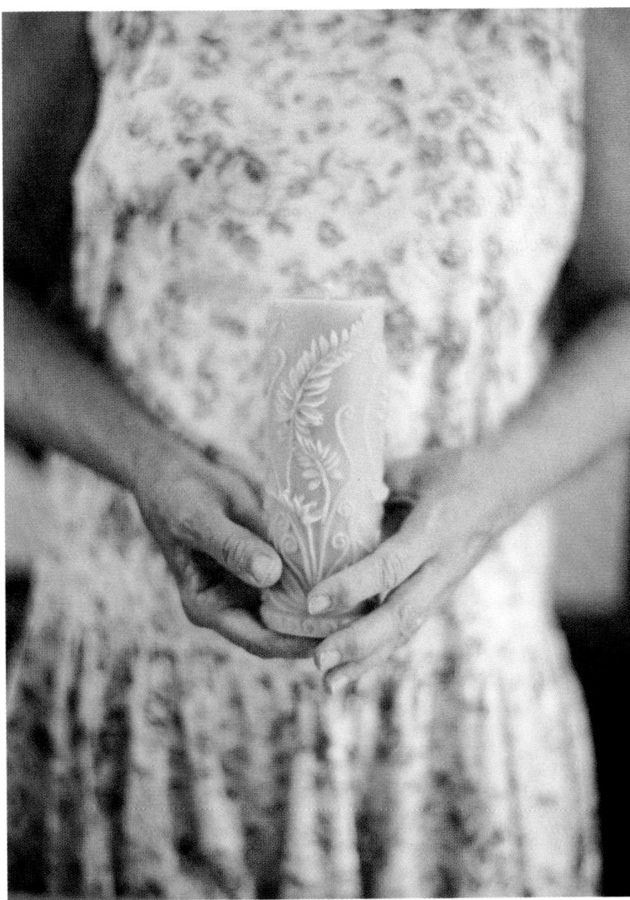

Making Goat Milk Soap

My sister Frances started off as a pre-med major at Smith College, and through a series of curvy life events, she's now an acupuncturist and owns a company that creates body care products. She makes all kinds of beautiful soaps that last a very long time, smell incredible, and are very moisturizing for the skin. I pulled her in for this project, which is a bit time-consuming but very rewarding and a great project for holiday gifts. (If you want to skip making this soap yourself and just buy Frances' soaps or other products, including her popular mustache wax, see the Resources section at the back of the book.)

This goat milk soap is a cold-process soap—unlike a hot-process soap, it doesn't need to be heated in a slow cooker or double boiler. Making a batch takes one to two hours, and it needs an additional four to six weeks to cure before it can be used or gifted. The curing process allows time for the water to completely evaporate, resulting in a harder, longer-lasting bar of soap.

This basic recipe uses oils you can buy at your local market—the high olive oil content yields a very mild bar. The recipe makes enough for a 9-by-12-inch loaf of soap that's 2 inches thick, so if you don't have a soap mold, you can use a baking pan instead.

The first time you make soap can be a bit of a wild ride, but once you get the basics down and begin to experiment, the opportunities for creativity are endless.

You will need:

TOOLS

- *A medium saucepan*
- *A candy or oil thermometer, or an infrared thermometer*
- *A kitchen scale*
- *Glass or Pyrex measuring cups*
- *A medium glass bowl*
- *Rubber gloves*
- *Plastic goggles*
- *Heatproof stirring spoons*
- *A soap mold (see Resources for where to buy) or a 9-by-12-inch baking pan*
- *Freezer paper, if you're using a baking pan or the soap mold requires it*
- *An immersion blender*
- *A spatula (for smoothing the soap) or a chopstick or spoon (for adding texture)*
- *Isopropyl alcohol (at least 90%) in a spray bottle*
- *A chef's knife*
- *A cookie sheet*

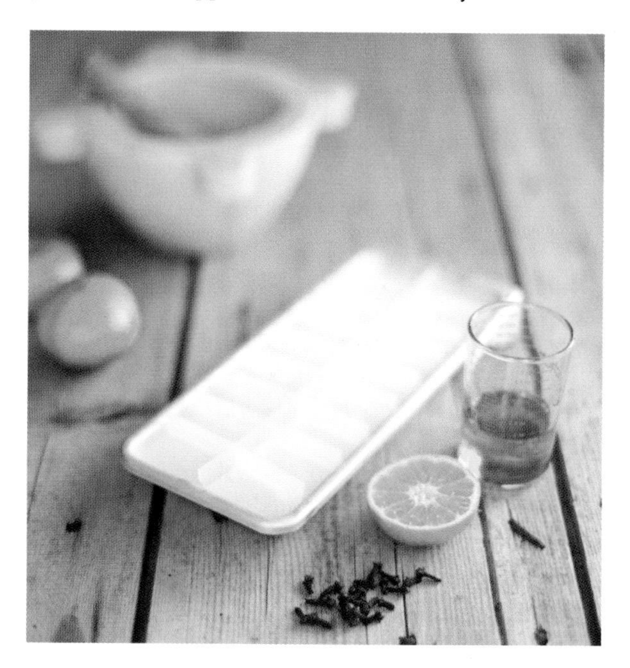

INGREDIENTS

- *8.4 ounces coconut oil*
- *19.6 ounces olive oil*
- *3.98 ounces lye*
- *9.8 ounces frozen goat milk*
- *1.6 ounces orange essential oil*
- *1 teaspoon ground cloves*

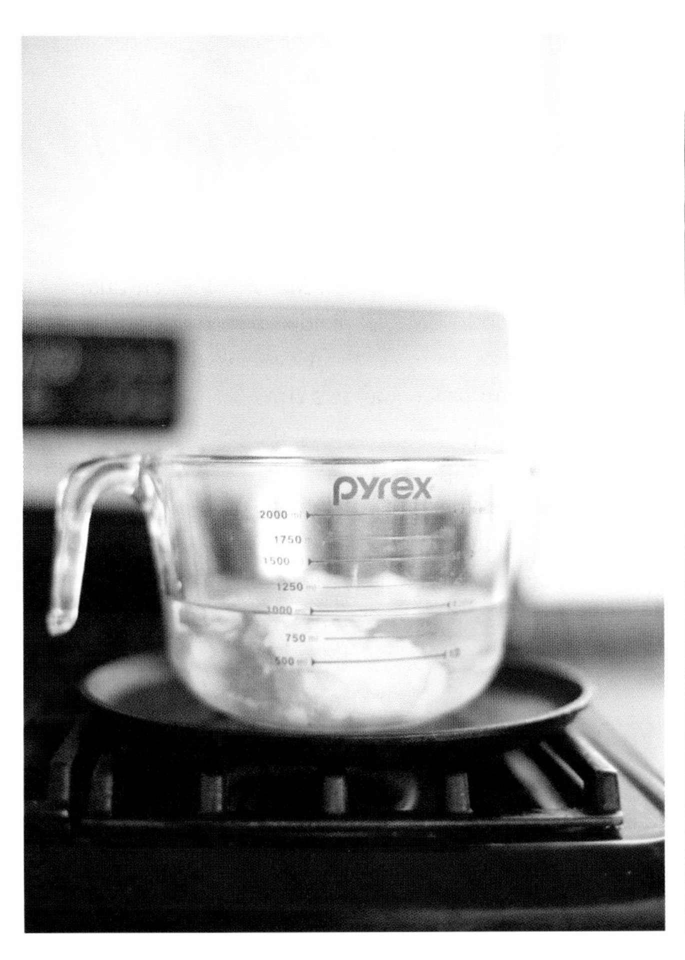

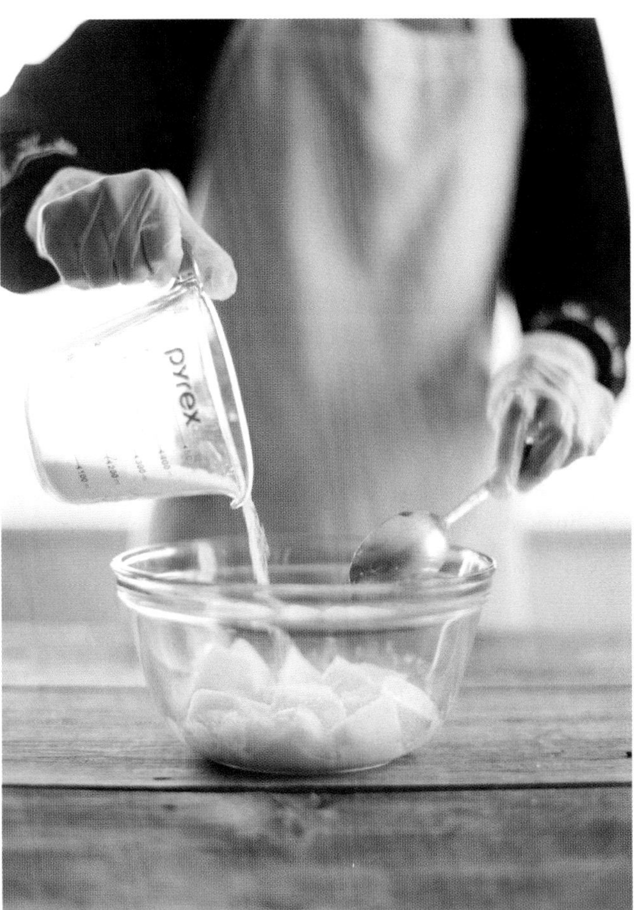

Melt the Base Oils and Make the Lye and Milk Solution

1. In a medium saucepan over medium-high heat, combine the coconut oil and olive oil and heat to about 110°F.

2. While the oils are gently melting, place the frozen goat milk cubes in a medium glass bowl. With protective gear on your hands, arms, and eyes, slowly pour about one-tenth of the lye onto the goat milk. This will cause a heat reaction. Stir as best you can and check the temperature. Be careful to not let it get above 90°F to 95°F or the milk will burn.

3. Continue adding the lye a little at a time, frequently checking the temperature. If brown spots start to form on the milk, it's a sign that the heat is too high and you need to add the lye more slowly. It should take about ten minutes to fully combine the lye and goat milk.

4. Once you've added all of the lye, let the lye and milk solution rest to reduce the temperature. A good temperature range to work with is between 90°F and 115°F.

MEASURING

The measurements in this recipe are all given by weight, not volume, so you'll need to weigh the ingredients on a kitchen scale. When using a digital scale, place the empty bowl or container on the scale first, set the scale to zero, then add the ingredient. Using exactly the amount of ingredient called for is critical for your soap to come out properly.

To measure the amount of frozen goat milk more precisely, pour the milk into ice cube trays and then freeze it—the small cubes make it easier to get the right amount of goat milk, and you can even cut the last cube in half if necessary to get the correct weight.

Combine the Base Oils, Lye Solution, and Other Ingredients and Pour the Soap into the Mold

1. If you are using a baking pan or plastic mold, line it with freezer paper. (Some molds don't require freezer paper; check with the manufacturer.)

2. Remove the saucepan of melted oils from heat and check the temperature.

3. When both the lye solution and base oils are below 115°F, slowly pour the lye solution into the melted oils. Add the orange essential oil and cloves.

4. With an immersion blender, mix the lye solution and base oils. Be sure to "burp" the immersion blender to avoid air bubbles, but generally keep the blender near the bottom of the bowl so the soap mixture doesn't splash out of the bowl. The mixture will soon become cloudy and then start to thicken to a runny, pudding-like consistency. If you want to add a colorant or exfoliant, do so now.

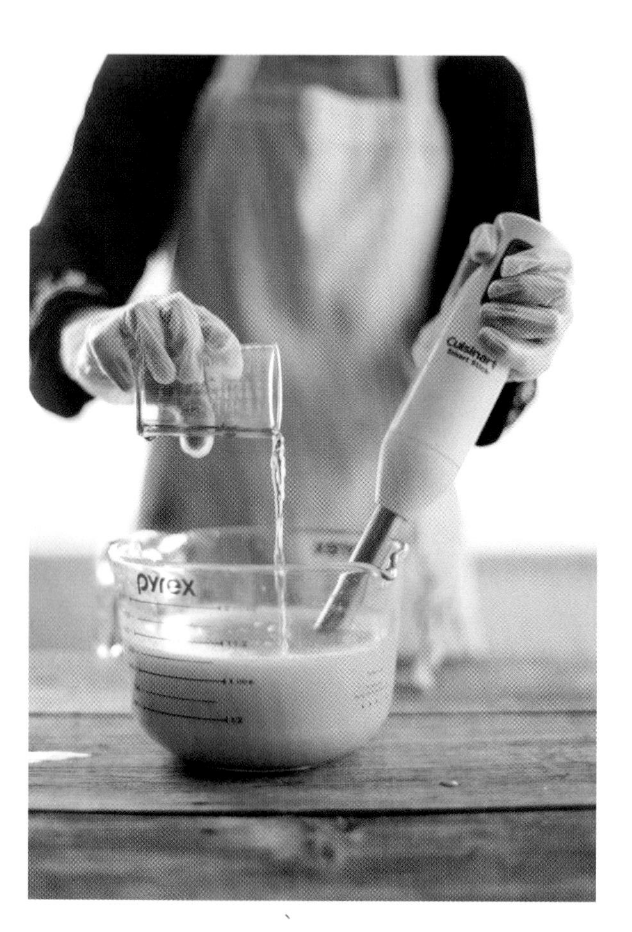

5. When you lift the blender out of the soap and it leaves marks on the surface, you've reached "trace," the point at which the oils and lye solution have emulsified. Stop here; do not overmix. If you do overmix, the mixture will become very thick and difficult to pour into the mold, and the final result will not look too pretty.

6. Pour the soap mixture into the mold or baking pan, using a spatula to get as much of the mixture out of the bowl as possible. Once the soap is in the mold, smooth out the top with the spatula or use a chopstick or spoon to give it a texture.

7. Spray the soap in the mold with the isopropyl alcohol. The scent will not stay, and the alcohol helps prevent a white substance called soda ash from forming on the top of the soap. Soda ash is perfectly harmless, but many people do not like the way it looks.

Unmold the Soap and Let It Cure

1. After about twenty-four to thirty-six hours, the soap will be hard to the touch. At this point, remove it from the mold.

2. Using a chef's knife, cut the soap into bars.

3. Place the bars on a cookie sheet lined with freezer paper and store them in a space with good ventilation. Allow the bars to cure for at least four to six weeks.

SAFETY ALERT

Although making soap is fun, it's not kid-friendly because it requires the use of lye (sodium hydroxide, or NaOH). Lye is a highly caustic substance that can cause severe burns if it's inhaled or makes contact with skin. It's extremely important to do this project in a well-ventilated room and wear rubber gloves and goggles. It's also wise to wear long sleeves and an apron to protect yourself from splashing. Use only glass or metal tools when making soap—the lye will eat away at wood and possibly even plastic.

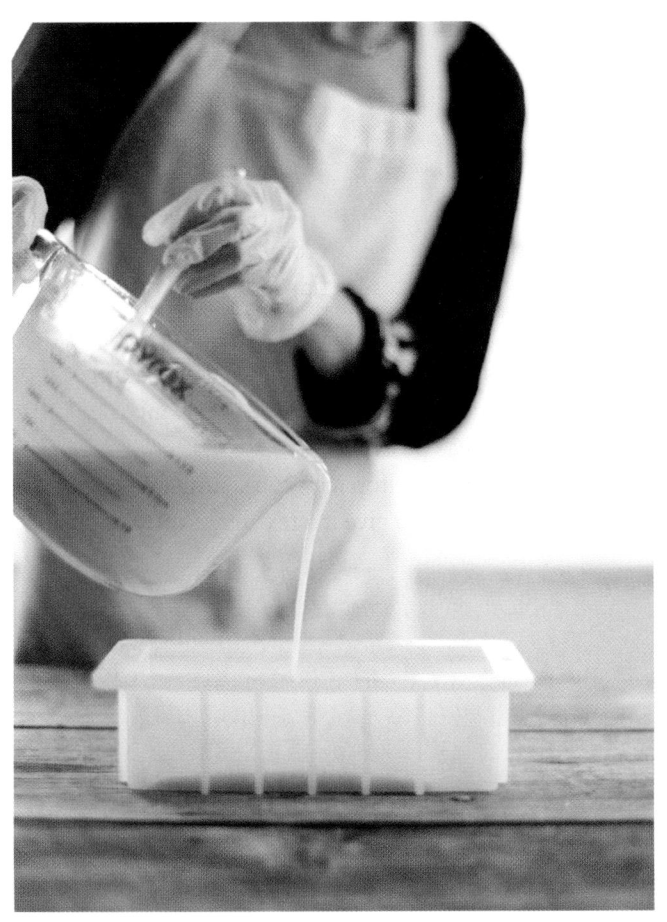
PYREX

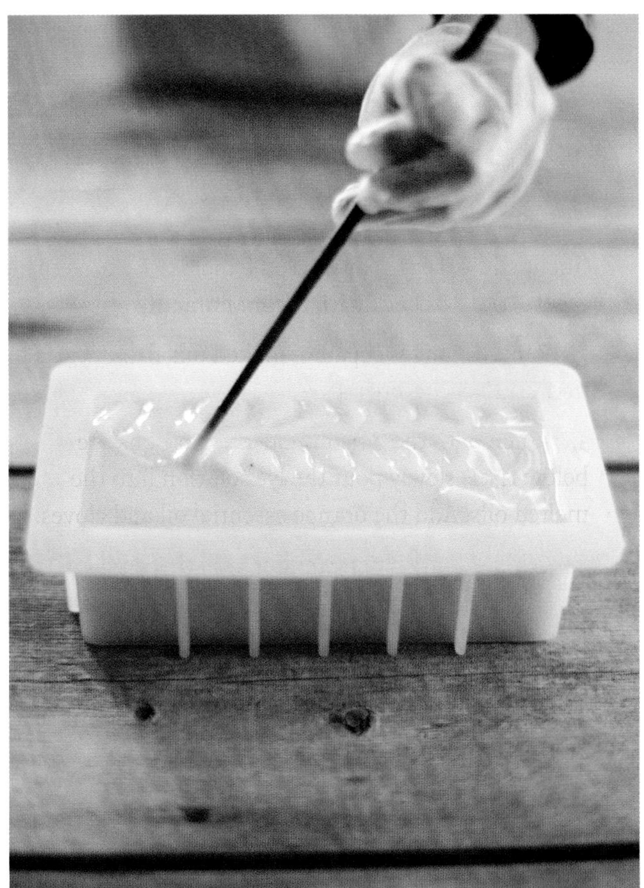

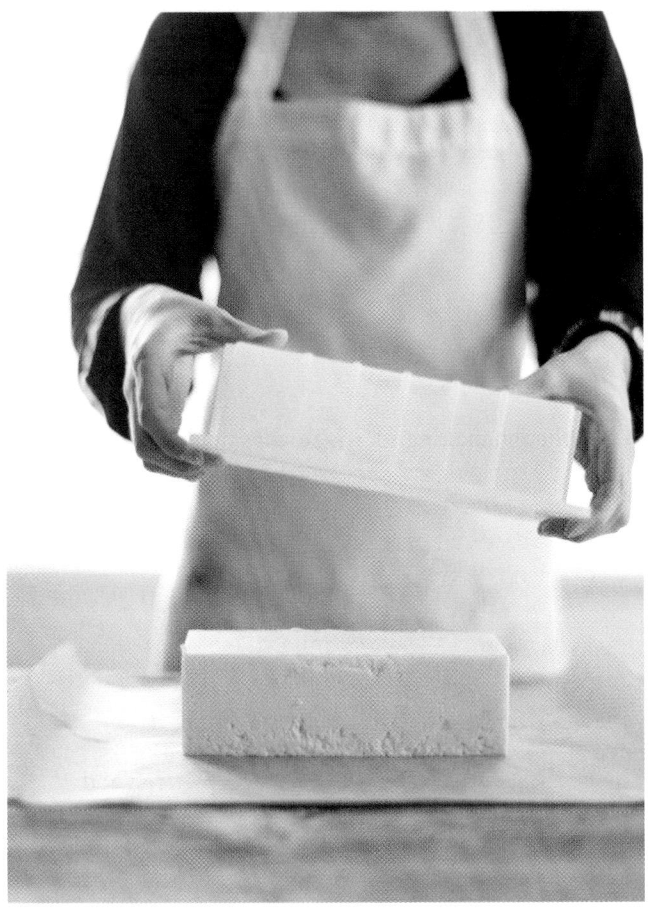

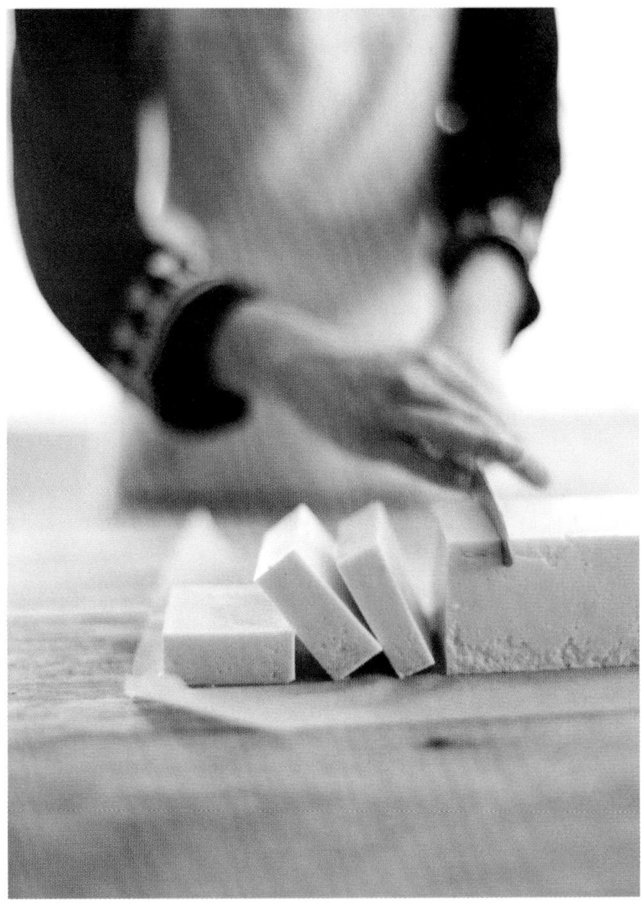

Giving Back

In our fast-paced, technology-driven world, we can be so focused on individual goals that we lose the sense of community that used to be an essential part of everyday life. Strong friendships, good relationships with neighbors, and ties to others in your town can make a big difference in both health and happiness. The good news is that there are lots of ways to reach out and help strengthen your community.

If your garden is doing well, share the wealth and take some to your neighbors. Or consider donating some to food pantries, which often have lots of canned items and dry goods but few fresh vegetables. At our farm, we host a program where folks with extra garden bounty drop it off with us; once a week, we add any CSA shares that have been donated by members as well as excess produce from our own farm, and we deliver it all to a meal center in a nearby town that desperately needs fresh vegetables. See if there's a similar program in your area, or consider starting one yourself!

Or try volunteering at a meal center, which can be both a great community-building exercise and a wonderful way to help those in need get a nutrient-dense, delicious meal. Think about getting a group together from your church or gym, or gather your neighbors and friends. It can be a lot of fun, as I discovered when I gathered a group from CrossFit Cape Ann, where I'm a nutrition consultant, to serve a meal at the Open Door Food Pantry in Gloucester, Massachusetts. We chopped farm-fresh cabbage, carrots, onions, and herbs for coleslaw, cooked mashed sweet potatoes, and sliced up some beautiful brisket provided by US Wellness Meats. The dessert was a simple, fresh fruit salad with mint. (See pages 171, 217, and 220 for the home-scale version of this meal.) The finished plate was something we were quite proud of! Our goal was to serve a nutritious meal that we would love to eat in our own homes or in a restaurant, and the clients seemed to agree that we succeeded. The whole experience was incredibly rewarding, and doing it with a group helped build friendships, too.

If you'd like to get your hands dirty and learn more about food production, think about volunteering at a local farm. Many hands make light work, and traditionally, events such as barn raisings were important gatherings for the entire community. Today, volunteering on a farm is a wonderful way to get active, spend the day outside, and meet people. I love the idea of a "weed dating" event—people weed on opposite sides of a row of crops while chatting to someone for a few minutes, then move down the row. Or, if you have a group full of strong, athletic people, why not form your own flash mob and help the farmer get weeds under control?

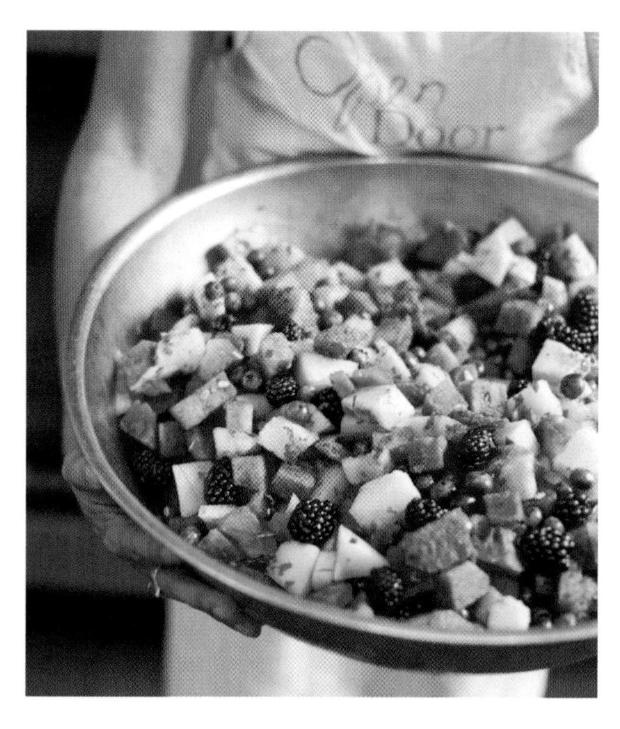

Paying It Forward

If you're like me, you're deeply saddened by our industrialized food system, which markets hyperpalatable, fluorescent-colored, sugar-dusted garbage as "fat-free" and "heart-healthy." This system also treats animals poorly, poisons the environment, and has led to the current obesity epidemic and nationwide health crisis. Trying to change this behemoth of a system can feel impossible, but we need not become overwhelmed or complacent. We can all do things to fix it.

First and most importantly, we can choose to opt out and instead engage in a decentralized food system that focuses on local, organic, sustainably grown food, that prioritizes the health of animals and the environment, and that respects those who labor to get that food to our plates. "Engaging in a decentralized food system" doesn't have to mean becoming a professional farmer (although if you do want to get into farming professionally, check out page 397 in the Resources section)—just growing a few vegetables in containers makes a difference. We can change the way we treat our property and make it useful and productive. Who needs a weed-free, monocropped lawn and ornamental shrubs when you can instead sustain a flock of chickens, or plant blueberries and fruit trees? Why not have backyards full of vegetables instead of chemical-filled pools? But if you're not yet ready to grow your own food, making a conscious effort to buy from local sustainable farms is a great start.

Let's also change the way we value the old-fashioned skills of homesteading and domesticity. They're becoming lost arts in our high-tech, specialized world. Let's value creativity and self-reliance more than compliance and conformity.

And finally, let's share the knowledge. When we include friends, neighbors, and youth in the hands-on act of growing and cooking nutrient-dense food, we're making a critical investment in society. The future generation needs to understand how to create a more resilient and sustainable food system, not one dependent on machines, petrochemical inputs and laboratory-grown proteins. Everybody needs to understand the vital importance of sustainability.

We need real food. It's not only good for our health, it's essential to the health of the planet. We just need to rethink why we're here and reframe what matters to us. The way forward may not be easy, but it's not as hard as we think, either. The rewards are more than worth it.

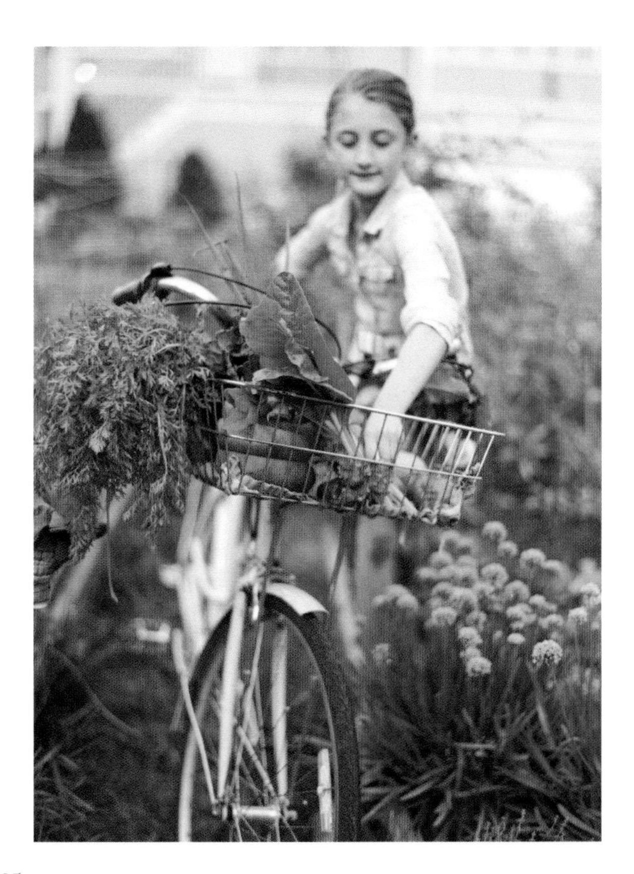

Resources

Informational Books and Websites

General

The Farm as Natural Habitat: Reconnecting Food Systems with Ecosystems, edited by Dana L. Jackson and Laura L. Jackson

The Unsettling of America: Culture and Agriculture, by Wendell Berry

The Vegetarian Myth: Food, Justice, and Sustainability, by Lierre Keith

You Can Farm, by Joel Salatin

Raising

The Backyard Homestead Guide to Raising Farm Animals, by Gail Damerow

Beekeeping for Dummies, by Howland Blackiston

The Family Cow, by Dirk van Loon

How to Build Animal Housing, by Carol Ekarius

Humane Livestock Handling, by Temple Grandin

Small-Scale Livestock Farming: A Grass-Based Approach for Health, Sustainability, and Profit, by Carol Ekarius

Storey's Guide to Raising Chickens, 3rd edition, by Gail Damerow

Storey's Guide to Raising Sheep, 4th edition, by Carol Ekarius and Paula Simmons

Storey's Guide to Raising Meat Goats, 2nd edition, by Maggie Sayer

Storey's Guide to Raising Dairy Goats, 4th edition, by Jerry Belanger

Toward Saving the Honeybee, by Gunther Hauk

Growing

The Apple Grower: A Guide for the Organic Orchardist, by Michael Phillips

Four-Season Harvest: Organic Vegetables from Your Home Garden All Year Long, 2nd edition, by Eliot Coleman

Gaia's Garden: A Guide to Home-Scale Permaculture, 2nd edition, by Toby Hemenway

The New Organic Grower: A Master's Manual of Tools and Techniques for the Home and Market Gardener, 2nd edition, by Eliot Coleman

The Organic Farming Manual, by Anne Larkin Hansen

The Rodale Book of Composting, edited by Deborah L. Martin and Grace Gershuny

Wild Plants I Have Known . . . and Eaten, by Russ Cohen

Cooking/Nutrition

All About Braising: The Art of Uncomplicated Cooking, by Molly Stevens

Balanced Bites, balancedbites.com

ChrisKresser.com

Death by Food Pyramid, by Denise Minger

Eat the Yolks, by Liz Wolfe

Evolutionary Psychology, evolutionarypsychiatry.blogspot.com

It Starts with Food, by Dallas and Melissa Hartwig

Mark's Daily Apple, marksdailyapple.com

The Paleo Manifesto, by John Durant

The Paleo Solution, by Robb Wolf

Practical Paleo, by Diane Sanfilippo

Real Food Liz, realfoodliz.com

RobbWolf.com

The 21-Day Sugar Detox, by Diane Sanfilippo

Your Personal Paleo Code, by Chris Kresser

Living

The Four Agreements: A Practical Guide to Personal Freedom, by Don Miguel Ruiz

Last Child in the Woods: Saving Our Children from Nature-Deficit Disorder, by Richard Louv

Make a Difference: America's Guide to Volunteering and Community Service, by Arthur I. Blaustein

The Mastery of Love: A Practical Guide to the Art of Relationship, by Don Miguel Ruiz

The Nature Connection: An Outdoor Workbook for Kids, Families, and Classrooms, by Clare Walker Leslie

Nature's Playground: Activities, Crafts, and Games to Encourage Children to Get Outdoors, by Fiona Danks and Jo Schofield

Radical Homemakers: Reclaiming Domesticity from a Consumer Culture, by Shannon Hayes

Your Money or Your Life: 9 Steps to Transforming Your Relationship with Money and Achieving Financial Independence, revised edition, by Vicki Robin, Joe Dominguez, and Monique Tilford

Learning Opportunities

The Sustainable Agriculture Education Association has a list of universities offering degree programs related to sustainable agriculture: sustainableaged.org/projects/degree-programs/

Worldwide Opportunities on Organic Farms, USA connects visitors with sustainable farms where they can help out and learn about sustainable agriculture: wwoofusa.org

The National Sustainable Agriculture Information Service, run by the National Center for Appropriate Technology, lists sustainable farming internships and apprenticeships: attra.ncat.org/attra-pub/internships/

The New Entry Sustainable Farming Project provides training for new farmers: nesfp.org

The Farm School teaches students to farm through hands-on experience: www.farmschool.org

Where to Find Supplies

Animal health

PBS Animal Health, pbsanimalhealth.com

Beekeeping

Brushy Mountain Bee Farm, brushymountainbeefarm.com

Bee Commerce, bee-commerce.com (includes helpful video tutorials)

Candlemaking

Lone Star Candle Supply, lonestarcandlesupply.com

Nature's Garden, naturesgardencandles.com

Cooking

Barefoot Provisions, barefootprovisions.com

Ingredients

While in general I recommend using homegrown or locally purchased ingredients, there are a few brands that I prefer to seek out.

Equal Exchange Coffee and Chocolate

Green and Black's Chocolate

Pure Indian Foods ghee

Red Boat fish sauce

Wright's Hickory Liquid Smoke

Taza Chocolate

Cast-iron cookware
Lodge Cast Iron, lodgemfg.com

Cider brewing supplies
Midwest Homebrewing and Winemaking Supplies, midwestsupplies.com

Desiccated liver powder
Radiant Life, radiantlifecatalog.com

Food storage
Ball canning jars, freshpreserving.com

LunchBots, lunchbots.com

Tattler Reusable Canning Lids, reusablecanninglids.com

Kombucha SCOBY, kefir grains, and other fermentation products
Cultures for Health, culturesforhealth.com

Seaweed
Ocean Approved Seaweed, oceanapproved.com

Electric fencing

Wellscroft Fence Systems, wellscroft.com

Seeds and farming supplies

Fedco Seeds, fedcoseeds.com

High Mowing Organic Seeds, highmowingseeds.com

Johnny's Selected Seeds, johnnyseeds.com

Nourse Farms, noursefarms.com

Seed Savers Exchange, seedsavers.org

Soapmaking

Phoenix Artisan Accoutrements, phoenixartisanaccoutrements.com

Soap Making Resource, soap-making-resource.com

Videos and How-Tos

Visit my blog, **SustainableDish.com**, for short films on a variety of topics, from rotational grazing and animal care to harvesting herbs.

How to build and assemble chicken coops and related items

How to Build Animal Housing, by Carol Ekarius

RootsCoopsAndMore.com

How to milk a cow
http://youtu.be/A0_9lHwDe40

How to process a chicken
http://youtu.be/7a0yO038A-k

How to process a rabbit
http://youtu.be/cNx07GFEXWw

How to start your own sweet potato slips
http://www.food-skills-for-self-sufficiency.com/sweet-potato-slips.html

How to trim hooves
http://youtu.be/Ya17IujktZM

Live feed of backyard chickens
HenCam.com

Find a Local Organic/Sustainable Farm

Local Harvest, localharvest.org

Eatwild, eatwild.com

Sources

The Problems with Modern Eating

American Academy of Child and Adolescent Psychiatry. "The Depressed Child." *Facts for Families* No. 4. Washington, DC: American Academy of Child and Adolescent Psychiatry, 2013. Web. http://www.aacap.org/aacap/Families_and_Youth/Facts_for_Families/Facts_for_Families_Pages/The_Depressed_Child_04.aspx

American Cancer Society. *Cancer Facts & Figures* 2014. Atlanta, GA: American Cancer Society, 2014. Web. http://www.cancer.org/acs/groups/content/@research/documents/webcontent/acspc-042151.pdf

Centers for Disease Control and Prevention. *National Diabetes Fact Sheet*, 2011. Atlanta, GA: U.S. Department of Health and Human Services, Centers for Disease Control and Prevention, 2011. Web. http://www.cdc.gov/diabetes/pubs/pdf/ndfs_2011.pdf

Centers for Disease Control and Prevention. *National Diabetes Statistics Report*, 2014. Atlanta, GA: U.S. Department of Health and Human Services, Centers for Disease Control and Prevention, 2014. Web. http://www.cdc.gov/diabetes/pubs/estimates14.htm

Cordain, Loren, et al. "Origins and Evolution of the Western Diet: Health Implications for the 21st Century." *American Journal of Clinical Nutrition* 81.2 (2005): 341–54.

"Data & Statistics." *Centers for Disease Control and Prevention*, 13 Nov. 2013. Web. http://www.cdc.gov/ncbddd/adhd/data.html

Davis, Steven L. "The Least Harm Principle May Require that Humans Consume a Diet Containing Large Herbivores, Not a Vegan Diet." *Journal of Agricultural and Environmental Ethics* 16 (2003): 387–94. https://ethik.univie.ac.at/fileadmin/user_upload/inst_ethik_wiss_dialog/Davis__S._2003_The_least_Harm_-_Anti_Veg_in_J._Agric._Ethics.pdf

Giovannucci, Daniele, et al. *Seeking Sustainability: COSA Preliminary Analysis of Sustainability Initiatives in the Coffee Sector.* International Institute for Sustainable Development, 2008. http://www.iisd.org/publications/seeking-sustainability-cosa-preliminary-analysis-sustainability-initiatives-coffee

Gurven, Michael, and Hillard Kaplan. "Longevity Among Hunter-Gatherers: A Cross-Cultural Examination." *Population and Development Review* 33.2 (2007): 321–65.

Haight, Colleen. "The Problem with Fair Trade Coffee." *Stanford Social Innovation Review* 9.3 (2011). http://www.ssireview.org/articles/entry/the_problem_with_fair_trade_coffee

Jacka, Felice N., et al. "The Association Between Habitual Diet Quality and the Common Mental Disorders in Community-Dwelling Adults: The Hordaland Health Study." *Psychosomatic Medicine* 73.6 (2011): 483–90.

Keith, Lierre. *The Vegetarian Myth: Food, Justice, and Sustainability.* Crescent City, CA: Flashpoint, 2009.

Kiple, Kenneth F., and Kriemhild Coneè Ornelas, eds. *The Cambridge World History of Food.* Cambridge, UK: Cambridge University Press, 2000.

Lange, J. R., B. E. Palis, D. C. Chang, S. J. Soong, and C. M. Balch. "Melanoma in Children and Teenagers: An Analysis of Patients from the National Cancer Database." *Journal of Clinical Oncology* 25.11 (2007): 1363–368.

National Center for Health Statistics. *Health, United States, 2013.* Hyattsville, MD: Centers for Disease Control and Prevention, U.S. Department of Health and Human Services, 2014. Web. http://www.cdc.gov/nchs/data/hus/hus13.pdf

Sonuga-Barke, Edmund J. S., et al. "Nonpharmacological Interventions for ADHD: Systematic Review and Meta-Analyses of Randomized Controlled Trials of Dietary and Psychological Treatments." *American Journal of Psychiatry* 170.3 (2013): 275–289. http://ajp.psychiatryonline.org/data/Journals/AJP/926441/275.pdf

Yoon, Paula W., et al. "Potentially Preventable Deaths from the Five Leading Causes of Death—United States, 2008–2010." *Morbidity and Mortality Weekly Report* 63.17 (2014): 369–374. Centers for Disease Control and Prevention. http://www.cdc.gov/mmwr/preview/mmwrhtml/mm6317a1.htm

The Sustainable Paleo Diet

Ehrenberg, Rachel, "Artificial Sweeteners May Tip Scales Toward Metabolic Problems." *Science News* 17 Sept. 2014. https://www.sciencenews.org/article/artificial-sweeteners-may-tip-scales-toward-metabolic-problems

Understanding Food Production

"2014 Poverty Guidelines." *Office of the Assistant Secretary for Planning and Evaluation (ASPE).* US Department of Health and Human Services. Web. http://aspe.hhs.gov/poverty/14poverty.cfm

CAFO: The Tragedy of Industrial Animal Factories. Web. http://www.cafothebook.org/

Final Report on the Status of Public and Private Efforts to Eliminate the Worst Forms of Child Labor (WFCL) in the Cocoa Sectors of Côte d'Ivoire and Ghana. Payson Center for International Development and Technology Transfer, Tulane University, 31 March 2011. Web. http://www.childlabor-payson.org/Tulane%20Final%20Report.pdf

"Low Wages." National Farm Worker Ministry. Web. http://nfwm.org/education-center/farm-worker-issues/low-wages/

Sustainable Seafood

Kresser, Chris. "Is Eating Fish Safe? A Lot Safer Than Not Eating Fish!" *ChrisKresser.com*, n.d. Web. http://chriskresser.com/is-eating-fish-safe-a-lot-safer-than-not-eating-fish

Mozaffarian, Dariush, and Eric B. Rimm. "Fish Intake, Contaminants, and Human Health: Evaluating the Risks and Benefits." *Journal of the American Medical Association* 296.15 (2006): 1885–1899. http://jama.jamanetwork.com/article.aspx?articleid=203640

Bees

Blackiston, Howland. *Beekeeping for Dummies.* Hoboken, NJ: Wiley, 2009.

Beyond Food: Having a Healthy Lifestyle

Pardi, Daniel. Interview by Joseph Mercola. *Dan's Plan*, 19 January 2014. Web. https://www.dansplan.com/blog/how-light-exposure-affects-health-an-interview-of-dan-by-dr-joseph-mercola/

Park, B.J., et al. "The Physiological Effects of Shinrin-Yoku (Taking in the Forest Atmosphere or Forest Bathing): Evidence from Field Experiments in 24 Forests Across Japan." *Environmental Health and Preventative Medicine*, 15.1 (2010): 18–26. http://link.springer.com/article/10.1007%2Fs12199-009-0086-9

Schnepf, Randy. *Consumers and Price Inflation.* Congressional Research Service, 13 Sept. 2013. Web. http://fas.org/sgp/crs/misc/R40545.pdf

WHERE TO FIND ME

Blog
Sustainable Dish, sustainabledish.com

Podcast
Modern Farm Girls

YouTube
SustainableDish

Instagram
@SustainableDish

Nutrition consultations
Radiance Nutrition, radiancenutrition.com

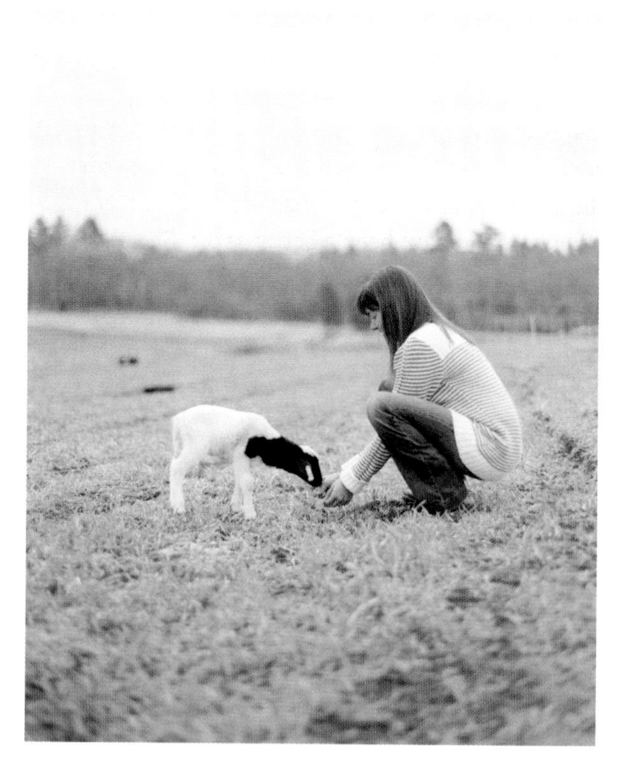

Acknowledgments

If my husband had not been so discontent with his corporate job, we would never have ended up with such an incredible life today. When I met him, he was a passionate environmentalist but was confused about which career path to take. After a brief stint in a suit and tie, he decided at age twenty-six to become an organic farmer. This decision changed our lives forever, and I'm so incredibly grateful for his dedication, passion, and honor, and I admire his humility. He's an incredible partner and father, and I'm thrilled to be raising our children with a dad who can teach them so much about life. Thank you, Andrew. I love you.

No one but Heidi Murphy of White Loft Studio could have made the photos in this book speak the way they do. The entire book was shot on film, not digital, and Heidi's photographs completely capture the essence of the food, the farm, and the life we live. Because she shot the vegetables as they came into season in order to capture them at their peak, Heidi had to visit the farm for more than thirty shoots over the course of one year. She took photos while camping with a broken leg, hauled her camera equipment in a boat to the island for the clambake, and was just such a trooper through the rain, mud, bugs, and all the other inconveniences that come with farm life. Nobody could have been a better sport. She also happened to have lost twenty pounds during the course of shooting this book, by changing her eating habits and going for long walks. I'm so happy to have helped her gain better health, and I'm in awe of the work she produced.

Thank you to my family for all of your support. I'd especially like to thank Gil Rodgers for spending time with the kids so Andrew and I could sneak away and work on the book. Also, thank you to my dad for sparking a love of food and adventure and for supporting my continuing education, and to my sister, Frances, who helped with the goat milk shoot and came on the Temenos trip. Thanks to Janet, my mother-in-law, for so many recipe suggestions. I also owe a huge debt of gratitude to my all-star kids, Anson and Phoebe, who came along on boats in the dark to clambakes, posed for numerous photos, and appeared in videos, all to help me spread the word about sustainability and health.

I have an incredible group of the coolest friends ever. Thank you, Kirsty Allore and your gorgeous children, for being in just about every chapter of the book and for opening up your cottage in Gloucester for the clambake. Thanks to Talie Kattwinkle for every conversation we've had, and for all of your help on the shoots as my personal fashion stylist. Thanks to Angus Beasley and Eric Adams for your help at the clambake. Thanks also to Diane Sills and Emily Williams for your help during the clambake and camping trip. You make a mean cocktail. Thank you, Chris Mountain, for your assistance during the pig roast and for accepting an orange kitty as payment. Thank you to Mary Manseur for your help with the beekeeping chapter, Don Zasada for the cow advice, Terry Golson for allowing us to shoot your beautiful chickens, and a huge thanks to Jennifer Hashley for your help with the rabbits chapter.

Huge thanks also to my mentor and friend, Robb Wolf, for all of your support for my numerous projects right from the day I met you. Much appreciation also goes out to Mathieu Lalonde for encouraging me through my nutrition education and answering all of my technical questions. Thank you to Emily Deans for your suggestions on the copy and for your texts (insert Beavis and Butthead laugh here). Thanks to Hayley and Bill Staley for connecting me with Erich to make this project happen, and to Diane Sanfilippo for your help with the title and support since the early days. Thanks to Dan McNamara and Charles Mayfield for your help with the hunting section. Thank you to Liz Wolfe for your humor, to Julie Mayfield for your friendship and encouragement, and to Melissa Joulwan, Katherine Morrison, Chris Kresser, Dallas and Melissa Hartwig, Dan Pardi, and countless others in the real-food community for your professional support. A special thanks also goes out to Michelle Tam and Henry Fong for being such great friends and rocks to lean on.

To Annette Lee, big props (literally!) for loaning me some of the gorgeous props for the shots. Thank you to the Lodge Company for sending me loads of cast iron cookware, which I absolutely love. Thank you to J Holt Pottery for the beautiful sheep and bird mugs. Thank you to Temenos Retreat Center for allowing us to take over your magical piece of earth for a couple of days.

This book would not have been possible without the opportunity our family has been given to live at Clark Farm. Thank you to Marjie Findlay and Geoff Freeman for your support. We are so honored to be the caretakers of such a special piece of land. To Frank Proctor, thank you for all you do at the farm, and for your help taste-testing recipes and smoking brisket. Huge gratitude also goes to Kristen Cummings and the rest of the crew for putting up with us and helping to make Clark Farm what it is.

Thanks to Justin Keane and the team at CrossFit Woodshed for your continued support with my books and my fitness goals.

Finally, thanks to Erich Krauss and Michelle Farrington; extra kudos to my editor, Erin Granville; and thanks to the rest of the team at Victory Belt for allowing me to write exactly the book I wanted to.

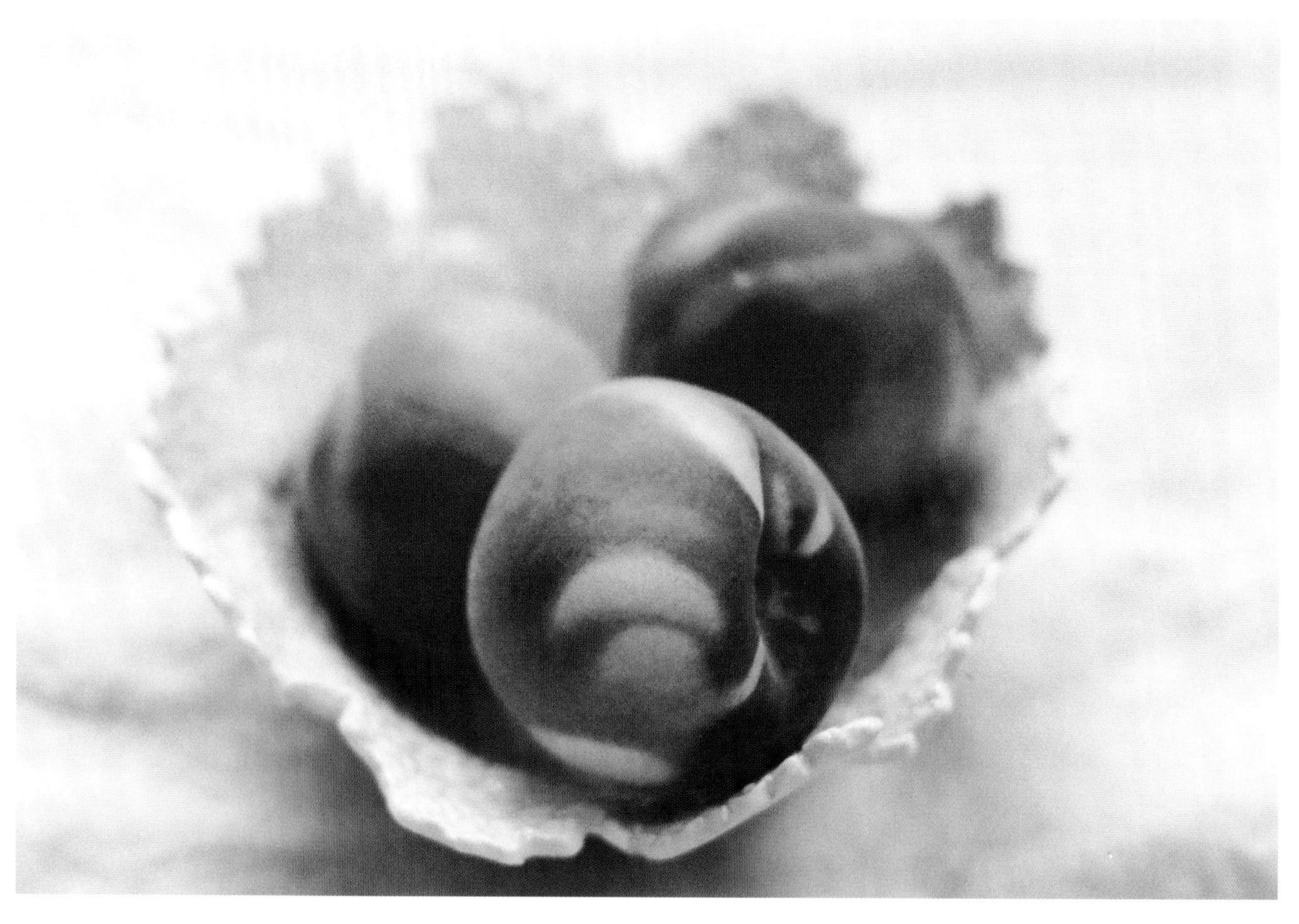

About the Authors

Diana Rodgers is a farmer and nutritionist and the best-selling author of *Paleo Lunches and Breakfasts on the Go*. On her blog, *Sustainable Dish*, and local television show of the same name, she explores which foods are optimal for both human nutrition and the environment. Diana also coproduces the podcast *Modern Farm Girls* with Liz Wolfe and produces videos about farming, cooking, nutrition, and life on her farm that can be found on her YouTube channel, *Sustainable Dish*. Diana lives on Clark Organic Farm, a working organic farm in Massachusetts, with her husband, Andrew, and two children.

Andrew Rodgers is the farm manager at Clark Farm in Carlisle, Massachusetts. He attended the master's program in soil science at the University of Massachusetts, Amherst, and ran Green Meadows Farm, a 230-acre organic farm in Hamilton, Massachusetts, for nearly ten years. When he's not farming, Andrew enjoys fishing and coaching baseball and softball.

Heidi Murphy is a Massachusetts-based photographer who runs White Loft Studio. When she's not shooting, Heidi can be found on the beach with her dog.

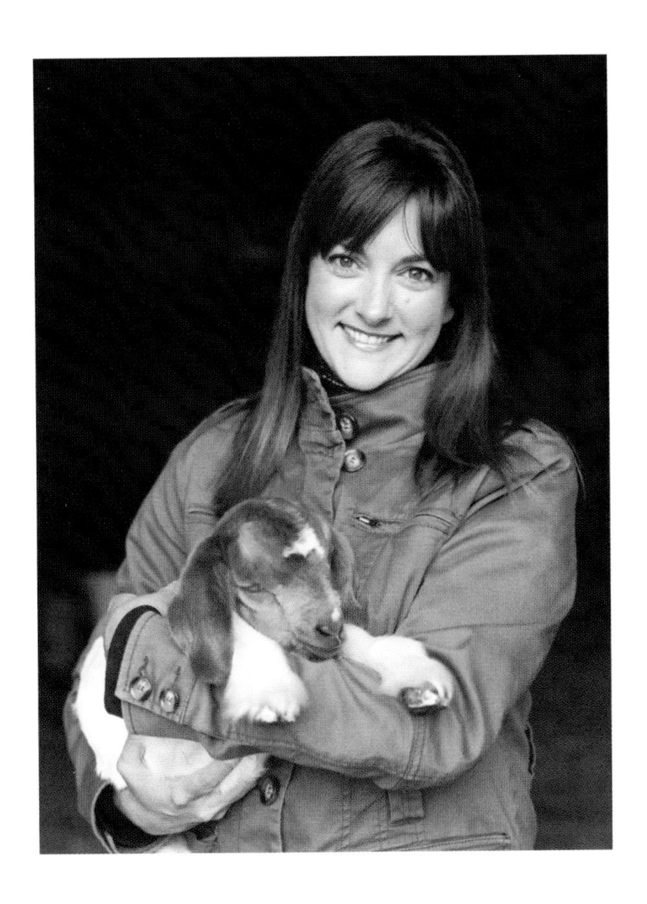

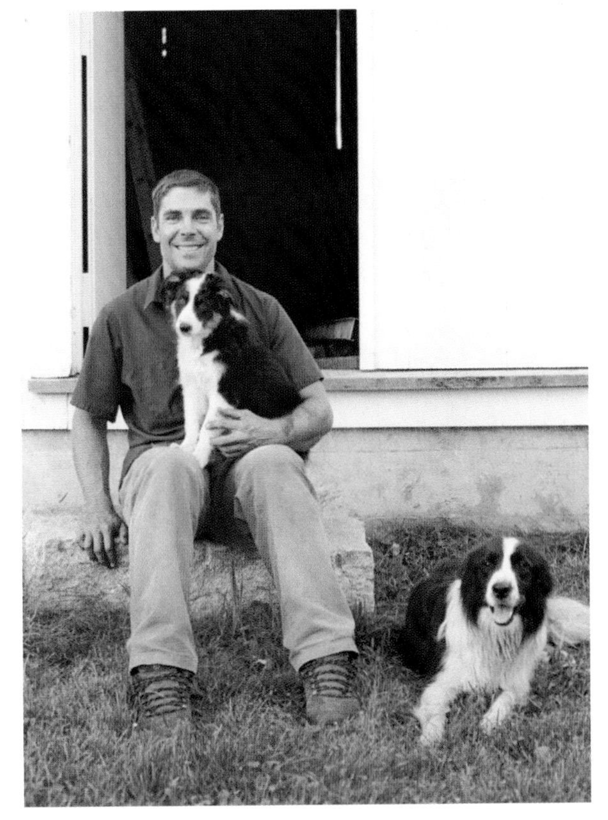

INDEX